W9-CEQ-371

Examination & Board Review

Medical Microbiology & Immunology

fifth edition

Warren Levinson, MD, PhD
Professor of Microbiology
Department of Microbiology and Immunology
University of California, San Francisco

Ernest Jawetz, MD, PhD
Professor of Microbiology and Medicine Emeritus
Department of Microbiology and Immunology
University of California, San Francisco

Appleton & Lange
Stamford, Connecticut

Notice: The authors and the publisher of this volume have taken care to make certain that the doses of drugs and schedules of treatment are correct and compatible with the standards generally accepted at the time of publication. Nevertheless, as new information becomes available, changes in treatment and in the use of drugs become necessary. The reader is advised to carefully consult the instructions and information material included in the package insert of each drug or therapeutic agent before administration. This advice is especially important when using, administering, or recommending new or infrequently used drugs. The authors and publisher disclaim all responsibility for any liability, loss, injury, or damage incurred as a consequence, directly or indirectly, of the use and application of any of the contents of this volume.

ISBN: 0-8385-6287-6
ISSN: 1042-8070

Acquisitions Editor: David A. Barnes
Senior Development Editor: Amanda M. Suver
Production Editor: Elizabeth C. Ryan
Associate Art Manager: Maggie Belis Darrow
Copy Editor: Yvonne Strong
Illustrators: ElectraGraphics, Inc., and Teshin Associates

ISBN 0-8385-6287-6

90000

9 780838 562871

PRINTED IN THE UNITED STATES OF AMERICA

Contents

Preface

This book is a concise review of the medically important aspects of microbiology. It covers both the basic and clinical aspects of bacteriology, virology, mycology, parasitology, and immunology. Its two major aims are (1) to assist those who are preparing for the USMLE (National Boards) and (2) to provide students who are presently taking medical microbiology courses with a brief and flexible source of information.

In this new edition, we present current, medically important information in the rapidly changing fields of microbiology and immunology. We have included updated information on such topics as human immunodeficiency virus, hepatitis viruses, and immunology. Our goal is to provide the reader with an accurate source of clinically relevant information at a level appropriate for those beginning their medical education.

These aims are achieved by utilizing several different formats, which should make the book useful to students with varying study objectives and learning styles:

(1) A narrative text for complete information.
(2) Summaries of important microorganisms for rapid review of essentials.
(3) Review questions at the end of each chapter.
(4) Sample questions in the USMLE (National Board) style, with answers provided after each group of questions.
(5) A USMLE (National Board) practice examination consisting of 160 questions with answers provided at the end of the examination.
(6) Clinical case discussions to illustrate the relevance of the material to patient problems.

In addition, the following specific features should be emphasized:

(1) The information is presented succinctly, with stress on making it clear, interesting, and up to date.
(2) There is strong emphasis in the text on the clinical application of microbiology and immunology to infectious diseases.
(3) In the clinical bacteriology and virology sections, the organisms are separated into major and minor pathogens. This allows the student to focus on the clinically most important microorganisms.
(4) Key information is summarized in useful review tables. Important concepts are illustrated by figures in color.
(5) The 583 USMLE (National Board) practice questions cover the important aspects of each of the subdisciplines on the USMLE—Bacteriology, Virology, Mycology, Parasitology, and Immunology. These practice questions are in the two formats used in the current USMLE. A separate section containing *extended* matching questions is included. In view of the emphasis placed on clinical relevance in the USMLE, another section provides questions set in a clinical case context.
(6) Brief summaries of medically important microorganisms are presented together in a separate section to facilitate access to the information and to encourage comparison of one organism with another.
(7) Ten clinical cases are presented as unknowns for the reader to analyze in a realistic, problem-solving way. These cases illustrate the importance of basic science information in clinical decision-making.

After teaching both medical microbiology and clinical infectious disease for many years, we believe that students appreciate a book that presents the essential information in a readable, interesting, and varied format. We hope you find this book meets those criteria.

San Francisco
May 1998

Warren E. Levinson, MD, PhD
Ernest Jawetz, MD, PhD

Acknowledgments

We gratefully acknowledge the thoughtful comments of Dr Bertie Argyris and Dr Candice McCoy, who reviewed the immunology section, and Dr Donald Heyneman, who reviewed the parasitology section. The excellent secretarial skills of Grace Stauffer and Bertha Cooke are greatly appreciated. We are indebted to our editor, Yvonne Strong, who ensured that the highest standards of grammar and style were met.

W. L. gratefully acknowledges the invaluable assistance of his wife, Barbara, in making this book become a reality.

W. L. dedicates this book to his father and mother, who instilled a love of scholarship, the joy of teaching, and the value of being organized.

Part I: Basic Bacteriology

Bacteria Compared With Other Microorganisms

1

AGENTS

The agents of human infectious diseases belong to five major groups of organisms: bacteria, fungi, protozoa, helminths, and viruses. The bacteria belong to the prokaryote kingdom, the fungi and protozoa are members of the kingdom of protists, and the helminths (worms) are classified in the animal kingdom (Table 1–1). The protists are distinguished from animals and plants by being either unicellular or relatively simple multicellular organisms. The helminths are complex multicellular organisms that are classified as metazoa within the animal kingdom. Taken together, the helminths and the protozoa are commonly called parasites. Viruses are quite distinct from other organisms. They are not cells but can replicate only within cells.

IMPORTANT FEATURES

Many of the essential characteristics of these organisms are described in Table 1–2. One salient feature is that bacteria, fungi, protozoa, and helminths are cellular whereas viruses are not. This distinction is based primarily on three criteria.

(1) Structure. Cells have a nucleus or nucleoid (see below) containing DNA; this is surrounded by cytoplasm, within which proteins are synthesized and energy is generated. Viruses have an inner core of genetic material (either DNA or RNA) but no cytoplasm, and so they depend on host cells to provide the machinery for protein synthesis and energy generation.

(2) Method of replication. Cells replicate either by binary fission or by mitosis, during which one parent cell divides to make two progeny cells while retaining its cellular structure. Prokaryotic cells, eg, bacteria, replicate by binary fission, whereas eukaryotic cells replicate by mitosis. In contrast, viruses disassemble, produce many copies of their nucleic acid and protein, and then reassemble into multiple progeny viruses. Furthermore, viruses must replicate within host cells, because, as mentioned above, they lack protein-synthesizing and energy-generating systems. With the exception of rickettsiae and chlamydiae, which are bacteria that also require living host cells for growth, bacteria can replicate extracellularly.

Table 1–1. Biologic relationships of pathogenic microorganisms.

Kingdom	Pathogenic Microorganisms	Type of Cells
Animal	Helminths	Eukaryotic
Plant	None	Eukaryotic
Protist	Protozoa Fungi	Eukaryotic Eukaryotic
Prokaryote	Bacteria	Prokaryotic
	Viruses	Noncellular

CHAPTER 1

Table 1–2. Comparison of medically important organisms.

Characteristic	Viruses	Bacteria	Fungi	Protozoa and Helminths
Cells	No	Yes	Yes	Yes
Approximate diameter (µm)[1]	0.02–0.2	1–5	3–10 (yeasts)	15–25 (trophozoites)
Nucleic acid	Either DNA or RNA	Both DNA and RNA	Both DNA and RNA	Both DNA and RNA
Type of nucleus	None	Prokaryotic	Eukaryotic	Eukaryotic
Ribosomes	Absent	70S	80S	80S
Mitochondria	Absent	Absent	Present	Present
Nature of outer surface	Protein capsid and lipoprotein envelope	Rigid wall containing peptidoglycan	Rigid wall containing chitin	Flexible membrane
Motility	None	Some	None	Most
Method of replication	Not binary fission	Binary fission	Budding or mitosis[2]	Mitosis

[1] For comparison, a human red blood cell has a diameter of 7 µm.
[2] Yeasts divide by budding, whereas molds divide by mitosis.
[3] Helminth cells divide by mitosis, but the organism reproduces itself by complex, sexual life cycles.

(3) Nature of the nucleic acid. Cells contain both DNA and RNA, whereas viruses contain either DNA or RNA but not both.

EUKARYOTES & PROKARYOTES

Cells have evolved into two fundamentally different types, **eukaryotic** and **prokaryotic,** which can be distinguished on the basis of their structure and the complexity of their organization. Fungi and protozoa are eukaryotic, whereas bacteria are prokaryotic.

(1) The eukaryotic cell has a true **nucleus** with multiple chromosomes surrounded by a nuclear membrane and uses a mitotic apparatus to ensure equal allocation of the chromosomes to progeny cells.

(2) The **nucleoid** of a prokaryotic cell consists of a single circular molecule of loosely organized DNA lacking a nuclear membrane and mitotic apparatus (Table 1–3).

In addition to the different types of nuclei, the two classes of cells are distinguished by several other criteria.

(1) Eukaryotic cells contain **organelles,** such as mitochondria and lysosomes, and larger (80S) ribosomes, whereas prokaryotes contain no organelles and smaller (70S) ribosomes.

(2) Most prokaryotes have a rigid external cell wall that contains **peptidoglycan,** a polymer of amino acids and sugars, as its unique structural component. Eukaryotes, on the other hand, do not contain

Table 1–3. Characteristics of prokaryotic and eukaryotic cells.

Characteristic	Prokaryotic Bacterial Cells	Eukaryotic Human Cells
DNA within a nuclear membrane	No	Yes
Mitotic division	No	Yes
DNA associated with histones	No	Yes
Chromosome number	One	More than one
Membrane-bound organelles such as mitochondria and lysosomes	No	Yes
Size of ribosome	70S	80S
Cell wall containing peptidoglycan	Yes	No

peptidoglycan. Either they are bound by a flexible cell membrane or, in the case of fungi, they have a rigid cell wall with chitin, a homopolymer of *N*-acetylglucosamine, typically forming the framework.

(3) The eukaryotic cell membrane contains **sterols,** whereas no prokaryote, except the wall-less *Mycoplasma,* has sterols in its membranes.

Another criterion by which these organisms can be contrasted is **motility.** Most protozoa and some bacteria are motile, whereas fungi and viruses are nonmotile. The protozoa are a heterogeneous group that possess three different organs of locomotion: flagella, cilia, and pseudopods. The motile bacteria move only by means of flagella.

Review Questions

1. What are the differences between bacteria and viruses?
2. Are bacteria prokaryotic or eukaryotic? What are the differences between prokaryotic and eukaryotic cells?
3. What are the similarities and the differences among bacteria, fungi, and protozoa?

Structure of Bacterial Cells

2

SHAPE & SIZE

Bacteria are classified by shape into three basic groups: **cocci, bacilli,** and **spirochetes** (Fig 2–1). Some bacteria are variable in shape and are said to be **pleomorphic** (many-shaped). The shape of a bacterium is determined by its rigid cell wall. The microscopic appearance of a bacterium is one of the most important criteria used in its identification.

In addition to their characteristic shapes, the arrangement of bacteria is important. For example, certain cocci occur in pairs **(diplococci),** some in chains **(streptococci),** and others in grapelike clusters **(staphylococci).** These arrangements are determined by the orientation and degree of attachment of the bacteria at the time of cell division.

Bacteria range in size from about 0.2 to 5 µm (Fig 2–2). The smallest bacteria (*Mycoplasma*) are

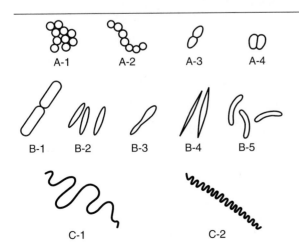

Figure 2–1. Bacterial morphology. **A:** Cocci: in clusters, eg, *Staphylococcus* (A-1); chains, eg, *Streptococcus* (A-2); in pairs with pointed ends, eg, *Streptococcus pneumoniae* (A-3); in pairs with kidney bean shape, eg, *Neisseria* (A-4). **B:** Rods: with square ends, eg, *Bacillus* (B-1); with rounded ends, eg, *Salmonella* (B-2); club-shaped, eg, *Corynebacterium* (B-3); fusiform, eg, *Fusobacterium* (B-4); comma-shaped, eg, *Vibrio* (B-5). **C:** Spirochetes: relaxed coil, eg, *Borrelia* (C-1); tightly coiled, eg, *Treponema* (C-2). (Modified and reproduced, with permission, from Joklik WK et al: *Zinsser Microbiology,* 20th ed. Appleton & Lange, 1992.)

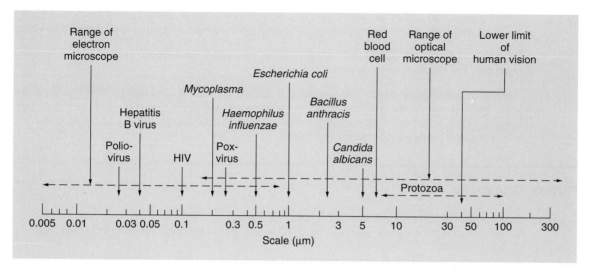

Figure 2–2. Sizes of representative bacteria, viruses, yeasts, protozoa, and human red cells. The bacteria range in size from *Mycoplasma,* the smallest, to *Bacillus anthracis,* one of the largest. The viruses range from poliovirus, one of the smallest, to poxviruses, the largest. Yeasts, such as *C albicans,* are generally larger than bacteria. Protozoa have many different forms and a broad size range. HIV, human immunodeficiency virus. (Modified and reproduced, with permission, from Joklik WK et al: *Zinsser Microbiology,* 20th ed. Appleton & Lange, 1992.)

about the same size as the largest viruses (poxviruses) and are the smallest organisms capable of existing outside the host. The longest bacteria rods approach the size of some yeasts and human red blood cells (7 μm).

STRUCTURE

The structure of a typical bacterium is illustrated in Fig 2–3, and the important features of each component are presented in Table 2–1.

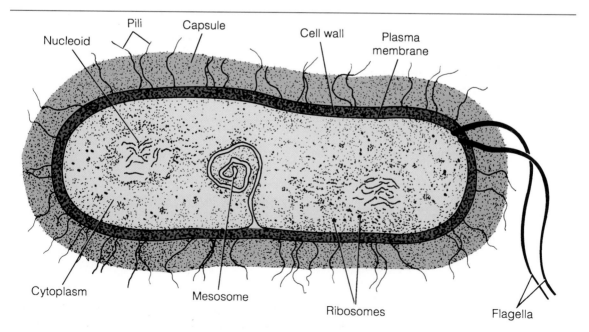

Figure 2–3. Bacterial structure. (Modified and reproduced, with permission, from Tortora G, Funk B, Case C: *Microbiology: An Introduction,* 5th ed. Benjamin/Cummings, 1995.)

Table 2–1. Bacterial structures.

Structure	Chemical Composition	Function
Essential components		
Cell wall		
Peptidoglycan	Sugar backbone with peptide side chains that are crosslinked	Gives rigid support, protects against osmotic pressure; is the site of action of penicillins and cephalosporins and is degraded by lysozyme.
Surface fibers of gram-positive bacteria	Teichoic acid	Major surface antigen but rarely used in laboratory diagnosis.
Outer membrane of gram-negative bacteria	Lipid A	Toxic component of endotoxin.
	Polysaccharide	Major surface antigen used frequently in laboratory diagnosis.
Cytoplasmic membrane	Lipoprotein bilayer without sterols	Site of oxidative and transport enzymes.
Ribosome	RNA and protein in 50S and 30S subunits	Protein synthesis; site of action of aminoglycosides, erythromycin, tetracyclines, and chloramphenicol.
Nucleoid	DNA	Genetic material.
Mesosome	Invagination of plasma membrane	Participates in cell division and secretion.
Periplasm	Space between plasma membrane and outer membrane	Contains many hydrolytic enzymes, including β-lactamases.
Nonessential components		
Capsule	Polysaccharide[1]	Protects against phagocytosis.
Pilus or fimbria	Glycoprotein	Two types: (1) mediates attachment to cell surfaces; (2) sex pilus mediates attachment of two bacteria during conjugation.
Flagellum	Protein	Motility.
Spore	Keratinlike coat, dipicolinic acid	Provides resistance to dehydration, heat, and chemicals.
Plasmid	DNA	Contains a variety of genes for antibiotic resistance and toxins.
Granule	Glycogen, lipids, polyphosphates	Site of nutrients in cytoplasm.
Glycocalyx	Polysaccharide	Mediates adherence to surfaces.

[1] Except in *Bacillus anthracis,* in which it is a polypeptide of D-glutamic acid.

Cell Wall   The cell wall is the outermost component common to all bacteria (except *Mycoplasma* species, which are bounded by a cell membrane, not a cell wall). Some bacteria have surface features external to the cell wall, such as a capsule, flagella, and pili, which are less common components and are discussed below.

The cell wall is a multilayered structure located external to the cytoplasmic membrane. It is composed of an inner layer of **peptidoglycan** (see p 6) surrounded by an outer membrane that varies in thickness and chemical composition depending upon the bacterial type (Fig 2–4). The peptidoglycan provides structural support and maintains the characteristic shape of the cell.

A. Cell Walls of Gram-Positive and Gram-Negative Bacteria: The structure, chemical composition, and thickness of the cell wall differ in gram-positive and gram-negative bacteria (box and Table 2–2).

(1) The peptidoglycan layer is much thicker in gram-positive than in gram-negative bacteria. Some gram-positive bacteria also have fibers of teichoic acid that protrude outside the peptidoglycan, whereas gram-negative bacteria do not.

(2) In contrast, the gram-negative organisms have a complex outer layer consisting of lipopolysaccharide, lipoprotein, and phospholipid. Lying between the outer-membrane layer and the cytoplasmic membrane in gram-negative bacteria is the **periplasmic space,** which is the site, in some species, of enzymes called beta-lactamases that degrade penicillins and other β-lactam drugs.

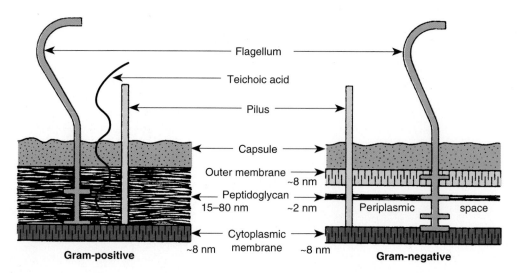

Figure 2–4. Cell walls of gram-positive and gram-negative bacteria. Note that the peptidoglycan in gram-positive bacteria is much thicker than in gram-negative bacteria. Note also that only gram-negative bacteria have an outer membrane containing endotoxin (lipopolysaccharide [LPS]) and have a periplasmic space where β-lactamases are found. Several important gram-positive bacteria, such as staphylococci and streptococci, have teichoic acids. (Reproduced, with permission, from Ingraham JL, Maaløe O, Neidhardt FC: *Growth of the Bacterial Cell,* Sinauer Associates, 1983.)

The cell wall has several other important properties:

(1) in gram-negative organisms, it contains **endotoxin,** a lipopolysaccharide (see pp 7 and 35);

(2) its polysaccharides and proteins are antigens that are useful in laboratory identification; and

(3) its **porin** proteins play a role in regulating the passage of small, hydrophilic molecules into the cell. Porin proteins in the outer membrane form a trimer that acts, usually nonspecifically, as a channel to allow the entry of essential substances such as sugars, amino acids, vitamins, and metals, as well as many antimicrobial drugs such as penicillins.

B. Cell Walls of Acid-Fast Bacteria: Mycobacteria, eg, *Mycobacterium tuberculosis,* have an unusual cell wall, resulting in their inability to be Gram-stained. These bacteria are said to be **"acid-fast,"** since they resist decolorization with acid-alcohol after being stained with carbolfuchsin. This property is related to the high concentration in the cell wall of lipids called mycolic acids.

In view of their importance, three components of the cell wall, ie, peptidoglycan, lipopolysaccharide, and teichoic acid, will be discussed in detail.

C. Peptidoglycan: Peptidoglycan is a complex, interwoven network that surrounds the entire cell and is composed of a single covalently linked macromolecule. It is found only in bacterial cell walls. It provides rigid support for the cell, is important in maintaining the characteristic shape of the cell, and allows the cell to withstand media of low osmotic pressure, such as water. A representative segment of the peptidoglycan layer is shown in Fig 2–5. The term "peptidoglycan" is derived from

Table 2–2. Comparison of cell walls of gram-positive and gram-negative bacteria.

Component	Gram-Positive Cells	Gram-Negative Cells
Peptidoglycan	Thicker; multilayer	Thinner; single layer
Teichoic acids	Yes	No
Lipopolysaccharide (endotoxin)	No	Yes

Gram Stain

This staining procedure, developed in 1884 by the Danish physician Christian Gram, is the most important procedure in microbiology. It separates most bacteria into two groups: the gram-positive bacteria, which stain blue, and the gram-negative bacteria, which stain red. The Gram stain involves the following four-step procedure.

(1) The crystal violet dye stains all cells blue.

(2) The iodine solution (a mordant) is added to form a crystal violet-iodine complex; all cells continue to appear blue.

(3) The organic solvent, such as acetone or ethanol, extracts the blue dye complex from the lipid-rich, thin-walled gram-negative bacteria to a greater degree than from the lipid-poor, thick-walled gram-positive bacteria. The gram-negative organisms appear colorless; the gram-positive bacteria remain blue.

(4) The red dye safranin stains the decolorized gram-negative cells red; the gram-positive bacteria remain blue.

Note that if step #2 is omitted and Gram's iodine is not added, gram-negative bacteria stain *blue* rather than pink, presumably because the organic solvent removes the crystal violet-iodine complex but not the crystal violet alone. Gram-positive bacteria also stain *blue* when Gram's iodine is not added.

The Gram stain is useful in two ways:

(1) in the identification of many bacteria, and

(2) in influencing the choice of antibiotic, since, in general, gram-positive bacteria are more susceptible to penicillin G than are gram-negative bacteria.

the peptides and the sugars (glycan) that make up the molecule. Synonyms for peptidoglycan are murein and mucopeptide.

Fig 2–5 illustrates the carbohydrate backbone, which is composed of alternating *N*-acetylmuramic acid and *N*-acetylglucosamine molecules. Attached to each of the muramic acid molecules is a tetrapeptide consisting of both D- and L-amino acids, the precise composition of which differs from one bacterium to another. Two of these amino acids are worthy of special mention: diaminopimelic acid, which is unique to bacterial cell walls, and D-alanine, which is involved in the cross-links between the tetrapeptides and in the action of penicillin. Note that this tetrapeptide contains the rare D-isomers of amino acids; most proteins contain the L-isomer. The other important component in this network is the peptide cross-link between the two tetrapeptides. The cross-links vary among species; in *Staphylococcus aureus,* for example, five glycines link the terminal D-alanine to the penultimate L-lysine.

Since peptidoglycan is present in bacteria but not in human cells, it is a good target for antibacterial drugs. Several of these drugs, such as the penicillins and cephalosporins, inhibit its synthesis (see Chapter 10).

The enzyme **lysozyme,** which is present in human tears, mucus, and saliva, can cleave the peptidoglycan backbone by breaking its glycosyl bonds, thereby contributing to the natural resistance of the host to microbial infection. Lysozyme-treated bacteria may swell and rupture as a result of the entry of water into the cells, which have a high internal osmotic pressure. However, if the lysozyme-treated cells are in a solution with the same osmotic pressure as that of the bacterial interior, they will survive as spherical forms, called protoplasts, surrounded only by a cytoplasmic membrane.

D. Lipopolysaccharide (LPS):   The LPS of the outer membrane of the cell wall of gram-negative bacteria is **endotoxin.** It is responsible for many of the features of disease, such as fever and shock (especially hypotension), caused by these organisms. It is called endotoxin because it is an integral part of

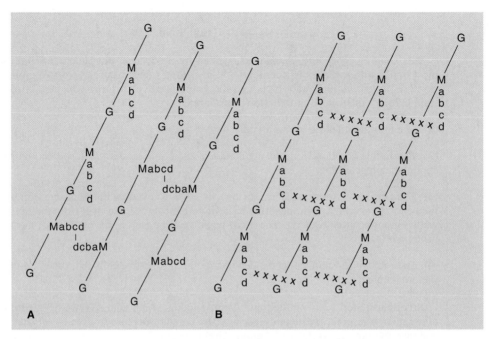

Figure 2–5. Peptidoglycan structure: *Escherichia coli* **(A)** has a different cross-link from that of *Staphylococcus aureus* **(B).** In *E coli,* c is cross-linked directly to d, whereas in *S aureus,* c and d are cross-linked by five glycines. However, in both organisms the terminal D-alanine is part of the linkage. M, muramic acid; G, glucosamine; a, L-alanine; b, D-glutamic acid; c, diaminopimelic acid **(A)** or L-lysine **(B);** d, D-alanine; x, pentaglycine bridge. (Modified and reproduced, with permission, from Joklik WK et al: *Zinsser Microbiology,* 20th ed. Appleton & Lange, 1992.)

the cell wall, in contrast to exotoxins, which are freely released from the bacteria. The pathologic effects of endotoxin are similar irrespective of the organism from which it is derived.

The LPS is composed of three distinct units (Fig 2–6):

(1) phospholipid called lipid A, which is responsible for the toxic effects;

(2) a core polysaccharide of five sugars linked through ketodeoxyoctulonate (KDO) to lipid A; and

(3) an outer polysaccharide consisting of up to 25 repeating units of three to five sugars. This outer polymer is the important somatic or O antigen of several gram-negative bacteria that is used to identify certain organisms in the clinical laboratory.

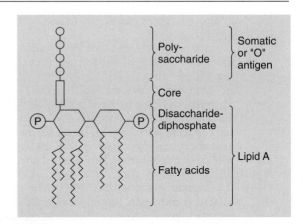

Figure 2–6. Endotoxin (LPS) structure. The O antigen polysaccharide is exposed on the exterior of the cell, whereas the lipid A faces the interior. (Modified and reproduced, with permission, from Brooks GF et al: *Medical Microbiology,* 19th ed. Appleton & Lange, 1991.)

E. Teichoic Acid: These polymers of glycerol phosphate or ribitol phosphate are located in the outer layer of the gram-positive cell wall. Some polymers of glycerol teichoic acid penetrate the peptidoglycan layer and are covalently linked to the lipid in the cytoplasmic membrane, in which case they are called **lipoteichoic acid;** others anchor to the muramic acid of the peptidoglycan. Teichoic acids are antigenic and induce antibodies that are species-specific. In staphylococci, teichoic acids mediate adherence of the organism to mucosal cells.

Cytoplasmic Membrane   Just inside the peptidoglycan layer of the cell wall lies the cytoplasmic membrane, which is composed of a phospholipid bilayer similar in microscopic appearance to that in eukaryotic cells. They are chemically similar, but eukaryotic membranes contain sterols whereas prokaryotes generally do not. The only prokaryotes that have sterols in their membranes are members of the genus *Mycoplasma.* The membrane has four important functions: (1) active transport of molecules into the cell, (2) energy generation by oxidative phosphorylation, (3) synthesis of precursors of the cell wall, and (4) secretion of enzymes and toxins.

Mesosome   This invagination of the cytoplasmic membrane is important during cell division, when it functions as the origin of the transverse septum that divides the cell in half and as the binding site of the DNA which will become the genetic material of each daughter cell.

Cytoplasm   The cytoplasm has two distinct areas when visualized in the electron microscope:

(1) an amorphous matrix that contains ribosomes, nutrient granules, metabolites, and plasmids; and

(2) an inner, nucleoid region composed of DNA.

A. Ribosomes: Bacterial ribosomes are the site of protein synthesis as in eukaryotic cells, but they differ from eukaryotic ribosomes in size and chemical composition. Bacterial ribosomes are 70S in size, with 50S and 30S subunits, whereas eukaryotic ribosomes are 80S in size, with 60S and 40S subunits. The differences in both the ribosomal RNAs and proteins constitute the basis of the selective action of several antibiotics that inhibit bacterial, but not human, protein synthesis (see Chapter 10).

B. Granules: The cytoplasm contains several different types of granules that serve as storage areas for nutrients and stain characteristically with certain dyes. For example, volutin is a reserve of high energy stored in the form of polymerized metaphosphate. It appears as a "metachromatic" granule, since it stains red with methylene blue dye instead of blue as one would expect.

C. Nucleoid: The nucleoid is the area of the cytoplasm in which DNA is located. The DNA of prokaryotes is a single, circular molecule that has a molecular weight of approximately 2×10^9 and contains about 2000 genes. (By contrast, human DNA has approximately 100,000 genes.) The nucleoid contains no nuclear membrane, no nucleolus, no mitotic apparatus, and no histones, so there is little resemblance to the eukaryotic nucleus. One major difference between bacterial DNA and eukaryotic DNA is that bacterial DNA has no introns whereas eukaryotic DNA does.

D. Plasmids: Plasmids are extrachromosomal, double-stranded, circular DNA molecules that are capable of replicating independently of the bacterial chromosome. Although plasmids are usually extrachromosomal, they can be integrated into the bacterial chromosome.

(1) Transmissible plasmids can be transferred from cell to cell by conjugation (see Chapter 4 for a discussion of conjugation). They are large (MW 40–100 million), since they contain about a dozen genes responsible for synthesis of the sex pilus and for the enzymes required for transfer. They are usually present in a few (one to three) copies per cell.

(2) Nontransmissible plasmids are small (MW 3–20 million), since they do not contain the transfer genes; they are frequently present in many (10–60) copies per cell.

Plasmids occur in both gram-positive and gram-negative bacteria, and several different types of plasmids can exist in one cell. Treatment with some compounds, such as acridine dyes, can "cure" bacteria of their plasmids in vitro.

The genes for the following functions and structures of medical importance are carried by plasmids:

(1) antibiotic resistance, which is mediated by a variety of enzymes;

(2) resistance to heavy metals such as mercury (the active component of some antiseptics, such as Merthiolate and Mercurochrome) and silver, which is mediated by a reductase enzyme;

(3) resistance to ultraviolet light, which is mediated by DNA repair enzymes;

(4) pili (fimbriae), which mediate the adherence of bacteria to epithelial cells; and

(5) exotoxins, including several enterotoxins.

Other plasmid-encoded products of interest are

(1) bacteriocins, which are toxins or enzymes that are produced by certain bacteria and are lethal for other bacteria;

(2) nitrogen fixation enzymes in *Rhizobium* in the root nodules of legumes;

(3) tumors caused by *Agrobacterium* in plants;

(4) several antibiotics produced by *Streptomyces;* and

(5) a variety of degradative enzymes that are produced by *Pseudomonas* and are capable of cleaning up environmental hazards such as oil spills and toxic chemical-waste sites.

E. Transposons: Transposons are pieces of DNA that move readily from one site to another, either within or between the DNAs of bacteria, plasmids, and bacteriophages. In view of their unusual ability to move, they are nicknamed "jumping genes." They can code for drug resistance enzymes, toxins, or a variety of metabolic enzymes, and they can either cause mutations in the gene into which they insert or alter the expression of nearby genes.

Transposons typically have four identifiable domains. On each end is a short DNA sequence of **inverted repeats,** which are involved in the integration of the transposon into the recipient DNA. The second domain is the gene for the transposase, which is the enzyme that mediates the excision and integration processes. The third region is the gene for the repressor that regulates the synthesis both of the transposase and of the gene product of the fourth domain, which, in many cases, is an enzyme mediating antibiotic resistance (Fig 2–7).

In contrast to plasmids or bacterial viruses, transposons are not capable of independent replication; they replicate as part of the recipient DNA. More than one transposon can be located in the DNA; for example, a plasmid can contain several transposons carrying drug resistance genes. **Insertion sequences** are a type of transposon that have fewer bases (800–1500 base pairs), since they do not code for their own integration enzymes. They can cause mutations at their site of integration and can be found in multiple copies at the ends of larger transposon units.

Figure 2–7. Transposon genes. This transposon is carrying a drug resistance gene. IR, inverted repeat. (Modified and reproduced, with permission, from Fincham JR: *Genetics.* Jones and Bartlett, 1983.)

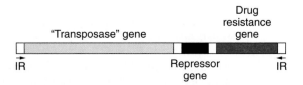

Specialized Structures Outside the Cell Wall

A. Capsule: The capsule is a gelatinous layer covering the entire bacterium. It is composed of polysaccharide, except in the anthrax bacillus, which has a capsule of polymerized D-glutamic acid. The sugar components of the polysaccharide vary from one species of bacteria to another and frequently determine the serologic type within a species. For example, there are 84 different serologic types of *Streptococcus pneumoniae,* which are distinguished by the antigenic differences of the sugars in the polysaccharide capsule.

The capsule is important for four reasons:

(1) It is a determinant of virulence of many bacteria, since it limits the ability of phagocytes to engulf the bacteria. Variants of encapsulated bacteria that have lost the ability to produce a capsule are usually nonpathogenic.

(2) Specific identification of an organism can be made by using antiserum against the capsular polysaccharide. In the presence of the homologous antibody, the capsule will swell greatly. This swelling phenomenon, which is used in the clinical laboratory to identify certain organisms, is called the **quellung reaction.**

(3) Capsular polysaccharides are used as the antigens in certain vaccines, since they are capable of eliciting protective antibodies. For example, the purified capsular polysaccharides of 23 types of *S pneumoniae* are present in the current vaccine.

(4) The capsule may play a role in the adherence of bacteria to human tissues, which is an important initial step in causing infection.

B. Flagella: Flagella are long, whiplike appendages that move the bacteria toward nutrients and other attractants, a process called **chemotaxis.** The long filament, which acts as a propeller, is composed of many subunits of a single protein, flagellin, arranged in several intertwined chains. The energy for movement, the **proton motive force,** is provided by adenosine triphosphate (ATP), derived from the passage of ions across the membrane.

Flagellated bacteria have a characteristic number and location of flagella: some bacteria have one, and others have many; in some the flagella are located at one end, and in others they are all over the outer surface. Only certain bacteria have flagella; many rods do, but most cocci do not and are therefore nonmotile. Spirochetes move by using a flagellumlike structure called the **axial filament,** which wraps around the spiral-shaped cell to produce an undulating motion.

Flagella are medically important for two reasons:

(1) Some species of motile bacteria, eg, *Escherichia coli* and *Proteus* species, are common causes of urinary tract infections. Flagella may play a role in pathogenesis by propelling the bacteria up the urethra into the bladder.

(2) Some species of bacteria, eg, *Salmonella* species, are identified in the clinical laboratory by the use of specific antibodies against flagellar proteins.

C. Pili (Fimbriae): Pili are hairlike filaments that extend from the cell surface. They are shorter and straighter than flagella and are composed of subunits of a protein, pilin, arranged in helical strands. They are found mainly on gram-negative organisms.

Pili have two important roles:

(1) They mediate the **attachment** of bacteria to specific receptors on the human cell surface, which is a necessary step in the initiation of infection for some organisms. Mutants of *Neisseria gonorrhoeae* that do not form pili are nonpathogens.

(2) A specialized kind of pilus, the sex pilus, forms the attachment between the male (donor) and the female (recipient) bacteria during conjugation (see Chapter 4).

D. Glycocalyx (slime layer): The glycocalyx is a polysaccharide coating that is secreted by many bacteria. It covers surfaces like a film and allows the bacteria to **adhere firmly** to various

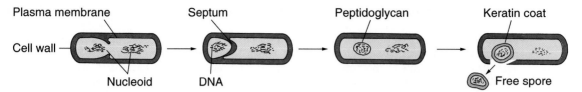

Figure 2–8. Bacterial spores. The spore contains the entire DNA genome of the bacterium surrounded by a thick, resistant coat. (Modified and reproduced, with permission, from Tortora G, Funk B, Case C: *Microbiology: An Introduction,* 5th ed. Benjamin/Cummings, 1995.)

structures, eg, skin, heart valves, and catheters. It also mediates adherence of certain bacteria, such as *Streptococcus mutans,* to the surface of teeth. This plays an important role in the formation of plaque, the precursor of dental caries.

Spores   These highly resistant structures are formed in response to adverse conditions by two genera of medically important gram-positive rods: the genus *Bacillus,* which includes the agent of anthrax, and the genus *Clostridium,* which includes the agents of tetanus and botulism. Spore formation (sporulation) occurs when nutrients, such as sources of carbon and nitrogen, are depleted (Fig 2–8). The spore forms inside the cell and contains bacterial DNA, a small amount of cytoplasm, cell membrane, peptidoglycan, very little water, and, most importantly, a thick, keratinlike coat that is responsible for the remarkable resistance of the spore to heat, dehydration, radiation, and chemicals. This resistance may be mediated by **dipicolinic acid,** a calcium ion chelator found only in spores.

Once formed, the spore has no metabolic activity and can remain dormant for many years. Upon exposure to water and the appropriate nutrients, specific enzymes degrade the coat; water and nutrients enter; and germination into a metabolizing, reproducing bacterial cell occurs. Note that this differentiation process is *not* a means of reproduction, since one cell produces one spore that germinates into one cell.

The medical importance of spores lies in their **extraordinary resistance to heat** and chemicals. As a result of their resistance to heat, sterilization cannot be achieved by boiling. Steam-heating under pressure (autoclaving) at 121 °C, usually for 30 minutes, is required to ensure the sterility of products for medical use. Spores are sometimes not seen in clinical specimens recovered from patients infected by spore-forming organisms, since the supply of nutrients is adequate.

Table 2–3 describes the medically important features of bacterial spores.

Table 2–3. Summary of important features of bacterial spores.

1. They are highly resistant to heating; ie, they are not killed by boiling at 100 °C. However, they are killed by raising the temperature to 121 °C in an autoclave.
2. They are highly resistant to many disinfectants. The resistance to chemicals and to heat is attributed to their thick keratinlike coats and to the absence of water.
3. They are produced only by members of two genera of bacteria of medical importance, *Bacillus* and *Clostridium,* both of which are gram-positive rods.
4. They are produced under conditions of nutritional deprivation, ie, when carbon or nitrogen sources are lacking. When nutritional sources are restored, the spores germinate to form vegetative bacterial cells.
5. They can survive for many years, especially in soil.
6. They exhibit no measurable metabolic activity.
7. They contain dipicolinic acid, a calcium chelator that is found virtually nowhere else in the biological world.

Review Questions

1. What is the structure of the bacterial cell wall? What is its function?
2. Where is the periplasmic space? What is its importance?
3. What are the differences between gram-positive and gram-negative cell walls?
4. What attribute of the cell wall of *Mycobacterium tuberculosis* makes it acid-fast?
5. What is the function of each step in the Gram stain procedure?
6. What is the structure of peptidoglycan? What is its function?

7. If certain bacteria are treated with lysozyme, a protoplast may result. What is the mode of action of lysozyme? What is a protoplast?
8. What is the importance of the lipopolysaccharide in the cell wall of gram-negative bacteria?
9. What are the similarities and differences between the cytoplasmic membranes of bacteria and eukaryotic cells?
10. What is the function of mesosomes?
11. How do bacterial ribosomes differ from eukaryotic ones?
12. How does the bacterial nucleoid differ from the nucleus of a eukaryotic cell?
13. What are plasmids? What is their function?
14. What are transposons? How do they differ from plasmids?
15. What is the function of (1) bacterial capsules, (2) bacterial flagella, and (3) pili?
16. What is the medical importance of bacterial spores? Describe the circumstances under which they form.

Growth

3

GROWTH CYCLE

Bacteria reproduce by **binary fission,** a process by which one parent cell divides to form two progeny cells. Because one cell gives rise to two progeny cells, bacteria are said to undergo exponential growth (logarithmic growth). The concept of exponential growth can be illustrated by the following relationship:

Number of cells	1	2	4	8	16
Exponential	2^0	2^1	2^2	2^3	2^4

Thus, one bacterium will produce 16 bacteria after four generations.

The doubling (generation) time of bacteria ranges from as little as 20 minutes for *Escherichia coli* to more than 24 hours for *Mycobacterium tuberculosis.* The exponential growth and the short doubling time of some organisms result in rapid production of very large numbers of bacteria. For example, one *E coli* organism will produce over 1000 progeny in about 3 hours and over 1 million in about 7 hours. The doubling time varies not only with the species but also with the amount of nutrients, the temperature, the pH, and other environmental factors.

The growth cycle of bacteria has four major phases. If a small number of bacteria are inoculated into a liquid nutrient medium and the bacteria are counted at frequent intervals, the typical phases of a standard growth curve can be demonstrated (Fig 3–1).

(1) The first is the **lag** phase, during which vigorous metabolic activity occurs but cells do not divide. This can last for a few minutes up to many hours.

(2) The **log** (logarithmic) phase is when rapid cell division occurs. Beta-lactam drugs, such as penicillin, act during this phase because the drugs are effective when cells are making peptidoglycan, ie, when they are dividing.

(3) The **stationary** phase occurs when nutrient depletion or toxic products cause growth to slow until the number of new cells produced balances the number of cells that die, resulting in a steady state. Cells grown in a special apparatus called a chemostat, into which fresh nutrients are added and from which waste products are removed continuously, can remain in the log phase and do not enter the stationary phase.

(4) The final phase is the **death** phase, which is marked by a decline in the number of viable bacteria.

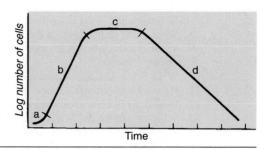

Figure 3–1. Growth curve of bacteria. **a,** lag phase; **b,** log phase; **c,** stationary phase; **d,** death phase. (Reproduced, with permission, from Joklik WK et al: *Zinsser Microbiology,* 20th ed. Appleton & Lange, 1992.)

AEROBIC & ANAEROBIC GROWTH

For most organisms, an adequate supply of oxygen enhances metabolism and growth. The oxygen acts as the hydrogen acceptor in the final steps of energy production catalyzed by the flavoproteins and cytochromes. Because the use of oxygen generates two toxic molecules, hydrogen peroxide (H_2O_2) and the free radical superoxide (O_2^-), bacteria require two enzymes to utilize oxygen. The first is **superoxide dismutase,** which catalyzes the reaction

$$2O_2^- + 2H^+ \rightarrow H_2O_2 + O_2$$

and the second is **catalase,** which catalyzes the reaction

$$2H_2O_2 \rightarrow 2H_2O + O_2$$

The response to oxygen is an important criterion for classifying bacteria and has great practical significance, because specimens from patients must be incubated in the proper atmosphere for the bacteria to grow.

(a) Some bacteria, such as *M tuberculosis,* are **obligate aerobes;** ie, they require oxygen to grow because their ATP-generating system is dependent on oxygen as the hydrogen acceptor.

(b) Other bacteria, such as *E coli,* are **facultative anaerobes (facultatives);** they utilize oxygen to generate energy by respiration if it is present, but they can use the fermentation pathway to synthesize ATP in the absence of sufficient oxygen.

(c) The third group of bacteria consists of the **obligate anaerobes,** such as *Clostridium tetani,* which cannot grow in the presence of oxygen because they lack either superoxide dismutase or catalase, or both. Obligate anaerobes vary in their response to oxygen exposure; some can survive but are not able to grow, whereas others are killed rapidly.

Review Questions

1. Draw and label a typical bacterial growth curve.
2. Distinguish among aerobic, facultative, and anaerobic growth.
3. Why do certain bacteria die in the presence of oxygen?

Genetics

The genetic material of a typical bacterium, *Escherichia coli,* consists of a single circular DNA molecule with a molecular weight of about 2×10^9 and composed of approximately 5×10^6 base pairs. This amount of genetic information can code for about 2000 proteins with an average molecular weight of 50,000. The DNA of the smallest free-living organism, the wall-less bacterium *Mycoplasma,* has a molecular weight of 5×10^8. Note that bacteria are **haploid,** since they have a single chromosome, in contrast to human cells, which are diploid. The DNA of human cells contains about 3×10^9 base pairs and can encode about 100,000 proteins.

MUTATIONS

A mutation is a change in the base sequence of DNA that usually results in insertion of a different amino acid into a protein and the appearance of an altered phenotype. Mutations result from three types of molecular changes:

(1) The first type is the **base substitution.** This occurs when one base is inserted in place of another. It takes place at the time of DNA replication, either because the DNA polymerase makes an error or because a mutagen alters the hydrogen bonding of the base being used as a template in such a manner that the wrong base is inserted. When the base substitution results in a codon that simply causes a different amino acid to be inserted, the mutation is called a **missense mutation;** when the base substitution generates a termination codon that stops protein synthesis prematurely, the mutation is called a **nonsense mutation.** Nonsense mutations almost always destroy protein function.

(2) The second type of mutation is the **frame shift mutation.** This occurs when one or more base pairs are added or deleted, which shifts the reading frame on the ribosome and results in incorporation of the wrong amino acids "downstream" from the mutation and in the production of an inactive protein.

(3) The third type of mutation occurs when **transposons** or **insertion sequences** are integrated into the DNA. These newly inserted pieces of DNA can cause profound changes in the genes into which they insert and in adjacent genes.

Mutations can be caused by chemicals, radiation, or viruses. Chemicals act in several different ways.

(1) Some, such as nitrous acid and alkylating agents, alter the existing base so that it forms a hydrogen bond preferentially with the wrong base; for example, adenine would no longer pair with thymine but with cytosine.

(2) Some chemicals, such as 5-bromouracil, are base analogues, since they resemble normal bases. Because the bromine atom has an atomic radius similar to that of a methyl group, 5-bromouracil can be inserted in place of thymine (5-methyluracil). However, 5-bromouracil has less hydrogen-bonding fidelity than does thymine, and so it binds to guanine with greater frequency. This results in a transition from an A-T base pair to a G-C base pair, thereby producing a mutation. The antiviral drug iododeoxyuridine acts as a base analogue of thymidine.

(3) Some chemicals, such as benzpyrene, which is found in tobacco smoke, bind to the existing DNA bases and cause frame shift mutations. These chemicals, which are frequently carcinogens as well as mutagens, intercalate between the adjacent bases, thereby distorting and offsetting the DNA sequence.

X-rays and ultraviolet light can cause mutations also.

(1) X-rays have high energy and can damage DNA in three ways: (a) by breaking the covalent bonds that hold the ribose phosphate chain together, (b) by producing free radicals that can attack the bases, and (c) by altering the electrons in the bases and thus changing their hydrogen bonding.

(2) Ultraviolet radiation, which has lower energy than x-rays, causes the cross-linking of the adjacent pyrimidine bases to form dimers. This cross-linking, for example, of adjacent thymines to form a thymine dimer, results in inability of the DNA to replicate properly.

Certain viruses, such as the bacterial virus Mu (mutator bacteriophage), cause a high frequency of mutations when their DNA is inserted into the bacterial chromosome. Since the viral DNA can insert into many different sites, mutations in various genes can occur. These mutations are either frame shift mutations or deletions.

Conditional-lethal mutations are of medical interest, since they may be useful in vaccines, eg, influenza vaccine. The word "conditional" indicates that the mutation is expressed only under certain conditions. The most important conditional-lethal mutations are the temperature-sensitive ones. Temperature-sensitive organisms can replicate at a relatively low, permissive temperature, eg, 32 °C, but cannot grow at a higher, restrictive temperature, eg, 37 °C. This behavior is due to a mutation that causes an amino acid change in an essential protein, allowing it to function normally at 32 °C but not at 37 °C because of an altered conformation at the higher temperature. An example of a conditional-lethal mutant of medical importance is a strain of influenza virus currently used in an experimental vaccine. This vaccine contains a virus that cannot grow at 37 °C and hence cannot infect the lungs and cause pneumonia, but it can grow at 32 °C in the nose, where it can replicate and induce immunity.

TRANSFER OF DNA WITHIN BACTERIAL CELLS

Transposons transfer DNA from one site on the bacterial chromosome to another site or to a plasmid. They do so by synthesizing a copy of their DNA and inserting the copy at another site in the bacterial chromosome or the plasmid. The structure and function of transposons are described in Chapter 2, and their role in antimicrobial drug resistance is described in Chapter 11.

Transfer of DNA within bacteria also occurs by **"programmed rearrangements"** (Fig 4–1). These gene rearrangements account for many of the antigenic changes seen in *Neisseria gonorrhoeae* and in *Borrelia recurrentis*, the cause of relapsing fever. (They also occur in trypanosomes which are discussed in Chapter 52.) A programmed rearrangement consists of the movement of a gene from a "silent" storage site

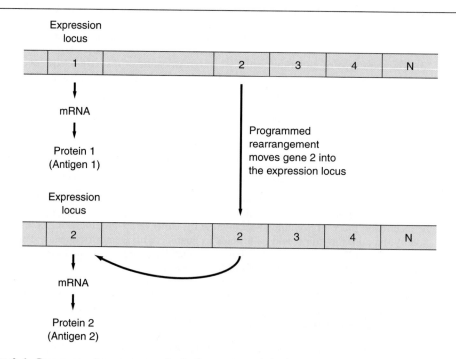

Figure 4–1. Programmed rearrangements. In the top part of the figure, the gene for protein 1 is in the expression locus and the mRNA for protein 1 is synthesized. At a later time, a copy of gene 2 is made and inserted into the expression locus. By moving only the copy of the gene, the cell always keeps the original DNA for use in the future. When the DNA of gene 2 is inserted, the DNA of gene 1 is excised and degraded.

Table 4–1. Comparison of conjugation, transduction, and transformation.

Transfer Procedure	Process	Type of Cells Involved	Nature of DNA Transferred
Conjugation	DNA transferred from one bacterium to another	Prokaryotic	Chromosomal or plasmid
Transduction	DNA transferred by a virus from one cell to another	Prokaryotic	Any gene in generalized transduction; only certain genes in specialized transduction
Transformation	Purified DNA taken up by a cell	Prokaryotic or eukaryotic (eg, human)	Any DNA

where the gene is not expressed to an "active" site where transcription and translation occur. There are many silent genes that encode variants of the antigens and the insertion of a new gene into the active site in a sequential, repeated "programmed" manner is the source of the consistent antigenic variation. These movements are not induced by an immune response but have the effect of allowing the organism to evade it.

TRANSFER OF DNA BETWEEN BACTERIAL CELLS

The transfer of genetic information from one cell to another can occur by three methods: conjugation, transduction, and transformation (Table 4–1). From a medical viewpoint, the most important consequence of DNA transfer is that antibiotic resistance genes are spread from one bacterium to another by these processes.

(1) Conjugation is the mating of two bacterial cells during which DNA is transferred from the donor to the recipient cell (Fig 4–2). The mating process is controlled by an **F (fertility) plasmid** (F factor), which carries the genes for the proteins required for conjugation. One of the most important proteins is pilin, which forms the **sex pilus** (conjugation tube). Mating begins when the pilus of the donor male bacterium carrying the F factor (F^+) attaches to a receptor on the surface of the recipient female bacterium, which does not contain an F factor (F^-). The cells are then drawn into direct contact by "reeling in" the pilus. After an enzymatic cleavage of the F factor DNA, one strand is transferred across the conjugal bridge into the recipient cell. The process is completed by synthesis of the complementary strand to form a double-stranded F factor plasmid in both the donor and recipient

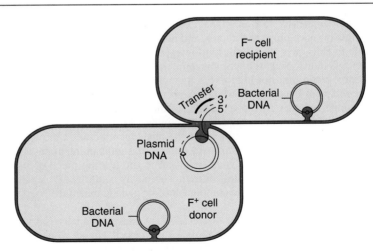

Figure 4–2. Conjugation. An F plasmid is being transferred from an F^+ donor bacterium to an F^- recipient. The transfer is at the contact site made by the sex pilus. The new plasmid in the recipient bacterium is composed of one parental strand (solid line) and one newly synthesized strand (dashed line). The previously existing plasmid in the donor bacterium now consists of one parental strand (solid line) and one newly synthesized strand (dashed line). Both plasmids are drawn with only a short region of newly synthesized DNA (dashed lines), but at the end of DNA synthesis, both the donor and the recipient contain a complete copy of the plasmid DNA. (Modified and reproduced, with permission, from Stanier RY, Doudoroff M, Adelberg EA: *The Microbial World,* 3rd ed. Copyright © 1970. By permission of Prentice-Hall, Inc., Englewood Cliffs, NJ.)

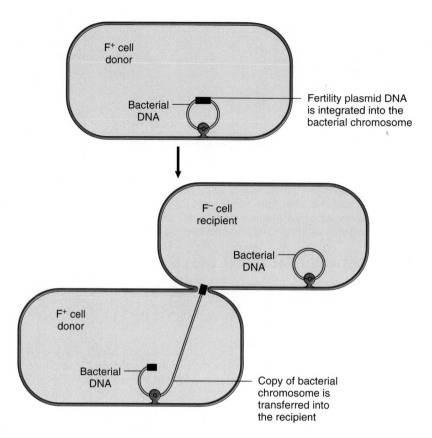

Figure 4–3. High frequency recombination. In the top part of the figure, a fertility (F) plasmid has integrated into the bacterial chromosome. In the bottom part, the F plasmid mediates the transfer of the bacterial chromosome of the donor into the recipient bacteria.

cells. The recipient is now an F⁺ male cell that is capable of transmitting the plasmid further. Note that in this instance only the F factor, and not the bacterial chromosome, has been transferred.

Some F⁺ cells have their F plasmid integrated into the bacterial DNA and thereby acquire the capability of transferring the chromosome into another cell. These cells are called **Hfr (high-frequency recombination)** cells (Fig 4–3). During this transfer, the single strand of DNA that enters the recipient F⁻ cell contains a piece of the F factor at the leading end followed by the bacterial chromosome and then by the remainder of the F factor. The time required for complete transfer of the bacterial DNA is approximately 100 minutes. Most matings result in the transfer of only a portion of the donor chromosome, because the attachment between the two cells can break. The donor cell genes that are transferred vary, since the F plasmid can integrate at several different sites in the bacterial DNA. The bacterial genes adjacent to the leading piece of the F factor are the first and therefore the most frequently transferred. The newly acquired DNA can recombine into the recipient's DNA and become a stable component of its genetic material.

(2) Transduction is the transfer of cell DNA by means of a bacterial virus **(bacteriophage, phage)** (Fig 4–4). During the growth of the virus within the cell, a piece of bacterial DNA is incorporated into the virus particle and is carried into the recipient cell at the time of infection. Within the recipient cell, the phage DNA can integrate into the cell DNA and the cell can acquire a new trait, a process called **lysogenic conversion** (see the end of chapter 29). This process can change a nonpathogenic organism into a pathogenic one. Diphtheria toxin, botulinum toxin, cholera toxin, and erythrogenic toxin (*Streptococcus pyogenes*) are encoded by bacteriophages and can be transferred by transduction.

There are two types of transduction, generalized and specialized. The **generalized** type occurs when the virus carries a segment from any part of the bacterial chromosome. This occurs because the cell DNA is fragmented after phage infection and pieces of cell DNA the same size as the viral

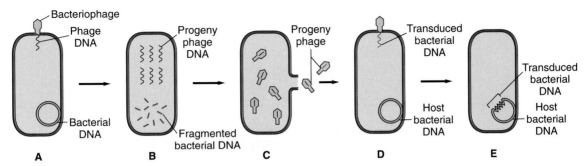

Figure 4–4. Transduction. **A:** A bacteriophage infects a bacterium, and phage DNA enters the cell. **B:** The phage DNA replicates, and the bacterial DNA fragments. **C:** The progeny phage assemble and are released; most contain phage DNA, and a few contain bacterial DNA. **D:** Another bacterium is infected by a phage containing bacterial DNA. **E:** The transduced bacterial DNA integrates into host DNA, and the host acquires a new trait. Figure 29–7 illustrates the integration of phage DNA into the bacterial chromosome.

DNA are incorporated into the virus particle at a frequency of about one in every 1000 virus particles. The **specialized** type occurs when the bacterial virus DNA that has integrated into the cell DNA is excised and carries with it an adjacent part of the cell DNA. Since most lysogenic (temperate) phages integrate at specific sites in the bacterial DNA, the adjacent cellular genes that are transduced are usually specific to that virus.

(3) Transformation is the transfer of DNA itself from one cell to another. This occurs by either of the two following methods. In nature, dying bacteria may release their DNA, which may be taken up by recipient cells. There is little evidence that this natural process plays a significant role in disease. In the laboratory, an investigator may extract DNA from one type of bacteria and introduce it into genetically different bacteria. When purified DNA is injected into the nucleus of a eukaryotic cell, the process is called **transfection.** Transfection is frequently used in genetic engineering procedures.

The experimental use of transformation has revealed important information about DNA. In 1944, it was shown that DNA extracted from encapsulated "smooth" pneumococci could transform nonencapsulated "rough" pneumococci into encapsulated smooth organisms. This demonstration that the "transforming principle" was DNA marked the first evidence that DNA was the genetic material.

RECOMBINATION

Once the DNA is transferred from the donor to the recipient cell by one of the three processes just described, it can integrate into the host cell chromosome by recombination. There are two types of recombination:

(1) homologous recombination, in which two pieces of DNA that have extensive homologous regions pair up and exchange pieces by the processes of breakage and reunion, and

(2) nonhomologous recombination, in which little, if any, homology is necessary.

Different genetic loci govern these two types, and so it is presumed that different enzymes are involved. Although it is known that a variety of endonucleases and ligases are involved, the precise sequence of events is unknown.

Review Questions

1. Describe the chromosomal DNA of a typical bacterium. Compare it with plasmid DNA.
2. What are the three main types of mutations?
3. How do base analogues, eg, iododeoxyuridine, and ultraviolet radiation cause mutations?
4. What is a conditional-lethal mutation?
5. What is conjugation? How does an Hfr cell differ from an F$^+$ cell? What is the medical importance of conjugation?

6. What is transduction? Why is it important?
7. How does transformation differ from transduction and conjugation?

5

Classification of Medically Important Bacteria

Table 5–1. Classification of medically important bacteria.

Characteristics	Genus	Representative Diseases
I. Rigid, thick-walled cells		
A. Free-living (extracellular bacteria)		
1. Gram-positive		
a. Cocci	Streptococcus	Pneumonia, pharyngitis, cellulitis
	Staphylococcus	Abscess of skin and other organs
b. Spore-forming rods		
(1) Aerobic	Bacillus	Anthrax
(2) Anaerobic	Clostridium	Tetanus, gas gangrene, botulism
c. Non-spore-forming rods		
(1) Nonfilamentous	Corynebacterium	Diphtheria
	Listeria	Meningitis
(2) Filamentous	Actinomyces	Actinomycosis
	Nocardia	Nocardiosis
2. Gram-negative		
a. Cocci	Neisseria	Gonorrhea, meningitis
b. Rods		
(1) Facultative		
(a) Straight		
(i) Respiratory organisms	Haemophilus	Meningitis
	Bordetella	Whooping cough
	Legionella	Pneumonia
(ii) Zoonotic organisms	Brucella	Brucellosis
	Francisella	Tularemia
	Pasteurella	Cellulitis
	Yersinia	Plague
(iii) Enteric and related organisms	Escherichia	Urinary tract infection, diarrhea
	Enterobacter	Urinary tract infection
	Serratia	Pneumonia
	Klebsiella	Pneumonia, urinary tract infection
	Salmonella	Enterocolitis, typhoid fever
	Shigella	Enterocolitis
	Proteus	Urinary tract infection
(b) Curved	Campylobacter	Enterocolitis
	Helicobacter	Gastritis, peptic ulcer
	Vibrio	Cholera
(2) Aerobic	Pseudomonas	Pneumonia, urinary tract infection
(3) Anaerobic	Bacteroides	Peritonitis
3. Acid-fast	Mycobacterium	Tuberculosis, leprosy
B. Non-free-living (obligate intracellular parasites)	Rickettsia	Rocky Mountain spotted fever, typhus, Q fever
	Chlamydia	Urethritis, trachoma, psittacosis
II. Flexible, thin-walled cells (spirochetes)	Treponema	Syphilis
	Borrelia	Lyme disease
	Leptospira	Leptospirosis
III. Wall-less cells	Mycoplasma	Pneumonia

The current classification of bacteria is based primarily on morphologic and biochemical characteristics. A scheme that divides the medically important organisms by genus is shown in Table 5–1. For pedagogic purposes this classification scheme deviates from those derived from strict taxonomic principles in two ways:

(1) only organisms that are described in this book in the section on medically important bacteria are included; and

(2) because there are so many gram-negative rods, they are divided into three categories: respiratory organisms, zoonotic organisms, and enteric and related organisms.

The initial criterion used in the classification is the nature of the cell wall; ie, is it rigid, flexible, or absent? Bacteria with rigid, thick walls can be subdivided into free-living bacteria, which are capable of growing on laboratory medium in the absence of human or other animal cells, and non-free-living bacteria, which are obligate intracellular parasites and therefore can grow only within human or other animal cells. The free-living organisms are further subdivided according to shape and staining reaction into a variety of gram-positive and gram-negative cocci and rods with different oxygen requirements and spore-forming abilities. Bacteria with flexible, thin walls (the spirochetes) and those without cell walls (the mycoplasmas) form separate units.

Review Question

Describe the criteria used to classify bacteria.

Normal Flora

6

Normal flora is the term used to describe the various bacteria and fungi that are **permanent residents** of certain body sites, especially the skin, oropharynx, colon, and vagina (Tables 6–1 and 6–2). The two other major groups of microorganisms, the viruses and parasites, are usually not considered members of the normal flora, although they can be present in asymptomatic individuals. The members of the normal flora vary in both number and kind from one site to another. Although the normal flora extensively populates many areas of the body, the internal organs usually are sterile. Areas such as the central nervous system, blood, lower bronchi and alveoli, liver, spleen, kidneys, and bladder are free of all but the occasional transient organism.

There is a distinction between the presence of these organisms and the **carrier state.** In a sense we all are carriers of microorganisms, but that is not the normal use of the term in the medical context. The term "carrier" implies that an individual harbors a potential pathogen and therefore can be a source of infection of others. It is most frequently used in reference to asymptomatic infection or to a patient who has recovered from a disease but continues to carry the organism and may shed it for a long period. When an organism establishes more than a temporary relationship, the host is said to be **colonized** by that organism.

The members of the normal flora play a role both in the maintenance of health and in the causation of disease in three significant ways.

(1) They can cause disease, especially in immunocompromised and debilitated individuals. Although these organisms are nonpathogens in their usual anatomic location, they can be pathogens in other parts of the body.

Table 6–1. Summary of the members of normal flora and their anatomic locations.

Members of the Normal Flora[1]	Anatomic Location
Bacteroides species	Colon, throat, vagina
Candida albicans	Mouth, colon, vagina
Clostridium species	Colon
Corynebacterium species (diphtheroids)	Nasopharynx, skin, vagina
Escherichia coli and other coliforms	Colon, vagina, outer urethra
Gardnerella vaginalis	Vagina
Haemophilus species	Nasopharynx, conjunctiva
Lactobacillus species	Mouth, colon, vagina
Neisseria species	Mouth, nasopharynx
Pseudomonas aeruginosa	Colon, skin
Staphylococcus aureus	Nose, skin
Staphylococcus epidermidis	Skin, nose, mouth, vagina, urethra
Streptococcus faecalis (enterococcus)	Colon
Viridans streptococci	Mouth, nasopharynx

[1] In alphabetical order.

(2) They constitute a protective host defense mechanism. The nonpathogenic resident bacteria occupy ecologic niches, and so pathogens have difficulty in multiplying efficiently. If the normal flora is suppressed, pathogens may grow and cause disease.

(3) They may serve a nutritional function. The intestinal bacteria produce several B vitamins and vitamin K. Poorly nourished people who are treated with oral antibiotics can suffer vitamin deficiencies as a result of the reduction in the normal flora. However, since germ-free animals are well nourished, the normal flora is not essential for proper nutrition.

NORMAL FLORA OF THE SKIN

The predominant organism is *Staphylococcus epidermidis,* which is a nonpathogen on the skin but can cause disease when it reaches certain sites such as artificial heart valves. It is found on the skin much more frequently than its pathogenic relative, *Staphylococcus aureus* (Table 6–2). There are about 10^3–10^4 organisms/cm^2 of skin. Most of them are located superficially in the stratum corneum, but some are found in the hair follicles and act as a reservoir to replenish the superficial flora after hand washing. Anaerobic organisms, such as *Peptococcus* and *Propionibacterium,* are situated in the deeper follicles in the dermis, where oxygen tension is low.

NORMAL FLORA OF THE RESPIRATORY TRACT

A wide spectrum of organisms colonize the nose, throat, and mouth, but the lower bronchi and alveoli typically contain few, if any, organisms. The nose is colonized by a variety of streptococcal and staphylococcal species, the most significant of which is the pathogen *S aureus.* Occasional outbreaks of disease due to this organism, particularly in the newborn nursery, can be traced to nasal, skin, or perianal carriage by personnel.

The throat contains a mixture of viridans streptococci, *Neisseria* species, and *S epidermidis* (Table 6–2). These nonpathogens are inhibitory to the growth of the pathogens *Streptococcus pyogenes, Neisseria meningitidis,* and *S aureus,* respectively.

In the mouth, viridans streptococci make up about half of the bacteria. *Streptococcus mutans,* a member of the viridans group, is of special interest since it is found in large numbers (10^{10}/g) in dental plaque, the precursor of caries. The plaque on the enamel surface is composed of gelatinous, high-molecular-weight glucans secreted by the bacteria. The entrapped bacteria produce a large amount of acid, which demineralizes the enamel and initiates caries. The viridans streptococci are

Table 6–2. Medically important members of the normal flora.

Location	Important Organisms[1]	Less Important Organisms[2]
Skin	Staphylococcus epidermidis	Staphylococcus aureus, Corynebacterium (diphtheroids), various streptococci, Pseudomonas aeruginosa, anaerobes (eg, Peptococcus), yeasts (eg, Candida albicans)
Nose	Staphylococcus aureus[3]	S epidermidis, Corynebacterium (diphtheroids), various streptococci
Mouth	Viridans streptococci	Various streptococci, Eikenella corrodens
Dental plaque	Streptococcus mutans	Prevotella intermedia, Porphyromonas gingivalis
Gingival crevices	Various anaerobes, eg, Bacteroides, Fusobacterium, streptococci, Actinomyces	
Throat	Viridans streptococci	Various streptococci (including Streptococcus pyogenes and S pneumoniae), Neisseria species, Haemophilus influenzae, S epidermidis
Colon	Bacteroides fragilis, Escherichia coli	Bifidobacterium, Eubacterium, Fusobacterium, Lactobacillus, various aerobic gram-negative rods, Enterococcus faecalis and other streptococci, Clostridium
Vagina	Lactobacillus, E coli,[3] group B streptococci[3]	Various streptococci, various gram-negative rods, B fragilis, Corynebacterium (diphtheroids), C albicans
Urethra		S epidermidis, Corynebacterium (diphtheroids), various streptococci, various gram-negative rods, eg, E coli[3]

[1] Organisms that are medically significant or present in large numbers.
[2] Organisms that are less medically significant or present in smaller numbers.
[3] These organisms are not part of the normal flora in this location but are important colonizers.

also the leading cause of subacute bacterial (infective) endocarditis. These organisms can enter the bloodstream at the time of dental surgery and attach to damaged heart valves. *Eikenella corrodens,* also part of the normal oral flora, causes skin and soft tissue infections associated with human bites and "clenched-fist" injuries, ie, injuries to the hand that occur during fist fights.

Anaerobic bacteria, such as species of *Bacteroides, Fusobacterium, Clostridium,* and *Peptostreptococcus,* are found in the gingival crevices, where the oxygen concentration is very low. If aspirated, these organisms can cause lung abscesses, especially in debilitated patients with poor dental hygiene. In addition, the gingival crevices are the natural habitat of *Actinomyces israelii,* an anaerobic actinomycete that can cause abscesses of the jaw, lungs, or abdomen.

NORMAL FLORA OF THE INTESTINAL TRACT

In normal fasting people, the stomach contains few organisms because of its low pH and its enzymes. The small intestine usually contains small numbers of streptococci, lactobacilli, and yeasts, particularly *Candida albicans.* Larger numbers of these organisms are found in the terminal ileum.

The colon is the major location of bacteria in the body. Roughly 20% of the feces consists of bacteria, approximately 10^{11} organisms/g. The major bacteria found in the colon are listed in Table 6–3.

The normal flora of the intestinal tract plays a significant role in extraintestinal disease. For example, *Escherichia coli* is the leading cause of urinary tract infections and *Bacteroides fragilis* is an important cause of peritonitis associated with perforation of the intestinal wall following trauma, appendicitis, or diverticulitis. Other organisms include *Streptococcus faecalis* (also known as *Enterococcus faecalis*), which causes urinary tract infections and endocarditis, and *Pseudomonas aeruginosa,* which can cause various infections, particularly in hospitalized patients with decreased host defenses. *P aeruginosa* is present in 10% of normal stools, as well as in soil and water.

Antibiotic therapy, for example with clindamycin, can suppress the predominant normal flora, thereby allowing a rare organism such as the toxin-producing *Clostridium difficile* to overgrow and cause a severe colitis. Administration of certain antibiotics, such as neomycin orally, prior to gastrointestinal surgery to "sterilize" the gut leads to a marked reduction of the normal flora for several days, followed by a gradual return to normal levels.

Table 6–3. Major bacteria found in the colon.

Bacterium[1]	Number/g of Feces	Important Pathogen
Bacteroides, especially *B fragilis*	10^{10}–10^{11}	Yes
Bifidobacterium	10^{10}	No
Eubacterium	10^{10}	No
Coliforms	10^{7}–10^{8}	Yes
Enterococcus, especially *E faecalis*	10^{7}–10^{8}	Yes
Lactobacillus	10^{7}	No
Clostridium, especially *C perfringens*	10^{6}	Yes

NORMAL FLORA OF THE GENITOURINARY TRACT

The vaginal flora of adult women consists primarily of *Lactobacillus* species (Table 6–2). Lactobacilli are responsible for producing the acid that keeps the pH of the adult woman's vagina low. Before puberty and after menopause, when estrogen levels are low, lactobacilli are rare and the vaginal pH is high. Lactobacilli appear to prevent the growth of potential pathogens, since their suppression by antibiotics can lead to overgrowth by *C albicans.*

The vagina is located close to the anus and can be colonized by members of the fecal flora. For example, women who are prone to recurrent urinary tract infections harbor organisms such as *E coli* and *Enterobacter* in the introitus. About 15–20% of women of childbearing age carry group B streptococci in the vagina. This organism is an important cause of sepsis and meningitis of the newborn and is acquired during passage through the birth canal.

Urine in the bladder is sterile in the normal person, but during passage through the outermost portions of the urethra it often becomes contaminated with *S epidermidis,* coliforms, diphtheroids, and nonhemolytic streptococci. The area around the urethras of women and uncircumcised men contains secretions that carry *Mycobacterium smegmatis,* an acid-fast organism.

Review Questions

1. What is the difference between the terms "normal flora" and "carrier state"?
2. What are the major organisms of the skin and of the oropharynx? With which diseases are they particularly associated?
3. Describe the important anaerobes and facultative anaerobes in the normal flora of the colon.
4. If the normal flora of the colon is suppressed by certain antibiotics, which disease can result? What is its pathogenesis?
5. What is the importance of the lactobacilli that are part of the vaginal normal flora?
6. The vaginas of some women are colonized by *Escherichia coli.* What is the significance of this observation? If the organisms were group B streptococci, what would be the significance?
7. If a urine culture grew many colonies of *Staphylococcus epidermidis,* what would be your interpretation?

Pathogenesis

7

A microorganism is a **pathogen** if it is capable of causing disease; however, some organisms are frequently pathogens, whereas others cause disease rarely. **Opportunistic** pathogens are those that rarely if ever cause disease in immunocompetent people but can cause serious infections in immunocompromised patients. These opportunists are frequently members of the body's normal flora. The origin of the term "opportunistic" refers to the ability of the organism to take the opportunity offered by reduced host defenses to cause disease. **Virulence** is a quantitative measure of pathogenicity and is measured by the number of organisms required to cause disease. The 50% lethal dose (LD_{50}) is the number of organisms needed to kill half the hosts, and the 50% infectious dose (ID_{50}) is the number needed to cause infection in half the hosts. The **infectious dose** of an organism required to cause disease varies greatly among the pathogenic bacteria. For example, *Shigella* and *Salmonella* both cause diarrhea by infecting the gastrointestinal tract but the infectious dose of *Shigella* is less than 100 organisms whereas the infectious dose of *Salmonella* is on the order of 100,000 organisms. The infectious dose of bacteria depends primarily on their **"virulence factors,"** for example, whether their pili allow them to adhere well to mucous membranes, whether they produce exotoxins or endotoxins, whether they possess a capsule to protect them from phagocytosis, and whether they can survive various nonspecific host defenses such as acid in the stomach.

There are two uses of the word **"parasite."** Within the context of this chapter, the term refers to the parasitic relationship of the bacteria to the host cells; that is, the presence of the bacteria are **detrimental** to the host cells. Bacteria that are human pathogens can be thought of, therefore, as parasites. Some bacterial pathogens are **obligate intracellular parasites,** eg, *Chlamydia* and *Rickettsia,* because they can grow only within host cells. Many bacteria are facultative parasites because they can grow within cells, outside cells, or on bacteriologic media. The other use of the term "parasite" refers to the protozoa and the helminths, which are discussed in Part VI of this book.

TYPES OF BACTERIAL INFECTIONS

Bacteria cause disease by two major mechanisms: (1) **toxin production** and (2) **invasion** and **inflammation.** Toxins fall into two general categories: **exotoxins** and **endotoxins.** Exotoxins are polypeptides released by the cell, whereas endotoxins are lipopolysaccharides, which form an integral part of the cell wall. Endotoxins occur only in gram-negative rods and cocci; are not actively released from the cell; and cause fever, shock, and other generalized symptoms. Both exotoxins and endotoxins by themselves can cause symptoms; the presence of the bacteria in the host is not required. Invasive bacteria, on the other hand, grow to large numbers locally and induce an inflammatory response consisting of erythema, edema, warmth, and pain. Invasion and inflammation are discussed below in the section entitled Determinants of Bacterial Pathogenesis.

Many, but not all, infections are communicable, ie, are spread from host to host. For example, tuberculosis is communicable, as it is spread from person to person via airborne droplets produced by coughing; but botulism is not, as the exotoxin produced by the organism in the contaminated food affects only those eating that food. If a disease is highly communicable, the term "contagious" is applied.

An infection is **epidemic** if it occurs much more frequently than usual; it is **pandemic** if it has a worldwide distribution. An **endemic** infection is constantly present at a low level in a specific population. In addition to infections that result in overt symptoms, many are **inapparent** or **subclinical** and can be detected only by demonstrating a rise in antibody titer or isolating the organism. Some infections result in a **latent** state, after which reactivation of the growth of the organism and recurrence of symptoms may occur. Certain other infections lead to a **chronic carrier** state, in which the organisms continue to grow with or without producing symptoms in the host. Chronic carriers, eg, Typhoid Mary, are an important source of infection of others and hence are a public health hazard.

The determination of whether an organism recovered from a patient is actually the cause of the disease involves an awareness of two phenomena: normal flora and colonization. Members of the normal flora are permanent residents of the body and vary in type according to anatomic site (see Chapter 6). When an organism is obtained from a patient's specimen, the question of whether it is a member of the normal flora is important in interpreting the finding. **Colonization** refers to the presence of a new organism that is neither a member of the normal flora nor the cause of symptoms. It can be a difficult clinical dilemma to distinguish between a pathogen and a colonizer, especially in specimens obtained from the respiratory tract, such as throat cultures and sputum cultures.

STAGES OF BACTERIAL PATHOGENESIS

Most bacterial infections are acquired from an external source, and for those, the stages of infection are as described below. Some bacterial infections are caused by members of the normal flora and, as such, are not transmitted directly prior to the onset of infection.

A generalized sequence of the stages of infection is as follows:

(1) Transmission from an external source into the portal of entry

(2) Evasion of primary host defenses such as skin or stomach acid

(3) Adherence to mucous membranes, usually by bacterial pili

(4) Colonization by growth of the bacteria at the site of adherence

(5) Disease symptoms caused by toxin production or invasion accompanied by inflammation

(6) Host responses, both nonspecific and specific (immunity), during steps 3, 4, and 5

(7) Progression or resolution of the disease

DETERMINANTS OF BACTERIAL PATHOGENESIS

1. Transmission

Although some infections are caused by members of the normal flora, most are acquired by transmission from external sources. Pathogens exit the infected patient most frequently from the respiratory and gastrointestinal tracts; hence, transmission to the new host usually occurs via airborne respiratory droplets or fecal contamination of food and water. Organisms can also be transmitted by sexual contact, urine, skin contact, blood transfusions, contaminated needles, or biting insects. The major bacterial diseases **transmitted by ticks** in the United States are Lyme disease, Rocky Mountain spotted fever, ehrlichiosis, relapsing fever, and tularemia.

There are four important portals of entry: respiratory tract, gastrointestinal tract, genital tract, and skin (Table 7–1). The important bacterial diseases transmitted by foods are listed in Table 7–2, and those transmitted by insects are listed in Table 7–3. The specific mode of transmission of each organism is described in the subsequent section devoted to that organism.

Animals can also be an important source of organisms that infect humans. They can be either the source (**reservoir**) or the mode of transmission (**vector**) of certain organisms. Diseases for which animals are the reservoirs are called **zoonoses.** The important zoonotic diseases caused by bacteria are listed in Table 7–4.

2. Adherence to Cell Surfaces

Certain bacteria have specialized structures, eg, **pili,** or produce substances, eg, **capsules** or **glycocalyces,** that allow them to adhere to the surface of human cells, thereby enhancing their ability to cause disease. These adherence mechanisms are essential for organisms that attach to mucous mem-

Table 7–1. Portals of entry of some common pathogens.

Portal of Entry	Pathogen	Type of Organism[1]	Disease
Respiratory tract	Streptococcus pneumoniae	B	Pneumonia
	Neisseria meningitidis	B	Meningitis
	Haemophilus influenzae	B	Meningitis
	Mycobacterium tuberculosis	B	Tuberculosis
	Influenza virus	V	Influenza
	Rhinovirus	V	Common cold
	Epstein-Barr virus	V	Infectious mononucleosis
	Coccidioides immitis	F	Coccidioidomycosis
	Histoplasma capsulatum	F	Histoplasmosis
Gastrointestinal tract	Shigella dysenteriae	B	Dysentery
	Salmonella typhi	B	Typhoid fever
	Vibrio cholerae	B	Cholera
	Hepatitis A virus	V	Infectious hepatitis
	Poliovirus	V	Poliomyelitis
	Trichinella spiralis	P	Trichinosis
Skin	Clostridium tetani	B	Tetanus
	Rickettsia rickettsii	B	Rocky Mountain spotted fever
	Rabies virus	V	Rabies
	Trichophyton rubrum	F	Tinea pedis (athlete's foot)
	Plasmodium vivax	P	Malaria
Genital tract	Neisseria gonorrhoeae	B	Gonorrhea
	Treponema pallidum	B	Syphilis
	Chlamydia trachomatis	B	Urethritis
	Candida albicans	F	Vaginitis

[1] B, bacterium; V, virus; F, fungus; P, parasite.

branes; mutants that lack these mechanisms are often nonpathogenic. For example, the **pili** of *Neisseria gonorrhoeae* and *Escherichia coli* mediate the attachment of the organisms to the urinary tract epithelium and the **glycocalyx** of *Staphylococcus epidermidis* and certain viridans streptococci allows the organisms to adhere strongly to the endothelium of heart valves.

Foreign bodies, such as artificial heart valves and artificial joints, predispose to infections. Bacteria can adhere to these surfaces, but phagocytes adhere poorly owing to the absence of selectins and other binding proteins on the artificial surface (see Chapter 8).

3. Invasion and Inflammation

One of the two main mechanisms by which bacteria cause disease is **invasion** of tissue followed by **inflammation.** (The inflammatory response is described in Chapter 8.) Several enzymes secreted by invasive bacteria play a role in pathogenesis. Among the most prominent are

(1) collagenase and **hyaluronidase,** which degrade collagen and hyaluronic acid, respectively, thereby allowing the bacteria to spread through subcutaneous tissue; they are especially important in cellulitis caused by *Streptococcus pyogenes;*

(2) coagulase, which is produced by *Staphylococcus aureus* and accelerates the formation of a fibrin clot from its precursor, fibrinogen (this clot may protect the bacteria from phagocytosis by walling off the infected area and by coating the organisms with a layer of fibrin);

(3) immunoglobulin A (IgA) protease, which degrades IgA, allowing the organism to adhere to mucous membranes, and is produced chiefly by *N gonorrhoeae, Haemophilus influenzae,* and *Streptococcus pneumoniae;* and

(4) leukocidins, which can destroy both neutrophilic leukocytes and macrophages.

In addition to these enzymes, several virulence factors contribute to invasiveness by limiting the ability of the host defense mechanisms, especially phagocytosis, to operate effectively.

Table 7–2. Bacterial diseases transmitted by foods.

Bacterium	Typical Food	Main Reservoir	Disease
A. Diarrheal diseases			
Gram-positive cocci			
Staphylococcus aureus	Custard-filled pastries; potato, egg, or tuna fish salad	Humans	Food poisoning, especially vomiting
Gram-positive rods			
Bacillus cereus	Reheated rice	Soil	Diarrhea
Clostridium perfringens	Cooked meat, stew, and gravy	Soil, animals, or humans	Diarrhea
Gram-negative rods			
Escherichia coli	Various foods and water	Humans	Diarrhea
Escherichia coli O157:H7 strain	Undercooked meat	Cattle	Hemorrhagic colitis
Salmonella enteritidis	Poultry, meats, and eggs	Domestic animals, especially poultry	Diarrhea
Shigella species	Various foods and water	Humans	Diarrhea (dysentery)
Vibrio cholerae	Various foods, eg, seafood, and water	Humans	Diarrhea
Vibrio parahaemolyticus	Seafood	Warm salt water	Diarrhea
Campylobacter jejuni	Various foods	Domestic animals	Diarrhea
Yersinia enterocolitica	Various foods	Domestic animals	Diarrhea
B. Nondiarrheal diseases			
Gram-positive rods			
Clostridium botulinum	Improperly canned vegetables, smoked fish	Soil	Botulism
Listeria monocytogenes	Unpasteurized milk products	Cows	Sepsis in neonate or mother
Gram-negative rods			
Vibrio vulnificus	Seafood	Warm salt water	Sepsis
Brucella species	Meat	Domestic animals	Brucellosis
Francisella tularensis	Meat	Rabbits	Tularemia
Mycobacteria			
Mycobacterium bovis	Milk	Cows	Intestinal tuberculosis

(a) The most important of these antiphagocytic factors is the **capsule** external to the cell wall of several important pathogens such as *S pneumoniae* and *Neisseria meningitidis.* The polysaccharide capsule prevents the phagocyte from adhering to the bacteria; anticapsular antibodies allow more effective phagocytosis to occur (a process called **opsonization**) (see p 41). The vaccines against *S pneumoniae, H influenzae,* and *N meningitidis* contain capsular polysaccharides that induce protective anticapsular antibodies.

(b) A second group of antiphagocytic factors are the cell wall proteins of the gram-positive cocci, such as the M protein of the group A streptococci (*S pyogenes*) and protein A of *S aureus.* The M protein is antiphagocytic, and protein A binds to IgG and prevents the activation of complement. These virulence factors are summarized in Table 7–5.

Bacteria can cause two types of inflammation: **pyogenic** and **granulomatous.** In pyogenic (pus-producing) inflammation, neutrophils are the predominant cells. Some of the most important pyo-

Table 7–3. Bacterial diseases transmitted by insects.

Bacterium	Insect	Reservoir	Disease
Gram-negative rods			
Yersinia pestis	Rat fleas	Rodents, eg, rats, prairie dogs	Plague
Francisella tularensis	Ticks *(Dermacentor)*	Many animals, eg, rabbits	Tularemia
Spirochetes			
Borrelia burgdorferi	Ticks *(Ixodes)*	Mice	Lyme disease
Borrelia recurrentis	Lice	Humans	Relapsing fever
Rickettsias			
Rickettsia rickettsii	Ticks *(Dermacentor)*	Dogs, rodents, and ticks *(Dermacentor)*	Rocky Mountain spotted fever
Rickettsia prowazekii	Lice	Humans	Epidemic typhus
Ehrlichia chafeensis	Ticks *(Dermacentor)*	Dogs	Ehrlichiosis

genic bacteria are the cocci listed in Table 7–5. In granulomatous inflammation, macrophages and T cells predominate. The most important organism in this category is *Mycobacterium tuberculosis.* No bacterial enzymes or toxins that induce granulomas have been identified. Rather, it appears that bacterial antigens stimulate the cell-mediated immune system, resulting in sensitized T-lymphocyte and macrophage activity. Phagocytosis by macrophages kills most of the bacteria, but some survive and grow within the macrophages in the granuloma.

Several bacterial and fungal pathogens typically invade, survive, and grow within reticuloendothelial cells. They are "intracellular" pathogens and commonly cause granulomatous lesions. The best-known of these bacteria belong to the genera *Mycobacterium, Legionella, Brucella,* and *Listeria.* The best-known fungus is *Histoplasma.* These organisms are not obligate intracellular parasites, which distinguishes them from *Chlamydia* and *Rickettsia.* They can be cultured on microbiologic media in the laboratory but prefer an intracellular location within the body. The precise mechanism by which these bacteria survive intracellularly is unclear, but some of them, eg, *Legionella,* inhibit the fusion of lysosomes with phagosomes, thereby avoiding the degradative enzymes in the lysosomes.

The invasion of cells by bacteria is dependent on the interaction of specific bacterial surface proteins called **invasins** and specific cellular receptors belonging to the integrin family of transmembrane adhesion proteins. The movement of bacteria into the cell is a function of actin microfilaments. Once inside the cell, these bacteria typically reside within cell vacuoles such as phagosomes. Some remain there, others migrate into the cytoplasm, and some move from the cytoplasm into adjacent cells through tunnels formed from actin. Infection of the surrounding cells in this manner allows the bacteria to evade host defenses.

4. Toxin Production

The second major mechanism by which bacteria cause disease is the production of toxins. A comparison of the main features of **exotoxins** and **endotoxins** is shown in Table 7–6.

Exotoxins Exotoxins are produced by several gram-positive and gram-negative bacteria, in contrast to endotoxins, which are present only in gram-negative bacteria. The essential characteristic of exotoxins is that they are **secreted** by the bacteria, whereas endotoxin is a component of the cell wall. Exotoxins are polypeptides whose genes are frequently located on plasmids or lysogenic bacterial viruses (bacteriophages).

Exotoxins are among the **most toxic** substances known. For example, the fatal dose of tetanus toxin for a human is estimated to be less than 1 μg. Because some purified exotoxins can reproduce all aspects of the disease, we can conclude that certain bacteria play no other role in pathogenesis than to synthesize the exotoxin. Exotoxin polypeptides are good antigens and induce the synthesis of protective antibodies called antitoxins, some of which are useful in prevention or treatment of diseases such as botulism and tetanus. When treated with formaldehyde (or acid or heat), the exotoxin polypeptides are converted into **toxoids,** which are used in protective vaccines because they retain their antigenicity but have lost their toxicity.

Table 7–4. Zoonotic diseases caused by bacteria.

Bacterium	Main Reservoir	Mode of Transmission	Disease
Gram-positive rods			
Bacillus anthracis	Domestic animals	Direct contact	Anthrax
Listeria mono-cytogenes	Domestic animals	Ingestion of unpasteurized milk products	Sepsis in neonate or mother
Erysipelothrix rhusiopathiae	Fish	Direct contact	Erysipeloid
Gram-negative rods			
Bartonella henselae	Cats	Skin scratch	Cat scratch disease
Brucella species	Domestic animals	Ingestion of unpasteurized milk products; contact with animal tissues	Brucellosis
Campylobacter jejuni	Domestic animals	Ingestion of contaminated meat	Diarrhea
Escherichia coli O157:H7	Cattle	Fecal-oral	Hemorrhagic colitis
Francisella tularensis	Many animals, especially rabbits	Tick bite, direct contact	Tularemia
Pasteurella multocida	Cats	Cat bite	Cellulitis
Salmonella enteritidis	Poultry, eggs, and cattle	Fecal-oral	Diarrhea
Yersinia enterocolitica	Domestic animals	Fecal-oral	Diarrhea
Yersinia pestis	Rodents, especially rats and prairie dogs	Rat flea bite	Sepsis
Mycobacteria			
Mycobacterium bovis	Cows	Ingestion of unpasteurized milk products	Intestinal tuberculosis
Spirochetes			
Borrelia burgdorferi	Mice	Tick bite (Ixodes)	Lyme disease
Leptospira inter-rogans	Rats and dogs	Urine	Leptospirosis
Chlamydiae			
Chlamydia psittaci	Psittacine birds	Inhalation of aerosols	Psittacosis
Rickettsiae			
Rickettsia rickettsii	Rats and dogs	Tick bite (Dermacentor)	Rocky Mountain spotted fever
Coxiella burnetti	Sheep	Inhalation of aerosols of amniotic fluid	Q fever
Ehrlichia chafeensis	Dogs	Tick bite (Dermacentor)	Ehrlichiosis

Many exotoxins have an **A-B subunit** structure; the A (or active) subunit possesses the toxic activity, and the B (or binding) subunit is responsible for binding the exotoxin to specific receptors on the membrane of the human cell. Important exotoxins that have an **A-B subunit** structure include diphtheria toxin, tetanus toxin, botulinum toxin, cholera toxin, and the enterotoxin of *E coli* (Fig 7–1).

The A subunit of several important exotoxins acts by **ADP-ribosylation;** ie, the A subunit is an enzyme that catalyzes the addition of ADP-ribose to the target protein in the human cell. The addition of ADP-ribose to the target protein often inactivates it but can also hyperactivate it, either of which can cause the symptoms of disease. For example, diphtheria toxin and *Pseudomonas* exotoxin A ADP-ribosylate elongation factor-2, thereby inactivating it and resulting in the inhibition of protein synthesis. On the other hand, cholera toxin and *E coli* toxin ADP-ribosylate G_s protein, thereby activating it. This causes an increase in adenylate cyclase activity, a consequent increase in the amount of cyclic AMP, and the production of watery diarrhea. Pertussis toxin is an interesting variation on the theme. It ADP-ribosylates G_i protein and inactivates it. Inactivation of the inhibitory G proteins turns on adenylate cyclase, causing an increase in the amount of cyclic AMP, which plays a role in causing the symptoms of whooping cough.

Table 7–5. Surface virulence factors important for bacterial pathogenesis.

Organism	Virulence Factor	Used in Vaccine	Comments
Gram-positive cocci			
Streptococcus pneumoniae	Polysaccharide capsule	Yes	Determines serotype
Streptococcus pyogenes	M protein	No	Determines serotype[1]
Staphylococcus aureus	Protein A	No	Binds to Fc region of IgG and prevents activation of complement
Gram-negative cocci			
Neisseria meningitidis	Polysaccharide capsule	Yes	Determines serotype
Gram-positive rods			
Bacillus anthracis	Polypeptide capsule	No	. . .
Gram-negative rods			
Haemophilus influenzae	Polysaccharide capsule	Yes	Determines serotype
Klebsiella pneumoniae	Polysaccharide capsule	No	. . .
Escherichia coli	Protein pili	No	Causes adherence
Salmonella typhi	Polysaccharide capsule	No	Not important for other salmonellae
Yersinia pestis	V and W proteins	No	. . .

[1] Do not confuse the serotype with the grouping of streptococci, which is determined by the polysaccharide in the cell wall.

The mechanisms of action of the important exotoxins produced by toxigenic bacteria are described below and summarized in Table 7–7.

A. Gram-positive bacteria

The exotoxins produced by gram-positive bacteria have several different mechanisms of action and produce different clinical effects. Some important exotoxins include diphtheria toxin, which inhibits protein synthesis by inactivating elongation factor-2; tetanus toxin and botulinum toxin, which are neurotoxins that prevent the release of neurotransmitters; and toxic shock syndrome toxin, which acts as a superantigen causing the release of large amounts of cytokines from helper T cells and macrophages. The mechanisms of action and the clinical effects of exotoxins produced by gram-positive bacteria are described below.

(1) As shown in Fig 7–1, diphtheria toxin, produced by *Corynebacterium diphtheriae,* inhibits protein synthesis by ADP-ribosylation of elongation factor 2 (EF-2).* The exotoxin activity depends on two functions mediated by different domains of the molecule. The toxin is synthesized as a single polypeptide (MW 62,000) that is nontoxic because the active site of the enzyme is masked (Fig 7–2). A single proteolytic "nick" plus reduction of the sulfhydryl bonds yields two active polypeptides. Fragment A, a 22,000-molecular-weight peptide at the amino-terminal end of the exotoxin, is an enzyme that catalyzes the transfer of ADP-ribose from nicotinamide adenine dinucleotide (NAD) to EF-2, thereby inactivating it. The ADP-ribosylation of EF-2 freezes the translocation complex, and protein synthesis stops. The reaction is as follows:

$$\text{EF-2} + \text{NAD} \rightarrow \text{EF-2–ADP-ribose} + \text{Nicotinamide}$$

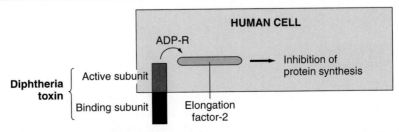

Figure 7–1. Mode of action of diphtheria toxin. The toxin binds to the cell surface via its binding subunit, and the active subunit enters the cell. The active subunit is an enzyme that catalyzes the addition of ADP-ribose (ADP-R) to elongation factor-2 (EF-2). This inactivates EF-2, and protein synthesis is inhibited.

Pseudomas aeruginosa exotoxin has the same mode of action.

Table 7–6. Main features of exotoxins and endotoxins.

Property	Comparison of Properties	
	Exotoxin	**Endotoxin**
Source	Certain species of some gram-positive and gram-negative bacteria	Cell wall of most gram-negative bacteria
Secreted from cell	Yes	No
Chemistry	Polypeptide	Lipopolysaccharide
Location of genes	Plasmid or bacteriophage	Bacterial chromosome
Toxicity	High (fatal dose on the order of 1 μg)	Low (fatal dose on the order of hundreds of micrograms)
Clinical effects	Various effects (see text)	Fever, shock
Mode of action	Various modes (see text)	Includes TNF and interleukin-1
Antigenicity	Induces high-titer antibodies called antitoxins	Poorly antigenic
Vaccines	Toxoids used as vaccines	No toxoids formed and no vaccine available
Heat stability	Destroyed rapidly at 60 °C (except staphylococcal enterotoxin)	Stable at 100 °C for 1 hour
Typical diseases	Tetanus, botulism, diphtheria	Meningococcemia, sepsis by gram-negative rods

Table 7–7. Important bacterial exotoxins.

Bacterium	Disease	Mode of Action	Toxoid Vaccine
Gram-positive			
Corynebacterium diphtheriae	Diphtheria	Inactivates EF-2 by ADP-ribosylation	Yes
Clostridium tetani	Tetanus	Blocks release of the inhibitory neurotransmitter glycine	Yes
Clostridium botulinum	Botulism	Blocks release of acetylcholine	Yes[1]
Clostridium difficile	Pseudomembranous colitis	Exotoxin B is cytotoxic to enterocytes	No
Clostridium perfringens	Gas gangrene	Alpha toxin is a lecithinase. Enterotoxin is a superantigen	No
Bacillus anthracis	Anthrax	One of the toxins is an adenylate cyclase	No
Staphylococcus aureus	Toxic shock	Is a superantigen; binds to class II MHC protein and T cell receptor; induces IL-1 and IL-2	No
Streptococcus pyogenes	Scarlet fever	Is a superantigen; action similar to toxic shock syndrome toxin of S aureus	No
Gram-negative			
Escherichia coli	1. Watery diarrhea	Labile toxin stimulates adenylate cyclase by ADP-ribosylation; stable toxin stimulates guanylate cyclase.	No
	2. Bloody diarrhea	Verotoxin is cytotoxic to enterocytes	No
Vibrio cholerae	Cholera	Stimulates adenylate cyclase by ADP-ribosylation	No
Bordetella pertussis	Whooping cough	Stimulates adenylate cyclase by ADP-ribosylation	No[2]

[1] For high-risk individuals only.
[2] An acellular vaccine is available but is not considered to be a toxoid vaccine.

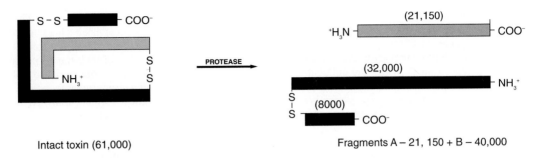

Figure 7–2. Diphtheria exotoxin. Intact extracellular toxin binds to a eukaryotic cell by its B region (dark fragment). After proteolytic cleavage and reduction of the disulfide bond, the A region (light fragment) containing the ribosylating enzyme is activated. (Modified and reproduced, with permission, from Pappenheimer AM Jr: Interaction of protein toxins with mammalian cell membranes. In *Microbiology—1979.* Schlessinger D [editor]. American Society for Microbiology, 1979.)

Fragment B, a 40,000-molecular-weight peptide at the carboxy-terminal end, binds to receptors on the outer membrane of eukaryotic cells and mediates transport of fragment A into the cells.

To summarize, the exotoxin binds to cell membrane receptors via a region near its carboxyl end. The toxin is transported across the membrane, and the proteolytic nick and reduction of the disulfide bonds occur. This releases the active fragment A, which inactivates EF-2. The enzymatic activity is specific for EF-2; no other protein is ADP-ribosylated. The specificity is due to the presence in EF-2 of a unique amino acid, a modified histidine called diphthamide. The reaction occurs in all eukaryotic cells; there is no tissue or organ specificity. Prokaryotic and mitochondrial protein synthesis is not affected, because a different, nonsusceptible elongation factor is involved. The enzyme activity is remarkably potent; a single molecule of fragment A will kill a cell within a few hours. Other organisms whose exotoxins act by ADP-ribosylation are *E coli, Vibrio cholerae,* and *Bordetella pertussis.*

The *tox* gene, which codes for the exotoxin, is carried by a temperate bacteriophage. As a result, only *C diphtheriae* strains lysogenized by this phage cause diphtheria. (Nonlysogenized *C diphtheriae* can be found in the throats of some healthy people.) Regulation of exotoxin synthesis is controlled by the interaction of iron in the medium with a *tox* gene repressor synthesized by the bacterium. As the concentration of iron increases, the iron-repressor complex inhibits the transcription of the *tox* gene.

(2) Tetanus toxin, produced by *Clostridium tetani,* is a **neurotoxin** that prevents release of the inhibitory neurotransmitter glycine. When the inhibitory neurons are nonfunctional, the excitatory neurons are unopposed, leading to muscle spasms and a spastic paralysis. Tetanus toxin (tetanospasmin) is composed of two polypeptide subunits encoded by plasmid DNA. The heavy chain of the polypeptide binds to gangliosides in the membrane of the neuron; the light chain is a protease that degrades the protein(s) responsible for the release of the inhibitory neurotransmitter. The toxin released at the site of the peripheral wound may travel either by retrograde axonal transport or in the bloodstream to the anterior horn and interstitial neurons of the spinal cord. Blockage of release of the inhibitory transmitter leads to convulsive contractions of the voluntary muscles best exemplified by spasm of the jaw and neck muscles ("lockjaw").

(3) Botulinum toxin, produced by *Clostridium botulinum,* is a **neurotoxin** that blocks the release of acetylcholine at the synapse, producing a flaccid paralysis. The toxin is encoded by the genes of a temperate bacteriophage. Approximately 1 µg is lethal for humans; it is one of the most toxic compounds known. The toxin is composed of two polypeptide subunits held together by disulfide bonds. One of the subunits binds to a receptor on the neuron; the other subunit is a protease that degrades the protein(s) responsible for the release of acetylcholine.

(4) Two exotoxins are produced by *Clostridium difficile* both of which are involved in the pathogenesis of pseudomembranous colitis. Exotoxin A is an enterotoxin that causes watery diarrhea. Exotoxin B is a **cytotoxin** that damages the colonic mucosa and causes pseudomembranes to form. Exotoxin B can disaggregate actin filaments in the cytoskeleton.

(5) Multiple toxins are produced by *Clostridium perfringens* and other species of clostridia that cause gas gangrene. A total of 7 lethal factors and 5 enzymes have been characterized, but no species of *Clostridium* makes all 12 products. The best-characterized is the **alpha toxin,** which is a **lecithinase** that hydrolyzes lecithin in the cell membrane, resulting in widespread cell death. The other four enzymes are collagenase, protease, hyaluronidase, and deoxyribonuclease (DNase). The seven lethal toxins are a heterogeneous group with hemolytic and necrotizing activity.

Certain strains of *C perfringens* produce an enterotoxin that causes watery diarrhea. This enterotoxin acts as a superantigen similar to the enterotoxin of *S aureus* (see below).

(6) Three exotoxins are produced by *Bacillus anthracis,* the agent of anthrax: edema factor, protective antigen, and lethal factor. Edema factor is an adenylate cyclase that requires protective antigen for its entry into human cells. The bacterial adenylate cyclase raises the cAMP concentration within the cell, resulting in loss of chloride ions and water and consequent edema formation in the tissue. The mode of action of lethal factor is unknown.

(7) Toxic shock syndrome toxin (TSST) is produced by certain strains of *Staphylococcus aureus.* TSST binds directly to class II major histocompatibility (MHC) proteins without intracellular processing. This complex interacts with the β-chain of the T cell receptor of many helper T cells (see the discussion of superantigens in Chapter 58). This causes the release of large amounts of interleukins, especially interleukin-1 and interleukin-2. They produce many of the signs and symptoms of toxic shock. The staphylococcal enterotoxins that cause food poisoning have a similar mode of action.

(8) Erythrogenic toxin, produced by *Streptococcus pyogenes,* causes the rash characteristic of scarlet fever. Its mechanism of action is similar to that of TSST; ie, it acts as a superantigen (see above). The DNA that codes for the toxin resides on a temperate bacteriophage. Nonlysogenic bacteria do not cause scarlet fever, although they can cause pharyngitis.

B. Gram-negative bacteria

The exotoxins produced by gram-negative bacteria also have several different mechanisms of action and produce different clinical effects. Two very important exotoxins are the enterotoxins of *E coli* and *V cholerae* (cholera toxin), which induce an increase in the amount of cyclic AMP within the enterocyte, resulting in watery diarrhea. The mechanisms of action and the clinical effects of exotoxins produced by gram-negative bacteria are described below.

(1) The **heat-labile enterotoxin** produced by *E coli* causes **watery, nonbloody diarrhea** by stimulating **adenylate cyclase** activity in cells in the small intestine (Fig 7–3). The resulting increase in the concentration of cyclic adenosine monophosphate (cAMP) causes excretion of the chloride ion, inhibition of sodium ion absorption, and significant fluid and electrolyte loss into the lumen of the gut. The heat-

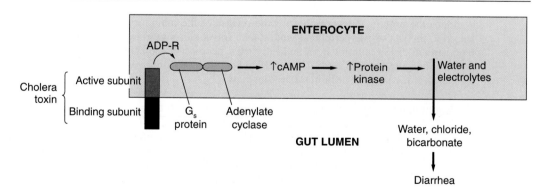

Figure 7–3. Mode of action of *E coli* and *V cholerae* enterotoxins. The enterotoxin, eg, cholera toxin, binds to the surface of the enterocyte via its binding subunit. The active subunit is an enzyme that catalyzes the addition of ADP-ribose (ADP-R) to the G_S regulatory protein. This activates adenylate cyclase to overproduce cAMP. As a consequence, cAMP-dependent protein kinase activity increases, and water and electrolytes leave the enterocyte, causing watery diarrhea.

labile toxin, which is inactivated at 65 °C for 30 minutes, is composed of two subunits, a B subunit, which binds to a ganglioside receptor in the cell membrane, and an A subunit, which enters the cell and mediates the transfer of ADP-ribose from NAD to a stimulatory coupling protein (G_s protein). This locks the G_s protein in the "on" position, thereby continually stimulating adenylate cyclase to synthesize cAMP. The genes for the heat-labile toxin and for the heat-stable toxin (see below) are carried on plasmids.

In addition to the labile toxin, there is a **heat-stable toxin,** which is a polypeptide that is not inactivated by boiling for 30 minutes. The heat-stable toxin affects cGMP rather than cAMP. It stimulates guanylate cyclase and thus increases the concentration of cGMP, which inhibits the reabsorption of sodium ions and causes diarrhea.

Verotoxin is an exotoxin produced by strains of *E coli* with the O157:H7 serotype. These strains cause **bloody diarrhea** and are the cause of outbreaks associated with eating undercooked hamburger in fast-food restaurants. The toxin is named for its cytotoxic effect on Vero (monkey) cells in culture. The toxin inactivates protein synthesis by removing adenine from the 28S rRNA in the large subunit of the human ribosome. The enterotoxin produced by *Shigella* and the toxin ricin, which is produced by the *Ricinus* plant, have the same mode of action as does verotoxin. (Ricin coupled to monoclonal antibody to human tumor antigens has been used experimentally to kill human cancer cells.)

(2) The enterotoxins produced by *V cholerae,* the agent of cholera (see Chapter 18), and *Bacillus cereus,* a cause of diarrhea, act in a manner similar to that of the heat-labile toxin of *E coli* (Fig 7–3).

(3) Pertussis toxin, produced by *Bordetella pertussis,* the cause of whooping cough, is an exotoxin that enhances adenylate cyclase activity by catalyzing the transfer of ADP-ribose from NAD to an inhibitory G protein that regulates adenylate cyclase. Inactivation of this inhibitory regulator results in the stimulation of adenylate cyclase activity and a consequent increase in the amount of cyclic AMP within the affected cells. Pertussis toxin also causes the marked **lymphocytosis** seen in patients with pertussis. The toxin inhibits signal transduction by all chemokine receptors, resulting in an inability of lymphocytes to enter lymphoid tissue (spleen, lymph nodes) and consequently, in an increase in their number in the blood (see the discussion of chemokines in Chapter 58).

Endotoxins   Endotoxins are integral parts of the cell walls of both gram-negative rods and cocci, in contrast to exotoxins, which are released from the cell (Table 7–6). In addition, several other features distinguish these substances. Endotoxins are **lipopolysaccharides (LPS),** whereas exotoxins are polypeptides; the enzymes that produce the lipopolysaccharide are encoded by genes on the bacterial chromosome, rather than by plasmid or bacteriophage DNA, which usually encodes the exotoxins. The toxicity of endotoxins is low in comparison with that of exotoxins. All endotoxins produce the same generalized effects of **fever** and **shock,** although the endotoxins of some organisms are more effective than those of others (Fig 7–4). Endotoxins are weakly antigenic; they induce

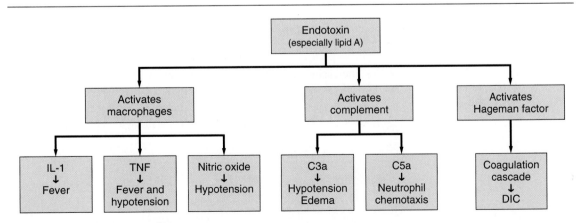

Figure 7–4. Mode of action of endotoxin. Endotoxin is the most important cause of septic shock, which is characterized primarily by fever, hypotension, and disseminated intravascular coagulation (DIC). Endotoxin causes these effects by activating three critical processes: (1) activating macrophages to produce interleukin-1 (IL-1), tumor necrosis factor (TNF), and nitric oxide; (2) activating complement to produce C3a and C5a; and (3) activating Hageman factor, an early component of the coagulation cascade.

protective antibodies so poorly that multiple episodes of toxicity can occur. No toxoids have been produced from endotoxins, and endotoxins are not used as antigens in any available vaccine.

The findings of fever and hypotension are salient features of **septic shock.** The endotoxins of gram-negative bacteria are the best-established causes of septic shock, but surface molecules of gram-positive bacteria (which do not have endotoxins) can also cause septic shock (see below). Two features of septic shock are interesting:

(1) Septic shock is different from toxic shock. In septic shock, the bacteria are in the bloodstream, whereas in toxic shock, it is the toxin that is circulating in the blood. The clinical importance of this observation is that in septic shock, blood cultures are usually positive, whereas in toxic shock, they are usually negative.

(2) Septic shock can cause the death of a patient even though antibiotics have killed the bacteria in the patient's blood, ie, the blood cultures have become negative. This occurs because septic shock is mediated by cytokines, such as tumor necrosis factor and interleukin-1 (see below), that continue to act even though the bacteria that induced the cytokines are no longer present.

The structure of the LPS is shown in Fig 2–6. The toxic portion of the molecule is **lipid A,** which is composed of disaccharides with several fatty acids attached. β-Hydroxymyristic acid is always one of the fatty acids and is found only in lipid A. The other fatty acids differ according to species. The polysaccharide core in the middle of the molecule protrudes from the surface of the bacteria and has the same chemical composition within members of a genus. The repeat unit of sugars on the exterior differs in each species and frequently differs between strains of a single species. It is an important antigen of some gram-negative rods ("O" or somatic antigen) and is composed of three, four, or five sugars repeated up to 25 times. Because the number of permutations of this array is very large, many antigenic types exist. For example, more than 1500 antigenic types have been identified for *Salmonella.*

The biologic effects of endotoxin (Table 7–8) include:

(1) fever due to the release by macrophages of endogenous pyrogen (interleukin-1), which acts on the hypothalamic temperature-regulatory center;

(2) hypotension, shock, and impaired perfusion of essential organs owing to bradykinin-induced vasodilation, increased vascular permeability, and decreased peripheral resistance (nitric oxide, a potent vasodilator, also causes hypotension);

(3) disseminated intravascular coagulation due to activation of the coagulation system through Hageman factor (factor XII), resulting in thrombosis, a petechial or purpuric rash, and tissue ischemia;

(4) activation of the alternative pathway of the complement cascade, resulting in inflammation and tissue damage; and

(5) activation of macrophages, increasing their phagocytic ability, and activation of many clones of B lymphocytes, increasing antibody production. (Endotoxin is a polyclonal activator of B cells, but not T cells.)

Table 7–8. Effects of endotoxin.

Clinical Findings[1]	Mediator or Mechanism
Fever	Interleukin-1
Hypotension (shock)	Bradykinin, nitric oxide
Inflammation	Alternative pathway of complement (C3a, C5a)
Coagulation (DIC)[2]	Activation of Hageman factor

[1] Tumor necrosis factor triggers many of these reactions.
[2] DIC, disseminated intravascular coagulation.

The evidence that endotoxin causes these effects comes from the following two findings: (1) purified lipopolysaccharide, free of the organism, reproduces the effects; and (2) antiserum against endotoxin can mitigate or block these effects.

Endotoxins do not cause these effects directly. Rather, they elicit the production of host factors such as **interleukin-1** and **cachectin*** **(tumor necrosis factor, TNF)** from macrophages.† TNF is the **central mediator** because purified recombinant TNF reproduces the effects of endotoxin and antiserum against TNF blocks the effects of the endotoxin.

Endotoxins can cause a pyrogenic response in the patient if they are present in intravenous fluids. In the past, intravenous fluids were sterilized by autoclaving, which killed any organisms present but resulted in the release of endotoxins that were not heat-inactivated. For this reason, these fluids are now sterilized by filtration, which physically removes the organism without releasing its endotoxin. The contamination of intravenous fluids by endotoxin is detected by a test based on the observation that nanogram amounts of endotoxin can clot extracts of the horseshoe crab, *Limulus.*

Endotoxinlike pathophysiologic effects can occur in **gram-positive** bacteremic infections (eg, *S aureus* and *S pyogenes* infections) as well. Since endotoxin is absent in these organisms, other cell wall components, eg, teichoic acid or peptidoglycan, probably cause the release of TNF and interleukin-1 from macrophages.

TYPICAL STAGES OF AN INFECTIOUS DISEASE

A typical acute infectious disease has four stages:

(1) the **incubation period,** which is the time between the acquisition of the organism (or toxin) and the beginning of symptoms (this time varies from hours to days to weeks depending on the organism);

(2) the **prodrome period,** during which nonspecific symptoms such as fever, malaise, and loss of appetite occur;

(3) the **specific-illness period,** during which the overt characteristic signs and symptoms of the disease occur; and

(4) the **recovery period,** during which the illness abates and the patient returns to the healthy state.

After the recovery period, some individuals become chronic carriers of the organisms and may shed them while remaining clinically well. Others may develop a **latent infection,** which can recur either in the same form as the primary infection or manifesting different signs and symptoms. Although many infections cause symptoms, many others are **subclinical;** ie, the individual remains asymptomatic although infected with the organism.

DID THE ISOLATED ORGANISM ACTUALLY CAUSE THE DISEASE?

Because people harbor microorganisms as members of the permanent normal flora and as transient passengers, this can be an interesting and sometimes confounding question. The answer depends on the situation. One type of situation relates to the problems of a disease for which no agent has been identified and a candidate organism has been isolated. This is the problem that Robert Koch faced in 1877 when he was among the first to try to determine the cause of an infectious disease, namely anthrax in cattle and tuberculosis in humans. His approach led to the formulation of **"Koch's postulates,"** which are criteria that he proposed must be satisfied to confirm the causal role of an organism. These criteria are as follows:

(1) the organism must be isolated from every patient with the disease;

(2) the organism must be isolated free from all other organisms and grown in pure culture in vitro;

---

*Cachectin also causes cachexia by inhibiting the synthesis of lipoprotein lipase in fat cells.
†Endotoxin (LPS) induces these factors by first binding to LPS-binding protein in the serum. This complex then binds to CD14, a receptor on the surface of the macrophage. This stimulates the macrophage to synthesize IL-1, TNF, and other factors.

(3) the pure organism must cause the disease in a healthy, susceptible animal; and

(4) the organism must be recovered from the inoculated animal.

The second type of situation pertains to the practical, everyday problem of a specific diagnosis of a patient's illness. In this instance, the signs and symptoms of the illness usually suggest a constellation of possible causative agents. The recovery of an agent in *sufficient numbers* from the *appropriate specimen* is usually sufficient for an etiologic diagnosis. This approach can be illustrated with two examples: (1) in a patient with a sore throat, the presence of a few beta-hemolytic streptococci is insufficient for a microbiologic diagnosis, whereas the presence of many would be sufficient; and (2) in a patient with fever, alpha-hemolytic streptococci in the throat are considered part of the normal flora, whereas the same organisms in the blood are likely to be the cause of bacterial endocarditis.

In some infections, no organism is isolated from the patient and the diagnosis is made by detecting a rise in antibody titer to an organism. For this purpose, the titer (amount) of antibody in the second or late serum sample should be at least 4 times the titer (amount) of antibody in the first or early serum sample.

Review Questions

1. What are the main differences between exotoxins and endotoxins?
2. What are the mechanisms of action of the exotoxins of (a) *Corynebacterium diphtheriae,* (b) *Clostridium tetani,* (c) *Clostridium botulinum,* (d) *Escherichia coli* (enterotoxin), (e) *Vibrio cholerae,* (f) *Clostridium perfringens* (alpha toxin), and (g) *Staphylococcus aureus?*
3. What is the chemical nature of endotoxin? What are its main physiologic effects? What host factors mediate its action?
4. What role do the capsular polysaccharide, M protein, A protein, and pili play in pathogenesis?
5. What enzymes and other factors play a role in the invasiveness of certain bacteria?
6. What is the mechanism by which certain bacteria cause granuloma formation?
7. What is the difference between the incubation and prodrome periods of an infectious disease?

8

Host Defenses

Host defenses are composed of two complementary, frequently interacting systems: (1) **nonspecific** defenses, which protect against microorganisms in general, and (2) **specific** natural and acquired immunity, which protects against a particular microorganism. The nonspecific defenses can be classified into three major categories: (1) physical barriers, such as intact skin and mucous membranes; (2) phagocytic cells, such as neutrophils, macrophages, and natural killer cells; and (3) proteins, such as complement, lysozyme, and interferon. Fig 8–1 shows the role of several components of the nonspecific defenses in the early response to bacterial infection. The specific defenses are mediated by antibodies and T lymphocytes. Chapter 57 describes these host defenses in more detail.

NONSPECIFIC DEFENSES

Skin & Mucous Membranes   **Intact skin** is the first line of defense against many organisms. In addition to the physical barrier presented by skin, the fatty acids secreted by sebaceous glands in the skin have antibacterial and antifungal activity. The increased fatty acid production that occurs at puberty is thought to explain the increased resistance to ringworm fungal infections that occurs at that time. The low pH of the skin (between pH 3 and 5), which is due to these fatty acids, also has an antimicrobial effect. Although many organisms live on or in the skin as members of the normal flora, they are harmless as long as they do not enter the body.

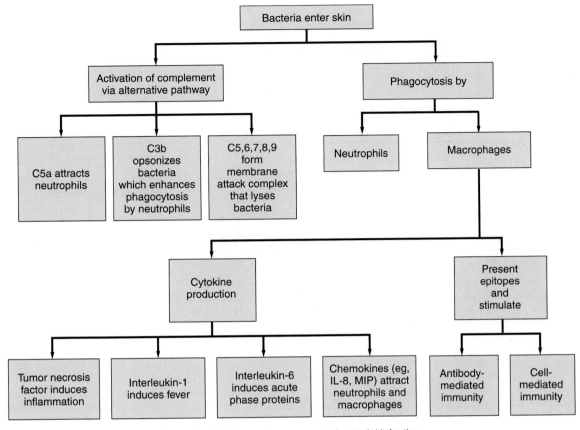

Figure 8–1. Early host responses to bacterial infection.

A second important defense is the mucous membrane of the respiratory tract, which is lined with cilia and covered with mucus. The coordinated beating of the cilia drives the mucus up to the nose and mouth, where the trapped bacteria can be expelled. This mucociliary apparatus, the **"ciliary elevator,"** can be damaged by alcohol, cigarette smoke, and viruses; the damage predisposes the host to bacterial infections. Other protective mechanisms of the respiratory tract involve alveolar macrophages, lysozyme in tears and mucus, hairs in the nose, and the cough reflex, which prevents aspiration into the lungs.

The nonspecific protection in the gastrointestinal tract includes hydrolytic enzymes in saliva, acid in the stomach, and various degradative enzymes and macrophages in the small intestine. The vagina of adult women is protected by the low pH generated by lactobacilli that are part of the normal flora.

The bacteria of the normal flora of the skin, nasopharynx, colon, and vagina occupy these ecologic niches, preventing pathogens from multiplying in these sites. The importance of the normal flora is appreciated in the occasional case when antimicrobial therapy suppresses these beneficial organisms, thereby allowing organisms such as *Clostridium difficile* and *Candida albicans* to cause diseases such as pseudomembranous colitis and vaginitis, respectively.

Inflammatory Response & Phagocytosis The presence of foreign bodies such as bacteria within the body provokes a protective inflammatory response (Fig 8–2). This response is characterized by the clinical findings of redness, swelling, warmth, and pain at the site of infection. These signs are due to increased blood flow, increased capillary permeability, and the escape of fluid and cells into the tissue spaces. The increased permeability is due to several chemical mediators, of which **histamine, prostaglandins,** and **leukotrienes** are the most important. **Bradykinin** is an important mediator of pain. Of the cells that appear at the site, neutrophils and macrophages, both of which perform phagocytic functions, arrive early. Neutrophils predominate in acute pyogenic infections, whereas macrophages are more prevalent in chronic or granulomatous infections. The impor-

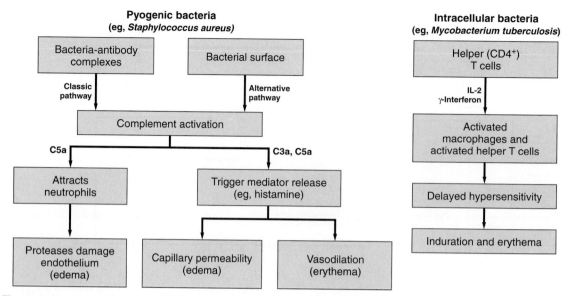

Figure 8–2. Inflammation. The inflammatory response can be caused by two different mechanisms. **Left:** Pyogenic bacteria, eg, *S aureus,* cause inflammation via antibody- and complement-mediated mechanisms. **Right:** intracellular bacteria, eg, *M tuberculosis,* cause inflammation via cell-mediated mechanisms.

tance of the inflammatory response in limiting infection is emphasized by the ability of anti-inflammatory agents such as corticosteroids to lower resistance to infection.

Certain proteins, known collectively as the "acute-phase response," are also produced early in inflammation, mainly by the liver. The best known of these are **C-reactive protein** and **mannose-binding protein,** which bind to the surface of bacteria and enhance the activation of the alternative pathway of complement (see Chapter 58). **Lipopolysaccharide (endotoxin)-binding protein** is another important acute-phase protein that is produced in response to gram-negative bacteria.

Other small polypeptides called **chemokines** attract neutrophils and macrophages to the site of the infection. Interleukin-8 is a chemokine that attracts primarily neutrophils, whereas MCP-1, MIP, and RANTES are attractants for macrophages and monocytes (see Chapter 58).

As part of the inflammatory response, bacteria are engulfed (phagocytized) by polymorphonuclear neutrophils (PMNs) and macrophages. PMNs make up approximately 60% of the leukocytes in the blood, and their numbers increase significantly during infection (leukocytosis). It should be noted, however, that in certain bacterial infections such as typhoid fever, a decrease in the number of leukocytes (leukopenia) is found. The increase in PMNs is caused by the production of granulocyte-stimulating factors (G-CSF and GM-CSF [see Chapter 58]) by macrophages soon after infection.

The process of phagocytosis can be divided into three steps: migration, ingestion, and killing. Migration of PMNs to the site of the organisms is due to chemotactic factors, such as complement component C5a and kallikrein, which—in addition to being chemotactic—is the enzyme that catalyzes the formation of bradykinin. Adhesion of PMNs to the endothelium at the site of infection is mediated first by the interaction of the PMNs with **selectin** proteins on the endothelium and then by the interaction of **integrin** proteins called LFA proteins, located on the PMN surface, with ICAM proteins on the endothelial cell surface.* ICAM proteins on the endothelium are increased by inflammatory mediators, such as interleukin-1 (IL-1) and tumor necrosis factor (TNF) (see Chapter 58), which are produced by macrophages in response to the presence of bacteria. The increase in the level of ICAM proteins ensures that PMNs selectively adhere to the site of infection. Increased permeability of capillaries as a result of histamine, kinins, and prostaglandins† allows PMNs to migrate through the capillary wall to reach the bacteria. This migration is called **diapedesis** and takes several minutes to occur.

---

* LFA proteins and ICAM proteins mediate adhesion between many types of cells. These proteins are described in more detail in Chapter 58.

† The anti-inflammatory action of aspirin is the result of its ability to inhibit cyclooxygenase, thus reducing the synthesis of prostaglandins.

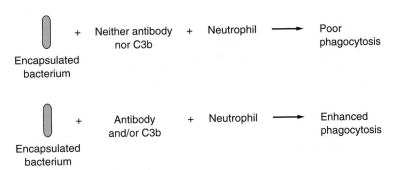

Figure 8–3. Opsonization. **_Top:_** An encapsulated bacterium is poorly phagocytized by a neutrophil in the absence of either antibody or C3b. **_Bottom:_** In the presence of either antibody or C3b or both, the bacterium is opsonized; ie, it is made more easily phagocytized by the neutrophil.

The bacteria are ingested by the invagination of the PMN cell membrane around the bacteria to form a vacuole (**phagosome**). This engulfment is enhanced by the binding of IgG antibodies (**opsonins**) to the surface of the bacteria, a process called **opsonization** (Fig 8–3). The C3b component of complement enhances opsonization. (The outer cell membranes of both PMNs and macrophages have receptors both for the Fc portion of IgG and for C3b.) Even in the absence of antibody, the C3b component of complement, which can be generated by the "alternative" pathway, can opsonize. This is particularly important for bacterial and fungal organisms whose polysaccharides activate the alternative pathway.

At the time of engulfment, a new metabolic pathway, known as the **respiratory burst,** is triggered; this results in the production of two microbicidal agents, the superoxide radical and hydrogen peroxide. These highly reactive compounds are synthesized by the following reactions:

$$O_2 + 1e^- \rightarrow O_2^-$$
$$2O_2^- + 2H^+ \rightarrow H_2O_2 + O_2$$

In the first reaction, molecular oxygen is reduced by an electron to form the superoxide radical, which is weakly bactericidal. In the next step, the enzyme superoxide dismutase catalyzes the formation of hydrogen peroxide from two superoxide radicals. Hydrogen peroxide is more toxic than superoxide but is not effective against catalase-producing organisms such as staphylococci.

The killing of the organism within the phagosome is a two-step process that consists of degranulation followed by production of **hypochlorite** ions (see below), which are probably the most important microbicidal agents. In degranulation, the two types of granules in the cytoplasm of the neutrophil fuse with the phagosome, emptying their contents in the process. These granules are lysosomes that contain a variety of enzymes essential to the killing and degradation that occur within the phagolysosome.

(1) The larger lysosomal granules, which constitute about 15% of the total, contain the important enzyme myeloperoxidase, as well as lysozyme and several other degradative enzymes. (Myeloperoxidase, which is green, makes a major contribution to the color of pus.)

(2) The smaller granules, which make up the remaining 85%, contain lactoferrin and ʼnal degradative enzymes such as proteases, nucleases, and lipases. Lysosomal granules ʼ to the extracellular space as well as into the phagosome. Outside the cell, the degrʼ attack structures too large to be phagocytized, such as fungal mycelia, as ʼ teria.

The actual killing of the microorganisms occurs by a varieʼ categories: oxygen-dependent and oxygen-independenʼ mechanism is the production of the highly reactive bʼ to the following reaction:

In this reaction, chloride ion plus H_2O_2, which was produced by the respiratory burst, yields hypochlorite ion in the presence of myeloperoxidase. Hypochlorite by itself damages cell walls but can also react with H_2O_2 to produce singlet oxygen, which damages cells by reacting with double bonds in the fatty acids of membrane lipids.

Rare individuals are genetically deficient in myeloperoxidase, yet their defense systems can kill bacteria, albeit more slowly. In these persons, the respiratory burst that produces H_2O_2 and superoxide ion seems to be sufficient, but with two caveats: if an organism produces catalase, H_2O_2 will be ineffective, and if an organism produces superoxide dismutase, superoxide ion will be ineffective.

The oxygen-independent mechanisms are important under anaerobic conditions. These mechanisms involve lactoferrin, which chelates iron from the bacteria; lysozyme, which degrades peptidoglycan in the bacterial cell wall; cationic proteins, which damage bacterial membranes; and low pH.

Macrophages also migrate, engulf, and kill bacteria by using essentially the same processes as PMNs do, but there are several differences.

(1) Macrophages do not possess myeloperoxidase and so cannot make hypochlorite ion; however, they do produce H_2O_2 and superoxide by respiratory burst.

(2) Certain organisms such as the agents of tuberculosis, brucellosis, and toxoplasmosis are preferentially ingested by macrophages rather than PMNs and may remain viable and multiply within these cells; granulomas formed during these infections contain many of these macrophages.

(3) Macrophages secrete plasminogen activator, an enzyme that converts the proenzyme plasminogen to the active enzyme plasmin, which dissolves the fibrin clot.

The importance of phagocytosis as a host defense mechanism is emphasized by the following observations.

(1) Repeated infections occur in children with genetic defects in the phagocytic process. Two examples of these defects are chronic granulomatous disease, in which the phagocyte cannot kill the ingested bacteria owing to a defect in NADPH oxidase and a resultant failure to generate H_2O_2; and Chédiak-Higashi syndrome, in which abnormal lysosomal granules that cannot fuse with the phagosome are formed, so that even though bacteria are ingested, they survive.

(2) Frequent infections occur in patients whose PMN count drops below 500/µL as a result of immunosuppressive drugs or irradiation. These infections are frequently caused by opportunistic organisms, ie, organisms that rarely cause disease in people with normal immune systems.

Fever   Infection causes a rise in the body temperature that is attributed to **endogenous pyrogen** (interleukin-1) released from macrophages. Fever may be a protective response, since a variety of bacteria and viruses grow more slowly at elevated temperatures.

SPECIFIC IMMUNITY

There are two types of immunity directed against specific organisms: natural immunity, which exists in the absence of exposure to the organisms, and acquired immunity, which results either from exposure to the organism (active immunity) or from receipt of preformed antibody made in another host (passive immunity).

Natural Immunity   Certain species have natural immunity against a particular organism. For example, *Shigella*, the bacterium that causes dysentery, is unable to infect nonprimates; only humans and chimpanzees are affected. In addition, some racial groups are more resistant to certain organisms; eg, light-skinned people are one-tenth as likely to develop the disseminated form of the fungal disease coccidioidomycosis as are dark-skinned people. The age of an individual is also a significant factor. Generally, very young and very old people are most susceptible to infection, but for some viruses such as poliomyelitis, young children get inapparent infections, whereas older children contract severe disease. The basis for the differences seen with polio is unknown.

Acquired Immunity   **Passive acquired immunity** is temporary protection against an organism and is acquired by receiving serum containing preformed antibodies from another person or animal. Passive immunization occurs normally in the form of immunoglobulins passed through the placenta (IgG) or breast milk (IgA) from mother to child. This protection is very important during the early days of life, when the child has a reduced capacity to mount an active response.

Passive immunity has the important advantage that its protective abilities are present immediately, whereas active immunity has a delay of a few days to a few weeks depending on whether it is a primary or secondary response. However, passive immunity has the important disadvantage that the antibody concentration decreases fairly rapidly as the proteins are degraded, so that protection usually lasts for only a month or two. The administration of preformed antibodies can be lifesaving in certain diseases, such as botulism and tetanus, that are caused by powerful exotoxins. Serum globulins, given intravenously, have been used to treat impending endotoxic shock in patients with gram-negative rod sepsis and as a prophylactic measure in patients with hypogammaglobulinemia or bone marrow transplants. In addition, they can mitigate the symptoms of certain diseases such as hepatitis caused by hepatitis A virus, but they appear to have little effect on bacterial diseases with an invasive form of pathogenesis.

Active acquired immunity is protection based on exposure to the organism in the form of overt disease, subclinical infection, ie, an infection without symptoms, or a vaccine. This protection has a slower onset but longer duration than passive immunity. An important advantage of active immunity is that an **anamnestic (secondary)** response occurs; ie, there is a rapid response of large amounts of antibody to an antigen that the immune system has previously encountered. Active immunity is mediated by both immunoglobulins and T cells:

(1) Immunoglobulins protect against organisms by a variety of mechanisms: neutralization of toxins, lysis of bacteria in the presence of complement, opsonization of bacteria to facilitate phagocytosis, and interference with adherence of bacteria and viruses to cell surfaces. If the level of IgG drops below 400 mg/dL (normal = 1000–1500), the risk of pyogenic infections caused by bacteria such as staphylococci increases.

(2) T cells mediate a variety of reactions including cytotoxic destruction of virus-infected cells and bacteria, activation of macrophages, and delayed hypersensitivity. T cells also help B cells to produce antibody against many, but not all, antigens.

Review Questions

1. How do the skin and mucous membranes protect against infection?
2. Which cells and proteins are involved in the pyogenic inflammatory response? in the granulomatous inflammatory response?
3. Describe the three steps involved when a neutrophil phagocytizes a bacterium.
4. What is the clinically observed effect of having defective or too few phagocytes?
5. What is the difference between passive and active immunity? What are the advantages and disadvantages of each?

9

Laboratory Diagnosis

In the diagnosis of a disease, several important steps precede the actual laboratory work, namely (1) choosing the appropriate specimen to examine, which requires an understanding of the pathogenesis of the infection; (2) obtaining the specimen properly to avoid contamination from the normal flora; (3) transporting the specimen promptly to the laboratory or storing it correctly; and (4) providing essential information to guide the laboratory personnel.

In general, there are three approaches to the laboratory work:

(1) *observing* the organism in the microscope after staining;

(2) *obtaining* a pure culture of the organism by inoculating it onto a bacteriologic medium; and

(3) *identifying* the organism by using biochemical reactions, growth on selective media, or specific antibody reactions. Which of these approaches are used and in what sequence depend on the type of specimen and organism. After the organism is grown in pure culture, its sensitivity to various antibiotics is determined by procedures described in Chapter 11.

In addition to these bacteriologic procedures, many diagnoses are made by serologic testing, which determines the presence of antibodies specific for the organism. In most cases, a 4-fold rise in antibody titer between the acute- and convalescent-phase serum samples is considered to be significant.

BACTERIOLOGIC METHODS

Blood Cultures   Blood cultures are performed most often when sepsis, endocarditis, osteomyelitis, meningitis, or pneumonia is suspected. The organisms most frequently isolated from blood cultures are two gram-positive cocci, *Staphylococcus aureus* and *Streptococcus pneumoniae,* and three gram-negative rods, *Escherichia coli, Klebsiella pneumoniae,* and *Pseudomonas aeruginosa.*

It is important to obtain at least three 10-mL blood samples in a 24-hour period, because the number of organisms can be small and their presence intermittent. The site for venipuncture must be cleansed with 2% iodine to prevent contamination by members of the flora of the skin, usually *Staphylococcus epidermidis.* The blood obtained is added to 100 mL of a rich growth medium such as brain-heart infusion broth. Whether one or two bottles are inoculated varies among hospitals. If two bottles are used, one is kept under anaerobic conditions and the other is not. If one bottle is used, the low oxygen tension at the bottom of the bottle permits anaerobes to grow.

Blood cultures are checked for turbidity or for CO_2 production daily for 7 days or longer. If growth occurs, Gram stain, subculture, and antibiotic sensitivity tests are performed. If no growth is observed after 1 or 2 days, blind subculturing onto other media may reveal organisms. Cultures should be held for 14 days when infective endocarditis, fungemia, or infection by slow-growing bacteria, eg, *Brucella,* is suspected.

Throat Cultures   Throat cultures are used primarily to detect the presence of group A beta-hemolytic streptococci (*Streptococcus pyogenes*), an important and treatable cause of pharyngitis. They are also used when diphtheria, gonococcal pharyngitis, or thrush (*Candida*) is suspected.

When the specimen is being obtained, the swab should touch not only the posterior pharynx but both tonsils or tonsillar fossae as well. The material on the swab is inoculated onto a blood agar plate and streaked to obtain single colonies. If colonies of beta-hemolytic streptococci are found after 24 hours of incubation at 35 °C, a bacitracin disk is used to determine whether the organism is likely to be a group A streptococcus. If growth is inhibited around the disk, it is a group A streptococcus; if not, it is a non-group A beta-hemolytic streptococcus.

Sputum Cultures   Sputum cultures are performed primarily when pneumonia, tuberculosis, or lung abscess is suspected. The most frequent cause of community-acquired pneumonia is *S pneumoniae,* whereas gram-negative rods, such as *K pneumoniae,* are common causes of hospital-acquired pneumonias.

It is important that the specimen for culture really be sputum, not saliva. Examination of a Gram-stained smear of the specimen frequently reveals whether the specimen is satisfactory. A reliable specimen has more than 25 leukocytes and fewer than 10 epithelial cells per 100× field. An unreliable sample can be misleading and should be rejected by the laboratory. If the patient cannot cough and the need for a microbiologic diagnosis is strong, induction of sputum, transtracheal aspirate, bronchial lavage, or lung biopsy may be necessary. Because these procedures bypass the normal flora of the upper airway, they are more likely to provide an accurate microbiologic diagnosis. A preliminary assessment of the cause of the pneumonia can be made by Gram stain if large numbers of typical organisms are seen.

Culture of the sputum on blood agar frequently reveals characteristic colonies, and identification is made by various serologic or biochemical tests. Cultures of *Mycoplasma* are infrequently done; diagnosis is usually confirmed by a rise in antibody titer. If tuberculosis is suspected, an acid-fast stain should be done immediately and the sputum cultured on special media, which are incubated for at least 6 weeks. In diagnosing aspiration pneumonia and lung abscesses, anaerobic cultures are important.

Spinal Fluid Cultures   Spinal fluid cultures are performed primarily when meningitis is suspected. Spinal fluid specimens from cases of encephalitis, brain abscess, and subdural empyema usually show negative cultures. The most frequent causes of acute bacterial meningitis are three encapsulated organisms: *Neisseria meningitidis, S pneumoniae,* and *Haemophilus influenzae.*

Because acute meningitis is a medical emergency, the specimen should be taken immediately to the laboratory. The Gram-stained smear of the sediment of the centrifuged sample guides the immediate empirical treatment. If organisms resembling *N meningitidis, H influenzae,* or *S pneumoniae* are seen, the quellung test or immunofluorescence with specific antisera can identify the organism rapidly. Cultures are done on blood and on chocolate agar and incubated at 35 °C in a 5% CO_2 atmosphere. Hematin and nicotinamide adenine dinucleotide (NAD) (factors X and V, respectively) are added to enhance the growth of *H influenzae.*

In cases of subacute meningitis, *Mycobacterium tuberculosis* and the fungus *Cryptococcus neoformans* are the most common organisms isolated. Acid-fast stains of the spinal fluid should be performed, although *M tuberculosis* may not be seen, because it can be present in small numbers. The fluid should be cultured and the cultures held for a minimum of 6 weeks. *C neoformans,* a budding yeast with a prominent capsule, can be seen in spinal fluid when India ink is used.

Immunologic tests to detect the presence of capsular antigen in the spinal fluid can be used to identify *N meningitidis, S pneumoniae, H influenzae,* group B streptococci, *E coli,* and *C neoformans.* The two tests most frequently used are latex particle agglutination and counterimmunoelectrophoresis.

Stool Cultures   Stool cultures are performed primarily for cases of enterocolitis. The most frequent bacterial pathogens causing diarrhea in the United States are *Shigella, Salmonella,* and *Campylobacter.*

A direct microscopic examination of the stool can be informative from two points of view: (1) a methylene blue stain that reveals many leukocytes indicates that an invasive organism rather than a toxigenic one is involved; and (2) a Gram stain may reveal large numbers of certain organisms, such as staphylococci, clostridia, or campylobacters. Gram's stain of the stool is not usually done, because the large numbers of bacteria in the normal flora of the colon make the interpretation difficult.

For culture of *Salmonella* and *Shigella,* a selective, differential medium such as MacConkey or eosin-methylene blue (EMB) agar is used. These media are selective because they allow gram-negative rods to grow but inhibit many gram-positive organisms. Their differential properties are based on the fact that *Salmonella* and *Shigella* do not ferment lactose, whereas many other enteric gram-negative rods do. If non-lactose-fermenting colonies are found, a triple sugar iron (TSI) agar slant is used to distinguish *Salmonella* from *Shigella.* Some species of *Proteus* resemble *Salmonella* on TSI agar but can be distinguished because they produce the enzyme urease, whereas *Salmonella* does not. The organism is further identified as either a *Salmonella* or a *Shigella* species by the use of specific antisera to the organism's cell wall O antigen in an agglutination test. This is usually done in hospital laboratories, but precise identification of the species is performed in public health laboratories.

Campylobacter jejuni is cultured on antibiotic-containing media, eg, Skirrow's agar, at 42 °C in an atmosphere containing 5% O_2 and 10% CO_2. It grows well under these conditions, unlike many other intestinal pathogens. Although the techniques are available, stool cultures are infrequently performed for organisms such as *Yersinia enterocolitica, Vibrio parahaemolyticus,* and enteropathic or toxigenic *E coli.* Despite the presence of large numbers of anaerobes in feces, they are rarely pathogens in the intestinal tract, and anaerobic cultures of stool specimens are therefore unnecessary.

Urine Cultures

Urine cultures are performed primarily when pyelonephritis or cystitis is suspected. By far the most frequent cause of urinary tract infections is *E coli.* Other common agents are *Enterobacter, Proteus,* and *Streptococcus faecalis* (the enterococcus).

Urine in the bladder of a healthy person is sterile, but it acquires organisms of the normal flora as it passes through the distal portion of the urethra. To avoid these organisms, a midstream specimen, voided after washing the external orifice, is used for urine cultures. In special situations, suprapubic aspiration or catheterization may be required to obtain a specimen. Because urine is a good culture medium, it is essential that the cultures be done within 1 hour after collection or stored in a refrigerator at 4 °C for no more than 18 hours.

It is commonly accepted that a bacterial count of at least 100,000/mL must be found to conclude that significant bacteriuria is present (in asymptomatic persons). There is evidence that as few as 100/mL are significant in symptomatic patients. For this determination to be made, quantitative or semiquantitative cultures must be performed. There are several techniques. (1) A calibrated loop that holds 0.001 mL of urine can be used to streak the culture. (2) Serial 10-fold dilutions can be made and samples from the dilutions streaked. (3) A screening procedure suitable for the physician's office involves an agar-covered "paddle" that is dipped into the urine. After the paddle is incubated, the density of the colonies is compared with standard charts to obtain an estimate of the concentration of bacteria.

Genital Tract Cultures

Genital tract cultures are performed primarily on specimens from individuals with an abnormal discharge or on specimens from asymptomatic contacts of a person with a sexually transmitted disease. One of the most important pathogens in the genital tract is *Neisseria gonorrhoeae.* The laboratory diagnosis of gonorrhea is made by microscopic examination of a Gram-stained smear and by culture of the organism.

Specimens are obtained by swabbing the urethral canal (for men), the cervix (for women), or the anal canal (for men and women). A urethral discharge from the penis is frequently used. Because *N gonorrhoeae* is very delicate, the specimen should be inoculated directly onto a Thayer-Martin chocolate agar plate or onto a special transport medium (eg, Trans-grow).

Gram-negative diplococci found *intracellularly* within neutrophils on a smear of a urethral discharge from a man have over 90% probability of being *N gonorrhoeae.* Because smears are less reliable when made from swabs of the endocervix and anal canal, cultures are necessary. The finding of only *extracellular* diplococci suggests that these neisseriae may be members of the normal flora and that the patient may have nongonococcal urethritis.

Nongonococcal urethritis and cervicitis are also extremely common infections. The most frequent cause is *Chlamydia trachomatis,* which cannot grow on artificial medium but must be grown in living cells. For this purpose, cultures of human cells or the yolk sacs of embryonated eggs are used. The finding of typical intracytoplasmic inclusions when using Giemsa's stain or fluorescent antibody is diagnostic.

Treponema pallidum, the agent of syphilis, cannot be cultured, and so diagnosis is made by microscopy and serology. The presence of motile spirochetes with typical morphologic features seen by darkfield microscopy of the fluid from a painless genital lesion is sufficient for the diagnosis. The serologic tests fall into two groups: the nontreponemal antibody tests such as the Venereal Disease Research Laboratory (VDRL) or rapid plasma reagin (RPR) test, and the treponemal antibody tests such as the fluorescent treponemal antibody-absorption (FTA-ABS) test. These tests are described on pp 48 and 135.

Wound & Abscess Cultures

A great variety of organisms are involved in wound and abscess infections. The bacteria most frequently isolated differ according to the anatomic site and predisposing factors. Abscesses of the brain, lungs, and abdomen are frequently caused by anaerobes such as *Bacteroides fragilis* and gram-positive cocci such as *S aureus* and *Streptococcus pyogenes.* Traumatic open-wound infections are caused primarily by members of the soil flora such as *Clostridium perfringens;* surgical-wound infections are usually due to *S aureus.* Infections of dog or cat bites are commonly due to *Pasteurella multocida,* whereas human bites primarily involve the mouth anaerobes.

Because anaerobes are frequently involved in these types of infection, it is important to place the specimen in anaerobic collection tubes and transport it promptly to the laboratory. Many of these infections are due to multiple organisms, including mixtures of anaerobes and nonanaerobes, and for that reason it is important to culture the specimen on several different media under different atmospheric conditions. The Gram stain can provide valuable information regarding the range of organisms under consideration.

IMMUNOLOGIC METHODS

These methods are described in more detail in Chapter 64. However, it is of interest here to present information on how serologic reactions aid the microbiologic diagnosis. There are essentially two basic approaches: (1) using known antibody to identify the microorganism, and (2) using known antigens to detect antibodies in the patient's serum.

Identification of an Organism with Known Antiserum

A. Capsular Swelling (Quellung) Reaction: Several bacteria can be identified *directly* in clinical specimens by this reaction, which is based on the microscopic observation that the capsule swells in the presence of homologous antiserum. Antisera against the following organisms are available: all serotypes of *S pneumoniae* (Omniserum), *H influenzae* type b, and *N meningitidis* groups A and C.

B. Slide Agglutination Test: Antisera can be used to identify *Salmonella* and *Shigella* by causing agglutination (clumping) of the unknown organism. Antisera directed against the cell wall O antigens of *Salmonella* and *Shigella* are commonly used in hospital laboratories. Antisera against the flagellar H antigens and the capsular Vi antigen of *Salmonella* are used in public health laboratories for epidemiologic purposes.

C. Latex Agglutination Test: Latex beads coated with specific antibody are agglutinated in the presence of the homologous bacteria or antigen. This test is used to determine the presence of the capsular antigen of *H influenzae, N meningitidis,* several species of streptococci, and the yeast *Cryptococcus neoformans.*

D. Counter-immunoelectrophoresis Test: In this test, the unknown bacterial antigen and a known specific antibody move toward each other in an electrical field. If they are homologous, a precipitate forms within the agar matrix. Because antibodies are positively charged at the pH of the test, only negatively charged antigens, usually capsular polysaccharides, can be assayed. The test can be used to detect the presence in the spinal fluid of the capsular antigens of *H influenzae, N meningitidis, S pneumoniae,* and group B streptococci.

E. Enzyme-Linked Immunosorbent Assay: In this test, a specific antibody to which an easily assayed enzyme has been linked is used to detect the presence of the homologous antigen. Because several techniques have been devised to implement this principle, the specific steps used cannot be detailed here (see Chapter 64). This test is useful in detecting a wide variety of bacterial, viral, and fungal infections.

F. Fluorescent-Antibody Tests: A variety of bacteria can be identified by exposure to known antibody labeled with fluorescent dye, which is detected visually in the ultraviolet microscope. Various methods can be used, such as the direct and indirect techniques (see Chapter 64).

Identification of Serum Antibodies with Known Antigens

A. Slide or Tube Agglutination Test: In this test, serial 2-fold dilutions of a sample of the patient's serum are mixed with standard bacterial suspensions. The highest dilution of serum capable of agglutinating the bacteria is the titer of the antibody. As with most tests of a patient's antibody, at least a 4-fold rise in titer between the early and late samples must be demonstrated for a diagnosis to be made. This test is used primarily to aid in the diagnosis of typhoid fever, brucellosis, tularemia, plague, leptospirosis, and rickettsial diseases.

B.   Serologic Tests for Syphilis: The detection of antibody in the patient's serum is frequently used to diagnose syphilis, because *T pallidum* does not grow on laboratory media. There are two kinds of tests.

(1) The nontreponemal tests use a cardiolipin-lecithin-cholesterol mixture as the antigen, not an antigen of the organism. Cardiolipin (diphosphatidylglycerol) is a lipid extracted from normal beef heart. Flocculation (clumping) of the cardiolipin occurs in the presence of antibody to *T pallidum*. The VDRL and RPR tests are non-treponemal tests commonly used as screening procedures. They are not specific for syphilis but are inexpensive and easy to perform.

(2) The treponemal tests use *T pallidum* as the antigen. The two most widely used treponemal tests are the FTA-ABS and the MHA-TP (microhemagglutination-*Treponema pallidum*) tests. In the FTA-ABS test, the patient's serum sample, which has been absorbed with treponemes other than *T pallidum* to remove nonspecific antibodies, is reacted with nonviable *T pallidum* on a slide. Fluorescein-labeled antibody against human immunoglobulin G (IgG) is then used to determine whether IgG antibody against *T pallidum* is bound to the organism. In the MHA-TP test, the patient's serum sample is reacted with sheep erythrocytes coated with antigens of *T pallidum*. If antibodies are present, hemagglutination occurs.

C.   Cold Agglutinin Test: Patients with *Mycoplasma pneumoniae* infections develop autoimmune antibodies that agglutinate human red blood cells in the cold (4 °C) but not at 37 °C. These antibodies occur in certain diseases other than *Mycoplasma* infections; thus, false-positive results can occur.

Review Questions

1. Why is the skin treated with 2% iodine before a blood culture specimen is taken?
2. What criteria are used to determine whether a sputum specimen is satisfactory?
3. What immunologic tests can be done on spinal fluid to provide a rapid diagnosis?
4. What is the purpose of EMB agar in stool cultures? What is the basis of its action?
5. In urine cultures, the number of organisms present as well as the kind is determined. Why?
6. Describe the microscopic findings in a urethral exudate from a patient with gonorrhea.
7. What test is performed to analyze the fluid from a chancre in a case of primary syphilis? Why?
8. What is the basis for the serologic tests for syphilis?

10

Antimicrobial Drugs: Mechanisms of Action

The most important concept underlying antimicrobial therapy is **selective toxicity,** ie, selective inhibition of the growth of the microorganism without damage to the host. Selective toxicity is achieved by exploiting the differences between the metabolism and structure of the microorganism and the corresponding features of human cells. For example, penicillins and cephalosporins are effective antibacterial agents because they prevent the synthesis of peptidoglycan, thereby inhibiting bacterial but not human cell growth.

Table 10–1. Modes of action of important antibacterial and antifungal drugs.

Mechanism of Action	Drugs
Inhibition of cell wall synthesis Inhibition of cross-linking (transpeptidation) of peptidoglycan	Penicillins, cephalosporins, imipenem, aztreonam
Inhibition of other steps in peptidoglycan synthesis	Vancomycin, cycloserine, bacitracin
Inhibition of protein synthesis Action on 50S ribosomal subunit	Chloramphenicol, erythromycin, clindamycin
Action on 30S ribosomal subunit	Tetracyclines and aminoglycosides
Inhibition of nucleic acid synthesis Inhibition of nucleotide synthesis	Sulfonamides, trimethoprim
Inhibition of DNA synthesis	Quinolones
Inhibition of mRNA synthesis	Rifampin
Alteration of cell membrane function Antibacterial activity	Polymyxin
Antifungal activity	Amphotericin B, nystatin, ketoconazole
Uncertain site of action Various mechanisms proposed	Isoniazid, metronidazole, pentamidine, griseofulvin, ethambutol, pyrazinamide

There are four major sites in the bacterial cell that are sufficiently different from the human cell that they serve as the basis for the action of clinically effective drugs: cell wall, ribosomes, nucleic acids, and cell membrane (Table 10–1).

There are far more antibacterial drugs than antiviral drugs. This is a consequence of the difficulty of designing a drug that will selectively inhibit viral replication. Because viruses use many of the normal cellular functions of the host in their growth, it is not easy to develop a drug that specifically inhibits viral functions and does not damage the host cell.

Broad spectrum antibiotics are those active against several types of microorganisms, eg, tetracyclines are active against many Gram-negative rods, chlamydiae, mycoplasmas, and rickettsiae. **Narrow spectrum** antibiotics are those active against one or very few types, eg, vancomycin is primarily used against certain Gram-positive cocci, namely staphylococci and enterococci.

Bactericidal & Bacteriostatic Activity

In some clinical situations, it is essential to use a bactericidal drug rather than a bacteriostatic one. A bactericidal drug kills bacteria, whereas a bacteriostatic drug inhibits their growth but does not kill them. The salient features of the behavior of bacteriostatic drugs are that (1) the bacteria can grow again when the drug is withdrawn, and (2) host defense mechanisms, such as phagocytosis, are required to kill the bacteria. Bactericidal drugs are particularly useful in certain infections, eg, those that are immediately life-threatening; those in patients whose polymorphonuclear leukocyte count is below 500/μL; and endocarditis, in which phagocytosis is limited by the fibrinous network of the vegetations and bacteriostatic drugs do not effect a cure.

Mechanisms of Action

INHIBITION OF CELL WALL SYNTHESIS

Penicillins Penicillins (and cephalosporins) act by inhibiting **transpeptidases,** the enzymes that catalyze the final cross-linking step in the synthesis of peptidoglycan (see Fig 2–5). For example, in

Staphylococcus aureus, transpeptidation occurs between the amino group on the end of the pentaglycine cross-link and the terminal carboxyl group of the D-alanine on the tetrapeptide side chain. Since the stereochemistry of penicillin is similar to that of a dipeptide, D-alanyl-D-alanine, it can bind to the active site of the transpeptidase and inhibit its activity.

There are two additional factors involved in the action of penicillin.

(a) The first is that penicillin binds to a variety of receptors in the bacterial cell membrane and cell wall called **penicillin-binding proteins (PBPs).** Some PBPs are transpeptidases; the function of others is unknown. Changes in PBPs are in part responsible for an organism's becoming resistant to penicillin.

(b) The second factor is that **autolytic enzymes** called murein hydrolases (murein is a synonym for peptidoglycan) are activated in penicillin-treated cells and degrade the peptidoglycan. Some bacteria, eg, strains of *S aureus,* are **tolerant** to the action of penicillin, since these autolytic enzymes are not activated. A tolerant organism is one that is inhibited but not killed by a drug that is usually bactericidal, such as penicillin (see Chapter 11).

Penicillin-treated cells die by rupture as a result of the influx of water into the high-osmotic-pressure interior of the bacterial cell. If the osmotic pressure of the medium is raised about 3-fold, by the addition of sufficient KCl for example, rupture will not occur and the organism can survive as a protoplast. Exposure of the bacterial cell to lysozyme, which is present in human tears, results in degradation of the peptidoglycan and osmotic rupture similar to that caused by penicillin.

Penicillin is bactericidal, but it kills cells only when they are growing. When cells are growing, new peptidoglycan is being synthesized and transpeptidation occurs. However, in nongrowing cells, no new cross-linkages are required and penicillin is inactive.

Penicillins (and cephalosporins) are called β-**lactam** drugs because of the importance of the β-lactam ring (Fig 10–1). An intact ring structure is essential for antibacterial activity; cleavage of the ring by

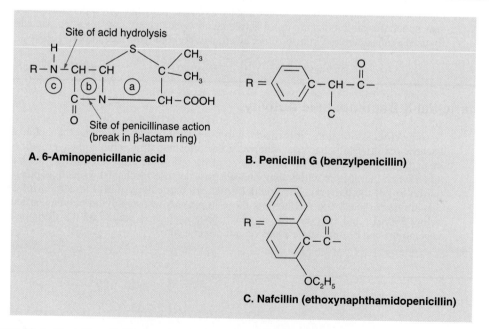

Figure 10–1. Penicillins. ***A:*** The 6-aminopenicillanic acid nucleus is composed of a thiazolidine ring (a), a β-lactam ring (b), and an amino group (c). The sites of inactivation by stomach acid and by penicillinase are indicated. ***B:*** The benzyl group, which forms benzylpenicillin (penicillin G) when attached at R. ***C:*** The large aromatic ring substituent that forms nafcillin, a β-lactamase-resistant penicillin, when attached at R. The large ring blocks the access of β-lactamase to the β-lactam ring.

penicillinases (β-lactamases) inactivates the drug. The most important naturally occurring compound is benzylpenicillin (penicillin G), which is composed of the 6-aminopenicillanic acid nucleus that all penicillins have in common, plus a benzyl side chain (Fig 10–1).

Benzylpenicillin is one of the most widely used and effective antibiotics. However, it has three disadvantages, all of which have been successfully overcome by chemical modification of the side chain. These disadvantages are (1) limited effectiveness against many gram-negative rods; (2) hydrolysis by gastric acids, so that it cannot be taken orally; and (3) inactivation by β-lactamases. There is a fourth disadvantage, common to all penicillins, which has *not* been overcome: hypersensitivity, especially anaphylaxis, in some recipients of the drug.

The effectiveness of penicillins against gram-negative rods has been increased by a series of chemical changes in the side chain (Table 10–2). It can be seen that ampicillin and amoxicillin have activity against several gram-negative rods that the earlier penicillins do not have. However, these drugs are not useful against *Pseudomonas aeruginosa* and *Klebsiella pneumoniae*. Hence, other penicillins were introduced. Generally speaking, as the activity against gram-negative bacteria increases, the activity against gram-positive bacteria decreases.

The second important disadvantage—acid hydrolysis in the stomach—also has been addressed by modification of the side chain. The site of acid hydrolysis is the amide bond between the side chain and penicillanic acid nucleus (Fig 10–1). Minor modifications of the side chain in that region, such as addition of an oxygen (to produce penicillin V) or an amino group (to produce ampicillin), prevent hydrolysis and allow the drug to be taken orally.

The inactivation of penicillin G by β-lactamases is another important disadvantage, especially in the treatment of *S aureus* infections. Access of the enzyme to the β-lactam ring is blocked by modification of the side chain with the addition of large aromatic rings containing bulky methyl or ethyl groups (methicillin, oxacillin, nafcillin, etc; Fig 10–1). Another defense against β-lactamases is inhibitors such as clavulanic acid and sulbactam. These are structural analogues of penicillin that have little antibacterial activity but bind strongly to β-lactamases and thus protect the penicillin. Combinations, such as amoxicillin and clavulanic acid (Augmentin), are in clinical use. Some bacteria resistant to these combinations have been isolated from patient specimens.

Generally speaking, penicillins are nontoxic at clinically effective levels. The major disadvantage of these compounds is hypersensitivity, which is estimated to occur in 1–10% of patients. The hypersensitivity reactions include anaphylaxis, skin rashes, hemolytic anemia, nephritis, and drug fever. Anaphylaxis, the most serious complication, occurs in 0.5% of patients. Death due to anaphylaxis occurs in 0.002% (1:50,000) of patients.

Cephalosporins Cephalosporins are β-lactam drugs that act in the same manner as penicillins; ie, they are bactericidal agents that inhibit the cross-linking of peptidoglycan. The structures, however, are different: The cephalosporins have a six-membered ring adjacent to the β-lactam ring and are substituted in two places on the 7-aminocephalosporanic acid nucleus (Fig 10–2), whereas penicillins have a five-membered ring and are substituted in only one place.

Table 10–2. Activity of selected penicillins.

Drug	Major Organisms[1]
Penicillin G	Gram-positive cocci, gram-positive rods, *Neisseria*, spirochetes such as *Treponema pallidum*, and many anaerobes (except *Bacteroides fragilis*) but none of the gram-negative rods listed below
Ampicillin or amoxicillin	Certain gram-negative rods, such as *Haemophilus influenzae*, *Escherichia coli*, *Proteus*, *Salmonella*, and *Shigella* but not *Pseudomonas aeruginosa*
Carbenicillin or ticarcillin	*P aeruginosa*, especially when used in synergistic combination with an aminoglycoside
Piperacillin	Similar to carbenicillin but with greater activity against *P aeruginosa* and *Klebsiella pneumoniae*
Nafcillin or dicloxacillin	Penicillinase-producing *Staphylococcus aureus*

[1] The spectrum of activity is intentionally incomplete. It is simplified for the beginning student to illustrate the expanded coverage of gram-negative organisms with successive generations and does not cover all possible clinical uses.

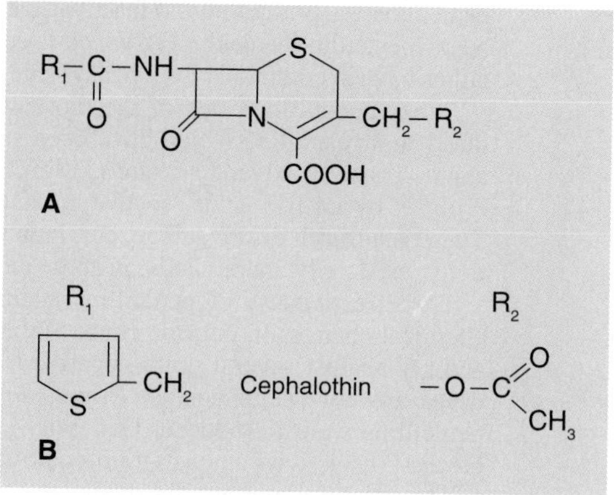

Figure 10–2. Cephalosporins. **A:** The 7-aminocephalosporanic acid nucleus. **B:** The two R groups in the drug cephalothin.

Similar to the penicillins, new cephalosporins were synthesized with expansion of activity against gram-negative rods as the goal. Cephalosporins are effective against a broad range of organisms, are generally well tolerated, and produce fewer hypersensitivity reactions than do the penicillins. Despite the structural similarity, a patient allergic to penicillin has only about a 10% chance of being hypersensitive to cephalosporins also. Cephalosporins are the products of molds of the genus *Cephalosporium,* except for a few, such as cefoxitin, which is made by the actinomycete *Streptomyces.*

Carbapenems   Carbapenems are β-lactam drugs that are structurally different from penicillins and cephalosporins. For example, imipenem (*N*-formimidoylthienamycin), the currently used carbapenem, has a methylene group in the ring in place of the sulfur (Fig 10–3). Imipenem has the widest spectrum of activity of the β-lactam drugs. It has excellent bactericidal activity against many gram-positive, gram-negative, and anaerobic bacteria. It is effective against most gram-positive cocci, eg, streptococci and staphylococci; gram-negative cocci, eg, *Neisseria;* many gram-negative rods, eg, *Enterobacteriaceae, Pseudomonas,* and *Haemophilus;* and various anaerobes, eg, *Bacteroides* and *Clostridium.* It is prescribed in combination with cilistatin, which is an inhibitor of dehydropeptidase, a kidney enzyme that inactivates imipenem. Imipenem is not activated by most β-lactamases.

Monobactams   Monobactams are also β-lactam drugs that are structurally different from penicillins and cephalosporins. Monobactams are characterized by a β-lactam ring without an adjacent sulfur-containing ring structure; ie, they are monocyclic (Fig 10–3). Aztreonam, currently the most useful monobactam, has excellent activity against many gram-negative rods, such as Enterobacteriaceae and *Pseudomonas,* but is inactive against gram-positive and anaerobic bacteria. It is resistant

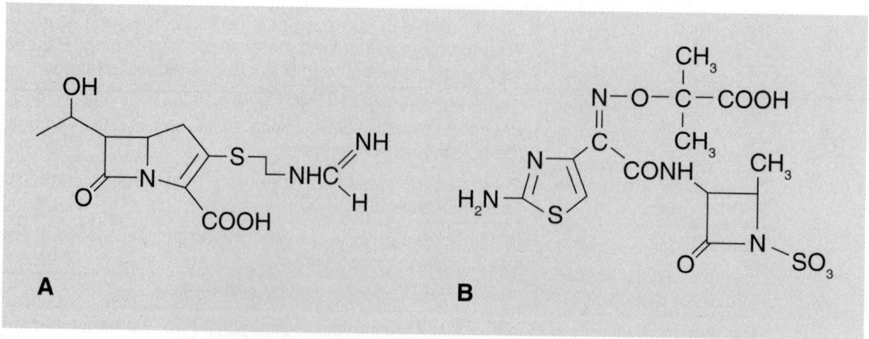

Figure 10–3. A: Imipenem. **B:** Aztreonam.

to most β-lactamases. It is very useful in patients who are hypersensitive to penicillin, because there is no cross-reactivity.

Vancomycin, Cycloserine, & Bacitracin   These three drugs inhibit cell wall synthesis by blocking the formation of precursors. Vancomycin binds to the D-alanyl-D-alanine portion of the pentapeptide to prevent the precursor subunit (muramic acid, pentapeptide, and glucosamine) from being incorporated into the growing peptidoglycan. Vancomycin is a bactericidal agent whose most important use is in the treatment of infections by *S aureus* strains that are resistant to the penicillinase-resistant penicillins such as nafcillin. Vancomycin-resistant mutants of *S aureus* are rare and are not clinically important.

Cycloserine is a structural analogue of D-alanine that inhibits the synthesis of the D-alanyl-D-alanine dipeptide. It is used as a second-line drug in the treatment of tuberculosis.

Bacitracin is a cyclic polypeptide antibiotic that prevents the dephosphorylation of the phospholipid that carries the peptidoglycan subunit across the cell membrane. This blocks the regeneration of the lipid carrier and inhibits cell wall synthesis. Bacitracin is a bactericidal drug useful in the treatment of superficial skin infections but too toxic for systemic use.

INHIBITION OF PROTEIN SYNTHESIS

Several drugs inhibit protein synthesis in bacteria without significantly interfering with protein synthesis in human cells. This selectivity is due to the differences between bacterial and human ribosomal proteins, RNAs, and associated enzymes. Bacteria have 70S* ribosomes with 50S and 30S subunits, whereas human cells have 80S ribosomes with 60S and 40S subunits. Chloramphenicol, erythromycin, and clindamycin act on the 50S subunit, whereas tetracyclines and aminoglycosides act on the 30S subunit. A summary of the modes of action of these drugs is presented in Table 10–3, and a summary of their clinically useful activity is presented in Table 10–4.

1.   Drugs That Act on the 30S Subunit

Aminoglycosides   Aminoglycosides are bactericidal drugs especially useful against many gram-negative rods. Certain aminoglycosides are used against other organisms; eg, streptomycin is used in the multiple-drug therapy of tuberculosis, and gentamicin is used in combination with penicillin G against enterococci. Aminoglycosides are named for the amino sugar component of the molecule, which is connected by a glycosidic linkage to other sugar derivatives (Fig 10–4).

The two important modes of action of aminoglycosides have been documented best for streptomycin; other aminoglycosides probably act similarly. Both **inhibition of the "initiation complex"** and **misreading of messenger RNA** (mRNA) occur; the former is probably more important for the bactericidal activity of the drug. An initiation complex composed of a streptomycin-treated 30S subunit, a 50S subunit, and mRNA will not function—ie, no peptide bonds are formed, no polysomes are made, and a frozen "streptomycin monosome" results. Misreading of the triplet codon of mRNA

Table 10–3. Mode of action of antibiotics that inhibit protein synthesis.

Antibiotic	Ribosomal Subunit	Mode of Action	Bactericidal or Bacteriostatic
Aminoglycosides	30S	Blocks functioning of initiation complex and causes misreading of mRNA	Bactericidal
Tetracyclines	30S	Blocks tRNA binding to ribosome	Bacteriostatic
Chloramphenicol	50S	Blocks peptidyltransferase	Both[1]
Erythromycin	50S	Blocks translocation	Primarily bacteriostatic
Clindamycin	50S	Blocks peptide bond formation	Primarily bacteriostatic

[1] Chloramphenicol can be either bactericidal or bacteriostatic, depending on the organism.

* S stands for Svedberg units, a measure of sedimentation rate in a density gradient. The rate of sedimentation is proportionate to the mass of the particle.

Table 10–4. Spectrum of activity of antibiotics that inhibit protein synthesis.

Antibiotic	Clinically Useful Activity	Comments
Aminoglycosides		
Streptomycin	Tuberculosis, tularemia, plague, brucellosis	Ototoxic and nephrotoxic.
Gentamicin and tobramycin	Many gram-negative rod infections including *Pseudomonas aeruginosa*	Most widely used aminoglycosides.
Amikacin	Same as gentamicin and tobramycin	Effective against some organisms resistant to gentamicin and tobramycin.
Neomycin	Preoperative bowel preparation	Too toxic to be used systemically; use orally since not absorbed.
Tetracyclines	Rickettsial and chlamydial infections, *Mycoplasma pneumoniae*	Not given during pregnancy or to young children.
Chloramphenicol	*Haemophilus influenzae* meningitis, typhoid fever, anaerobic infections (especially *Bacteroides fragilis*)	Bone marrow toxicity limits use to severe infections.
Erythromycin	Pneumonia caused by *Mycoplasma* and *Legionella,* infections by gram-positive cocci in penicillin-allergic patients	Toxicity uncommon.
Clindamycin	Anaerobes such as *Clostridium perfringens* and *Bacteroides fragilis*	Pseudomembranous colitis is a major side effect.

so that the wrong amino acid is inserted into the protein also occurs in streptomycin-treated bacteria. The site of action on the 30S subunit includes both a ribosomal protein and the ribosomal RNA (rRNA). As a result of inhibition of initiation and misreading, membrane damage occurs and the bacterium dies. (In 1993, another possible mode of action was described, namely, that aminoglycosides inhibit ribozyme-mediated self-splicing of rRNA.)

Aminoglycosides have certain limitations in their use: (1) They have a toxic effect both on the kidneys and on the auditory and vestibular portions of the eighth cranial nerve. To avoid toxicity, serum levels of the drug, blood urea nitrogen, and creatinine should be measured. (2) They are poorly absorbed from the gastrointestinal tract and cannot be given orally. (3) They penetrate the spinal fluid poorly and must be given intrathecally in the treatment of meningitis. (4) They are ineffective against anaerobes, because their transport into the bacterial cell requires oxygen.

Tetracyclines Tetracyclines are a family of antibiotics with bacteriostatic activity against a variety of gram-positive and gram-negative bacteria, mycoplasmas, chlamydiae, and rickettsiae. They inhibit protein synthesis by binding to the 30S ribosomal subunit and **blocking the aminoacyl transfer RNA (tRNA) from entering the acceptor site** on the ribosome. However, the selective

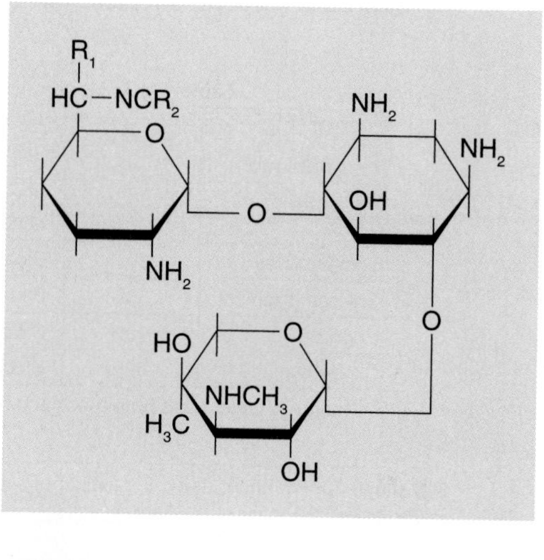

Figure 10–4. Aminoglycosides. Aminoglycosides consist of amino sugars joined by a glycosidic linkage. The structure of gentamicin is shown.

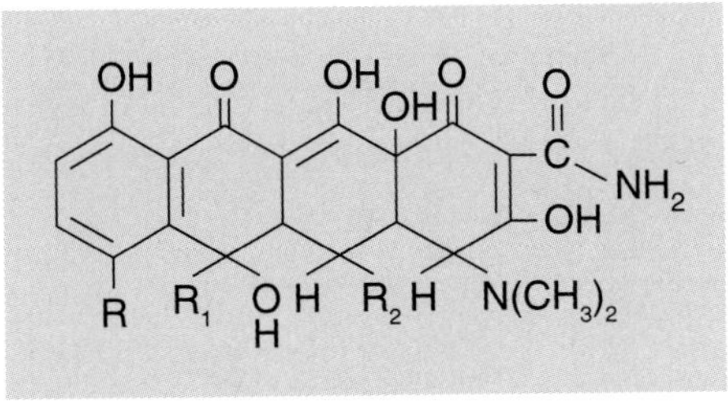

Figure 10–5. Tetracycline structure. The four-ring structure is depicted with its three R sites. Chlortetracycline, for example, has R = Cl, R_1 = CH_3, and R_2 = H.

action of tetracycline on bacteria is not at the level of the ribosome, as tetracycline in vitro will inhibit protein synthesis equally well in purified ribosomes from both bacterial and human cells. Its selectivity is based on its greatly increased uptake into susceptible bacterial cells compared with human cells.

Tetracyclines, as the name indicates, have four cyclic rings with different substituents at the three R groups (Fig 10–5). The various tetracyclines (eg, doxycycline, minocycline, oxytetracycline) have similar antimicrobial activity but different pharmacologic properties. In general, tetracyclines have low toxicity but are associated with two significant difficulties. One is suppression of the normal flora of the intestinal tract, which can lead to diarrhea and overgrowth by drug-resistant bacteria and fungi. The other is brown staining of the teeth of fetuses and young children owing to deposition of the drug in developing teeth; tetracyclines are avid calcium chelators. For this reason, tetracycline is contraindicated for use in pregnant women and in children under age 8 years.

2. Drugs That Act on the 50S Subunit

Chloramphenicol Chloramphenicol is active against a broad range of organisms, including gram-positive and gram-negative bacteria (including anaerobes). It is bacteriostatic against certain organisms, such as *Salmonella typhi*, but has bactericidal activity against the three important encapsulated organisms that cause meningitis: *Haemophilus influenzae*, *Streptococcus pneumoniae*, and *Neisseria meningitidis*.

Chloramphenicol inhibits protein synthesis by binding to the 50S ribosomal subunit and **blocking the action of peptidyltransferase;** this prevents the synthesis of new peptide bonds. It inhibits bacterial protein synthesis selectively, because it binds to the catalytic site of the transferase in the 50S bacterial ribosomal subunit but not to the transferase in the 60S human ribosomal subunit. Chloramphenicol inhibits protein synthesis in the mitochondria of human cells to some extent, since mitochondria have a 50S subunit (mitochondria are thought to have evolved from bacteria). This inhibition may be the cause of the dose-dependent toxicity to the bone marrow (discussed below).

Chloramphenicol is a comparatively simple molecule with a nitrobenzene nucleus (Fig 10–6). Nitrobenzene itself is a bone marrow depressant, and so the nitrobenzene portion of the molecule may be involved in the hematologic problems reported with this drug. The most important side effect of chloramphenicol is bone marrow toxicity, of which there are two distinct types. One is a dose-dependent suppression, which is more likely to occur in patients on high doses for long periods and which is reversible when administration of the drug is stopped. The other is aplastic anemia, which is caused by an idiosyncratic reaction to the drug. This reaction is not dose-dependent, can occur weeks after administration of the drug has been stopped, and is not reversible. Fortunately, this reaction is rare, occurring in about 1:30,000 patients.

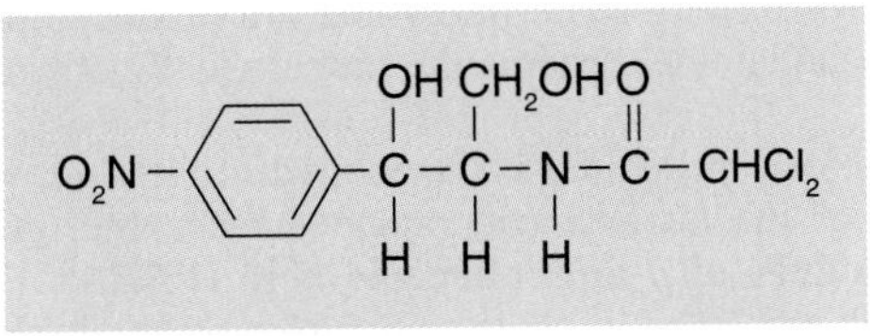

Figure 10–6. Chloramphenicol.

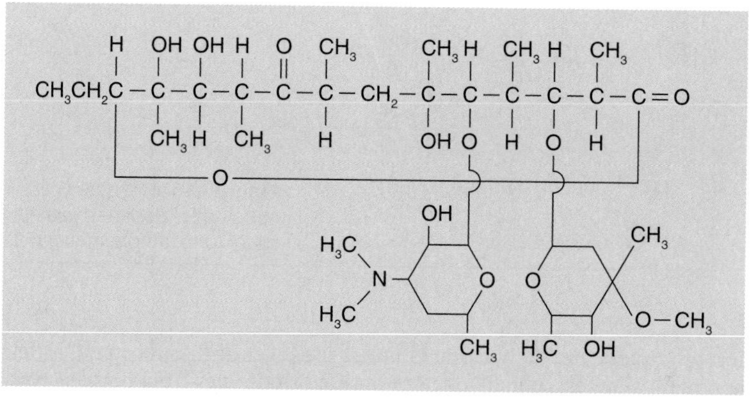

Figure 10–7. Erythromycin.

Erythromycin   Erythromycin is a bacteriostatic drug with a wide spectrum of activity. It is the treatment of choice for pneumonia caused by *Legionella* (a gram-negative rod) and *Mycoplasma* (a wall-less bacterium) and is also an effective alternative against a variety of infections caused by gram-positive cocci in penicillin-allergic patients.

Erythromycin binds to the 50S subunit and blocks the translocation step by preventing the release of the uncharged tRNA from the donor site after the peptide bond is formed. It has a macrolide structure composed of a large 13-carbon ring to which two sugars are attached by glycosidic linkages (Fig 10–7). Erythromycin is one of the least toxic drugs, with only some gastrointestinal distress associated with oral use.

Two derivatives of erythromycin, azithromycin and clarithromycin, have the same mechanism of action as erythromycin but are effective against a broader range of organisms and have a longer half-life so need to be taken only once or twice a day.

Clindamycin   The most useful clinical activity of this bacteriostatic drug is against anaerobes, both gram-positive bacteria such as *Clostridium perfringens* and gram-negative bacteria such as *Bacteroides fragilis.*

Clindamycin binds to the 50S subunit and blocks peptide bond formation by an undetermined mechanism. Its specificity for bacteria arises from its inability to bind to the 60S subunit of human ribosomes.

The most important side effect of clindamycin is pseudomembranous colitis, which, in fact, can occur with virtually any antibiotic, whether taken orally or parenterally. The pathogenesis of this potentially severe complication is suppression of the bowel normal flora by the drug and overgrowth of a drug-resistant strain of *Clostridium difficile.* The organism secretes an exotoxin that produces the pseudomembrane in the colon.

INHIBITION OF NUCLEIC ACID SYNTHESIS

1.   Inhibition of Precursor Synthesis

Sulfonamides   Either alone or in combination with trimethoprim, sulfonamides are useful in a variety of bacterial diseases such as *Escherichia coli* urinary tract infections, otitis media caused by *S pneumoniae* or *H influenzae* in children, shigellosis, nocardiosis, and chancroid. In combination, they are also the drugs of choice for two protozoan diseases, toxoplasmosis and *Pneumocystis* pneumonia. The sulfonamides are a large family of bacteriostatic drugs that are produced by chemical synthesis. In 1935, the parent compound, sulfanilamide, became the first clinically effective antimicrobial agent.

The mode of action of sulfonamides is to block the synthesis of tetrahydrofolic acid, which is required as a methyl donor in the synthesis of the nucleic acid precursors adenine, guanine, and thymine. Sulfonamides are **structural analogues of p-aminobenzoic acid (PABA).** PABA condenses with a pteridine compound to form dihydropteroic acid, a precursor of tetrahydrofolic acid

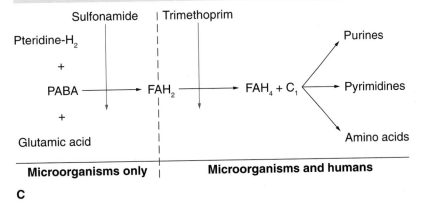

Figure 10–8. Sulfonamide and trimethoprim. **A:** Comparison of PABA (left) and sulfonamide (right). **B:** Trimethoprim. **C:** Inhibition of the folic acid pathway by sulfonamide and trimethoprim (FAH_2 = dihydrofolate; FAH_4 = tetrahydrofolate). (Modified and reproduced, with permission, from Corcoran JW, Hahn FE [editors]: *Mechanism of Action of Antimicrobial and Antitumor Agents.* Vol. 3 of: *Antibiotics.* Springer-Verlag, 1975.)

(Fig 10–8). Sulfonamides compete with PABA for the active site of the enzyme dihydropteroate synthetase. This competitive inhibition can be overcome by an excess of PABA.

The basis of the selective action of sulfonamides on bacteria is that many bacteria synthesize their folic acid from PABA-containing precursors, whereas human cells require preformed folic acid as an exogenous nutrient, since they lack the enzymes to synthesize it. Human cells therefore bypass the step at which sulfonamides act. Bacteria that can use preformed folic acid are similarly resistant to sulfonamides.

The *p*-amino group on the sulfonamide is essential for its activity. Modifications are therefore made on the sulfonic acid side chain.

Sulfonamides are inexpensive and cause side effects uncommonly. Drug fever, rashes, and bone marrow suppression can occur.

Trimethoprim   Trimethoprim also inhibits the production of tetrahydrofolic acid but by a mechanism different from that of the sulfonamides; ie, it inhibits the enzyme **dihydrofolate reductase** (Fig 10–8). Its specificity for bacteria is based on its much greater affinity for bacterial reductase than for the human enzyme.

Trimethoprim is used most frequently together with sulfamethoxazole. Note that both drugs act on the same pathway—but at different sites—to inhibit the synthesis of tetrahydrofolate. The advantages of the combination are that (1) bacterial mutants resistant to one drug will be inhibited by the other and that (2) the two drugs can act **synergistically**—ie, when used together, they cause significantly greater inhibition than the sum of the inhibition caused by each drug separately.

Trimethoprim-sulfamethoxazole is clinically useful in the treatment of urinary tract infections, *Pneumocystis* pneumonia, and shigellosis. It also is used for prophylaxis in granulopenic patients to prevent opportunistic infections.

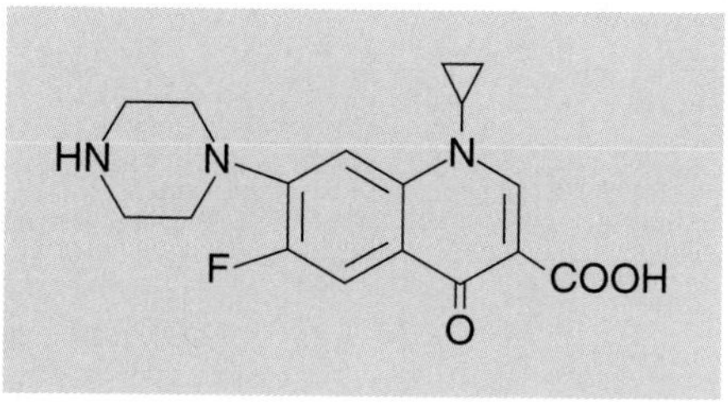

Figure 10–9. Ciprofloxacin. The triangle indicates a cyclopropyl group.

2. Inhibition of DNA Synthesis

Quinolones Quinolones are bactericidal drugs that block bacterial DNA synthesis by inhibiting **DNA gyrase (topoisomerase).** The fluoroquinolones, ciprofloxacin (Fig 10–9), norfloxacin, ofloxacin, and others are active against a broad range of organisms that cause infections of the lower respiratory tract, intestinal tract, urinary tract, and skeletal and soft tissues. Fluoroquinolones should not be given to pregnant women and young children, because they damage growing bone. Nalidixic acid, which is not a fluoroquinolone, is much less active and is used only for the treatment of urinary tract infections. Quinolones are not recommended for children and pregnant women because they damage growing cartilage.

Flucytosine Flucytosine (fluorocytosine, 5-FC) is an antifungal drug that inhibits DNA synthesis. It is a nucleoside analogue that is metabolized to fluorouracil, which inhibits thymidylate synthetase, thereby limiting the supply of thymidine. It is used in combination with amphotericin B in the treatment of disseminated cryptococcal or candidal infections, especially cryptococcal meningitis. It is not used alone, because resistant mutants emerge very rapidly.

3. Inhibition of mRNA Synthesis

Rifampin Rifampin is used primarily for the treatment of tuberculosis in combination with other drugs and for prophylaxis in close contacts of patients with meningitis caused by either *N meningitidis* or *H influenzae*. It is also used in combination with other drugs in the treatment of prosthetic-valve endocarditis caused by *Staphylococcus epidermidis*. With the exception of the short-term prophylaxis of meningitis, rifampin is given in combination with other drugs, since resistant mutants appear at a high rate when it is used alone.

The selective mode of action of rifampin is based on **blocking mRNA synthesis** by bacterial RNA polymerase without affecting the RNA polymerase of human cells. Rifampin is red, and the urine, saliva, and sweat of patients taking rifampin often turn orange; this is disturbing but harmless. Rifampin is excreted in high concentration in saliva, which accounts for its success in the prophylaxis of bacterial meningitis, as the organisms are carried in the throat.

Rifabutin, a rifampin derivative with the same mode of action as rifampin, is useful in the prevention of disease caused by *Mycobacterium avium-intracellulare* in patients with severely reduced numbers of helper T cells, eg, AIDS patients.

ALTERATION OF CELL MEMBRANE FUNCTION

1. Bacterial

There are few antimicrobial compounds that act on the cell membrane, because the structural and chemical similarities of bacterial and human cell membranes make it difficult to provide sufficient selective toxicity.

Polymyxins Polymyxins are a family of polypeptide antibiotics of which the clinically most useful compound is polymyxin E (colistin). It is active against gram-negative rods, especially *P aeruginosa*. Polymyxins are cyclic peptides composed of 10 amino acids, 6 of which are diaminobutyric acid. The positively charged free amino groups act like a cationic detergent to disrupt the phospholipid structure of the cell membrane.

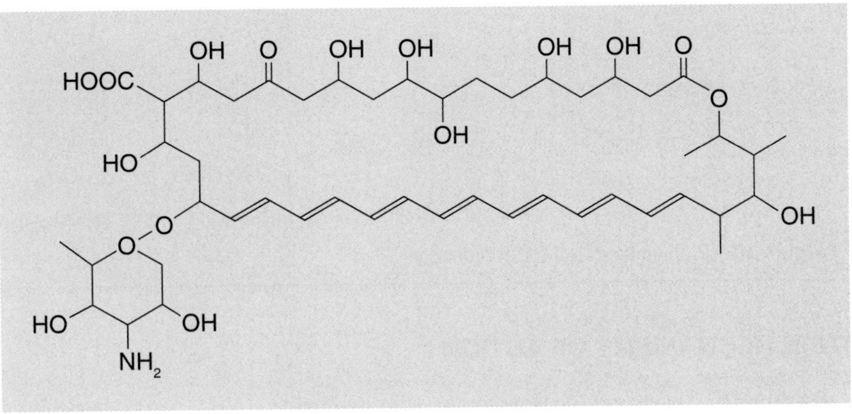

Figure 10–10. Amphotericin B.

2. Fungal

Amphotericin B & Nystatin   Amphotericin B, the most important antifungal drug, is used in the treatment of a variety of disseminated fungal diseases. It is classified as a polyene compound, because it has a series of seven unsaturated double bonds in its macrolide ring structure (*poly* means many, and *-ene* is a suffix indicating the presence of double bonds; Fig 10–10). It disrupts the cell membrane of fungi owing to its affinity for **ergosterol,** a component of fungal membranes but not of bacterial or human cell membranes. Fungi resistant to amphotericin B have rarely been recovered from patient specimens. Amphotericin B has significant renal toxicity; serum creatinine is used to monitor the dose. Fever, chills, nausea, and vomiting are common side effects.

Nystatin is another polyene antifungal agent, which, because of its toxicity, is used topically for infections caused by the yeast *Candida.*

Azoles   Azoles are antifungal drugs that act by **inhibiting ergosterol synthesis.** They block cytochrome P-450-dependent demethylation of lanosterol, the precursor of ergosterol. Fluconazole, ketoconazole, and itraconazole are used to treat systemic fungal diseases; clotrimazole and miconazole are used only topically, because they are too toxic to be given systemically. The two nitrogen-containing azole rings of fluconazole can be seen in Fig 10–11.

Ketoconazole is useful in the treatment of blastomycosis, chronic mucocutaneous candidiasis, coccidioidomycosis, and skin infections caused by dermatophytes. Fluconazole is useful in the treatment of candidal and cryptococcal infections. Itraconazole is used to treat histoplasmosis and blastomycosis. Miconazole and clotrimazole, two other imidazoles, are useful for topical therapy of *Candida* infections and dermatophytoses. Fungi resistant to the azole drugs have rarely been recovered from patient specimens.

Fluconazole

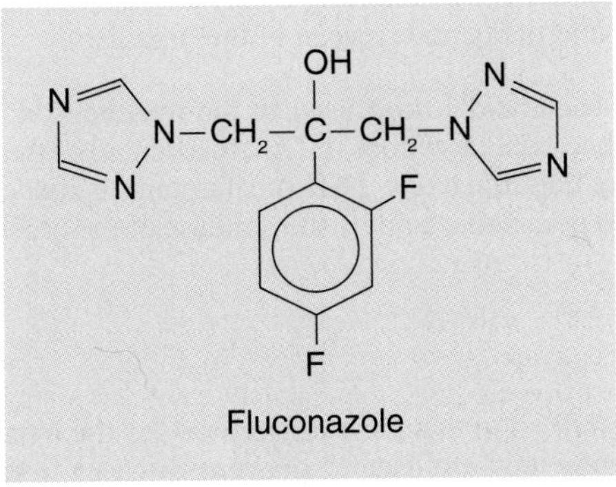

Figure 10–11. Fluconazole.

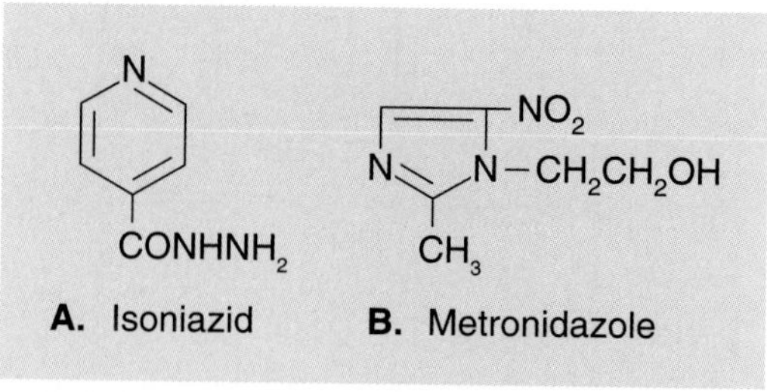

Figure 10–12. Isoniazid and metronidazole.

UNCERTAIN MECHANISMS OF ACTION

Isoniazid   Isoniazid, or isonicotinic acid hydrazide (INH), is a bactericidal drug highly specific for *Mycobacterium tuberculosis* and other mycobacteria. It is used in combination with other drugs to treat tuberculosis and by itself to prevent tuberculosis in exposed persons. Because it penetrates human cells well, it is effective against the organisms residing within macrophages. The structure of isoniazid is shown in Fig 10–12.

Despite its widespread use and its availability for over 30 years, its mode of action is unclear. The most likely possibility is that it inhibits mycolic acid synthesis, which explains why it is specific for mycobacteria and relatively nontoxic for humans. The active drug is probably a metabolite formed by the action of catalase-peroxidase, because deletion of the gene for these enzymes results in resistance to the drug. Its main side effect is liver toxicity. It is given with pyridoxine to prevent neurologic complications.

Metronidazole   Metronidazole (Flagyl) is bactericidal against anaerobic bacteria. (It is also effective against certain protozoa such as *Giardia* and *Trichomonas*.) This drug has two possible mechanisms of action, and it is unclear which is the more important. The first, which explains its specificity for anaerobes, is its ability to act as an **electron sink.** By accepting electrons, the drug deprives the organism of required reducing power. In addition, when electrons are acquired, the drug ring is cleaved and a toxic intermediate is formed. The precise nature of the intermediate and its action is unknown. The structure of metronidazole is shown in Fig 10–12.

The second mode of action of metronidazole relates to its ability to inhibit DNA synthesis. The drug binds to DNA and causes strand breakage, which prevents its proper functioning as a template for DNA polymerase.

Pentamidine   Pentamidine is active against fungi and protozoa. It is widely used to prevent or treat pneumonia caused by *Pneumocystis carinii*. It inhibits DNA synthesis by an unknown mechanism.

Griseofulvin   Griseofulvin is an antifungal drug that is useful in the treatment of hair and nail infections caused by dermatophytes. It binds to tubulin in microtubules and may act by preventing formation of the mitotic spindle.

Ethambutol   Ethambutol is a bacteriostatic drug active against *Mycobacterium tuberculosis* and many of the atypical mycobacteria. It is thought to act by inhibiting the synthesis of arabinogalactan, which is the linker between the mycolic acids and the peptidoglycan of the organism.

Pyrazinamide   Pyrazinamide (PZA) is a bactericidal drug used in the treatment of tuberculosis but not in the treatment of most atypical mycobacterial infections. PZA is particularly effective against semidormant organisms in the lesion, which are not affected by INH or rifampin. Its mode of action is unclear, but to be active, it must be converted to pyrazinoic acid by the amidase of the organism.

CHEMOPROPHYLAXIS

In most instances, the antimicrobial agents described in this chapter are used for the *treatment* of infectious diseases. However, there are times when they are used to **prevent** diseases from occurring,

Table 10–5. Chemoprophylactic use of drugs described in this chapter.

Drug	Use	Number of Chapter for Additional Information
Penicillin	1. Prevent recurrent pharyngitis in those who have had rheumatic fever	15
	2. Prevent syphilis in those exposed to *T pallidum*	24
Ampicillin	Prevent neonatal sepsis and meningitis in children born of mothers carrying group B streptococci	15
Ceftriaxone	Prevent gonorrhea in those exposed to *N gonorrhoeae*	16
Rifampin	Prevent meningitis in those exposed to *N meningitidis* and *H influenzae*	16, 19
Isoniazid	Prevent progression of *M tuberculosis* in those recently infected	21
Erythromycin	Prevent pertussis in those exposed to *B pertussis*	19
Tetracycline	Prevent plague in those exposed to *Y pestis*	20
Fluconazole	Prevent cryptococcal meningitis in AIDS patients	50
Clotrimazole	Prevent thrush in AIDS patients and in others with reduced cell-mediated immunity	50
Trimethoprim-sulfamethoxazole	Prevent *Pneumocystis* pneumonia in AIDS patients	52
Pentamidine	Prevent *Pneumocystis* pneumonia in AIDS patients	52

a process called **chemoprophylaxis.** Chemoprophylaxis is used in three circumstances: prior to surgery, in immunocompromised patients, and in people with normal immunity who have been exposed to certain pathogens. Table 10–5 describes the drugs and the situations in which they are used. For more information, see the chapters on the individual organisms.

Review Questions

1. What is the basis for the selective ability of the following drugs to affect bacteria but not human cells: (a) penicillins, (b) cephalosporins, (c) aminoglycosides, (d) tetracyclines, (e) erythromycin, (f) chloramphenicol, (g) sulfonamides, (h) rifampin.
2. What is the mode of action of each of the above drugs?
3. What is the difference between a bactericidal and a bacteriostatic drug?
4. What is the essential portion of the penicillin and cephalosporin molecules?
5. Why are sulfonamides and trimethoprim used in combination to treat certain infections?
6. Why is rifampin frequently given in combination with other drugs?
7. Why is amphotericin B selectively active against fungal and not bacterial or human cells?
8. What is the likely reason that isoniazid is selectively active against *Mycobacterium tuberculosis?*

11 Antimicrobial Drugs: Resistance

There are three major mechanisms that mediate bacterial resistance to drugs. (1) Bacteria produce enzymes that **inactivate the drug;** eg, β-lactamases can inactivate penicillins and cephalosporins by cleaving the β-lactam ring of the drug. (2) Bacteria **synthesize modified targets** against which the drug has no effect; eg, a mutant protein in the 30S ribosomal subunit can result in resistance to streptomycin, and a methylated 23S rRNA can result in resistance to erythromycin. (3) Bacteria **alter their permeability** so that an effective intracellular concentration of the drug is not achieved; eg, tetracycline is concentrated less in resistant bacteria than in susceptible ones.

Most drug resistance is due to a genetic change in the organism, either a chromosomal **mutation** or the acquisition of a **plasmid** or **transposon.** Nongenetic changes, which are of lesser importance, are discussed on p 65.

Hospital-acquired infections are significantly more likely to be caused by antibiotic-resistant organisms than are community-acquired infections. This is especially true for hospital infections caused by *Staphylococcus aureus* and enteric gram-negative rods such as *Escherichia coli* and *Pseudomonas aeruginosa.* Antibiotic-resistant organisms are common in the hospital setting because widespread antibiotic use in hospitals selects for these organisms. Furthermore, hospital strains are often resistant to multiple antibiotics. This is usually due to the acquisition of plasmids carrying several genes that encode the enzymes which mediate resistance.

Table 11–1 describes certain medically important bacteria and the main drugs to which they are resistant. Note that these bacteria are resistant to other drugs as well, but, for simplicity, only the most characteristic drugs are listed.

GENETIC BASIS OF RESISTANCE

Chromosome-Mediated Resistance Chromosomal resistance is due to a mutation in the gene that codes for either the target of the drug or the transport system in the membrane that controls the uptake of the drug. The frequency of spontaneous mutations usually ranges from 10^{-7} to 10^{-9}, which is much lower than the frequency of acquisition of resistance plasmids. Therefore, chromosomal resistance is less of a clinical problem than is plasmid-mediated resistance.

Table 11–1. Important bacteria that exhibit significant drug resistance.

Type of Bacteria	Clinically Significant Drug Resistance
Gram-positive cocci	
Staphylococcus aureus	Penicillin G, nafcillin
Streptococcus pneumoniae	Penicillin G
Enterococcus faecalis	Penicillin G, aminoglycosides, vancomycin
Gram-negative cocci	
Neisseria gonorrhoeae	Penicillin G
Gram-positive rods	
None	
Gram-negative rods	
Haemophilus influenzae	Ampicillin
Pseudomonas aeruginosa	β-Lactams,[1] aminoglycosides
Enterobacteriaceae[2]	β-Lactams,[2] aminoglycosides
Mycobacteria	
M tuberculosis[3]	Isoniazid, rifampin
M avium-intracellulare	Isoniazid, rifampin, and many others

[1] β-Lactams are penicillins and cephalosporins.
[2] The family Enterobacteriaceae includes bacteria such as *Escherichia coli, Enterobacter cloacae, Klebsiella pneumoniae,* and *Serratia marcescens.*
[3] Some strains of *M tuberculosis* are resistant to more than two drugs.

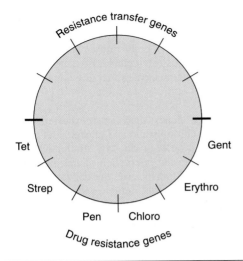

Figure 11–1. Resistance plasmid (R plasmid, R factor). Most resistance plasmids have two sets of genes: (1) resistance transfer genes that encode the sex pilus and other proteins which mediate transfer of the plasmid DNA during conjugation and (2) drug resistance genes that encode the proteins which mediate drug resistance. The bottom half of the figure depicts, from left to right, the genes that encode resistance to tetracycline, streptomycin, penicillin (β-lactamase), chloramphenicol, erythromycin, and gentamicin.

The treatment of certain infections with two or more drugs is based on the following principle. If the frequency that a bacterium mutates to become resistant to antibiotic A is 10^{-7} (1 in 10 million) and the frequency that the same bacterium mutates to become resistant to antibiotic B is 10^{-8} (1 in 100 million), then the chance that the bacterium will become resistant to both antibiotics (assuming that the antibiotics act by different mechanisms) is the product of the two probabilities or 10^{-15}. It is therefore highly unlikely that the bacterium will become resistant to *both* antibiotics. Stated another way, although an organism may be resistant to one antibiotic, it is likely that it will be effectively treated by the other antibiotic.

Plasmid-Mediated Resistance   Plasmid-mediated resistance is very important from a clinical point of view for three reasons:

(1) it occurs in many different species, especially gram-negative rods;

(2) plasmids frequently mediate resistance to multiple drugs; and

(3) plasmids have a high rate of transfer from one cell to another, usually by conjugation.

Resistance plasmids (resistance factors, R factors) are extrachromosomal, circular, double-stranded DNA molecules that carry the genes for a variety of enzymes that can degrade antibiotics and modify membrane transport systems (Fig 11–1). Table 11–2 describes the most important mechanisms of resistance for several important drugs.

In addition to producing drug resistance, R factors have two very important properties: (1) They can replicate independently of the bacterial chromosome, so that a cell can contain many copies; and (2) they can be transferred not only to cells of the same species but also to other species and genera. Note that this conjugal transfer is under the control of the genes of the R plasmid and not of the F (fertility) plasmid, which governs the transfer of the bacterial chromosome (see Chapter 4).

R factors exist in two broad size categories: large plasmids with molecular weights of about 60 million and small ones with molecular weights of about 10 million. The large plasmids are conjuga-

Table 11–2. R-factor-mediated resistance mechanisms.

Drug	Mechanism of Resistance
Penicillins and cephalosporins	β-Lactamase cleavage of β-lactam ring
Aminoglycosides	Modification by acetylation, adenylylation, or phosphorylation
Chloramphenicol	Modification by acetylation
Erythromycin	Change in receptor by methylation of rRNA
Tetracycline	Reduced uptake or increased export
Sulfonamides	Active export out of the cell and reduced affinity of enzyme

tive R factors, which contain the extra DNA to code for the conjugation process, whereas small R factors are not conjugative and contain only the resistance genes.

In addition to conveying antibiotic resistance, R factors impart two other traits: (1) resistance to metal ions (eg, they code for an enzyme that reduces mercuric ions to elemental mercury); and (2) resistance to certain bacterial viruses by coding for restriction endonucleases that degrade the DNA of the infecting bacteriophages.

Transposon-Mediated Resistance **Transposons** are genes that are transferred either within or between larger pieces of DNA such as the bacterial chromosome and plasmids. A typical drug resistance transposon is composed of three genes flanked on both sides by shorter DNA sequences, usually a series of inverted repeated bases that mediate the interaction of the transposon with the larger DNA (see Fig 2–7). The three genes code for (1) transposase, the enzyme that catalyzes excision and reintegration of the transposon; (2) a repressor that regulates synthesis of the transposase; and (3) the drug resistance gene.

SPECIFIC MECHANISMS OF RESISTANCE

Penicillins & Cephalosporins There are several mechanisms of resistance to these drugs. Cleavage by β-lactamases (penicillinases and cephalosporinases) is by far the most important (see Fig 10–1). β-Lactamases produced by various organisms have different properties. For example, staphylococcal penicillinase is inducible by penicillin and is secreted into the medium. In contrast, some β-lactamases produced by several gram-negative rods are constitutively produced, are located in the periplasmic space near the peptidoglycan, and are not secreted into the medium. The β-lactamases produced by various gram-negative rods have different specificities; some are more active against cephalosporins, others against penicillins. Clavulanic acid and sulbactam are penicillin analogues that bind strongly to β-lactamases and inactivate them. Combinations of these inhibitors and penicillins, eg, clavulanic acid and amoxicillin (Augmentin), can overcome resistance mediated by many but not all β-lactamases.

Resistance to penicillins can also be due to changes in the **penicillin-binding proteins** in the bacterial cell membrane. These changes account for both the low-level and the high-level resistance exhibited by *Streptococcus pneumoniae* to penicillin G and for the resistance of *Staphylococcus aureus* to nafcillin and other β-lactamase-resistant penicillins. The relative resistance of *Enterococcus faecalis* to penicillins may be due to altered penicillin-binding proteins. Low-level resistance of *Neisseria gonorrhoeae* to penicillin is attributed to **poor permeability** to the drug. High-level resistance is due to the presence of a plasmid coding for penicillinase.

Some isolates of *S aureus* demonstrate yet another form of resistance, called **tolerance**, in which growth of the organism is inhibited by penicillin but the organism is not killed. This is attributed to a failure of activation of the autolytic enzymes, murein hydrolases, which degrade the peptidoglycan.

Vancomycin Resistance to vancomycin is caused by a change in the peptide component of peptidoglycan from D-alanine:D-alanine, which is the normal binding site for vancomycin, to D-alanine:D-lactate, which is not recognized by the drug. Vancomycin-resistant strains of enterococci have been recovered from clinical specimens. Rare isolates of *S aureus* that exhibit resistance to vancomycin have also been recovered from patient specimens.

Aminoglycosides Resistance to aminoglycosides occurs by three mechanisms: (1) modification of the drugs by plasmid-encoded phosphorylating, adenylylating, and acetylating enzymes (the most important mechanism); (2) chromosomal mutation, eg, a mutation in the gene that codes for the target protein in the 30S subunit of the bacterial ribosome; and (3) decreased permeability of the bacterium to the drug.

Tetracyclines Resistance to tetracyclines is the result of failure of the drug to reach an inhibitory concentration inside the bacteria. This is due to plasmid-encoded processes that either reduce uptake of the drug or **enhance its transport** out of the cell.

Chloramphenicol Resistance to chloramphenicol is due to a plasmid-encoded acetyltransferase that acetylates the drug, thus inactivating it.

Erythromycin   Resistance to erythromycin is due primarily to a plasmid-encoded enzyme that methylates the 23S rRNA, thereby blocking binding of the drug.

Sulfonamides   Resistance to sulfonamides is mediated primarily by two mechanisms: (1) a plasmid-encoded transport system that **actively exports** the drug out of the cell; and (2) a chromosomal mutation in the gene coding for the target enzyme, dihydropteroate synthetase, which reduces the binding affinity of the drug.

Quinolones   Resistance to quinolones is due primarily to chromosomal mutations that modify the bacterial DNA gyrase. Resistance can also be caused by changes in bacterial outer-membrane proteins that result in reduced uptake of drug into the bacteria.

Rifampin   Resistance to rifampin is due to a chromosomal mutation in the gene for the β subunit of the bacterial RNA polymerase, resulting in ineffective binding of the drug. Resistance occurs at high frequency (10^{-5}), and so rifampin is not prescribed alone for the *treatment* of infections. It is used alone for the *prevention* of certain infections because it is administered for only a short time (see Table 10–5).

Isoniazid   Resistance of *Mycobacterium tuberculosis* to isoniazid is due to mutations in the organism's catalase-peroxidase gene. Catalase or peroxidase enzyme activity is required for activation of isoniazid to the active drug within the organism.

Ethambutol   Resistance of *M tuberculosis* to ethambutol is due to mutations in the gene that encodes arabinosyl transferase, the enzyme that synthesizes the arabinogalactan in the organism's cell wall.

Pyrazinamide   Resistance of *M tuberculosis* to pyrazinamide (PZA) is due to mutations in the gene that encodes bacterial amidase, the enzyme that converts PZA to the active form of the drug, pyrazinoic acid.

NONGENETIC BASIS OF RESISTANCE

There are several nongenetic reasons for the failure of drugs to inhibit the growth of bacteria.

(1) Bacteria can be walled off within an abscess cavity that the drug cannot penetrate effectively. Surgical drainage is therefore a necessary adjunct to chemotherapy.

(2) Bacteria can be in a resting state, ie, not growing; they are therefore insensitive to cell wall inhibitors such as penicillins and cephalosporins. Similarly, *M tuberculosis* can remain dormant in tissues for many years, during which time it is insensitive to drugs. If host defenses are lowered and the bacteria begin to multiply, they are again susceptible to the drugs, indicating that a genetic change did not occur.

(3) Under certain circumstances, organisms that would ordinarily be killed by penicillin can lose their cell walls, survive as **protoplasts,** and be insensitive to cell-wall-active drugs. Later, if such organisms resynthesize their cell walls, they are fully susceptible to these drugs.

(4) Several artifacts can make it appear that the organisms are resistant, eg, administration of the wrong drug or the wrong dose, failure of the drug to reach the appropriate site in the body (a good example is the poor penetration into spinal fluid by several early-generation cephalosporins), or failure of the patient to take the drug.

SELECTION OF RESISTANT BACTERIA BY OVERUSE AND MISUSE OF ANTIBIOTICS

Serious outbreaks of diseases caused by gram-negative rods resistant to multiple antibiotics have occurred in many developing countries. In North America, many hospital-acquired infections are caused by multiple resistant organisms. There are three main focal points of overuse and misuse of

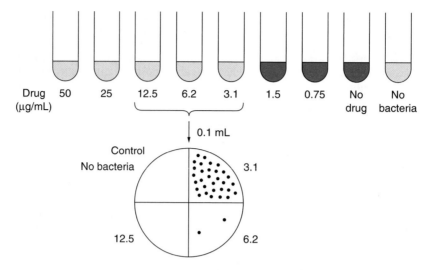

Figure 11–2. Determination of minimal inhibitory concentration (MIC) and minimal bactericidal concentration (MBC). In the top part of the figure, the patient's organism is added to tubes containing decreasing amounts of the antibiotic. After incubation at 37 °C overnight, growth of the bacteria is observed visually. The lowest concentration of drug that inhibits growth, ie, 3.1 μg/mL, is the MIC. However, at this point, it is not known whether the bacteria have been killed or whether the drug has only inhibited their growth. To determine whether that concentration of drug is bactericidal, ie, to determine its MBC, an aliquot (0.1 mL) from the tubes is plated on an agar plate that does not contain any drug. The concentration of drug that inhibits at least 99.9% of the bacterial colonies, ie, 6.2 μg/mL, is the MBC.

antibiotics that increase the likelihood of these problems by enhancing the selection of resistant mutants:

(1) Some physicians use multiple antibiotics when one would be sufficient, prescribe unnecessarily long courses of antibiotic therapy, use antibiotics in self-limited infections for which they are not needed, and overuse antibiotics for prophylaxis before and after surgery.

(2) In many countries, antibiotics are sold over the counter to the general public; this practice encourages the inappropriate and indiscriminate use of the drugs.

(3) Antibiotics are used in animal feed to prevent infections and promote growth. This selects for resistant organisms in the animals and may contribute to the pool of resistant organisms in humans.

ANTIBIOTIC SENSITIVITY TESTING

Minimal Inhibitory Concentration For many infections, the results of sensitivity testing are important in the choice of antibiotic. These results are commonly reported as the **minimal inhibitory concentration (MIC),** which is defined as the lowest concentration of drug that inhibits the growth of the organism. The MIC is determined by inoculating the organism isolated from the patient into a series of tubes or cups containing two-fold dilutions of the drug (Fig 11–2). After incubation at 35 °C for 18 hours, the lowest concentration of drug that prevents visible growth of the organism is the MIC. This provides the physician with a precise concentration of drug to guide the choice of both the drug and the dose.

A second method of determining antibiotic sensitivity is the disk diffusion method, in which disks impregnated with various antibiotics are placed on the surface of an agar plate that has been inoculated with the organism isolated from the patient (Fig 11–3). After incubation at 35 °C for 18 hours, during which time the antibiotic diffuses outward from the disk, the diameter of the zone of inhibition is determined. The size of the zone of inhibition is compared with standards to determine the sensitivity of the organism to the drug.

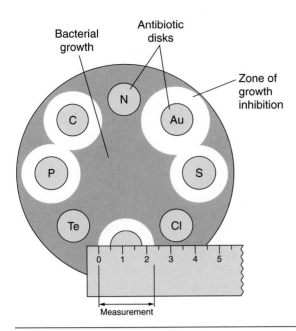

Figure 11–3. Antibiotic sensitivity testing. A zone of inhibition surrounds several antibiotic-containing disks. A zone of a certain diameter or greater indicates that the organism is sensitive. Some resistant organisms will grow all the way up to the disk, eg, disk N. (Modified and reproduced, with permission, from Wistreich GA, Lechtman MD: *Laboratory Exercises in Microbiology,* 5th ed. Macmillan, 1984.)

Minimal Bactericidal Concentration   For certain infections, such as endocarditis, it is important to know the concentration of drug that actually kills the organism rather than the concentration that merely inhibits growth. This concentration, called the **minimal bactericidal concentration (MBC),** is determined by taking a small sample (0.01 or 0.1 mL) from the tubes used for the MIC assay and spreading it over the surface of a drug-free blood agar plate (Fig 11–2). Any organisms that were inhibited but not killed now have a chance to grow, because the drug has been diluted significantly. After incubation at 35 °C for 48 hours, the lowest concentration that has reduced the number of colonies by 99.9%, compared with the drug-free control, is the MBC. Bactericidal drugs usually have an MBC equal or very similar to the MIC, whereas bacteriostatic drugs usually have an MBC significantly higher than the MIC.

Serum Bactericidal Activity   In the treatment of endocarditis, it can be useful to determine whether the drug is effective by assaying the ability of the drug in the patient's serum to kill the organism. This test, called the **serum bactericidal activity,** is performed in a manner similar to that of the MBC determination, except that it is a serum sample from the patient, rather than a standard drug solution, that is diluted in 2-fold steps. After a standard inoculum of the organism has been added and the mixture incubated at 35 °C for 18 hours, a small sample is subcultured onto blood agar plates, and the serum dilution that kills 99.9% of the organisms is determined. Clinical experience has shown that a peak* serum bactericidal activity of 1:8 or 1:16 is adequate for successful therapy of endocarditis.

β-Lactamase Production   For severe infections caused by certain organisms, such as *S aureus* and *Haemophilus influenzae,* it is important to know as soon as possible whether the organism isolated from the patient is producing β-lactamase. For this purpose, rapid assays for the enzyme can be used that yield an answer in a few minutes, as opposed to an MIC test or a disk diffusion test, both of which take 18 hours.

A commonly used procedure is the chromogenic β-lactam method, in which a colored β-lactam drug is added to a suspension of the organisms. If β-lactamase is made, hydrolysis of the β-lactam ring causes the drug to turn a different color in 2–10 minutes. Disks impregnated with a chromogenic β-lactam can also be used.

---

* One of the variables in this test is whether the serum is drawn shortly after the drug has been administered (at the "peak concentration") or shortly before the next dose is due (at the "trough"). Another is the inoculum size.

USE OF ANTIBIOTIC COMBINATIONS

The main concept underlying the use of antimicrobial agents is to select the *single* best drug whenever possible, because this minimizes side effects. However, there are several instances in which two or more drugs are commonly given:

(1) to treat serious infections before the identity of the organism is known;

(2) to achieve a synergistic inhibitory effect against certain organisms; and

(3) to prevent the emergence of resistant organisms (if bacteria become resistant to one drug, the second drug will kill them, thereby preventing the emergence of resistant strains).

Two drugs can interact in one of several ways (Fig 11–4). They are usually indifferent to each other, ie, additive only. Sometimes there is a **synergistic** interaction, in which the effect of the two drugs together is significantly greater than the sum of the effects of the two drugs acting separately. Rarely, the effect of the two drugs together is **antagonistic,** and the result is significantly lower activity than the sum of the activities of the two drugs alone.

A synergistic effect can result from a variety of mechanisms. For example, the combination of a penicillin and an aminoglycoside such as gentamicin has a synergistic action against enterococci *(E faecalis),* because penicillin damages the cell wall sufficiently to enhance the entry of aminoglycoside. When given alone, neither drug is effective. A second example is the combination of a sulfonamide with trimethoprim. In this instance, the two drugs act on the same metabolic pathway, so that if one drug does not inhibit folic acid synthesis sufficiently, the second drug provides effective inhibition by blocking a subsequent step in the pathway.

Although antagonism between two antibiotics is unusual, one example is clinically important. This involves the use of penicillin G combined with the bacteriostatic drug tetracycline in the treatment of meningitis caused by *S pneumoniae.* Antagonism occurs because the tetracycline inhibits the growth of the organism, thereby preventing the bactericidal effect of penicillin G, which kills growing organisms only.

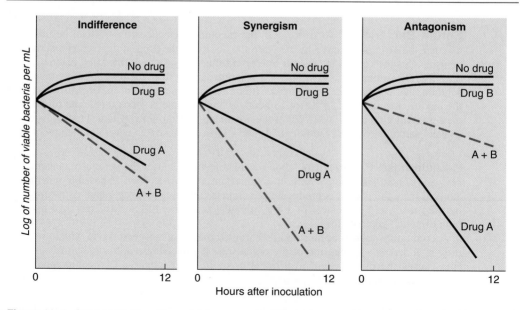

Figure 11–4. Drug interaction. The solid lines represent the response of bacteria to drug A alone, drug B alone, or no drug. The dotted lines represent the response to drug A and drug B together.

Review Questions

1. What are the similarities and differences between chromosome- and plasmid-mediated resistance to antimicrobial drugs?
2. How is plasmid-mediated resistance transmitted from one bacterium to another?
3. How does an R plasmid (R factor) differ from an F plasmid?
4. What are the characteristics of transposons that mediate antibiotic resistance?
5. What are the specific mechanisms of resistance to the following drugs: (a) penicillins, (b) cephalosporins, (c) aminoglycosides, (d) tetracyclines, (e) chloramphenicol, (f) erythromycin, (g) sulfonamides, (h) rifampin?
6. How are (a) the MIC test and (b) the MBC test performed, and what information is obtained?
7. What is the basis for the synergistic effect of penicillin and streptomycin against enterococci?

Bacterial Vaccines

12

Bacterial diseases can be prevented by the use of immunizations that induce either active or passive immunity. **Active** immunity is induced by vaccines prepared from bacteria or their products. This chapter will present a summary of the types of vaccines (Table 12–1); detailed information regarding each vaccine is located in the chapters on the specific organisms. **Passive** immunity is provided by the administration of preformed antibody in preparations called immune globulins. The immune globulins useful against bacterial diseases are described below. **Passive-active** immunity involves giving both immune globulins to provide immediate protection and a vaccine to provide long-term protection. This approach is described below in the section on tetanus antitoxin.

Active immunity Bacterial vaccines are composed of capsular polysaccharides, inactivated protein exotoxins (toxoids), killed bacteria, or live attenuated bacteria. The available bacterial vaccines and their indications are as follows.

A. Capsular Polysaccharide Vaccines

(1) *Streptococcus pneumoniae* vaccine contains the capsular polysaccharides of the 23 most prevalent types. It is recommended for persons over 60 years of age and patients of any age with chronic diseases such as diabetes and cirrhosis or with compromised spleen function or splenectomy.

(2) *Neisseria meningitidis* vaccine contains capsular polysaccharide of four important types (A, C, W-135, and Y). It is given when there is a high risk of meningitis, eg, during an outbreak, when military recruits enter boot camp, or for travelers to areas where meningitis is hyperendemic.

(3) *Haemophilus influenzae* vaccine contains the type b polysaccharide conjugated to diphtheria toxoid or other carrier protein. It is given to children between the ages of 2 and 15 months to prevent meningitis. The capsular polysaccharide alone is a poor immunogen in young children, but coupling it to a carrier protein greatly enhances its immunogenicity. A combined vaccine consisting of this vaccine plus the diphtheria, pertussis, and tetanus (DPT) vaccines is available.

B. Toxoid Vaccines

(1) *Corynebacterium diphtheriae* vaccine contains the toxoid (formaldehyde-treated exotoxin). Immunization against diphtheria is indicated for every child and is given in three doses at 2, 4, and 6 months of age, with boosters given 1 year later and at intervals thereafter.

Table 12–1. Current bacterial vaccines (1998).

Usage	Bacterium	Disease	Antigen
Common usage	*Corynebacterium diphtheriae*	Diphtheria	Toxoid
	Clostridium tetani	Tetanus	Toxoid
	Bordetella pertussis	Whooping cough	Killed organisms or acellular (purified proteins)
	Haemophilus influenzae	Meningitis	Capsular polysaccharide conjugated to carrier protein, eg, diphtheria toxoid
	Streptococcus pneumoniae	Pneumonia	Capsular polysaccharide
Special situations	*Neisseria meningitidis*	Meningitis	Capsular polysaccharide
	Salmonella typhi	Typhoid fever	Killed or live organisms
	Vibrio cholerae	Cholera	Killed organisms
	Yersinia pestis	Plague	Killed organisms
	Bacillus anthracis	Anthrax	Partially purified proteins
	Mycobacterium bovis (BCG)	Tuberculosis	Live organisms
	Francisella tularensis	Tularemia	Live organisms
	Rickettsia prowazekii	Typhus	Killed organisms
	Coxiella burnetii	Q fever	Killed organisms

(2) *Clostridium tetani* vaccine contains tetanus toxoid and is given to everyone both early in life and later as boosters for protection against tetanus.

C.   Whole Bacterial or Purified Protein Vaccines

(1) There are two types of *B pertussis* vaccines: one containing killed bacteria and the other containing purified proteins from the organism (acellular vaccine). The acellular vaccine is now recommended in the United States. The vaccine is indicated for every child as a protection against whooping cough. It is usually given in combination with diphtheria and tetanus toxoids (DPT vaccine).

(2) *Bacillus anthracis* vaccine contains "protective antigen" purified from the organism. It is given to persons whose occupations place them at risk of anthrax.

(3) *Salmonella typhi* vaccine contains killed organisms and is indicated for persons living in high-risk areas for typhoid fever and for those in close contact with infected patients and carriers. A live, attenuated vaccine is available also.

(4) *Vibrio cholerae* vaccine contains killed organisms and is given to persons traveling to areas where cholera is endemic.

(5) *Yersinia pestis* vaccine contains killed organisms and is indicated for persons at high risk of contracting plague.

(6) The vaccine against tuberculosis contains a live, attenuated strain of *Mycobacterium bovis* called BCG and is recommended for children at high risk of exposure to active tuberculosis in some countries.

(7) The vaccine against tularemia contains live, attenuated *Francisella tularensis* organisms and is used primarily in people who are exposed in their occupation, such as laboratory personnel, veterinarians, and hunters.

(8) The vaccine against typhus contains killed organisms and is used primarily to immunize members of the armed forces.

(9) The vaccine against Q fever contains killed organisms and is used to immunize those who are at high risk of being exposed to animals infected with *Coxiella burnetii*.

Passive Immunity Antitoxins (immune globulins) can be used for either the treatment or prevention of certain bacterial diseases. The following preparations are available.

(1) Tetanus antitoxin is used both in the treatment of tetanus and in its prevention (prophylaxis). In treatment, the goal is to neutralize any unbound toxin to prevent the disease from getting worse, so the antitoxin should be given promptly. In prevention, the antitoxin is given to inadequately immunized persons with contaminated ("dirty") wounds. The antitoxin is made in humans to avoid hypersensitivity reactions. In addition to the antitoxin, these people should receive tetanus toxoid. This is an example of **passive-active** immunity. The toxoid and the antitoxin should be given at different sites in the body to prevent the antitoxin from neutralizing the toxoid.

(2) Botulinum antitoxin is used in the treatment of botulism. The antitoxin can neutralize unbound toxin to prevent the disease from progressing, so the antitoxin should be given promptly. It contains antibodies against botulinum toxins A, B, and E, the most commonly occurring types. The antitoxin is made in horses, so hypersensitivity may be a problem.

(3) Diphtheria antitoxin is used in the treatment of diphtheria. The antitoxin can neutralize unbound toxin to prevent the disease from progressing, so the antitoxin should be given promptly. The antitoxin is made in horses, so hypersensitivity may be a problem.

Review Question

What is the nature of the antigen in the vaccines against each of the following organisms: (a) *Streptococcus pneumoniae*, (b) *Haemophilus influenzae*, (c) *Corynebacterium diphtheriae*, (d) *Clostridium tetani*, (e) *Bordetella pertussis*, (f) *Mycobacterium tuberculosis?*

Sterilization & Disinfection 13

Sterilization is the killing or removal of *all* microorganisms, including bacterial spores, which are highly resistant. Sterilization is usually carried out by autoclaving, which consists of exposure to steam at 121 °C under a pressure of 15 lb/in² for 15 minutes. Surgical instruments that can be damaged by moist heat are usually sterilized by exposure to ethylene oxide gas, and most intravenous solutions are sterilized by filtration.

Disinfection is the killing of many, but not all, microorganisms. For adequate disinfection, pathogens must be killed but some organisms and bacterial spores may survive. Disinfectants vary in their tissue-damaging properties from the corrosive phenol-containing compounds, which should be used only on inanimate objects, to less toxic materials such as ethanol and iodine, which can be used on skin surfaces. Chemicals used to kill microorganisms on the surface of skin and mucous membranes are called **antiseptics.**

Rate of Killing of Microorganisms

Death of microorganisms occurs at a certain rate dependent primarily upon two variables: the concentration of the killing agent and the length of time it is applied. The rate of killing is defined by the relationship

$$N \propto 1/CT$$

which shows that the number of survivors, N, is inversely proportionate to the concentration of the agent, C, and the time of application of the agent, T. Collectively, CT is often referred to as the dose. Stated alternatively, the number of microorganisms killed is directly proportionate to CT. The relationship is usually stated in terms of survivors, as they are easily measured by colony formation. Death is defined as the inability to reproduce. In certain circumstances, the physical remains of dead bacteria can still cause problems (see p 37).

Chemical Agents

Chemicals vary greatly in their ability to kill microorganisms. A quantitative measure of this variation is expressed as the **phenol coefficient,** which is the ratio of the concentration of phenol to the concentration of the agent required to cause the same amount of killing under the standard conditions of the test.

Chemical agents act primarily by one of three mechanisms: disruption of the lipid-containing cell membrane, modification of proteins, or modification of DNA. Each of the following chemical agents has been classified into one of the three categories, but some of the chemicals act by more than one mechanism.

DISRUPTION OF CELL MEMBRANES

Alcohols   Ethanol is widely used to clean the skin prior to an immunization or venipuncture. It acts mainly by disorganizing the lipid structure in membranes but denatures proteins as well. Ethanol requires the presence of water for maximal activity; ie, it is far more effective at 70% than at 100%.

Detergents   Detergents are "surface-active" agents composed of a long-chain, lipid-soluble, hydrophobic portion and a polar hydrophilic group, which can be a cation, an anion, or a nonionic group. These surfactants interact with the lipid in the cell membrane through their hydrophobic chain and with the surrounding water through their polar group and thus disrupt the membrane. Quaternary ammonium compounds, eg, benzalkonium chloride, are cationic detergents widely used for skin antisepsis.

Phenols   Phenol was the original disinfectant used in the operating room by Lister in the 1860s, but it is rarely used as a disinfectant today because it is too caustic. Hexachlorophene, which is a biphenol with six chlorine atoms, is used in germicidal soaps, but concern over possible neurotoxicity has limited its use. Another phenol derivative is cresol (methylphenol), the active ingredient in Lysol. Phenols not only damage membranes but also denature proteins.

MODIFICATION OF PROTEINS

Chlorine   Chlorine is used as a disinfectant to purify the water supply and to treat swimming pools. It is also the active component of hypochlorite (bleach, Clorox), which is used as a disinfectant in the home and in hospitals. Chlorine is a powerful oxidizing agent that kills by cross-linking essential sulfhydryl groups in enzymes to form the inactive disulfide.

Iodine   Iodine is the most effective skin antiseptic used in medical practice. It is supplied in two forms:

(1) Tincture of iodine (2% solution of iodine and potassium iodide in ethanol) is used to prepare the skin prior to blood culture. Because tincture of iodine can be irritating to the skin, it should be removed with alcohol.

(2) Iodophors are complexes of iodine with detergents that are frequently used to prepare the skin prior to surgery because they are less irritating than tincture of iodine. Iodine, like chlorine, is an oxidant that inactivates sulfhydryl-containing enzymes. It also binds specifically to tyrosine residues in proteins.

Heavy Metals   Mercury and silver have the greatest antibacterial activity of the heavy metals and are the most widely used in medicine. They act by binding to sulfhydryl groups, thereby blocking enzymatic activity. Thimerosal (Merthiolate) and merbromin (Mercurochrome), which contain mercury, are used as skin antiseptics. Silver nitrate drops are useful in preventing gonococcal ophthalmia neonatorum. Silver sulfadiazine is used to prevent infection of burn wounds.

Hydrogen Peroxide   Hydrogen peroxide is used as an antiseptic to clean wounds and to disinfect contact lenses. Its effectiveness is limited by the organism's ability to produce catalase, an enzyme that degrades H_2O_2. (The bubbles produced when peroxide is used on wounds are formed by oxygen arising from the breakdown of H_2O_2 by tissue catalase.) Hydrogen peroxide is an oxidizing agent that attacks sulfhydryl groups, thereby inhibiting enzymatic activity.

Formaldehyde & Glutaraldehyde   Formaldehyde, which is available as a 37% solution in water (Formalin), denatures proteins and nucleic acids. Both proteins and nucleic acids contain essential $-NH_2$ and $-OH$ groups, which are the main sites of alkylation by the hydroxymethyl group of formaldehyde. Glutaraldehyde, which has two reactive aldehyde groups, is 10 times more effective than formaldehyde and is less toxic. In hospitals, it is used to sterilize respiratory therapy equipment.

Ethylene Oxide   Ethylene oxide gas is used extensively in hospitals for the sterilization of heat-sensitive materials such as surgical instruments and plastics. It kills by alkylating both proteins and nucleic acids; ie, the hydroxyethyl group attacks the reactive hydrogen atoms on essential amino and hydroxyl groups.

Acids & Alkalis   Strong acids and alkalis kill by denaturing proteins. Although most bacteria are susceptible, it is important to note that *Mycobacterium tuberculosis* and other mycobacteria are relatively resistant to 2% NaOH, which is used in the clinical laboratory to liquefy sputum prior to culturing the organism. Weak acids, such as benzoic, propionic, and citric acids, are frequently used as food preservatives because they are bacteriostatic. The action of these acids is partially a function of the organic moiety, eg, benzoate, as well as the low pH.

MODIFICATION OF NUCLEIC ACIDS

A variety of dyes not only stain microorganisms but also inhibit their growth. One of these is crystal violet (gentian violet), which is used as a skin antiseptic. Its action is based on binding of the positively charged dye molecule to the negatively charged phosphate groups of the nucleic acids. Malachite green, a triphenylamine dye like crystal violet, is a component of Löwenstein-Jensen's medium, which is used to grow *M tuberculosis*. The dye inhibits the growth of unwanted organisms in the sputum during the 6-week incubation period.

Physical Agents

The physical agents act either by imparting energy in the form of heat or radiation or by removing organisms through filtration.

HEAT

Heat energy can be applied in three ways: in the form of moist heat (either boiling or autoclaving) or dry heat or by pasteurization. In general, heat kills by denaturing proteins, but membrane damage and enzymatic cleavage of DNA may also be involved. Moist heat sterilizes at a lower temperature than dry heat, since water aids in the disruption of noncovalent bonds, eg, hydrogen bonds, which hold protein chains together in their secondary and tertiary structures.

Moist-heat sterilization, usually **autoclaving,** is the most frequently used method of sterilization. Because bacterial **spores are resistant to boiling** (100 °C at sea level), they must be exposed to a higher temperature; this cannot be achieved unless the pressure is increased. For this purpose, an autoclave chamber is used in which steam, at a pressure of 15 lb/in^2, reaches a temperature of 121 °C and is held for 15–20 minutes. This kills even the highly heat-resistant spores of *Clostridium botulinum,* the cause of botulism, with a margin of safety.

Sterilization by dry heat, on the other hand, requires temperatures in the range of 180 °C for 2 hours. This process is used primarily for glassware and is less frequently used than autoclaving.

Pasteurization, which is used primarily for milk, consists of heating the milk to 62 °C for 30 minutes followed by rapid cooling. ("Flash" pasteurization at 72 °C for 15 seconds is frequently used.) This is sufficient to kill the vegetative cells of the milk-borne pathogens, eg, *M bovis, Salmonella, Streptococcus, Listeria,* and *Brucella,* but not to sterilize the milk.

RADIATION

The two types of radiation used to kill microorganisms are **ultraviolet (UV) light and x-rays.** The greatest antimicrobial activity of UV light occurs at 250–260 nm, which is the wavelength region of maximum absorption by the purine and pyrimidine bases of DNA. The most significant lesion caused by UV irradiation is the formation of thymine dimers, but addition of hydroxyl groups to the bases also occurs. As a result, DNA replication is inhibited and the organism cannot grow. Cells have repair mechanisms against UV-induced damage that involve either cleavage of dimers in the presence of visible light (photoreactivation) or excision of damaged bases, which is not dependent upon visible light (dark repair). The use of UV irradiation in medicine is limited, as UV radiation can damage the cornea and skin.

X-rays have higher energy and penetrating power than UV radiation and kill mainly by the production of free radicals, eg, production of hydroxyl radicals by the hydrolysis of water. These highly reactive radicals can break covalent bonds in DNA, thereby killing the organism. Sulfhydryl-containing compounds, such as the amino acid cysteine, can protect DNA from free-radical attack. Another mechanism is a direct hit on a covalent bond in DNA, resulting in chain breakage, but this is probably less important than the mechanism involving free radicals.

X-rays kill vegetative cells readily, but spores are remarkably resistant, probably owing to their lower water content. X-rays are used in medicine for sterilization of heat-sensitive items, such as sutures and surgical gloves, and plastic items, such as syringes.

FILTRATION

Filtration is the preferred method of sterilizing certain solutions, eg, those with heat-sensitive components. In the past, solutions for intravenous use were autoclaved, but heat-resistant endotoxin in the cell walls of the dead gram-negative bacteria caused fever in recipients of the solutions. Therefore, solutions are now filtered to make them **"pyrogen-free"** prior to autoclaving.

The most commonly used filter is composed of nitrocellulose and has a pore size of 0.22 μm. This size will retain all bacteria and spores. Filters work by physically trapping particles larger than the pore size and by retaining somewhat smaller particles due to electrostatic attraction of the particles to the filters.

Review Questions

1. What is the difference between sterilization and disinfection?
2. What are the mechanisms of action of the following agents: (a) ethanol, (b) detergents, (c) iodine, (d) formaldehyde, (e) UV light?
3. How is pasteurization performed, and what does it accomplish?

Part II: Clinical Bacteriology

Overview of the Major Pathogens & Introduction to Anaerobic Bacteria

14

OVERVIEW OF THE MAJOR PATHOGENS

The major bacterial pathogens are presented in Table 14–1 and described in Chapters 15–26. So that the reader may concentrate on the important pathogens, the bacteria that are less medically important are described in a separate chapter (see Chapter 27).

Table 14–1 is divided into organisms that are readily Gram-stained and those that are not. The readily stained organisms fall into four categories: gram-positive cocci, gram-negative cocci, gram-positive rods, and gram-negative rods. Since there are so many kinds of gram-negative rods, they have been divided into three groups:

(1) organisms associated with the enteric tract,

(2) organisms associated with the respiratory tract, and

(3) organisms from animal sources (zoonotic bacteria).

For ease of understanding, the organisms associated with the enteric tract are further subdivided into three groups: (1) pathogens both inside and outside the enteric tract, (2) pathogens inside the enteric tract, and (3) pathogens outside the enteric tract.

As is true of any classification dealing with biologic entities, this one is not entirely precise. For example, *Campylobacter* causes enteric tract disease but frequently has an animal source. Nevertheless, despite some uncertainties, subdivision of the large number of gram-negative rods into these functional categories should be helpful to the reader.

The organisms that are not readily Gram-stained fall into six major categories: *Mycobacterium* species, which are acid-fast rods; *Mycoplasma* species, which have no cell wall and so do not stain with Gram's stain; *Treponema* and *Leptospira* species, which are spirochetes too thin to be seen when stained with Gram's stain; and *Chlamydia* and *Rickettsia* species, which stain well with Giemsa's stain or other special stains but poorly with Gram's stain. *Chlamydia* and *Rickettsia* species are obligate intracellular parasites, whereas members of the other four genera are not.

Table 14–2 presents the 10 most common "notifiable" bacterial diseases in the United States for 1995 as compiled by the Centers for Disease Control and Prevention. Note that only notifiable diseases are included and that certain common conditions such as streptococcal pharyngitis and chlamydial infection are not included. Two sexually transmitted diseases, chlamydial infection and gonorrhea, are by far the most common diseases listed, followed by salmonellosis, shigellosis, and tuberculosis in the top five.

INTRODUCTION TO ANAEROBIC BACTERIA

Important Properties Anaerobes are characterized by their ability to grow only in an atmosphere containing less than 20% oxygen; ie, they grow poorly if at all in room air. They are a heterogeneous group composed of bacteria that can barely grow in 20% oxygen to those that can grow

Table 14–1. Major bacterial pathogens.

Type of Organism	Genus
Readily Gram-stained	
Gram-positive cocci	*Staphylococcus, Streptococcus, Enterococcus*
Gram-negative cocci	*Neisseria*
Gram-positive rods	*Corynebacterium, Listeria, Bacillus, Clostridium, Actinomyces, Nocardia*
Gram-negative rods	
Enteric tract organisms	
Pathogenic inside and outside tract	*Escherichia, Salmonella*
Pathogenic primarily inside tract	*Shigella, Vibrio, Campylobacter, Helicobacter*
Pathogenic outside tract	*Klebsiella-Enterobacter-Serratia* group, *Pseudomonas, Proteus-Providencia-Morganella* group, *Bacteroides*
Respiratory tract organisms	*Haemophilus, Legionella, Bordetella*
Organisms from animal sources	*Brucella, Francisella, Pasteurella, Yersinia*
Not readily Gram-stained	
Not obligate intracellular parasites	*Mycobacterium, Mycoplasma, Treponema, Leptospira*
Obligate intracellular parasites	*Chlamydia, Rickettsia*

only in less than 0.02% oxygen. Table 14–3 describes the optimal oxygen requirements for several representative groups of organisms. The obligate aerobes, such as *Pseudomonas aeruginosa,* grow best in the 20% oxygen of room air and not at all under anaerobic conditions. Facultative anaerobes such as *Escherichia coli* can grow well under either circumstance. Aerotolerant organisms such as *Clostridium histolyticum* can grow to some extent in air but multiply much more rapidly in a lower oxygen concentration. Microaerophilic organisms such as *Campylobacter jejuni* require a reduced oxygen concentration (approximately 5%) to grow optimally. The obligate anaerobes such as *Bacteroides fragilis* and *Clostridium perfringens* require an almost total absence of oxygen. Many anaerobes use nitrogen as the terminal electron acceptor rather than oxygen.

The precise reason why the growth of anaerobes is inhibited by oxygen is not understood, but several factors are probably involved (see Chapter 3). One important aspect is the production of toxic compounds, such as H_2O_2 and superoxides, and the reduced amount (or absence of) catalase and superoxide dismutase in anaerobes to detoxify them. A second factor is oxidation of essential sulfhydryl groups in enzymes without sufficient reducing power to regenerate them.

In addition to oxygen concentration, the oxidation-reduction potential (E_h) of a tissue is an important determinant of the growth of anaerobes. Areas with low E_h, such as the periodontal pocket, dental plaque, and colon, support the growth of anaerobes well. Crushing injuries that result in devitalized tissue owing to impaired blood supply produce a low E_h, allowing anaerobes to grow and cause disease.

Table 14–2. The 10 most common notifiable bacterial diseases in the United States in 1995.[1]

Disease	Number of Cases
Chlamydial infections	477,638
Gonorrhea	392,848
Salmonellosis	45,970
Shigellosis	32,080
Tuberculosis	22,860
Syphilis, primary and secondary	16,500
Lyme disease	11,700
Pertussis	5,137
E coli O157 infections	2,139
Legionellosis	1,241

[1]The latest year for which complete data are available.

Table 14–3. Optimal oxygen requirements of representative bacteria.

Bacterial Type	Representative Organism	Growth Under Following Conditions	
		Aerobic	Anaerobic
Obligate aerobes	*Pseudomonas aeruginosa*	3 +	0
Facultative anaerobes	*Escherichia coli*	4 +	3 +
Aerotolerant organisms	*Clostridium histolyticum*	1 +	4 +
Microaerophiles	*Campylobacter jejuni*	0	1 +[1]
Obligate anaerobes	*Bacteroides fragilis*	0	4 +

[1] *C jejuni* grows best (3 +) in 5% O_2 plus 10% CO_2. It is also called **capnophilic** in view of its need for CO_2 for optimal growth.

Anaerobes of Medical Interest   The anaerobes of medical interest are presented in Table 14–4. It can be seen that they include both rods and cocci and both gram-positive and gram-negative organisms. The rods are divided into the spore formers, eg, *Clostridium,* and the non-spore formers, eg, *Bacteroides.* In this book, three genera of anaerobes are described as major bacterial pathogens, namely *Clostridium, Actinomyces,* and *Bacteroides. Streptococcus* is a genus of major pathogens, consisting of both anaerobic and facultative organisms. The remaining anaerobes are less important and are discussed in Chapter 27.

Clinical Infections   Many of the medically important anaerobes are part of the normal human flora. As such, they are nonpathogens in their normal habitat and cause disease only when they leave those sites. The two prominent exceptions to this are *Clostridium botulinum* and *Clostridium tetani,* the agents of botulism and tetanus, respectively, which are soil organisms. *C perfringens,* another important human pathogen, is found in the colon and in the soil.

Diseases caused by members of the anaerobic normal flora are characterized by abscesses, which are most frequently located in the brain, lungs, female genital tract, biliary tract, and other intra-abdominal sites. Most abscesses contain more than one organism, either multiple anaerobes or a mixture of anaerobes plus facultative anaerobes. It is thought that the facultative anaerobes consume sufficient oxygen to allow the anaerobes to flourish.

Three important findings on physical examination that arouse suspicion of an anaerobic infection are a foul-smelling discharge, gas in the tissue, and necrotic tissue. In addition, infections in the setting of pulmonary aspiration, bowel surgery, abortion, cancer, or human and animal bites frequently involve anaerobes.

Laboratory Diagnosis   Two aspects of microbiologic diagnosis of an anaerobic infection are important even before the specimen is cultured: (1) obtaining the appropriate specimen, and (2) rapidly transporting the specimen under anaerobic conditions to the laboratory. An appropriate specimen is one that does not contain members of the normal flora to confuse the interpretation. For example, specimens such as blood, pleural fluid, pus, and transtracheal aspirates are appropriate, but sputum and feces are not.

In the laboratory, the cultures are handled and incubated under anaerobic conditions. In addition to the usual diagnostic criteria of Gram's stain, morphology, and biochemical reactions, the special

Table 14–4. Anaerobic bacteria of medical interest.

Morphology	Gram Stain	Genus
Spore-forming rods	+	*Clostridium*
	–	None
Non-spore-forming rods	+	*Actinomyces, Bifidobacterium, Eubacterium, Lactobacillus, Propionibacterium*
	–	*Bacteroides, Fusobacterium*
Non-spore-forming cocci	+	*Peptococcus, Peptostreptococcus, Streptococcus*
	–	*Veillonella*

technique of gas chromatography is important. In this procedure, organic acids such as formic, acetic, and propionic acids are measured.

Treatment In general, surgical drainage of the abscess plus administration of antimicrobial drugs are indicated. Drugs that are commonly used to treat anaerobic infections are penicillin G, cefoxitin, chloramphenicol, clindamycin, and metronidazole. Note, however, that many isolates of the important pathogen *B fragilis* produce β-lactamase and so are resistant to penicillin.

Review Questions

1. Why is the growth of anaerobes inhibited in the presence of oxygen?
2. *Clostridium* and *Bacteroides* are two genera of medically important organisms. What are two significant differences between these organisms?
3. What are the characteristics of anaerobic infections?

15

Gram-Positive Cocci

There are two medically important genera: *Staphylococcus* and *Streptococcus*. They are nonmotile and do not form spores.

STAPHYLOCOCCUS

Diseases *Staphylococcus aureus* causes abscesses, various pyogenic infections (eg, endocarditis and osteomyelitis), food poisoning, and toxic shock syndrome. *Staphylococcus epidermidis* can cause endocarditis, and *Staphylococcus saprophyticus* causes urinary tract infections.

Important Properties Staphylococci are spherical gram-positive cocci arranged in irregular **grapelike clusters.** All staphylococci produce **catalase,** whereas no streptococci do (catalase degrades H_2O_2 into O_2 and H_2O).

Three species of staphylococci are human pathogens: *S aureus, S epidermidis,* and *S saprophyticus* (Table 15–1). Of the three, *S aureus* is by far the most important. *S aureus* is distinguished from the others primarily by **coagulase** production (coagulase clots citrated plasma). Furthermore, it usually ferments mannitol and hemolyzes blood, whereas the others do not.

S aureus has several important cell wall components and antigens.

(1) Protein A is the major protein in the cell wall. It is an important virulence factor, since it binds to the Fc portion of IgG at the complement-binding site thereby preventing the activation of comple-

Table 15–1. Staphylococci of medical importance.

Species	Coagulase Production	Typical Hemolysis	Important Features[1]
S aureus	+	Beta	Protein A on cell surface; suppurative lesions.
S epidermidis	–	None	Sensitive to novobiocin; common member of skin flora.
S saprophyticus	–	None	Resistant to novobiocin; sometimes causes urinary tract infections.

[1] All staphylococci are catalase-positive.

ment. As a consequence, no C3b is produced, and the opsonization and phagocytosis of the organisms are greatly reduced. Protein A is used in certain tests in the clinical laboratory because it binds to IgG and forms a "coagglutinate" with antigen-antibody complexes.

(2) Teichoic acids are polymers of ribitol phosphate. They mediate adherence of the staphylococci to mucosal cells. Antibodies to teichoic acids develop in certain staphylococcal infections, eg, endocarditis.

(3) Surface receptors for specific staphylococcal bacteriophages permit the "phage typing" of strains for epidemiologic purposes. Teichoic acids make up part of these receptors.

Transmission   Staphylococci are found primarily in the normal human flora. *S epidermidis* is regularly present on normal **skin** and mucous membranes. *S aureus* is often found in the **nose** and sometimes on the skin, especially in hospital staff and patients. Additional sources of staphylococcal infection are shedding from human lesions and fomites contaminated by these lesions. Disease production is favored by a heavily contaminated environment (eg, family members with boils) and a compromised immune system.

Pathogenesis   Staphylococci cause disease both by producing toxins and by multiplying in tissue and causing inflammation. The typical lesion of *S aureus* infection is an **abscess**. Abscesses undergo central necrosis and usually drain to the outside (eg, furuncles and boils), but organisms may disseminate via the bloodstream as well.
  Several important toxins and enzymes are produced by *S aureus*.

(1) Enterotoxin is a protein that causes vomiting and watery, nonbloody diarrhea. It acts by stimulating the release of large amounts of interleukin-1 and interleukin-2. It is fairly heat-resistant and so is usually not inactivated by brief cooking. There are six immunologic types of enterotoxin, types A–F.

(2) Toxic shock syndrome toxin (TSST) causes toxic shock, especially in tampon-using menstruating women or in individuals with wound infections. Toxic shock also occurs in patients with nasal packing used to stop bleeding from the nose. It is indistinguishable from enterotoxin F. TSST is a superantigen and causes toxic shock by stimulating the release of large amounts of IL-1, IL-2, and TNF (see the discussions of exotoxins in Chapter 7 and superantigens in Chapter 58).

(3) Exfoliatin is a protein produced by staphylococci of phage group II, which causes "scalded-skin" syndrome in young children. Exfoliatin is also a superantigen.

(4) Several toxins can kill leukocytes (leukocidins) and cause necrosis of tissues in vivo. Of these, the most important is **alpha toxin,** which causes marked necrosis of the skin and hemolysis. The cytotoxic effect of alpha toxin is attributed to the formation of holes in the cell membrane and the consequent loss of low-molecular-weight substances from the damaged cell.

(5) The enzymes include **coagulase,** fibrinolysin, hyaluronidase, proteases, nucleases, and lipases.

Clinical Findings   The important clinical manifestations caused by *S aureus* can be divided into two groups: inflammatory and toxin-mediated. In the following list, the first six are inflammatory in origin whereas the last three are toxin-mediated.

A. *S aureus*

1. Inflammatory
(1) skin infections, including impetigo, furuncles, carbuncles, paronychia, cellulitis, surgical wound infections, eyelid infections (blepharitis), and postpartum breast infections (mastitis);

(2) septicemia (sepsis) can originate from any localized lesion, especially wound infection, or as a result of intravenous drug abuse;

(3) endocarditis on normal or prosthetic heart valves, especially right-sided endocarditis in intravenous drug users (prosthetic valve endocarditis is often caused by *S epidermidis*);

(4) osteomyelitis and arthritis, either hematogenous or traumatic; it is a very common cause of osteomyelitis and arthritis, especially in children;

(5) pneumonia in postoperative patients or following viral respiratory infection, especially influenza (staphylococcal pneumonia often leads to empyema);

(6) abscesses (metastatic) in any organ, after bacteremia;

2. Toxin-Mediated

(7) food poisoning (characterized by vomiting being more prominent than diarrhea) due to ingestion of enterotoxin, which is preformed in foods and hence has a short incubation period (1–8 hours);

(8) toxic shock syndrome, which includes fever, hypotension, a rash that goes on to desquamate, and multisystem involvement; and

(9) scalded skin syndrome, in which the superficial layers of the epidermis slough in response to the presence of exfoliatin.

B. *S epidermidis* and *S saprophyticus*

There are two coagulase-negative staphylococci of medical importance: *S epidermidis* and *S saprophyticus*. *S epidermidis* is part of the normal human flora on the skin and mucous membranes but can cause infections of intravenous catheters and prosthetic implants, eg, heart valves. *S epidermidis* is also a major cause of sepsis in neonates and of peritonitis in patients with renal failure who are undergoing peritoneal dialysis through an indwelling catheter. *S saprophyticus* causes urinary tract infections, particularly in sexually active young women. It is second to *E coli* as a cause of community-acquired urinary tract infections in this population.

Laboratory Diagnosis   Smears from staphylococcal lesions reveal gram-positive cocci in grapelike clusters. Cultures of *S aureus* typically yield golden-yellow colonies that are usually beta-hemolytic. *S aureus* is **coagulase-positive.** Mannitol-salt agar is a commonly used screening device for *S aureus*. Cultures of coagulase-negative staphylococci typically yield white colonies that are non-hemolytic. The two coagulase-negative staphylococci are distinguished by their reaction to the antibiotic novobiocin: *S epidermidis* is sensitive, whereas *S saprophyticus* is resistant. There are no generally useful serologic or skin tests.

Treatment   In the United States, 90% or more of *S aureus* strains are resistant to penicillin G. Most of them produce β-**lactamase** under control of transmissible plasmids. Such organisms can be treated with β-lactamase-resistant penicillins, eg, nafcillin or cloxacillin, some cephalosporins, or vancomycin. Treatment with a combination of a β-lactamase–sensitive penicillin, eg, amoxicillin, and a β-lactamase inhibitor, eg, clavulanic acid, is also useful. Some staphylococci are "methicillin-resistant" (or "nafcillin-resistant") by virtue of altered penicillin-binding proteins. Such organisms can produce sizable outbreaks of disease, especially in hospitals. The drug of choice for these staphylococci is vancomycin, to which gentamicin is sometimes added. In 1997, vancomycin-resistant *S aureus* was isolated from patients' specimens for the first time.

Some strains of staphylococci exhibit **tolerance;** ie, they can be inhibited by antibiotics but are not killed (the MBC/MIC ratio is very high). Tolerance may be due to failure of the drugs to inactivate inhibitors of autolytic enzymes that degrade the organism. Tolerant organisms should be treated with drug combinations (see Chapter 10).

Drainage (spontaneous or surgical) is the cornerstone of abscess treatment. Previous infection provides only partial immunity to reinfection.

S epidermidis is highly antibiotic resistant. The drug of choice is vancomycin to which either rifampin or an aminoglycoside can be added. *S saprophyticus* urinary tract infections can be treated with a quinolone, such as norfloxacin, or with trimethoprim-sulfamethoxazole.

Prevention   There is no effective immunization with toxoids or bacterial vaccines. Cleanliness, frequent hand-washing, and aseptic management of lesions help to control spread of *S aureus*. Persistent colonization of the nose by *S aureus* can be reduced by intranasal mupirocin or by oral antibiotics, such as ciprofloxacin or trimethoprim-sulfamethoxazole, but is difficult to eliminate completely. Shedders may have to be removed from high-risk areas, eg, operating rooms and newborn nurseries.

STREPTOCOCCUS

Streptococci of medical importance are listed in Table 15–2. All but one of these streptococci are discussed here; *Streptococcus pneumoniae* is discussed separately.

Diseases   Streptococci produce a wide variety of infections, ranging from pharyngitis and cellulitis to sepsis. They also can trigger immunologic disorders such as rheumatic fever and acute glomerulonephritis.

Important Properties   Streptococci are spherical gram-positive cocci usually arranged in chains or pairs. All streptococci are **catalase-negative,** whereas staphylococci are catalase-positive (Table 15–2).

One of the most important criteria for identification is the type of hemolysis.

(1) Alpha-hemolytic streptococci form a green zone around their colonies as a result of incomplete lysis of red blood cells in the agar.

(2) Beta-hemolytic streptococci form a clear zone around their colonies, since complete lysis of the red cells occurs. Beta-hemolysis is due to the production of enzymes (hemolysins) called streptolysin O and streptolysin S (see the Pathogenesis section below).

(3) Some streptococci are nonhemolytic (gamma-hemolysis).

There are two important antigens of beta-hemolytic streptococci:

(1) C carbohydrate determines the *group* of beta-hemolytic streptococci. It is located in the cell wall, and its specificity is determined by an amino sugar.

(2) M protein is the most important virulence factor and determines the *type* of group A beta-hemolytic streptococci. It protrudes from the outer surface of the cell and interferes with ingestion by phagocytes; ie, it is antiphagocytic. Antibody to M protein provides type-specific immunity. There are approximately 80 serotypes based on the M protein, which explains why multiple infections with *S pyogenes* can occur. Strains of *S pyogenes* that produce certain M protein types are **rheumatogenic,** ie, cause primarily rheumatic fever, whereas strains of *S pyogenes* that produce other M protein types are **nephritogenic,** ie, cause primarily acute glomerulonephritis.

The classification of streptococci is as follows.

A.   Beta-Hemolytic Streptococci: These are arranged into groups A–U (known as Lancefield groups) on the basis of antigenic differences in C carbohydrate. In the clinical laboratory, the group is determined by precipitin tests with specific antisera or by immunofluorescence.

Group A streptococci (*Streptococcus pyogenes*) are among the most important human pathogens. They are the most frequent bacterial cause of pharyngitis. They adhere to pharyngeal epithelium via

Table 15–2. Streptococci of medical importance.

Species	Lancefield Group	Typical Hemolysis	Diagnostic Features[1]
S pyogenes	A	Beta	Bacitracin-sensitive.
S agalactiae	B	Beta	Bacitracin-resistant; hippurate hydrolyzed.
S faecalis[2]	D	Alpha or beta or none	Growth in 6.5% NaCl.[3]
S bovis	D	Alpha or none	No growth in 6.5% NaCl.
S pneumoniae	NA[4]	Alpha	Bile-soluble; inhibited by optochin.
Viridans group	NA	Alpha	Not bile-soluble; not inhibited by optochin.

[1] All streptococci are catalase-negative.
[2] Now called *Enterococcus faecalis* and abbreviated enterococci; *S bovis* is a nonenterococcal group D organism.
[3] Both *S faecalis* and *S bovis* grow on bile-esculin agar, whereas other streptococci do not. They hydrolyze the esculin, and this results in a characteristic black discoloration of the agar.
[4] NA, not applicable.

pili covered with lipoteichoic acid and M protein. Many strains have a hyaluronic acid capsule that is antiphagocytic. They are usually **bacitracin-susceptible,** an important diagnostic criterion.

Group B streptococci (*Streptococcus agalactiae*) colonize the genital tract of some women and can cause neonatal meningitis and sepsis. They are usually bacitracin-resistant.

Group D streptococci include enterococci (eg, *Enterococcus faecalis,* formerly known as *Streptococcus faecalis*) and nonenterococci (eg, *Streptococcus bovis*). Enterococci grow in 6.5% NaCl and are not killed by penicillin G. They occur as part of the normal flora in the gut and are noted for their ability to cause urinary, biliary, and cardiovascular infections. Nonenterococci can produce similar infections but are inhibited by 6.5% NaCl and killed by penicillin G. Note that the hemolytic reaction of group D streptococci is variable: some are beta-hemolytic, whereas most are alpha-hemolytic or nonhemolytic.

Groups C, E, F, G, H, and K–U streptococci infrequently cause human disease.

Group N "lactic" streptococci produce normal souring of milk.

B. Non-Beta-Hemolytic Streptococci: Some produce no hemolysis; others produce alpha-hemolysis. The principal alpha-hemolytic organisms are *S pneumoniae* and the viridans group of streptococci. The viridans streptococci (eg, *Streptococcus mitis, S sanguis,* and *S mutans*) are *not* bile-soluble and *not* inhibited by optochin—in contrast to *S pneumoniae*. Viridans streptococci are part of the normal flora of the human pharynx and intermittently reach the bloodstream to cause infective endocarditis. *S mutans* synthesizes polysaccharides (dextrans) that are found in dental plaque and lead to dental caries.

Streptococcus intermedius and *Streptococcus anginosus* (also known as the *Streptococcus anginosus-milleri* group) are usually alpha-hemolytic or nonhemolytic, but some isolates are beta-hemolytic. They are found primarily in the mouth and colon.

C. Peptostreptococci: These grow under anaerobic or microaerophilic conditions and produce variable hemolysis. Peptostreptococci are members of the normal flora of the gut and the female genital tract and participate in mixed anaerobic infections.

Transmission Most streptococci are part of the normal flora of the human throat, skin, and intestines but produce disease when they gain access to tissues or blood. Viridans streptococci and *S pneumoniae* are found chiefly in the **oropharynx;** *S pyogenes* is found on the **skin** and in the oropharynx in small numbers; *S agalactiae* occurs in the **female genital tract;** and both the enterococci and anaerobic streptococci are located in the **lower intestinal tract.**

Pathogenesis Group A streptococci (*S pyogenes*) cause disease by three mechanisms: (1) **inflammation,** which is induced locally at the site of the organisms in tissue; (2) **exotoxin** production, which can cause widespread systemic symptoms in areas of the body where there are no organisms; and (3) **immunologic,** which occurs when antibody against a component of the organism cross-reacts with normal tissue or forms immune complexes that damage normal tissue (see the section on poststreptococcal diseases below).

Group A streptococci produce the following eight important toxins and enzymes:

A. Inflammation-Related Enzymes

(1) Streptokinase (fibrinolysin) activates plasminogen to form plasmin, which dissolves fibrin in clots, thrombi, and emboli.

(2) DNase (streptodornase) depolymerizes DNA in exudates or necrotic tissue. Antibody to DNase B develops during pyoderma; this can be used for diagnostic purposes. Streptokinase-streptodornase mixtures applied as a skin test give a positive reaction in most adults, indicating normal cell-mediated immunity.

(3) Hyaluronidase degrades hyaluronic acid, which is the ground substance of subcutaneous tissue. Hyaluronidase is known as **spreading factor** because it facilitates the rapid spread of *S pyogenes* in skin infections (cellulitis).

B. Toxins and Hemolysins

(4) Erythrogenic toxin causes the rash of scarlet fever. Its mechanism of action is similar to that of the toxic shock syndrome toxin (TSST) of *S aureus;* ie, it acts as a superantigen (see *S aureus,* above, and Chapter 58). It is produced only by certain strains of *Streptococcus pyogenes* lysogenized by a bacteriophage carrying the gene for the toxin. The injection of a skin test dose of erythrogenic toxin (Dick test) gives a positive result in persons lacking antitoxin (ie, susceptible persons).

(5) Streptolysin O is a hemolysin that is inactivated by oxidation (oxygen-labile). It causes beta-hemolysis only when colonies grow under the surface of a blood agar plate. It is antigenic, and antibody to it (ASO) develops after group A streptococcal infections. The titer of ASO antibody can be important in the diagnosis of rheumatic fever.

(6) Streptolysin S is a hemolysin that is not inactivated by oxygen (oxygen-stable). It is *not* antigenic but is responsible for beta-hemolysis when colonies grow on the surface of a blood agar plate.

(7) Pyrogenic exotoxin A is a toxin similar to staphylococcal **toxic shock syndrome toxin** (TSST). It has the same mode of action as does staphylococcal TSST; ie, it is a superantigen that causes the release of large amounts of cytokines from helper T cells and macrophages (see p 79 and Chapters 7 and 58).

(8) Exotoxin B is a protease that rapidly destroys tissue and is produced in large amounts by the strains of *S pyogenes* that cause necrotizing fasciitis.

Resistance or immunity to group A streptococci is due to type-specific antibody to **M protein.** Resistance to group B infection of neonates is due to transplacentally passed antibody developed by the mother.

Clinical Findings   *S pyogenes* causes three types of diseases: (1) **pyogenic** diseases such as pharyngitis and cellulitis, (2) **toxigenic** diseases such as scarlet fever and toxic shock syndrome, and (3) **immunologic** diseases such as rheumatic fever and acute glomerulonephritis. (See the section on poststreptococcal diseases, below.)

S pyogenes (group A beta-hemolytic streptococcus) is the most common bacterial cause of sore throat. **Pharyngitis** is characterized by inflammation, exudate, fever, leukocytosis, and tender cervical lymph nodes. If untreated, spontaneous recovery occurs in 10 days. However, it may extend to otitis, sinusitis, mastoiditis, and meningitis. If the infecting streptococci produce erythrogenic toxin and the host lacks antitoxin, scarlet fever may result. Rheumatic fever may occur, especially following pharyngitis. *S pyogenes* also causes another toxin-mediated disease, streptococcal toxic shock syndrome, which has clinical findings similar to those of staphylococcal toxic shock syndrome (see p 80).

Group A streptococci can enter skin defects to produce **cellulitis,** erysipelas, necrotizing fasciitis (streptococcal gangrene), lymphangitis, or bacteremia. They can enter the uterus after delivery to produce endometritis and sepsis (puerperal fever). Streptococcal pyoderma (impetigo) is a superficial infection of abraded skin that forms pus or crusts. It is communicable among children, especially in hot, humid climates. Glomerulonephritis may occur, especially following skin infections.

Group B streptococci cause **neonatal sepsis and meningitis.** The main predisposing factor is prolonged rupture of the membranes, ie, longer than 18 hours, in women who are colonized with the organism. Children born prior to 37 weeks' gestation have a greatly increased risk of disease.

Viridans streptococci (eg, *S mutans, S sanguis, S salivarius,* and *S mitis*) are the most common cause of infective **endocarditis.** They enter the bloodstream from the oropharynx, typically after dental surgery. Signs of endocarditis are fever, anemia, heart murmur, and embolic events. It is 100% fatal unless effectively treated with antimicrobial agents. About 10% of endocarditis cases are caused by enterococci, but any organism causing bacteremia may settle on deformed valves. At least three blood cultures are necessary to ensure recovery of the organism in more than 90% of cases.

Enterococci cause **urinary tract infections,** especially in hospitalized patients. Indwelling urinary catheters and urinary tract instrumentation are important predisposing factors. Enterococci also cause endocarditis, particularly in patients who have undergone gastrointestinal or urinary tract surgery or instrumentation. They also cause intra-abdominal and pelvic infections, typically in combination with anaerobes. *Streptococcus bovis,* a nonenterococcal group D streptococcus, causes **endocarditis,** especially in patients with carcinoma of the colon. This association is so strong that patients with *S bovis* bacteremia or endocarditis should be investigated for the presence of colonic carcinoma.

Streptococcus intermedius and *Streptococcus anginosus* cause dental, brain, and abdominal abscesses and endocarditis. Peptostreptococci participate in mixed anaerobic infections of the abdomen, pelvis, lungs, and brain.

Poststreptococcal (Nonsuppurative) Diseases   These are disorders in which a local infection with group A streptococci is followed weeks later by inflammation in an organ that was *not* infected by the streptococci. The inflammation is caused by an **immunologic** response to streptococcal M proteins that cross-react with human tissues. Some strains of *S pyogenes* bearing certain M proteins are nephritogenic and cause acute glomerulonephritis, and other strains bearing different M proteins are rheumatogenic and cause acute rheumatic fever.

A.   Acute Glomerulonephritis: Acute glomerulonephritis (AGN) typically occurs 2–3 weeks after skin infection by certain group A streptococcal types in children (eg, M protein type 49 causes AGN most frequently). AGN is more frequent after skin infections than after pharyngitis. The most striking clinical features are hypertension, edema of the face (especially periorbital edema) and ankles, and "smoky" urine (due to red cells in the urine). Most patients recover completely. Reinfection with streptococci rarely leads to recurrence of acute glomerulonephritis.

The disease is initiated by antigen-antibody complexes on the glomerular basement membrane, and soluble antigens from streptococcal membranes may be the inciting antigen. It can be prevented by early eradication of nephritogenic streptococci from skin colonization sites but *not* by administration of penicillin after onset of the symptoms.

B.   Acute Rheumatic Fever: Approximately 2 weeks after any type of group A streptococcal infection—usually pharyngitis—rheumatic fever, characterized by fever, migratory polyarthritis, and carditis, may develop. The carditis damages myocardial and endocardial tissue, especially the mitral and aortic valves. ASO titers and the erythrocyte sedimentation rate are elevated.

Rheumatic fever is due to an immunologic reaction between cross-reacting antibodies to certain streptococcal M proteins and antigens of joint and heart tissue. It is an autoimmune disease, greatly exacerbated by recurrence of streptococcal infections. If streptococcal infections are treated within 8 days after onset, rheumatic fever is usually prevented. After a heart-damaging attack of rheumatic fever, reinfection must be prevented by long-term prophylaxis. In the United States, fewer than 0.5% of group A streptococcal infections lead to rheumatic fever, but in developing tropical countries, the rate is higher than 5%.

Laboratory Diagnosis

A.   Microbiologic: Gram-stained smears are useless in streptococcal pharyngitis because viridans streptococci are members of the normal flora and cannot be visually distinguished from the pathogenic *S pyogenes.* However, stained smears from skin lesions or wounds that reveal streptococci are diagnostic. Cultures of swabs from the pharynx or lesion on blood agar plates show small, translucent beta-hemolytic colonies in 18–48 hours. If **inhibited by bacitracin** disk, they are likely to be group A streptococci. Group B streptococci are characterized by their ability to **hydrolyze hippurate** and by the production of a protein that causes enhanced hemolysis on sheep blood agar when combined with beta-hemolysin of *S aureus* (CAMP test). Group D streptococci **hydrolyze esculin in the presence of bile;** ie, they produce a black pigment on bile-esculin agar. The group D organisms are further subdivided: the enterococci **grow in hypertonic (6.5%) NaCl,** whereas the nonenterococci do not.

B.   Serologic: ASO titers are high soon after group A streptococcal infections. In patients suspected of having rheumatic fever, an **elevated ASO titer** is typically used as evidence of previous infection because throat cultures are often negative at the time the patient presents with rheumatic fever. Titers of anti-DNase B are high in group A streptococcal skin infections and serve as an indicator of prior streptococcal infection in patients suspected of having AGN.

Treatment   All group A streptococci are susceptible to penicillin G, but neither rheumatic fever nor AGN patients benefit from penicillin treatment *after* onset. In mild Group A streptococcal infections, oral penicillin V can be used. In penicillin-allergic patients, erythromycin or one of its long-acting derivatives, eg, azithromycin, can be used. Endocarditis caused by most viridans streptococci is curable by prolonged penicillin treatment. However, enterococcal endocarditis can be eradicated only by a penicillin combined with an aminoglycoside. Enterococci resistant to multiple drugs, eg, penicillin, aminoglycosides and vancomycin, have emerged. Nonenterococcal group D streptococci, eg, *S bovis,* are not highly resistant and can be treated with penicillin G. The drug of choice for group B streptococcal infections is penicillin G. Some strains may require higher doses of penicillin G or a combination of penicillin G and an aminoglycoside to eradicate the organism. Peptostreptococci can be treated with penicillin G.

Prevention   Rheumatic fever can be prevented by prompt treatment of group A streptococcal pharyngitis with penicillin. Prevention of streptococcal infections (usually with benzathine penicillin once each month for several years) in persons who have had rheumatic fever is important to prevent recurrence of the disease. There is no evidence that patients who have had AGN require similar penicillin prophylaxis.

Endocarditis caused by viridans streptococci can be prevented in patients with damaged heart valves who undergo invasive dental procedures by using amoxicillin perioperatively. Endocarditis caused by enterococci can be prevented in patients with damaged heart valves who undergo gastrointestinal or urinary tract procedures by using ampicillin and gentamicin perioperatively.

There are no vaccines available against these streptococcal infections.

STREPTOCOCCUS PNEUMONIAE

Diseases   Pneumococci cause pneumonia, bacteremia, meningitis, and infections of the upper respiratory tract such as otitis and sinusitis.

Important Properties   Pneumococci are gram-positive lancet-shaped cocci arranged in pairs (**diplococci**) or short chains. (The term "lancet-shaped" means that the diplococci are oval with somewhat pointed ends rather than being round.) On blood agar they produce alpha-hemolysis. In contrast to viridans streptococci, they are lysed by bile or deoxycholate and their growth is inhibited by optochin.

Pneumococci possess **polysaccharide capsules** of more than 85 antigenically distinct types. With type-specific antiserum, capsules swell (**quellung reaction**), and this can be used to identify the type. Capsules are virulence factors; ie, they interfere with phagocytosis and favor invasiveness. Specific antibody to the capsule opsonizes the organism, facilitates phagocytosis, and promotes resistance. Such antibody develops in humans as a result either of infection (asymptomatic or clinical) or of administration of polysaccharide vaccine. Capsular polysaccharide elicits primarily a B cell (ie, T-independent) response.

Transmission   Humans are the natural hosts for pneumococci; there is no animal reservoir. Pneumococcal infections are not considered to be communicable, since a proportion (5–50%) of the healthy population harbor virulent organisms in the oropharynx. Resistance is high in healthy young people, and disease results most often when predisposing factors (see below) are present.

Pathogenesis   Pneumococci produce no toxins known to play a role in pathogenesis. They do produce IgA protease that may enhance the organism's ability to colonize the mucosa of the upper respiratory tract. Pneumococci multiply in tissues and cause inflammation. When they reach alveoli, there is outpouring of fluid and red and white blood cells, resulting in consolidation of the lung. During recovery, pneumococci are phagocytized, mononuclear cells ingest debris, and the consolidation resolves.

Factors that lower resistance and predispose persons to pneumococcal infection include (1) alcohol or drug intoxication or other cerebral impairment that can depress the cough reflex and increase aspiration of secretions; (2) abnormality of the respiratory tract (eg, viral infections), pooling of mucus, bronchial obstruction, and respiratory tract injury due to irritants (which disturb the integrity and movement of the mucociliary blanket); (3) abnormal circulatory dynamics (eg, pulmonary congestion and heart failure); (4) **splenectomy;** and (5) certain chronic diseases such as sickle cell anemia and nephrosis. Trauma to the head that causes **leakage of spinal fluid** through the nose predisposes to pneumococcal meningitis.

Clinical Findings   Pneumonia often begins with a sudden chill, fever, cough, and pleuritic pain. Sputum is a red or brown "rusty" color. Bacteremia occurs in 15–25% of cases. Spontaneous recovery may begin in 5–10 days, and is accompanied by development of anticapsular antibodies. Pneumococci are a prominent cause of otitis media, sinusitis, purulent bronchitis, bacterial meningitis, and sepsis, especially in immunocompromised patients.

Laboratory Diagnosis   In sputum, pneumococci can be seen as predominant organisms in Gram-stained smears or in the quellung reaction with multitype antiserum. On blood agar, pneumococci form small **alpha-hemolytic** colonies. The colonies are **bile-soluble,** ie, are lysed by bile, and growth is **inhibited by optochin.** Blood cultures are positive in 15–25% of pneumococcal infections. Culture of cerebrospinal fluid is usually positive in meningitis. Because of the increasing numbers of strains resistant to penicillin, antibiotic sensitivity tests must be done on organisms isolated from serious infections.

Treatment   Most pneumococci are susceptible to penicillins and erythromycin. In severe pneumococcal infections, penicillin G is the drug of choice, whereas in mild pneumococcal infections, oral penicillin V can be used. In penicillin-allergic patients, erythromycin or one of its long-acting derivatives, eg, azithromycin, can be used. In the United States, about 25% of isolates exhibit low-level resistance to penicillin, primarily as a result of changes in penicillin-binding proteins. An increasing percentage of isolates, about 7% currently, show high-level resistance, which is attributed to multiple changes in penicillin-binding proteins. They do not produce β-lactamase.

Prevention   In spite of the efficacy of antimicrobial drug treatment, the mortality rate is high in elderly (ie, people over 65 years old), immunocompromised (especially splenectomized), or debilitated persons. They should be immunized with the polyvalent (23-type) **polysaccharide vaccine.** The vaccine is safe and fairly effective and provides long-lasting protection (at least 5 years). At present, booster doses are not recommended. Oral penicillin is given to young children with hypogammaglobulinemia or splenectomy because they are prone to pneumococcal infections and respond poorly to the vaccine.

Review Questions

1. What are the differences in appearance on Gram-stained smears between staphylococci, streptococci, and pneumococci?
2. What is the typical pathologic lesion caused by staphylococci?
3. What laboratory test distinguishes *Staphylococcus aureus* from *Staphylococcus epidermidis?*
4. Which staphylococcal species is usually associated with (a) endocarditis in drug addicts, (b) endocarditis in patients with prosthetic heart valves, (c) osteomyelitis, (d) lower urinary tract infections, and (e) carbuncle?
5. What is the pathogenesis of staphylococcal food poisoning?
6. What are the virulence factors produced by *S aureus,* and what is their postulated mode of action?
7. Many *S aureus* infections are unsuccessfully treated with benzylpenicillin (penicillin G). Why? Which two drugs can be used instead? Why?
8. Distinguish between the grouping and typing of streptococci.
9. Which streptococcal species is usually associated with (a) pharyngitis, (b) neonatal sepsis, (c) infective (subacute) endocarditis, (d) pyoderma, (e) urinary tract infection, (f) glomerulonephritis, and (g) rheumatic fever?
10. What is the role of hemolysis in the classification of streptococci?
11. What are the natural habitat and special growth characteristics of enterococci?
12. What is the role of each of the following virulence factors in the production of disease by *Streptococcus pyogenes?* (a) hyaluronidase; (b) M protein; (c) erythrogenic toxin.
13. Describe the pathogenesis of (a) rheumatic fever and (b) acute glomerulonephritis.
14. How is *Streptococcus pyogenes* (group A) distinguished from *Streptococcus agalactiae* (group B) in the clinical laboratory?
15. How are pneumococci (*Streptococcus pneumoniae*) and viridans streptococci distinguished in the clinical laboratory?
16. Pneumococci have many serologic types. What is the nature of the antigen, and what role does it play in pathogenesis?
17. What is the pathogenesis of pneumococcal pneumonia?
18. How can pneumococcal pneumonia and bacteremia be prevented?

Gram-Negative Cocci

16

NEISSERIA

Diseases   The genus *Neisseria* contains two important human pathogens: *Neisseria meningitidis* and *Neisseria gonorrhoeae*. *N meningitidis* mainly causes meningitis and meningococcemia. *N gonorrhoeae* causes gonorrhea, the second most common notifiable bacterial disease in the United States (Table 16–1). It also causes neonatal conjunctivitis (ophthalmia neonatorum) and pelvic inflammatory disease (PID).

Important Properties   Neisseriae are gram-negative cocci that resemble paired kidney beans.

(1) *N meningitidis* (meningococcus) has a prominent **polysaccharide capsule** that enhances virulence by its antiphagocytic action and induces protective antibodies. Meningococci are divided into at least 13 serologic groups based on the antigenicity of their capsular polysaccharides (Table 16–2).

(2) *N gonorrhoeae* (gonococcus) has no polysaccharide capsule but has multiple serotypes based on the antigenicity of its pilus protein. There is **marked antigenic variation** in the gonococcal pili as a result of chromosomal rearrangement; more than 100 serotypes are known. Gonococci have three outer membrane proteins (proteins I, II, and III). Protein II plays a role in attachment of the organism to cells and varies antigenically as well.

Neisseriae are gram-negative bacteria and contain endotoxin in their outer membrane. The endotoxin of *N meningitidis* is a lipo**poly**saccharide (LPS) similar to that found in many gram-negative rods, but the endotoxin of *N gonorrhoeae* is a lipo**oligo**saccharide (LOS). Both LPS and LOS contain lipid A, but LOS lacks the long repeating sugar side chains of LPS.

The growth of both organisms is inhibited by toxic trace metals and fatty acids found in certain culture media, eg, blood agar plates. They are therefore cultured on "chocolate" agar containing blood heated to 80 °C, which inactivates the inhibitors. Neisseriae are **oxidase-positive;** ie, they possess the enzyme cytochrome *c*. This is an important laboratory diagnostic test in which colonies exposed to phenylenediamine turn black as a result of oxidation of the reagent by the enzyme.

The genus *Neisseria* is one of several in the family *Neisseriaceae*. A separate genus contains the organism *Moraxella catarrhalis,* which is part of the normal throat flora and an occasional opportunistic cause of pneumonia. *M catarrhalis* and members of other genera, such as *Branhamella, Kingella,* and *Acinetobacter,* are described in Chapter 27. (*M catarrhalis* is the new name for *Branhamella catarrhalis.*)

1. Neisseria meningitidis

Pathogenesis & Epidemiology   Humans are the only natural hosts for meningococci. The organisms are transmitted by **airborne droplets;** they colonize the membranes of the nasopharynx and become part of the transient flora of the upper respiratory tract. Carriers are usually asympto-

Table 16–1. Neisseriae of medical importance.[1]

Species	Portal of Entry	Polysaccharide Capsule	Maltose Fermentation	β-Lactamase Production	Available Vaccine
N meningitidis (meningococcus)	Respiratory tract	+	+	None	+
N gonorrhoeae (gonococcus)	Genital tract	–	–	Some	–

[1] All neisseriae are oxidase-positive.

Table 16–2. Properties of the polysaccharide capsule of the meningococcus.[1]

(1) Enhances virulence by its antiphagocytic action
(2) Is the antigen that defines the serologic groups
(3) Is the antigen detected in the spinal fluid of patients with meningitis
(4) Is the antigen in the vaccine

[1] The same four features apply to the capsule of the pneumococcus and *Haemophilus influenzae*.

matic. From the nasopharynx, the organism can enter the bloodstream and spread to specific sites, such as the meninges or joints, or be disseminated throughout the body (meningococcemia). About 5% of people become chronic carriers and serve as a source of infection for others. The carriage rate can be as high as 35% in people who live in close quarters, eg, military recruits; this explains the high frequency of outbreaks of meningitis in the armed forces prior to the use of the vaccine. The carriage rate is also high in close (family) contacts of patients.

Three organisms cause more than 80% of cases of bacterial meningitis in persons over 2 months of age: *Haemophilus influenzae, Streptococcus pneumoniae,* and *N meningitidis.* Of these organisms, meningococci, especially those in group A, are most likely to cause epidemics of meningitis. As a cause of sporadic cases, meningococci rank second to *H influenzae* in causing meningitis in children aged 6 months to 6 years and are similar to *S pneumoniae* in the frequency of infections in adults.

Meningococci have three important virulence factors:

(1) a **polysaccharide capsule** that enables the organism to resist phagocytosis by polymorphonuclear leukocytes (PMNs);

(2) endotoxin (LPS), which causes fever, shock, and other pathophysiologic changes (in purified form, endotoxin can reproduce many of the clinical manifestations of meningococcemia); and

(3) an immunoglobulin A **(IgA) protease,** which, by cleaving secretory IgA, helps the bacteria to attach to the membranes of the upper respiratory tract.

Resistance to disease correlates with the presence of antibody to the capsular polysaccharide. Most carriers develop protective antibody titers within 2 weeks of colonization. Immunity is group-specific, and so it is possible to have protective antibodies to one group of organisms yet be susceptible to infection by organisms of the other groups. Complement is an important feature of the host defenses, because people with complement deficiencies, particularly in the **late-acting complement components** (C6–C9), have an increased incidence of meningococcal bacteremia.

Clinical Findings   The two most important manifestations of disease are **meningococcemia** and **meningitis.** The most severe form of meningococcemia is the life-threatening **Waterhouse-Friderichsen syndrome,** which is characterized by high fever, shock, widespread purpura, disseminated intravascular coagulation, and adrenal insufficiency. Bacteremia can result in the seeding of many organs, especially the meninges. The symptoms of meningococcal meningitis are those of a typical bacterial meningitis—namely fever, headache, stiff neck, and an increased level of PMNs in spinal fluid.

Laboratory Diagnosis   The principal laboratory procedures are smear and culture of blood and spinal fluid samples. A presumptive diagnosis of meningococcal meningitis can be made if gram-negative cocci are seen in a smear of spinal fluid. The organism grows best on chocolate agar incubated at 37 °C in a 5% CO_2 atmosphere. A presumptive diagnosis of *Neisseria* can be made if oxidase-positive colonies of gram-negative diplococci are found. The differentiation between *N meningitidis* and *N gonorrhoeae* is made on the basis of sugar fermentation: meningococci ferment maltose, whereas gonococci do not (both organisms ferment glucose). Immunofluorescence can also be used to identify these species. Tests for serum antibodies are not useful for clinical diagnosis. However, a procedure that can assist in the rapid diagnosis of meningococcal meningitis is the latex agglutination test, which detects capsular polysaccharide in the spinal fluid.

Treatment   Penicillin G is the treatment of choice for meningococcal infections. Strains resistant to penicillin have rarely emerged, but sulfonamide resistance is common.

Prevention   Chemoprophylaxis and immunization are both used to prevent meningococcal disease. Rifampin is used for prophylaxis in household and other close contacts. It is preferred because it is efficiently secreted into the saliva, in contrast to penicillin G. The meningococcal vaccine, which contains the capsular polysaccharides of group A, C, Y, and W-135 strains, is effective in preventing epidemics of meningitis and in reducing the carrier rate, especially in military personnel. The vaccine does not contain the group B polysaccharide, which is poorly immunogenic in humans.

2. *Neisseria gonorrhoeae*

Pathogenesis & Epidemiology   Gonococci, like meningococci, cause disease only in humans. The organism is usually transmitted **sexually;** newborns can be infected during birth. Because the gonococcus is quite sensitive to dehydration and cool conditions, sexual transmission favors its survival. Gonorrhea is usually symptomatic in men but often asymptomatic in women. Infections of the anorectal area and pharynx, as well as those of the genital tract, can act as the source of the organisms.

Pili constitute one of the most important virulence factors, because they mediate attachment to mucosal cell surfaces and are antiphagocytic. Piliated gonococci are usually virulent, whereas non-piliated strains are avirulent. Two virulence factors in the cell wall are **lipooligosaccharide** (a modified form of endotoxin), and the outer membrane proteins. The organism's **IgA protease** can hydrolyze secretory IgA, which could otherwise block attachment to the mucosa. Gonococci have no capsules.

The main host defenses against gonococci are antibodies (IgA and IgG), complement, and neutrophils. Antibody-mediated opsonization and killing within phagocytes occur, but repeated gonococcal infections are common primarily as a result of antigenic changes of pili and the outer membrane proteins.

Gonococci infect primarily the mucosal surfaces, eg, the urethra and vagina, but dissemination occurs. Certain strains of gonococci cause disseminated infections more frequently than others. These strains are characterized by three features: (1) resistance to the bactericidal action of serum; (2) marked sensitivity to penicillin; and (3) auxotrophy for arginine, uracil, and hypoxanthine; ie, for growth, they require that these substances be present in the medium.

The occurrence of a disseminated infection is a function not only of the strain of gonococcus but also of the effectiveness of the host defenses. Persons with a deficiency of the late-acting complement components (C6–C9) are at risk for disseminated infections, as are women during menses and pregnancy. Disseminated infections usually arise from asymptomatic infections, indicating that local inflammation may deter dissemination.

Clinical Findings   Gonococci cause both localized infections, usually in the genital tract, and disseminated infections with seeding of various organs. Gonorrhea in men is characterized primarily by urethritis accompanied by dysuria and a purulent discharge. In women, infection is located primarily in the endocervix, causing a purulent vaginal discharge and intermenstrual bleeding (cervicitis). The most frequent complication in women is an ascending infection of the uterine tubes (**salpingitis, PID**), which can result in **sterility** or ectopic pregnancy due to scarring of the tubes. Disseminated infections commonly manifest as arthritis, tenosynovitis or pustules. It is the most common cause of septic arthritis in sexually active adults.

Other infected sites include the anorectal area and the throat. Anorectal infections occur chiefly in women and homosexual men. They are frequently asymptomatic, but a bloody or purulent discharge (proctitis) can occur. In the throat, pharyngitis occurs but many patients are asymptomatic. In newborn infants, a purulent conjunctivitis (ophthalmia neonatorum) is the result of gonococcal infection acquired from the mother during passage through the birth canal. The incidence of gonococcal ophthalmia has declined markedly in recent years owing to the widespread use of prophylactic erythromycin eye ointment (or silver nitrate) given shortly after birth.

Other sexually transmitted infections, eg, syphilis and nongonococcal urethritis caused by *Chlamydia trachomatis,* can coexist with gonorrhea; therefore, appropriate diagnostic and therapeutic measures must be taken.

Laboratory Diagnosis   The diagnosis of localized infections depends on Gram staining and culture of the discharge. In **men,** the finding of gram-negative diplococci **within PMNs** in a sample of urethral discharge is sufficient for diagnosis. In **women,** the use of the Gram stain alone can be difficult to interpret, so cultures should be done. Gram stains on cervical specimens can be falsely positive because of the presence of Gram-negative diplococci in the normal flora and can be falsely negative because of the inability to see small numbers of gonococci when using the oil immersion lens. Cultures must also be used in diagnosing suspected pharyngitis or anorectal infections.

Specimens are cultured on Thayer-Martin medium, which is a chocolate agar containing antibiotics (vancomycin, colistin, trimethoprim, and nystatin) to suppress the normal flora, and are incubated at 37 °C in a 5% CO_2 atmosphere. The finding of an oxidase-positive colony composed of gram-negative diplococci is sufficient to diagnose *Neisseria.* Specific identification of the gonococcus can be made either by its fermentation of glucose (but not maltose) or by fluorescent-antibody staining.

Two rapid tests that detect the presence of gonococci in patient specimens are the ELISA, which detects gonococcal antigens, and the DNA probe assay, which detects gonococcal ribosomal genes. Serologic tests to determine the presence of antibody to gonococci are *not* useful for diagnosis.

Treatment   Ceftriaxone is the treatment of choice in uncomplicated gonococcal infections. Spectinomycin or ciprofloxacin should be used if the patient is allergic to penicillin. Because mixed infections with *C trachomatis* are common, tetracycline should be prescribed also. A follow-up culture should be done 1 week after completion of treatment to determine whether gonococci are still present.

Prior to the mid 1950s, all gonococci were highly sensitive to penicillin. Subsequently, isolates emerged with low-level resistance to penicillin and to other antibiotics such as tetracycline and chloramphenicol. This type of resistance is encoded by the bacterial chromosome and is due to reduced uptake of the drug or to altered binding sites rather than to enzymatic degradation of the drug. Then, in 1976, **penicillinase-producing (PPNG)** strains that exhibited high-level resistance were isolated from patients. Penicillinase is plasmid-encoded. PPNG strains are now common in many areas of the world including several urban areas in the United States, where approximately 10% of isolates are resistant.

Prevention   The prevention of gonorrhea involves the use of condoms and the prompt treatment of symptomatic patients and their contacts. Cases of gonorrhea must be reported to the public health department to ensure proper follow-up. A major problem is the detection of asymptomatic carriers. Gonococcal conjunctivitis in newborns is prevented most often by the use of erythromycin ointment. Silver nitrate drops are used less frequently. No vaccine is available.

Review Questions

1. What role does the polysaccharide capsule of *Neisseria meningitidis* play in pathogenesis?
2. *Neisseria gonorrhoeae* does not have a capsule, but it does have pili. What role do the pili play in pathogenesis?
3. Why is chocolate agar used to culture neisseriae?
4. What is the meaning of the statement, "Neisseriae are oxidase-positive"?
5. Meningococci colonize the oropharynx. How do they reach the meninges to cause meningitis?
6. What role does endotoxin play in meningococcal disease?
7. Which three organisms cause most of the cases of meningitis in persons over the age of 2 months?
8. What immunologic deficiency predisposes individuals to bacteremia caused by meningococci and gonococci?
9. How can meningococci and gonococci be distinguished in the clinical laboratory?
10. What means are available to prevent meningococcal meningitis?
11. What role does IgA protease play in gonococcal disease?
12. What is the risk to the newborn of gonorrhea in the mother?
13. What is the significance of finding gram-negative diplococci within neutrophils in a urethral exudate?

14. Why is Thayer-Martin medium used to culture gonococci?

15. Why does penicillin fail to cure gonorrhea in some patients?

Gram-Positive Rods

17

There are four medically important genera of gram-positive rods: *Bacillus, Clostridium, Corynebacterium,* and *Listeria. Bacillus* and *Clostridium* form spores, whereas *Corynebacterium* and *Listeria* do not. Members of the genus *Bacillus* are aerobic, whereas those of the genus *Clostridium* are anaerobic (Table 17–1).

Spore-Forming Gram-Positive Rods

BACILLUS

There are two medically important *Bacillus* species: *Bacillus anthracis* and *Bacillus cereus.*

1. Bacillus anthracis

Disease *B anthracis* causes anthrax, which is common in animals but rare in humans.

Important Properties *B anthracis* is a large gram-positive rod with square ends, frequently found in chains. Its antiphagocytic capsule is composed of D-glutamate. (This is unique—capsules of other bacteria are polysaccharides.) It is nonmotile, whereas other members of the genus are motile.

Transmission Spores of the organism persist in soil for years. Humans are infected by **spores on animal products** such as hides, bristles, and wool or by contact with sick animals. The portals of entry are the skin, mucous membranes, and respiratory tract.

Pathogenesis *B anthracis* invades the host and produces **anthrax toxin,** which has three components: protective antigen, lethal factor, and edema factor. Edema factor, an exotoxin, is an **adenylate cyclase** dependent on protective antigen for its binding and entry into the cell. Lethal factor in the presence of protective antigen is rapidly fatal for mice. The mode of action of lethal factor is unknown.

Clinical Findings The typical lesion is a painless ulcer with a black eschar (crust, scab). Local edema is striking. The lesion is called a **"malignant pustule."** Untreated cases progress to bac-

Table 17–1. Gram-positive rods of medical importance.

Genus	Anaerobic Growth	Spore Formation	Exotoxins Important in Pathogenesis
Bacillus	–	+	+
Clostridium	+	+	+
Corynebacterium	–	–	+
Listeria	–	–	–

teremia and death. "Woolsorter's disease" (pulmonary anthrax) is a life-threatening pneumonia caused by inhalation of spores.

Laboratory Diagnosis   Smears show large, gram-positive rods in chains. Spores are usually not seen in smears of exudate. Colonies form on blood agar aerobically. No serologic tests are useful.

Treatment   Penicillin G is the most effective treatment. No resistant strains have been isolated clinically.

Prevention   Soil contamination is prevented by sterilizing dead animals and animal products from areas of endemic infection. Protective clothing should be worn by persons at risk of exposure. Persons at high risk can be immunized with cell-free vaccine containing purified protective antigen as immunogen.

2. *Bacillus cereus*

Disease   *B cereus* causes food poisoning.

Transmission   Spores on grains such as rice survive steaming and rapid frying. The spores germinate when rice is kept warm for many hours (eg, **reheated fried rice**). The portal of entry is the gastrointestinal tract.

Pathogenesis   *B cereus* produces two enterotoxins. The mode of action of one of the enterotoxins is the same as that of cholera toxin; ie, it ADP-ribosylates a G protein, which stimulates adenylate cyclase and leads to an increased concentration of cyclic AMP within the enterocyte. The mode of action of the other enterotoxin is uncertain.

Clinical Findings   There are two syndromes: (1) one involves a short incubation period (4 hours) with nausea and vomiting and is similar to staphylococcal food poisoning; (2) the other involves a long incubation period (18 hours) with watery, nonbloody diarrhea and resembles clostridial gastroenteritis.

Laboratory Diagnosis   This is not usually done.

Treatment   Only symptomatic treatment is given.

Prevention   No specific means of prevention. Rice should not be kept warm for long periods.

CLOSTRIDIUM

There are four medically important *Clostridium* species: *C tetani, C botulinum, C perfringens* (which causes either gas gangrene or food poisoning), and *C difficile.* All clostridia are anaerobic, spore-forming, gram-positive rods.

1. *Clostridium tetani*

Disease   *C tetani* causes tetanus (lockjaw).

Transmission   Spores are widespread in soil. The portal of entry is usually a **wound** site, eg, where a nail penetrates the foot, but the spores also can be introduced during "skin-popping," a technique used by drug addicts to inject drugs into the skin. Germination of spores is favored by necrotic tissue and poor blood supply in the wound. Neonatal tetanus, in which the organism enters through a contaminated umbilicus or circumcision wound, is a major problem in some developing countries.

Pathogenesis   **Tetanus toxin** (tetanospasmin) is an exotoxin produced by vegetative cells at the wound site. This polypeptide toxin is carried intra-axonally (retrograde) to the central nervous system, where it binds to ganglioside receptors and blocks release of inhibitory mediators (eg, glycine) at spinal synapses. Tetanus toxin and botulinum toxin (see below) are among the most toxic substances known. They are proteases that cleave the proteins involved in mediator release.

Tetanus toxin has one antigenic type, unlike botulinum toxin, which has eight. There is therefore only one antigenic type of tetanus toxoid in the vaccine against tetanus.

Clinical Findings   Violent muscle spasms; **lockjaw** (trismus) due to rigid contraction of the jaw muscles, which prevents the mouth from opening; a characteristic grimace known as **"risus sardonicus";** and exaggerated reflexes occur. Respiratory failure ensues. A high mortality rate is associated with this disease.

Laboratory Diagnosis   There is no microbiologic or serologic diagnosis. Organisms are rarely isolated from the wound site. *C tetani* produces a **terminal spore,** ie, a spore at the end of the rod. This gives the organism the characteristic appearance of a "tennis racket."

Treatment   Tetanus immune globulin is used. Penicillin G or metronidazole is probably useful. An adequate airway must be maintained and respiratory support given. Benzodiazepines, eg, valium, should be given to prevent spasms.

Prevention   Tetanus is prevented by immunization with tetanus **toxoid** (formaldehyde-treated toxin) in childhood and every 10 years thereafter. When trauma occurs, the wound should be cleaned and debrided and tetanus toxoid booster should be given. If the wound is grossly contaminated, **tetanus immune globulin,** as well as the toxoid booster, should be given and penicillin administered. Tetanus immune globulin (tetanus antitoxin) is made in humans to avoid serum sickness reactions that occur when antitoxin made in horses is used. The administration of both immune globulins and tetanus toxoid (at different sites in the body) is an example of **passive-active immunity.**

2.   *Clostridium botulinum*

Disease   *C botulinum* causes botulism.

Transmission   Spores, widespread in soil, contaminate vegetables and meats. When these foods are canned or vacuum-packed without adequate sterilization, spores survive and germinate in the anaerobic environment. Toxin is produced within the canned food and **ingested preformed.** The highest-risk foods are (1) alkaline vegetables such as green beans, peppers, and mushrooms and (2) smoked fish. The toxin is relatively heat-labile; it is inactivated by boiling for several minutes. Thus, disease can be prevented by sufficient cooking.

Pathogenesis   **Botulinum toxin** is absorbed from the gut and carried via the blood to peripheral nerve synapses, where it blocks release of acetylcholine. It is a protease that cleaves the proteins involved in acetylcholine release. The toxin is a polypeptide encoded by a lysogenic phage. Along with tetanus toxin, it is among the most toxic substances known. There are eight immunologic types of toxin; types A, B, and E are the most common in human illness. Minute amounts of the toxin are effective in the treatment of certain spasmodic muscle disorders such as torticollis and blepharospasm.

Clinical Findings   Descending weakness and paralysis including diplopia, dysphagia, and respiratory muscle failure are seen. No fever is present. Two special clinical forms occur: (1) wound botulism, in which spores contaminate a wound, germinate, and produce toxin at the site; and (2) infant botulism, in which the organisms grow in the gut and produce toxins. Ingestion of honey containing the organism is implicated in transmission of infant botulism. Affected infants develop weakness or paralysis and may need respiratory support but usually recover spontaneously. Infant botulism accounts for about half of the cases of botulism in the United States. In the United States, wound botulism is associated with drug abuse, especially skin-popping with black tar heroin.

Laboratory Diagnosis   The organism is usually not cultured. Botulinum toxin is demonstrable in uneaten food and the patient's serum by mouse protection tests. Mice are inoculated with a sample of the clinical specimen and will die unless protected by antitoxin.

Treatment Trivalent antitoxin (types A, B, and E) is given, along with respiratory support. The antitoxin is made in horses, and serum sickness occurs in about 15% of antiserum recipients.

Prevention Proper sterilization of all canned and vacuum-packed foods is essential. Food must be adequately cooked to inactivate the toxin. Swollen cans must be discarded (clostridial proteolytic enzymes cause gas formation that swells cans).

3.   *Clostridium perfringens*

C perfringens causes two distinct diseases: gas gangrene and food poisoning.

A.   Gas Gangrene (Myonecrosis)*

Transmission Spores are located in the **soil;** vegetative cells are members of the **normal flora of the colon and vagina.** Gas gangrene is associated with war wounds, automobile and motorcycle accidents, and septic abortions.

Pathogenesis Organisms grow in traumatized tissue (especially muscle) and produce a variety of toxins. The most important is **alpha toxin** (lecithinase), which damages cell membranes, including those of erythrocytes, resulting in hemolysis. Degradative enzymes produce gas in tissues.

Clinical Findings Pain, edema, and cellulitis occur in the wound area. Crepitation indicates the presence of gas in tissues. Hemolysis and jaundice are common, as are blood-tinged exudates. Shock and death can ensue. Mortality rates are high.

Laboratory Diagnosis Smears of tissue and exudate samples show large gram-positive rods. Spores are not usually seen because they are formed primarily under nutritionally deficient conditions. The organisms are cultured anaerobically and then identified by sugar fermentation reactions and organic acid production. *C perfringens* colonies exhibit a double zone of hemolysis on blood agar. Egg yolk agar is used to demonstrate the presence of the lecithinase. Serologic tests are not useful.

Treatment Penicillin G is the antibiotic of choice. Wounds should be debrided.

Prevention Wounds should be cleansed and debrided. Penicillin may be given for prophylaxis.

B.   Food Poisoning

Transmission Spores are located in **soil** and can contaminate **food.** The heat-resistant spores survive cooking and germinate. The organisms grow to large numbers in reheated foods, especially meat dishes.

Pathogenesis During sporulation (spore formation) in the gastrointestinal tract, an **enterotoxin** is produced. The enterotoxin is identical to a protein in the spore coat. The mode of action of the enterotoxin is the same as that of the enterotoxin of *S aureus;* ie, it acts as a superantigen.

Clinical Findings The disease has an 8- to 16-hour incubation period and is characterized by watery diarrhea with cramps and little vomiting. It resolves in 24 hours.

Laboratory Diagnosis This is not usually done. There is no assay for the toxin. Large numbers of the organisms can be isolated from uneaten food.

Treatment Symptomatic treatment is given; no antimicrobial drugs are administered.

Prevention There are no specific preventive measures. Food should be adequately cooked to kill the organism.

---

* Gas gangrene is also caused by other histotoxic clostridia such as *C histolyticum, C septicum,* and *C novyi.*

4. *Clostridium difficile*

Disease   *C difficile* causes antibiotic-associated pseudomembranous colitis.

Transmission   The organism is carried in the **gastrointestinal tract** in approximately 3% of the general population. Up to 30% of hospitalized patients become colonized and this organism is therefore an important cause of nosocomial disease. It is transmitted by the fecal-oral route. The hands of hospital personnel are important intermediaries.

Pathogenesis   Antibiotics suppress drug-sensitive members of the normal flora, allowing *C difficile* to multiply and produce exotoxins A and B. Exotoxin A is an enterotoxin that causes an outpouring of fluid, resulting in watery diarrhea. Exotoxin B is a cytotoxin that causes damage to the colonic mucosa, leading to pseudomembrane formation. One of the diagnostic tests in the laboratory is based on the ability of exotoxin B to kill cell cultures. The mechanism of action of exotoxin B is to ADP-ribosylate a GTP-binding protein called Rho that causes depolymerization of actin in the cytoskeleton. The mechanism of action of exotoxin A is unknown. Clindamycin and ampicillin are two of many antibiotics that cause this disease. *C difficile* rarely invades the intestinal mucosa.

Clinical Findings   *C difficile* causes diarrhea, associated with **pseudomembranes** (yellow-white plaques) on the colonic mucosa. The diarrhea is usually not bloody, and neutrophils are found in the stool in about half of the cases. The pseudomembranes are visualized by sigmoidoscopy. Toxic megacolon can occur, and surgical resection of the colon may be necessary.

Laboratory Diagnosis   Exotoxin B is detected in filtrates of stool samples by its cytotoxic effect on cultured cells. It is identified by inhibition of cytotoxicity by specific antibody. Anaerobic culture is usually not done. An ELISA that detects both exotoxins A and B is available.

Treatment   The causative antibiotic should be withdrawn. Oral metronidazole or vancomycin should be given and fluids replaced. Metronidazole is preferred because using vancomycin may select for vancomycin-resistant enterococci. In many patients, treatment does not eradicate the carrier state and repeated episodes of colitis can occur.

Prevention   There are no vaccines or drugs. Antibiotics should be prescribed only when necessary.

Non–Spore-Forming Gram-Positive Rods

There are two important pathogens in this group: *Corynebacterium diphtheriae* and *Listeria monocytogenes.*

CORYNEBACTERIUM DIPHTHERIAE

Disease   *C diphtheriae* causes diphtheria. Other *Corynebacterium* species (diphtheroids) are implicated in opportunistic infections.

Important Properties   Corynebacteria are gram-positive rods that appear **club-shaped** (wider at one end) and are arranged in palisades or in V- or L-shaped formations. The rods have a beaded appearance. The beads consist of granules of highly polymerized polyphosphate, a storage mechanism for high-energy phosphate bonds. The granules stain **metachromatically;** ie, a dye that stains the rest of the cell blue will stain the granules red.

Transmission   Humans are the only natural host of *C diphtheriae.* Both toxigenic and nontoxigenic organisms reside in the upper respiratory tract and are transmitted by **airborne droplets.** The organism can also infect the skin at the site of a preexisting skin lesion. This occurs primarily in the tropics but can occur worldwide in indigent persons with poor skin hygiene.

Pathogenesis Although exotoxin production is essential for pathogenesis, invasiveness is also necessary because the organism must first establish and maintain itself in the throat. Diphtheria toxin inhibits protein synthesis by **ADP ribosylation of elongation factor 2** (EF-2). The toxin affects all eukaryotic cells regardless of tissue type but has no effect on the analogous factor in prokaryotic cells.

The toxin is a single polypeptide with two functional domains. One domain mediates binding of the toxin to glycoprotein receptors on the cell membrane. The other domain possesses enzymatic activity that cleaves nicotinamide from nicotinamide adenine dinucleotide (NAD) and transfers the remaining ADP-ribose to EF-2, thereby inactivating it. Other organisms whose exotoxins act by ADP ribosylation are listed on p 32.

The DNA that codes for diphtheria toxin is part of the genetic material of a temperate bacteriophage. During the lysogenic phase of viral growth, the DNA of this virus integrates into the bacterial chromosome and the toxin is synthesized. *C diphtheriae* cells that are not lysogenized by this phage do not produce exotoxin and are nonpathogenic.

The host response to *C diphtheriae* consists of

(1) local inflammation in the throat, with a fibrinous exudate that forms the tough, adherent, gray "pseudomembrane" characteristic of the disease; and

(2) antibody that can neutralize exotoxin activity by blocking the interaction of fragment B with the receptors, thereby preventing entry into the cell. The immune status of a person can be assessed by Schick's test. The test is performed by intradermal injection of 0.1 mL of purified standardized toxin. If the patient has no antitoxin, the toxin will cause inflammation at the site 4–7 days later. If no inflammation occurs, antitoxin is present and the patient is immune. The test is rarely performed in the United States except under special epidemiologic circumstances.

Clinical Findings Although diphtheria is rare in the United States, physicians should be aware of its most prominent sign, the thick, gray, adherent membrane over the tonsils and throat. The other aspects are nonspecific: fever, sore throat, and cervical adenopathy. There are three prominent complications:

(1) extension of the membrane into the larynx and trachea, causing airway obstruction;

(2) myocarditis accompanied by arrhythmias and circulatory collapse; and

(3) recurrent laryngeal nerve palsy.

Cutaneous diphtheria causes ulcerating skin lesions and does not cause systemic symptoms.

Laboratory Diagnosis Laboratory diagnosis involves both isolating the organism and demonstrating toxin production. It should be emphasized that the decision to treat with antitoxin is a clinical one and cannot wait for the laboratory results. A throat swab should be cultured on Löffler's medium, a **tellurite plate,** and a blood agar plate. The tellurite plate contains a tellurium salt that is reduced to elemental tellurium within the organism. The typical gray-black color of tellurium in the colony is a telltale diagnostic criterion. If *C diphtheriae* is recovered from the cultures, either animal inoculation or a gel diffusion precipitin test is performed to document toxin production.

Smears of the throat swab should be stained with both Gram's stain and methylene blue. Although the diagnosis of diphtheria cannot be made by examination of the smear, the finding of many tapered, pleomorphic gram-positive rods can be suggestive. The methylene blue stain is excellent for revealing the typical metachromatic granules.

Treatment The treatment of choice is **antitoxin,** which should be given immediately on the basis of clinical impression because there is a delay in laboratory diagnostic procedures. The toxin binds rapidly and irreversibly to cells and, once bound, cannot be neutralized by antitoxin. The function of antitoxin is therefore to neutralize unbound toxin in the blood. Because the antiserum is made in horses, the patient must be tested for hypersensitivity and medications for the treatment of anaphylaxis must be available.

Treatment with penicillin G or an erythromycin is recommended also, but neither is a substitute for antitoxin. Antibiotics inhibit growth of the organism, reduce toxin production, and decrease the incidence of chronic carriers.

Prevention   Diphtheria is very rare in the United States because children are immunized with **diphtheria toxoid** (usually given as a combination of diphtheria toxoid, tetanus toxoid, and killed pertussis organisms). Diphtheria toxoid is prepared by treating the exotoxin with formaldehyde. This treatment inactivates the toxic effect but leaves the antigenicity intact. Immunization consists of three doses given at 2, 4, and 6 months of age, with boosters at 1 and 6 years of age. Because immunity wanes, a booster every 10 years is recommended. Immunization does not prevent nasopharyngeal carriage of the organism.

LISTERIA MONOCYTOGENES

Diseases   *L monocytogenes* causes meningitis and sepsis in newborns and immunosuppressed adults.

Important Properties   *L monocytogenes* is a small gram-positive rod arranged in V- or L-shaped formations similar to corynebacteria. The organism exhibits an unusual **tumbling** movement that distinguishes it from the corynebacteria, which are nonmotile. Colonies on a blood agar plate produce a narrow zone of beta-hemolysis that resembles the hemolysis of some streptococci.

Pathogenesis   *Listeria* infections occur primarily in two clinical settings: (1) in the fetus or newborn as a result of transmission **across the placenta or during delivery;** and (2) in immunosuppressed adults, especially renal transplant patients. The organism is distributed worldwide in animals, plants, and soil. From these reservoirs, it is transmitted to humans by contact with animals or their feces, by unpasteurized milk, and by contaminated vegetables. In the United States, listeriosis is primarily a food-borne disease associated with eating unpasteurized cheese.

The pathogenesis of *Listeria* is dependent upon the organism's ability to invade mononuclear phagocytic cells. Because *Listeria* preferentially grows intracellularly, cell-mediated immunity is a more important host defense than humoral immunity. Suppression of cell-mediated immunity predisposes to *Listeria* infections. *L monocytogenes* can move from cell to cell by means of **"actin rockets,"** a filament of actin that contracts and propels the bacteria through the membrane of one human cell and into another. The organism produces listeriolysin O, a hemolysin similar to streptolysin O. It acts by producing holes in cell membranes.

Clinical Findings   Infection during pregnancy can cause abortion, premature delivery, or sepsis during the peripartum period. Newborns infected at the time of delivery can have acute meningitis 1–4 weeks later. The infected mother either is asymptomatic or has an influenzalike illness. *L monocytogenes* infections in immunocompromised adults can be either sepsis or meningitis. This organism also causes outbreaks of food-borne gastroenteritis in otherwise healthy individuals.

Laboratory Diagnosis   Laboratory diagnosis is made primarily by Gram stain and culture. The appearance of gram-positive rods resembling **diphtheroids** and the formation of small, gray colonies with a narrow zone of beta-hemolysis on a blood agar plate suggest the presence of *Listeria*. The isolation of *Listeria* is confirmed by the presence of motile organisms, which differentiate them from the nonmotile corynebacteria. Identification of the organism as *L monocytogenes* is made by sugar fermentation tests.

Treatment   Treatment consists of ampicillin with or without gentamicin. Trimethoprim-sulfamethoxazole is also effective. Resistant strains are rare.

Prevention   Prevention is difficult because there is no immunization. Limiting the exposure of immunosuppressed patients to potential sources such as infected animals and their products and contaminated vegetables is recommended.

Review Questions

1. How is the capsule of *Bacillus anthracis* different from that of most other bacteria?
2. What is the natural habitat of *B anthracis,* and how does it persist there for long periods?
3. How does *B anthracis* cause disease?

4. *Bacillus cereus* causes food poisoning. How is it transmitted? What is the pathogenesis?
5. How is tetanus acquired? What is its pathogenesis?
6. What are the three important components of tetanus prevention?
7. How is botulism acquired? What is its pathogenesis? How is it prevented?
8. *Clostridium perfringens* can cause gas gangrene. Under what circumstances does this occur, and what is the role of alpha toxin in the disease? How can the disease be prevented?
9. In an exudate from a patient with gas gangrene, what would you see on Gram's stain? How would you culture the organism?
10. What is the pathogenesis of food poisoning caused by *C perfringens?*
11. What is the pathogenesis of diarrhea caused by *Clostridium difficile?*
12. What is the appearance of *Corynebacterium diphtheriae* on Gram's stain?
13. What is the mechanism of action of diphtheria toxin?
14. Only lysogenized strains of *C diphtheriae* are pathogenic. Why?
15. Why is diphtheria rare in the United States?
16. What is the role of antitoxin in the treatment of diphtheria?
17. In which two population groups do *Listeria* infections primarily occur?
18. How is *Listeria monocytogenes* transmitted, and what is its mode of pathogenesis?

18

Gram-Negative Rods Related to the Enteric Tract

Overview

Gram-negative rods are a large group of diverse organisms. In this book, these bacteria are subdivided into three clinically relevant categories, each in a separate chapter, according to whether the organism is related primarily to the enteric or the respiratory tract or to animal sources (Table 18–1). Although this approach leads to some overlaps, it should be helpful because it allows general concepts to be emphasized.

Gram-negative rods related to the enteric tract include a large number of genera. These genera have therefore been divided into three groups depending on the major anatomic location of disease, namely (1) pathogens both within and outside the enteric tract, (2) pathogens primarily within the enteric tract, and (3) pathogens outside the enteric tract (Table 18–1).

The frequency with which the organisms related to the enteric tract cause disease in the United States is shown in Table 18–2. *Salmonella, Shigella,* and *Campylobacter* are frequent pathogens in the gastrointestinal tract, whereas *Escherichia, Vibrio,* and *Yersinia* are less so. Enterotoxigenic strains of *Escherichia coli* are a common cause of diarrhea in developing countries but are less com-

Table 18–1. Categories of gram-negative rods.

Chapter	Source of Site of Infection	Genus
18	Enteric tract	
	1. Both within and outside	*Escherichia, Salmonella*
	2. Primarily within	*Shigella, Vibrio, Campylobacter, Helicobacter*
	3. Outside only	*Klebsiella-Enterobacter-Serratia* group, *Proteus-Providencia-Morganella* group, *Pseudomonas, Bacteroides*
19	Respiratory tract	*Haemophilus, Legionella, Bordetella*
20	Animal sources	*Brucella, Francisella, Pasteurella, Yersinia*

Table 18–2. Frequency of diseases caused in the United States by gram-negative rods related to the enteric tract.

Site of Infection	Frequent Pathogens	Less-Frequent Pathogens
Enteric tract	Salmonella, Shigella, Campylobacter	Escherichia, Vibrio, Yersinia
Urinary tract	Escherichia	Enterobacter, Klebsiella, Proteus, Pseudomonas

mon in the United States. Urinary tract infections are caused primarily by *E coli;* the other organisms occur less commonly.

Patients infected with enteric pathogens such as *Shigella, Salmonella, Campylobacter,* and *Yersinia* have a high incidence of certain autoimmune diseases such as Reiter's syndrome (see Chapter 66). In addition, infection with *Campylobacter jejuni* predisposes to Guillain-Barré syndrome.

Before describing the specific organisms, it is appropriate to describe the family Enterobacteriaceae, to which many of these gram-negative rods belong.

ENTEROBACTERIACEAE & RELATED ORGANISMS

The *Enterobacteriaceae* is a large family of gram-negative rods found primarily in the colon of humans and other animals, many as part of the normal flora. These organisms are the major facultative anaerobes in the large intestine but are present in relatively small numbers compared with anaerobes such as *Bacteroides.* Although the members of the *Enterobacteriaceae* are classified together taxonomically, they cause a variety of diseases with different pathogenetic mechanisms. The organisms and some of the diseases they cause are listed in Table 18–5.

Members of this heterogeneous family are united both by their anatomic location and by the following four metabolic processes: (1) they are all facultative anaerobes; (2) they all ferment glucose (fermentation of other sugars varies); (3) none have cytochrome oxidase (ie, they are oxidase-negative); and (4) they reduce nitrates to nitrites as part of their energy-generating processes.

These four reactions can be used to distinguish the *Enterobacteriaceae* from another medically significant group of organisms, the nonfermenting gram-negative rods, the most important of which is *Pseudomonas aeruginosa.** P aeruginosa,* a significant cause of urinary tract infections and sepsis in

Table 18–3. Gram-negative rods causing diarrhea.

Species	Fever	Leukocytes in Stool	Infective Dose	Typical Bacteriologic or Epidemiologic Findings
Enterotoxin-mediated				
1. *Escherichia coli*	–	–	?	Ferments lactose.
2. *Vibrio cholerae*	–	–	10^7	Comma-shaped bacteria.
Invasive-inflammatory				
1. *Salmonella,* eg, *S typhimurium*	+	+	10^5	Does not ferment lactose.
2. *Shigella,* eg, *S dysenteriae*	+	+	10^2	Does not ferment lactose.
3. *Campylobacter jejuni*	+	+	10^4	Comma- or S-shaped bacteria; growth at 42 °C.
4. *Escherichia coli* (enteropathic strains)	+	+	?	
5. *Escherichia coli* O157:H7	+	–	?	Transmitted by undercooked hamburger; causes hemolytic-uremic syndrome.
Mechanism uncertain				
1. *Vibrio parahaemolyticus*[1]	+	+	?	Transmitted by seafood.
2. *Yersinia enterocolitica*[1]	+	+	10^8	Usually transmitted from pets, eg, puppies.

[1] Some strains produce enterotoxin, but its pathogenetic role is not clear.

*The other less frequently isolated organisms in this group are members of the following genera: *Achromobacter, Acinetobacter, Alcaligenes, Eikenella, Flavobacterium, Kingella,* and *Moraxella;* see Chapter 27.

Table 18–4. Gram-negative rods causing urinary tract infection[1] or sepsis.[2]

Species	Lactose Fermented	Features of the Organism
Escherichia coli	+	Colonies show metallic sheen on EMB agar.
Enterobacter cloacae	+	Often nosocomial and drug-resistant.
Klebsiella pneumoniae	+	Has large mucoid capsule and hence viscous colonies.
Serratia marcescens	–	Some strains produce red pigment; often nosocomial and drug-resistant.
Proteus mirabilis	–	Motility causes "swarming" on agar; produces urease.
Pseudomonas aeruginosa	–	Blue-green pigment and fruity odor produced; usually nosocomial and drug-resistant.

[1] Diagnosed by quantitative culture of urine.
[2] Diagnosed by culture of blood or pus.

hospitalized patients, does not ferment glucose or reduce nitrates, and is oxidase-positive. In contrast to the *Enterobacteriaceae,* it is a strict aerobe and derives its energy from oxidation, not fermentation.

Pathogenesis   All members of the *Enterobacteriaceae,* being gram-negative, contain endotoxin in their cell walls. In addition, several exotoxins are produced; eg, *E coli* and *Vibrio cholerae* secrete exotoxins, called enterotoxins, that activate adenylate cyclase within the cells of the small intestine, causing diarrhea (see Chapter 7).

Antigens   The antigens of several members of the *Enterobacteriaceae,* especially *Salmonella* and *Shigella,* are important; they are used for identification purposes both in the clinical laboratory and in epidemiologic investigations. The three surface antigens are as follows.

(1) The cell wall antigen (also known as the somatic or O antigen) is the outer polysaccharide portion of the lipopolysaccharide (see Fig 2–6). The O antigen, which is composed of repeating oligosaccharides consisting of three or four sugars repeated 15 or 20 times, is the basis for the serologic typing of many enteric rods. The number of different O antigens is very large; eg, there are approximately 1500 types of *Salmonella* and 150 types of *E coli.*

(2) The H antigen is on the flagellar protein. Only flagellated organisms, such as *Escherichia* and *Salmonella,* have H antigens, whereas the nonmotile ones, such as *Klebsiella* and *Shigella,* do not. The H antigens of certain *Salmonella* species are unusual because the organisms can reversibly alternate between two types of H antigens called phase 1 and phase 2. The organisms may use this change in antigenicity to evade the immune response.

(3) The capsular or K polysaccharide antigen is particularly prominent in heavily encapsulated organisms such as *Klebsiella.* The K antigen is identified by the quellung (capsular swelling) reaction in the presence of specific antisera and is used to serotype *E coli* and *Salmonella typhi* for epidemiologic purposes. In *S typhi,* the cause of typhoid fever, it is called the Vi (or virulence) antigen.

Table 18–5. Diseases caused by members of the *Enterobacteriaceae.*

Major Pathogen	Representative Diseases	Minor Related Genera
Escherichia	Urinary tract infection, traveler's diarrhea, neonatal meningitis	
Shigella	Dysentery	
Salmonella	Typhoid fever, enterocolitis	Arizona, Citrobacter, Edwardsiella
Klebsiella	Pneumonia, urinary tract infection	
Enterobacter	Pneumonia, urinary tract infection	Hafnia
Serratia	Pneumonia, urinary tract infection	
Proteus	Urinary tract infection	Providencia, Morganella
Yersinia	Plague, enterocolitis, mesenteric adenitis	

Table 18–6. Lactose fermentation by members of the *Enterobacteriaceae* and related organisms.

Fermentation	Genera
Occurs	*Escherichia, Klebsiella, Enterobacter*
Does not occur	*Shigella, Salmonella, Proteus, Pseudomonas*
Occurs slowly	*Serratia, Vibrio*

Laboratory Diagnosis Specimens suspected of containing members of the *Enterobacteriaceae* and related organisms are usually inoculated onto two media, a blood agar plate and a selective differential medium such as MacConkey's agar or eosin-methylene blue (EMB) agar. The *differential* ability of these latter media is based on **lactose fermentation,** which is the most important metabolic criterion used in the identification of these organisms (Table 18–6). On these media, the nonlactose fermenters, eg, *Salmonella* and *Shigella,* form colorless colonies, whereas the lactose fermenters form colored colonies. The *selective* effect of the media in suppressing unwanted gram-positive organisms is exerted by bile salts or bacteriostatic dyes in the agar.

An additional set of screening tests, consisting of triple sugar iron (TSI) agar and urea agar, is done prior to the definitive identification procedures. The rationale for the use of these media and the reactions of several important organisms are presented in the box and in Table 18–7. The results of the screening process are frequently sufficient to identify the genus of an organism; however, an array of 20 or more biochemical tests is required to identify the species.

Another valuable piece of information used to identify some of these organisms is their motility, which is dependent on the presence of flagella. *Proteus* species are very motile and characteristically **"swarm"** over the blood agar plate, obscuring the colonies of other organisms. Motility is also an important diagnostic criterion in the differentiation of *Enterobacter cloacae,* which is motile, from *Klebsiella pneumoniae,* which is nonmotile.

If the results of the screening tests suggest the presence of a *Salmonella* or *Shigella* strain, an agglutination test can be used to identify the genus of the organism and to determine whether it is a member of group A, B, C, or D.

Coliforms & Public Health Contamination of the public water supply system by sewage is detected by the presence of coliforms in the water. In a general sense, the term "coliform" includes not only *E coli* but also other inhabitants of the colon such as *Enterobacter* and *Klebsiella.* However, because only *E coli* is exclusively a large-intestine organism, whereas the others are found in the environment also, it is used as the indicator of fecal contamination. In water quality testing, *E coli* is identified by its ability to ferment lactose with the production of acid and gas, its ability to grow at 44.5 °C, and its characteristic colony type on EMB agar. An *E coli* colony count above 4/dL in municipal drinking water is indicative of unacceptable fecal contamination. Because *E coli* and the enteric pathogens are killed by chlorination of the drinking water, there is rarely a problem with meeting this standard. Disinfection of the public water supply is one of the most important advances of public health in this century.

Table 18–7. Triple sugar iron agar reactions.

Reactions[1]				Representative Genera
Slant	Butt	Gas	H$_2$S	
Acid	Acid	+	–	*Escherichia, Enterobacter, Klebsiella*
Alkaline	Acid	–	–	*Shigella, Serratia*
Alkaline	Acid	+	+	*Salmonella, Proteus*
Alkaline	Alkaline	–	–	*Pseudomonas*[2]

[1] Acid production causes the phenol red indicator to turn yellow; the indicator is red under alkaline conditions. The presence of black FeS in the butt indicates H$_2$S production. Not every species within the various genera will give the above appearance on TSI agar. For example, some *Serratia* strains can ferment lactose slowly and give an acid reaction on the slant.
[2] *Pseudomonas,* although not a member of the *Enterobacteriaceae,* is included in this table because its reaction on TSI agar is a useful diagnostic criterion.

Triple Sugar Iron Agar

The important components of this medium are ferrous sulfate and the three sugars glucose, lactose, and sucrose. The glucose is present in one-tenth the concentration of the other two sugars. The medium in the tube is produced so that there is a solid, poorly oxygenated area on the bottom, called the butt, and an angled, well-oxygenated area on top, called the slant. The organism is inoculated into the butt and across the surface of the slant.

The interpretation of the test is as follows: (1) If lactose (or sucrose) is fermented, a large amount of acid is produced, which turns the phenol red indicator yellow both in the butt and on the slant. Some organisms generate gases, which produce bubbles in the butt. (2) If lactose is not fermented but the small amount of glucose is, the oxygen-deficient butt will be yellow, but on the slant the acid will be oxidized to CO_2 and H_2O by the organism and the slant will be red (neutral or alkaline). (3) If neither lactose nor glucose is fermented, both the butt and the slant will be red. The slant can become a deeper red-purple (more alkaline) owing to the production of ammonia from the oxidative deamination of amino acids. (4) If H_2S is produced, the black color of ferrous sulfide is seen.

The reactions of some of the important organisms are presented in Table 18–7. Because several organisms can give the same reaction, TSI agar is only a screening device.

Urea Agar

The important components of this medium are urea and the pH indicator phenol red. If the organism produces urease, the urea is hydrolyzed to NH_3 and CO_2. Ammonia turns the medium alkaline, and the color of the phenol red changes from light orange to reddish purple. The important organisms that are urease-positive are *Proteus* species and *K pneumoniae*.

Antibiotic Therapy   The appropriate treatment for infections caused by members of the *Enterobacteriaceae* and related organisms must be individually tailored to the antibiotic sensitivity of the organism. Generally speaking, a wide range of antimicrobial agents are potentially effective, eg, some penicillins and cephalosporins, aminoglycosides, chloramphenicol, tetracyclines, quinolones, and sulfonamides. The specific choice usually depends upon the results of antibiotic sensitivity tests.

Note that many isolates of these enteric gram-negative rods are **highly antibiotic resistant** because of the production of β-lactamases and other drug-modifying enzymes. These organisms undergo conjugation frequently, at which time they acquire plasmids (R factors) that mediate multiple drug resistance.

Pathogens Both Within and Outside the Enteric Tract

ESCHERICHIA

Diseases   *E coli* is the most common cause of urinary tract infections and gram-negative rod sepsis. It is one of the two important causes of neonatal meningitis and the agent most frequently associated with "traveler's diarrhea," a watery diarrhea. Some strains of *E coli* are enterohemorrhagic and cause bloody diarrhea.

Important Properties   *E coli* is the most abundant facultative anaerobe in the colon and feces. It is, however, greatly outnumbered by the obligate anaerobes such as *Bacteroides*.

E coli **ferments lactose,** a property that distinguishes it from the two major intestinal pathogens, *Shigella* and *Salmonella*. It has three antigens that are used to identify the organism in epidemiologic investigations: the O or cell wall antigen, the H or flagellar antigen, and the K or capsular antigen. Because there are more than 150 O, 50 H, and 90 K antigens, the various combinations result in more than 1000 antigenic types of *E coli*. Specific serotypes are associated with certain diseases; eg, O55 and O111 cause outbreaks of neonatal diarrhea.

Pathogenesis   *E coli* has several clearly identified components that contribute to its ability to cause disease: pili, a capsule, endotoxin, and two exotoxins (enterotoxins).

A. Intestinal Tract Infection: The first step is the adherence of the organism to the cells of the jejunum and ileum by means of **pili** that protrude from the bacterial surface. Once attached, the bacteria synthesize **enterotoxins** (exotoxins that act in the enteric tract), which act on the cells of the jejunum and ileum to cause diarrhea. The toxins are strikingly cell-specific; the cells of the colon are not susceptible, probably because they lack receptors for the toxin. Enterotoxigenic strains of *E coli* can produce either or both of two enterotoxins.

(1) The high-molecular-weight, heat-labile toxin (LT) acts by stimulating **adenylate cyclase.** Both LT and cholera toxin act by catalyzing the addition of ADP-ribose to the G protein that stimulates the cyclase. The resultant increase in intracellular cyclic AMP (cAMP) concentration stimulates cAMP-dependent protein kinase, causing an outpouring of fluid, potassium, and chloride from the enterocytes.

(2) The other enterotoxin is a low-molecular-weight, heat-stable toxin (ST), which stimulates guanylate cyclase.

The enterotoxin-producing strains **do not cause inflammation,** do not invade the intestinal mucosa, and cause a watery, non-bloody diarrhea. However, certain strains of *E coli* are enteropathic (enteroinvasive) and cause disease not by enterotoxin formation but by invasion of the epithelium of the large intestine, causing bloody diarrhea (dysentery) accompanied by inflammatory cells (neutrophils) in the stool. Certain enterohemorrhagic strains of *E coli,* ie, those with the O157:H7 serotype, also cause bloody diarrhea but do not cause inflammation; therefore no neutrophils are found in the stool. These O157:H7 strains produce **verotoxin,** so called because it is toxic to Vero (monkey) cells in culture and presumably to the cells lining the colon. These strains are associated with outbreaks of diarrhea following ingestion of undercooked hamburger at fast-food restaurants. Some patients with bloody diarrhea caused by O157:H7 strains also have a life-threatening complication called hemolytic-uremic syndrome. This syndrome consists of a nonimmune hemolytic anemia, thrombocytopenia, and acute renal failure.

B. Systemic Infection: The other two structural components, the **capsule** and the **endotoxin,** play a more prominent role in the pathogenesis of systemic, rather than intestinal tract, disease. The capsular polysaccharide interferes with phagocytosis, thereby enhancing the organism's ability to cause infections in various organs. For example, *E coli* strains that cause neonatal meningitis usually have a specific capsular type called the K1 antigen. The endotoxin of *E coli* is the cell wall lipopolysaccharide, which causes several features of gram-negative sepsis such as fever, hypotension, and disseminated intravascular coagulation. Certain O serotypes of *E coli* preferentially cause urinary tract infections. These **uropathic** strains are characterized by pili with adhesin proteins that bind to specific receptors on the urinary tract epithelium. The binding site on these receptors consists of dimers of galactose **(Gal-Gal dimers).**

Clinical Findings   *E coli* causes a variety of diseases both within and outside the intestinal tract. It is the leading cause of community-acquired **urinary tract infections.** These occur primarily in women; this finding is attributed to three features that facilitate ascending infection into the bladder, namely a short urethra, the proximity of the urethra to the anus, and colonization of the vagina by members of the fecal flora. It is also the most frequent cause of nosocomial (hospital-acquired) urinary tract infections, which occur equally frequently in both men and women and are associated with the use of indwelling urinary catheters. Urinary tract infections can be limited to the bladder or extend up the collecting system to the kidneys. If only the bladder is involved, the disease is called cystitis, whereas infection of the kidney is called pyelonephritis. The most prominent symptoms of cystitis are pain (dysuria) and frequency of urination; pyelonephritis is characterized by fever, chills, and flank pain.

E coli is also a major cause, along with the group B streptococci, of **neonatal meningitis.** Exposure of the newborn to *E coli* and group B streptococci occurs during birth as a result of colonization of the vagina by these organisms in approximately 25% of pregnant women. *E coli* is the organism isolated most frequently from patients with hospital-acquired sepsis, which arises primarily from urinary, biliary, or peritoneal infections.

Diarrhea caused by **enterotoxigenic** *E coli* is usually **watery,** non-bloody, self-limited, and of short duration (1–3 days). It is frequently associated with travel (traveler's diarrhea, or "turista").* Infection with **enteropathogenic** *E coli,* on the other hand, results in a dysenterylike syndrome characterized by **bloody diarrhea,** abdominal cramping, and fever similar to that caused by *Shigella.* The O157:H7 strains of E coli also cause bloody diarrhea which can be complicated by **hemolytic-uremic syndrome.**

Laboratory Diagnosis   Specimens suspected of containing enteric gram-negative rods such as *E coli* are grown initially on a blood agar plate and on a differential medium, such as EMB agar or MacConkey's agar. *E coli,* which ferments lactose, forms pink colonies, whereas lactose-negative organisms are colorless. On EMB agar, *E coli* colonies have a characteristic **green sheen.** Some of the important features that help to distinguish *E coli* from other lactose-fermenting gram-negative rods are as follows: (1) it produces indole from tryptophan, (2) it decarboxylates lysine, (3) it utilizes acetate as its only source of carbon, and (4) it is motile. *E coli* O157:H7 does not ferment sorbitol, which serves as an important criterion that distinguishes it from other strains of *E coli.* The isolation of enterotoxigenic or enteropathogenic *E coli* from patients with diarrhea is not a routine diagnostic procedure.

Treatment   Treatment of *E coli* infections depends on the site of disease and the resistance pattern of the specific isolate. For example, an uncomplicated lower urinary tract infection can be treated for just 1–3 days with oral trimethoprim-sulfamethoxazole or an oral penicillin, eg, ampicillin. However, *E coli* sepsis requires treatment with parenteral antibiotics (eg, a third-generation cephalosporin, such as cefotaxime, with or without an aminoglycoside, such as gentamicin). For the treatment of neonatal meningitis, a combination of ampicillin and cefotaxime is usually given. Antibiotic therapy is usually *not* indicated in *E coli* diarrheal diseases. However, administration of trimethoprim-sulfamethoxazole or loperamide (Imodium) may shorten the duration of symptoms. Rehydration is typically all that is necessary in this self-limited disease.

Prevention   There is no specific prevention for *E coli* infections, such as active or passive immunization. However, various general measures can be taken to prevent certain infections caused by *E coli* and other organisms. For example, the incidence of urinary tract infections can be lowered by the judicious use and prompt withdrawal of catheters and, in recurrent infections, by prolonged prophylaxis with urinary antiseptic drugs, eg, nitrofurantoin. Some cases of sepsis can be prevented by prompt removal of or switching the site of intravenous lines. Traveler's diarrhea can sometimes be prevented by the prophylactic use of doxycycline, ciprofloxacin, trimethoprim-sulfamethoxazole, or Pepto-Bismol. Caution regarding uncooked foods and unpurified water while traveling in certain countries is also advisable.

SALMONELLA

Diseases   *Salmonella* species cause enterocolitis, enteric fevers such as typhoid fever, and septicemia with metastatic abscesses. They are one of the most common causes of bacterial enterocolitis in the United States.

Important Properties   Salmonellae are gram-negative rods that **do not ferment lactose** but do produce H_2S—features that are used in their laboratory identification. Their antigens—cell wall O, flagellar H, and capsular Vi (virulence)—are important for taxonomic and epidemiologic purposes. The O antigens, which are the outer polysaccharides of the cell wall, are used to subdivide the salmonellae into groups A–I. There are two forms of the H antigens, phases 1 and 2. Only one of the two H proteins is synthesized at any one time, depending on which gene sequence is in the correct alignment for transcription into mRNA. The Vi antigens are used primarily for the typing of *S typhi,* the agent of typhoid fever.

---

*Enterotoxigenic *E coli* is the most common cause of traveler's diarrhea, but other bacteria (eg., *Salmonella, Shigella, Campylobacter,* and *Vibrio* species), viruses such as Norwalk virus, and protozoa such as *Giardia* and *Cryptosporidium* species are also involved.

Prevention   There are no specific preventive measures, but many hospital-acquired urinary tract infections can be prevented by prompt removal of urinary catheters.

PSEUDOMONAS

Diseases   *Pseudomonas aeruginosa* causes infections (eg, sepsis, pneumonia, and urinary tract infections) primarily in patients with lowered host defenses. *Pseudomonas cepacia* (renamed *Burkholderia cepacia)* and *Pseudomonas maltophilia* (renamed *Xanthomonas maltophilia* and now called *Stenotrophomonas maltophilia*) also cause these infections, but much less frequently. *Pseudomonas pseudomallei,* the cause of melioidosis, is described in Chapter 27.

Important Properties   Pseudomonads are gram-negative rods that resemble the members of the *Enterobacteriaceae* but differ in that they are strict aerobes; ie, they derive their energy only by oxidation of sugars rather than by fermentation. Because they do not ferment glucose, they are called **"nonfermenters,"** in contrast to the members of the *Enterobacteriaceae,* which do ferment glucose. Oxidation involves electron transport by cytochrome *c;* ie, they are **oxidase-positive.**

Pseudomonads are able to grow in **water** containing only traces of nutrients, eg, tap water, and this favors their persistence in the hospital environment. *P aeruginosa* and *P cepacia* have a remarkable ability to withstand disinfectants; this accounts in part for their role in hospital-acquired infections. They have been found growing in hexachlorophene-containing soap solutions, in antiseptics, and in detergents.

P aeruginosa produces two pigments useful in clinical and laboratory diagnosis: (1) **pyocyanin,** which can **color the pus in a wound blue;** and (2) pyoverdin (fluorescein), a yellow-green pigment that fluoresces under ultraviolet light, a property that can be used in the early detection of skin infection in burn patients. In the laboratory, these **pigments diffuse into the agar, imparting a blue-green color** that is useful in identification. *P aeruginosa* is the only species of *Pseudomonas* that synthesizes pyocyanin.

Strains of *P aeruginosa* isolated from cystic fibrosis patients have a prominent slime layer (glycocalyx), which gives their colonies a very mucoid appearance. The slime layer mediates adherence of the organism to mucous membranes of the respiratory tract and prevents antibody from binding to the organism.

Pathogenesis & Epidemiology   *P aeruginosa* is found chiefly in soil and water, although approximately 10% of people carry it in the normal flora of the colon. It is found on the skin in moist areas and can colonize the upper respiratory tract of hospitalized patients. Its ability to grow in simple aqueous solutions has resulted in contamination of respiratory therapy and anesthesia equipment, intravenous fluids, and even distilled water.

P aeruginosa is primarily an opportunistic pathogen that causes infections in hospitalized patients, eg, those with extensive burns, in whom the skin host defenses are destroyed; those with chronic respiratory disease (eg, cystic fibrosis), in whom the normal clearance mechanisms are impaired; those who are immunosuppressed; those with neutrophil counts of less than 500/μL; and those with indwelling catheters. It causes 10–20% of hospital-acquired infections.

Both endotoxin and an exotoxin play important roles in pathogenesis. *P aeruginosa* produces exotoxin A, which inhibits eukaryotic protein synthesis by the same mechanism as diphtheria exotoxin, namely ADP ribosylation of elongation factor 2. The two pigments, pyocyanin and fluorescein, are nontoxic.

Clinical Findings   *P aeruginosa* can cause infections virtually anywhere in the body, but urinary tract infections, pneumonia (especially in **cystic fibrosis** patients), and wound infections (especially burns) predominate. From these sites, the organism can enter the blood, causing sepsis. The bacteria can spread to the skin where they cause black, necrotic lesions called **ecthyma gangrenosum.** Patients with *P aeruginosa* sepsis have a mortality rate of over 50%. A severe external otitis (malignant otitis externa) and other skin lesions (eg, folliculitis) occur in users of swimming pools and hot tubs in which the chlorination is inadequate. *P aeruginosa* is the most common cause of osteochondritis of the foot in those who sustain puncture wounds through the soles of gym shoes. Corneal infections caused by *P aeruginosa* are seen in contact lens users.

Laboratory Diagnosis   *P aeruginosa* grows as non-lactose-fermenting (colorless) colonies on MacConkey's or EMB agar. It is **oxidase-positive.** A typical metallic sheen of the growth on TSI agar, coupled with the blue-green pigment on ordinary nutrient agar and a fruity aroma, is sufficient to make a presumptive diagnosis. The diagnosis is confirmed by biochemical reactions. Identification for epidemiologic purposes is done by bacteriophage or pyocin* typing.

Treatment   Because *P aeruginosa* is **resistant to many antibiotics,** treatment must be tailored to the sensitivity of each isolate and monitored frequently; resistant strains can emerge during therapy. The treatment of choice is an antipseudomonal penicillin, eg, ticarcillin or piperacillin, plus an aminoglycoside, eg, gentamicin or amikacin. The drug of choice for infections caused by *Burkholderia cepacia* and *Stenotrophomonas maltophilia* is trimethoprim-sulfamethoxazole.

Prevention   Prevention of *P aeruginosa* infections involves keeping neutrophil counts above 500/μL, removing indwelling catheters promptly, taking special care of burned skin, and taking other similar measures to limit infection in patients with reduced host defenses.

BACTEROIDES

Diseases   *Bacteroides* is the most common cause of serious anaerobic infections, eg, sepsis, peritonitis, and abscesses. *Bacteroides fragilis* is the most frequent pathogen.

Important Properties   *Bacteroides* organisms are anaerobic, non-spore-forming, gram-negative rods. Of the 22 species of *Bacteroides,* three are human pathogens: *B fragilis,*† *Bacteroides melaninogenicus,* and *Bacteroides corrodens. Bacteroides melaninogenicus* was recently renamed *Prevotella melaninogenica,* but the former name is still commonly used.

Members of the *B fragilis* group are the predominant organisms in the human colon, numbering approximately 10^{11}/g of feces, and are found in the vagina of approximately 60% of women. *B melaninogenicus* and *B corrodens* occur primarily in the oral cavity.

Pathogenesis & Epidemiology   Because *Bacteroides* species are part of the normal flora, **infections are endogenous,** usually arising from a break in a mucosal surface, and are not communicable. These organisms cause a variety of infections, such as local abscesses at the site of a mucosal break, metastatic abscesses by hematogenous spread to distant organs, or lung abscesses by aspiration of oral flora.

Predisposing factors such as surgery, trauma, and chronic disease play an important role in pathogenesis. Local tissue necrosis, impaired blood supply, and growth of facultative anaerobes at the site contribute to anaerobic infections. The facultative anaerobes, such as *E coli,* utilize the oxygen, thereby reducing it to a level that allows the anaerobic *Bacteroides* strains to grow. As a result, many anaerobic infections contain a mixed facultative and anaerobic flora. This has important implications for therapy; both the facultative anaerobes and the anaerobes should be treated.

The polysaccharide capsule of *B fragilis* is an important virulence factor. Many of the symptoms of *Bacteroides* sepsis resemble those of sepsis caused by bacteria with endotoxin, but the lipopolysaccharide of *Bacteroides* is chemically different from the typical endotoxin. No exotoxins have been found.

Clinical Findings   The *B fragilis* group of organisms is most frequently associated with intra-abdominal infections, either peritonitis or localized abscesses. Pelvic abscesses and bacteremia occur as well. Oral, pharyngeal, and pulmonary abscesses are more commonly caused by *B melaninogenicus,* a member of the normal oral flora, but *B fragilis* is found in about 25% of lung abscesses. In general, *B fragilis* causes disease below the diaphragm whereas *B melaninogenicus* causes disease above the diaphragm.

Laboratory Diagnosis   *Bacteroides* species can be isolated anaerobically on blood agar plates containing kanamycin and vancomycin to inhibit unwanted organisms. They are identified by biochemical reactions (eg, sugar fermentations) and by production of certain organic acids (eg, formic,

---

*A pyocin is a type of bacteriocin produced by *P aeruginosa*. Different strains produce various pyocins, which can serve to distinguish the organisms.

†*B fragilis* is divided into five subspecies, the most important of which is *B fragilis* subsp *fragilis*. The other four subspecies are *B fragilis* subspp *distasonis, ovatus, thetaiotaomicron,* and *vulgatus*. It is proper, therefore, to speak of the *B fragilis* group rather than simply *B fragilis*.

acetic, and propionic acids), which are detected by gas chromatography. *B melaninogenicus* produces characteristic black colonies.

Treatment Members of the *B fragilis* group are resistant to penicillins, first-generation cephalosporins, and aminoglycosides, making them among the most antibiotic-resistant of the anaerobic bacteria. Penicillin resistance is the result of β-lactamase production. Metronidazole is the drug of choice, with cefoxitin, clindamycin, and chloramphenicol as alternatives. Aminoglycosides are frequently combined to treat the facultative gram-negative rods in mixed infections. By contrast, the drug of choice for *B melaninogenicus* infections is penicillin G, although β-lactamase producing strains have emerged. However, strains resistant to penicillin have been isolated from patients. Surgical drainage of abscesses usually accompanies antibiotic therapy, but lung abscesses often heal without drainage.

Prevention Prevention of *Bacteroides* infections centers on perioperative administration of a cephalosporin, frequently cefoxitin, for abdominal or pelvic surgery. There is no vaccine.

Review Questions

1. What are the important characteristics of the *Enterobacteriaceae?*
2. What are the differences between the O and H antigens of the *Enterobacteriaceae?*
3. What is the importance of lactose fermentation in distinguishing between certain members of the *Enterobacteriaceae?*
4. Why is the incidence of urinary tract infections caused by *Escherichia coli* higher in women than in men?
5. *E coli* is one of the two main causes of neonatal meningitis. What predisposes to this disease?
6. What is the pathogenesis of *E coli*-induced diarrhea?
7. *E coli* sepsis is frequently accompanied by shock. What is the pathogenesis of the shock?
8. Salmonellae can change their flagellar antigens by DNA rearrangement. What is the pathogenetic significance of this?
9. Is *Salmonella* enterocolitis caused by toxins or by invasion of the gut epithelium?
10. Is the infectious dose of *Salmonella* higher or lower than that of *Shigella?*
11. What is the pathogenesis of typhoid fever?
12. Where are salmonellae found in nature, and how are they transmitted?
13. In enteric fevers caused by salmonellae, what are the two most important cultures to perform?
14. Which measures are appropriate to prevent *Salmonella* infections?
15. What is the natural habitat and mode of transmission for *Shigella?*
16. Is *Shigella* enterocolitis caused by toxins or by invasion of the gut epithelium? Are fecal leukocytes usually found in shigellosis?
17. What is the appearance of *Vibrio cholerae* on Gram's stain?
18. What is the mode of action of cholera toxin?
19. Why is cholera more common in developing countries than in the United States?
20. What is the relative importance of fluid and electrolyte replacement and of antibiotics in the treatment of cholera?
21. What is the appearance of *Campylobacter* on Gram's stain?
22. What is the natural reservoir for *Campylobacter?* What is its mode of transmission?
23. How can *Campylobacter* infections be prevented?
24. Why are *Klebsiella, Enterobacter,* and *Serratia* grouped together? In general, which of these three generally cause(s) opportunistic infections?
25. *Klebsiella pneumoniae* has a very prominent capsule. What are two important functions of this capsule?
26. The O antigens of certain *Proteus* strains cross-react with which organisms in the Weil-Felix test?
27. *Proteus* species resemble *Salmonella* species on TSI agar but can be distinguished by the production of which enzyme?
28. *Proteus* species are motile and produce urease. How might these features contribute to pathogenesis?
29. *Pseudomonas* is not a member of the *Enterobacteriaceae.* What is the major metabolic feature that accounts for this?

30. Pus from wound infections caused by *Pseudomonas aeruginosa* can be blue. Why?
31. In the hospital, *P aeruginosa* is usually found in which environment?
32. Does a neutrophil count of less than 500/μL predispose to *P aeruginosa* infection? Is the organism an opportunist?
33. What is the natural habitat of *Bacteroides fragilis?*
34. Why do an impaired blood supply and the presence of *E coli* contribute to infection by *B fragilis?*
35. *B fragilis* infections frequently do not respond to penicillin G. Why?

19 Gram-Negative Rods Related to the Respiratory Tract

There are three medically important gram-negative rods typically associated with the respiratory tract, namely *Haemophilus influenzae, Legionella pneumophila,* and *Bordetella pertussis* (Table 19–1).

HAEMOPHILUS

Diseases *H influenzae* is the leading cause of meningitis in young children, but the incidence of meningitis has been greatly reduced in the last few years by the use of an effective vaccine (see the Prevention section below). It is also an important cause of upper respiratory tract infections (otitis media, sinusitis, and epiglottitis) and sepsis in children. It causes pneumonia in adults, particularly those with chronic obstructive lung disease. *Haemophilus ducreyi,* the agent of chancroid, is discussed in Chapter 27.

Important Properties *H influenzae* is a small gram-negative rod (coccobacillus) with a polysaccharide capsule. It is one of the three important **encapsulated pyogens,** along with the pneumococcus and the meningococcus. Serologic typing is based on the antigenicity of the capsular polysaccharide. Of the six serotypes, **type b** causes most of the severe, invasive diseases, such as meningitis and sepsis. The type b capsule is composed of polyribitol phosphate. Unencapsulated and therefore untypeable strains can also cause disease but are usually noninvasive. Growth of the organism on laboratory media requires the addition of two components, **heme (factor X)** and **NAD (factor V),** for adequate energy production.

Pathogenesis & Epidemiology *H influenzae* infects only humans; there is no animal reservoir. It enters the body through the **upper respiratory tract,** resulting in either asymptomatic colonization or infections such as otitis media, sinusitis, or pneumonia. The organism produces an IgA protease that degrades secretory IgA, thus facilitating attachment to the respiratory mucosa. After becoming established in the upper respiratory tract, the organism can enter the bloodstream and spread to the meninges. Meningitis is caused primarily by the encapsulated strains (95% of which possess the type b capsule), but nonencapsulated strains are frequently involved in otitis media, sinusitis, and pneumonia. Pathogenesis involves the antiphagocytic capsule and endotoxin; no exotoxin is produced.

Most infections occur in children between the ages of 6 months and 6 years, with a peak in the age group from 6 months to 1 year. This age distribution is attributed to a decline in maternal IgG in the child coupled with the inability of the child to generate sufficient antibody against the polysaccharide capsular antigen until the age of approximately 2 years.

Table 19–1. Gram-negative rods associated with the respiratory tract.

Species	Major Disease	Diagnosis	Factors X and V Required for Growth	Vaccine Available	Prophylaxis for Contacts
H influenzae	Meningitis	Culture.	+	+	Rifampin
L pneumophila	Pneumonia	Serology; culture not usually done.	–	–	None
B pertussis	Whooping cough	Clinical plus culture.	–	+	Erythromycin

Clinical Findings Meningitis caused by *H influenzae* cannot be distinguished on clinical grounds from that caused by other bacterial pathogens, eg, pneumococci or meningococci. The rapid onset of fever, headache, and stiff neck along with drowsiness is typical. Sinusitis and otitis media cause pain in the affected area, opacification of the infected sinus, and redness with bulging of the tympanic membrane. *H influenzae* is second only to the pneumococcus as a cause of these two infections. Rarely, **epiglottitis,** which can obstruct the airway, occurs. This life-threatening disease of young children is caused almost exclusively by *H influenzae.* Pneumonia in elderly adults, especially those with chronic respiratory disease, can be caused by untypeable strains of *H influenzae.*

Laboratory Diagnosis Laboratory diagnosis depends on isolation of the organism on heated-blood ("chocolate") agar enriched with two growth factors required for bacterial respiration, namely factor X (a heme compound) and factor V (NAD). The blood used in chocolate agar is heated to inactivate nonspecific inhibitors of *H influenzae* growth.

An organism that grows only in the presence of both growth factors is presumptively identified as *H influenzae;* other species of *Haemophilus,* such as *H parainfluenzae,* do not require both factors. Definitive identification can be made with either biochemical tests or the capsular swelling (quellung) reaction. Additional means of identifying encapsulated strains include fluorescent-antibody staining of the organism and counterimmunoelectrophoresis or latex agglutination tests, which detect the capsular polysaccharide.

Treatment The treatment of choice for *H influenzae* meningitis or other serious systemic infections is ceftriaxone. From 20 to 30% of *H influenzae* type b isolates produce a β-lactamase that degrades penicillinase-sensitive β-lactams such as ampicillin but not ceftriaxone. It is important to institute antibiotic treatment promptly, because the incidence of neurologic sequelae, eg, subdural empyema, is high. Untreated *H influenzae* meningitis has a fatality rate of approximately 90%. *H influenzae* upper respiratory tract infections, such as otitis media and sinusitis, are treated with either amoxicillin-clavulanate or trimethoprim-sulfamethoxazole.

Prevention The vaccine contains the capsular polysaccharide of *H influenzae* type b **conjugated to diphtheria toxoid** or other carrier protein. Depending upon the carrier protein, it is given some time between the ages of 2 and 15 months. This vaccine is **much more effective** in young children than the unconjugated vaccine and has reduced the incidence of meningitis caused by this organism by approximately 90% in immunized children. Meningitis in close contacts of the patient can be prevented by rifampin. Rifampin is used because it is secreted in the saliva to a greater extent than ampicillin. Rifampin decreases respiratory carriage of the organism, thereby reducing transmission.

LEGIONELLA

Disease *Legionella pneumophila* (and other legionellae) causes pneumonia, both in the community and in hospitalized immunocompromised patients. The genus is named after the famous outbreak of pneumonia among people attending the American Legion convention in Philadelphia in 1976 (Legionnaires' disease).

Important Properties Legionellae are gram-negative rods that **stain faintly with the standard Gram stain.** They do, however, have a gram-negative type of cell wall, and increasing the time of the safranin counterstain enhances visibility. In lung biopsy sections, they do not stain by the standard hematoxylin-and-eosin (H&E) procedure, and so special methods, such as the Dieterle silver impregnation stain, are used.

During the 1976 outbreak, initial attempts to grow the organisms on ordinary culture media failed. This is due to the organism's requirement for a high concentration of iron and cysteine; culture media supplemented with these nutrients will support growth.

L pneumophila causes approximately 90% of pneumonia attributed to legionellae. There are about 30 other *Legionella* species that cause pneumonia, but most of the remaining 10% of cases are caused by 2 species, *L micdadei* and *L bozemanii.*

Pathogenesis & Epidemiology   Legionellae are associated chiefly with **environmental water sources** such as air conditioners and water-cooling towers. Outbreaks of pneumonia in hospitals have been attributed to the presence of the organism in water taps, sinks, and showers. The portal of entry is the respiratory tract, and pathologic changes occur primarily in the lung.

The typical candidate for Legionnaires' disease is an older man who smokes and consumes substantial amounts of alcohol. Patients with AIDS, cancer, transplants (especially renal transplants), or those being treated with corticosteroids are predisposed to *Legionella* pneumonia, which indicates that cell-mediated immunity is the most important defense mechanism. Despite airborne transmission of the organism, person-to-person spread does *not* occur, as shown by the failure of secondary cases to occur in close contacts of patients.

Clinical Findings   The clinical picture can vary from a mild influenzalike illness to a severe pneumonia accompanied by mental confusion, nonbloody diarrhea, proteinuria, and microscopic hematuria. Although cough is a prominent symptom, sputum is frequently scanty and nonpurulent. Most cases resolve spontaneously in 7–10 days, but in older or immunocompromised patients the infection can be fatal.

Legionellosis is an **atypical pneumonia*** and must be distinguished from other similar pneumonias such as *Mycoplasma* pneumonia, viral pneumonia, psittacosis, and Q fever. Pontiac fever is a mild, flulike form of *Legionella* infection that does not result in pneumonia. The name "Pontiac" is derived from the city in Michigan that was the site of an outbreak in 1968.

Laboratory Diagnosis   Sputum Gram stains reveal many neutrophils but no bacteria. The organism **fails to grow on ordinary media** in a culture of sputum or blood, but it will grow on medium supplemented with iron and cysteine. Diagnosis usually depends on a significant increase in antibody titer in convalescent-phase serum by the indirect immunofluorescence assay. Detection of *L pneumophila* antigens in the urine is a rapid means of making a diagnosis. If tissue is available, it is possible to demonstrate *Legionella* antigens in infected lung tissue by using fluorescent-antibody staining. The cold-agglutinin titer does not rise in *Legionella* pneumonia, in contrast to pneumonia caused by *Mycoplasma.*

Treatment   Erythromycin (or erythromycin plus rifampin) is the treatment of choice. Erythromycin is effective not only against *L pneumophila* but also against *Mycoplasma pneumoniae* and *Streptococcus pneumoniae.* The organism frequently produces β-lactamase, and so penicillins and cephalosporins are less effective.

Prevention   Prevention involves reducing cigarette and alcohol consumption, eliminating aerosols from water sources, and reducing the incidence of *Legionella* in hospital water supplies by using high temperatures and hyperchlorination.

BORDETELLA

Disease   *Bordetella pertussis* causes whooping cough (pertussis).

Important Properties   *B pertussis* is a small, coccobacillary, encapsulated gram-negative rod.

Pathogenesis & Epidemiology   *B pertussis,* a pathogen **only for humans,** is transmitted by **airborne droplets.** The organisms attach to the ciliated epithelium of the upper respiratory tract but do not invade the underlying tissue. Decreased cilia activity and epithelial cell death occur. The mechanism of pathogenesis is uncertain, but several factors play a role.

---

*A pneumonia is atypical when its causative agent cannot be isolated on ordinary laboratory media or when its clinical picture does not resemble that of typical pneumococcal pneumonia.

(1) Attachment of the organism to the cilia of the epithelial cells is mediated by a protein on the pili called filamentous hemagglutinin (FHA). Antibody against the FHA inhibits attachment and protects against disease.

(2) Pertussis toxin stimulates adenylate cyclase by catalyzing the addition of ADP-ribose to the inhibitory subunit of the G protein complex. This results in prolonged stimulation of adenylate cyclase and a consequent rise in cAMP and in cAMP-dependent protein kinase activity. The toxin also has a domain that mediates its binding to target cell receptors. Antibodies against the toxin prevent the disease in experimental animals.

Pertussis toxin also causes a striking **lymphocytosis** in patients with pertussis. The toxin inhibits signal transduction by chemokine receptors, resulting in an inability of lymphocytes to enter lymphoid tissue (spleen, lymph nodes) and, consequently, an increase in their number in the blood (see the discussion of chemokines in Chapter 58).

(3) The organisms also synthesize and export adenylate cyclase. This enzyme, when taken up by phagocytic cells, eg, neutrophils, can inhibit their bactericidal activity. Bacterial mutants that lack cyclase activity are avirulent.

(4) Tracheal cytotoxin is a fragment of the bacterial peptidoglycan that damages ciliated cells of the respiratory tract. Its mode of action is uncertain.

Pertussis is a highly contagious disease that occurs primarily in infants and young children and has a worldwide distribution. It occurs infrequently in the United States because use of the vaccine is widespread.

Clinical Findings Whooping cough is an acute tracheobronchitis that begins with mild upper respiratory tract symptoms followed by the typical paroxysmal cough, which lasts from 1 to 4 weeks. The paroxysmal pattern is characterized by a series of hacking coughs, accompanied by production of copious amounts of mucus, that end with an inspiratory "whoop" as air rushes past the narrowed glottis. Despite the severity of the symptoms, the organism is restricted to the respiratory tract and blood cultures are negative. A pronounced leukocytosis with up to 70% lymphocytes is seen. Central nervous system anoxia and exhaustion can occur, although death is due mainly to pneumonia.

Laboratory Diagnosis The organism can be isolated from nasopharyngeal swabs taken during the paroxysmal stage. Bordet-Gengou* medium used for this purpose contains a high percentage of blood (20–30%) to inactivate inhibitors in the agar. Specific identification is made either by agglutination with specific antiserum or by fluorescent-antibody staining.

Treatment Erythromycin reduces the number of organisms in the throat and decreases the risk of secondary complications but has little influence on the course of the disease because the toxins have already damaged the respiratory mucosa. Supportive care, eg, oxygen therapy and suction of mucus, during the paroxysmal stage is important, especially in infants.

Prevention Whooping cough can be prevented by active immunization with either **killed** *B pertussis* organisms or the **acellular** vaccine containing purified proteins from the organism. The pertussis vaccine is usually given combined with diphtheria and tetanus toxoids in three doses beginning at 2 months of age. A booster at 12–15 months of age and another at the time of entering school are recommended. Because pertussis occurs primarily in children, booster immunizations for adults are not recommended. There is controversy about whether to continue using the killed vaccine, because it produces postvaccine encephalopathy at a rate of about one case per million doses administered.

An **acellular vaccine** consisting of five antigens purified from the organism is now recommended in the United States. The main immunogen in this vaccine is inactivated pertussis toxin (pertussis toxoid). The acellular vaccine has fewer side effects than the killed vaccine.

Erythromycin is useful in prevention of disease in exposed, unimmunized individuals. It should also be given to immunized children under the age of 4 who have been exposed, because vaccine-induced immunity is not completely protective.

---

*The French scientists who first isolated the organism in 1906.

Review Questions

1. Type b *Haemophilus influenzae* is responsible for most of the invasive disease caused by this species. What determines the serotype?
2. What are the three most common bacteria that cause meningitis? What important pathogenetic feature do they share?
3. Factors X (heme) and V (NAD) are required for *H influenzae* growth. Why?
4. What are two methods of preventing *H influenzae* meningitis?
5. Which two features of *Legionella pneumophila* account for the difficulty in isolating the organism during the 1976 outbreak at the American Legion Convention?
6. What is the natural habitat of *L pneumophila?* What is its usual mode of transmission?
7. What is the most common method of making the diagnosis of *L pneumophila* pneumonia in the clinical laboratory? Why?
8. What is the pathogenesis of whooping cough?
9. What is the nature of *Bordetella pertussis* vaccine? What are the problems associated with the vaccine?

20

Gram-Negative Rods Related to Animal Sources (Zoonotic Organisms)

Zoonoses are human diseases caused by organisms that are acquired from animals. There are bacterial, viral, fungal, and parasitic zoonoses. Some zoonotic organisms are acquired directly from the animal reservoir, while others are transmitted by vectors, such as mosquitoes or ticks.

There are four medically important gram-negative rods that have significant animal reservoirs: *Brucella* species, *Francisella tularensis, Yersinia pestis,* and *Pasteurella multocida* (Table 20–1).

BRUCELLA

Disease *Brucella* species cause brucellosis (undulant fever).

Important Properties Brucellae are small gram-negative rods without a capsule. The three major human pathogens and their animal reservoirs are *Brucella melitensis* (goats and sheep), *Brucella abortus* (cattle), and *Brucella suis* (pigs).

Pathogenesis & Epidemiology The organisms enter the body either by ingestion of **contaminated milk products** or **through the skin** by direct contact in an occupational setting such as an abattoir. They localize in the **reticuloendothelial system,** namely the lymph nodes, liver, spleen, and bone marrow. Many organisms are killed by macrophages, but some survive within these cells, where they are protected from antibody. The host response is granulomatous, with lymphocytes and epithelioid giant cells, which can progress to form focal abscesses and caseation. The mechanism of pathogenesis of these organisms is not well defined, except that endotoxin is involved; ie, when the O antigen polysaccharides are lost from the external portion of the endotoxin, the organism loses its virulence. No exotoxins are produced.

Imported cheese made from unpasteurized goats' milk produced in either Mexico or the Mediterranean region has been a source of *B melitensis* infection in the United States. The disease occurs worldwide but is rare in the United States, because pasteurization of milk kills the organism.

Table 20–1. Gram-negative rods associated with animal sources.

Species	Disease	Source of Human Infection	Mode of Transmission From Animal to Human	Diagnosis
Brucella species	Brucellosis	Pigs, cattle, goats, sheep	Dairy products; contact with animal tissues.	Serology
Francisella tularensis	Tularemia	Rabbits, deer, ticks	Contact with animal tissues; ticks.	Serology
Yersinia pestis	Plague	Rodents	Flea bite.	Immunofluorescence
Pasteurella multocida	Cellulitis	Cats, dogs	Cat or dog bite.	Wound culture

Clinical Findings   After an incubation period of 1–3 weeks, nonspecific symptoms resembling influenza occur. The undulating (rising-and-falling) fever pattern that gives the disease its name occurs in a minority of patients. Weakness and fatigue are marked. Enlarged lymph nodes, liver, and spleen are frequently found. *B melitensis* infections tend to be more severe and prolonged, whereas those caused by *B abortus* are more self-limited. Osteomyelitis is the most frequent complication. Secondary spread from person to person is rare.

Laboratory Diagnosis   Recovery of the organism requires the use of enriched culture media and incubation in 10% CO_2. The organisms can be presumptively identified by using a slide agglutination test with *Brucella* antiserum, and the species can be identified by biochemical tests. If organisms are not isolated, analysis of a serum sample from the patient for a rise in antibody titer to *Brucella* can be used to make a diagnosis. In the absence of an acute-phase serum specimen, a titer of at least 1:160 in the convalescent-phase serum sample is diagnostic.

Treatment   The treatment of choice is tetracycline plus gentamicin. There is no significant resistance to these drugs.

Prevention   Prevention of brucellosis involves pasteurization of milk, immunization of animals, and slaughtering of infected animals. There is no human vaccine.

FRANCISELLA

Disease   *Francisella tularensis* causes tularemia.

Important Properties   *F tularensis* is a small, pleomorphic gram-negative rod. It has a single serologic type.

Pathogenesis & Epidemiology   *F tularensis* is remarkable in the wide variety of animals that it infects and in the breadth of its distribution in the United States. It is enzootic (endemic in animals) in every state, but most human cases occur in the rural areas of Arkansas and Missouri. It has been isolated from more than 100 different species of **wild animals,** the most important of which are rabbits, deer, and a variety of rodents. The bacteria are transmitted among these animals by vectors such as **ticks,** mites, and lice, especially the *Dermacentor* ticks that feed on the blood of wild rabbits. The tick maintains the chain of transmission by passing the bacteria to its offspring by the transovarian route. In this process, the bacteria are passed through ovum, larva, and nymph stages to adult ticks capable of transmitting the infection.

Humans are accidental "dead-end" hosts who acquire the infection most often by being bitten by the vector or by having skin contact with the animal during removal of the hide. Rarely, the organism is ingested in infected meat, causing gastrointestinal tularemia, or is inhaled, causing pneumonia. There is no person-to-person spread. The main type of tularemia in the United States is tick-borne tularemia from a rabbit reservoir.

The organism enters through the skin, forming an ulcer at the site in most cases. It then localizes to the cells of the reticuloendothelial system, and granulomas are formed. Caseation necrosis and abscesses can also occur.

Clinical Findings   Presentation can vary from sudden onset of an influenzalike syndrome to prolonged onset of a low-grade fever and adenopathy. Approximately 75% of cases are the "ulceroglandular" type, in which the site of entry ulcerates and the regional lymph nodes are swollen and painful. Other, less frequent forms of tularemia include glandular, oculoglandular, typhoidal, gastrointestinal, and pulmonary. Disease usually confers lifelong immunity.

Laboratory Diagnosis   Attempts to culture the organism in the laboratory are rarely undertaken, because there is a high risk to laboratory workers of infection by inhalation and the special cysteine-containing medium required for growth is not usually available. The most frequently used diagnostic method is the agglutination test with acute- and convalescent-phase serum samples. Fluorescent-antibody staining of infected tissue can be used if available.

Treatment   Streptomycin is the drug of choice. There is no significant antibiotic resistance.

Prevention   Prevention involves avoiding both being bitten by ticks and handling wild animals. There is a live, attenuated bacterial vaccine that is given only to persons, such as fur trappers, whose occupation brings them into close contact with wild animals. This and the BCG vaccine for tuberculosis are the only two live bacterial vaccines for human use.

YERSINIA

Disease   *Yersinia pestis* is the cause of plague, also known as the black death, the scourge of the Middle Ages. It is also a 20th century disease, occurring in the western United States and in many other countries around the world. Two less important species, *Yersinia enterocolitica* and *Yersinia pseudotuberculosis,* are described in Chapter 27.

Important Properties   *Y pestis* is a small gram-negative rod that exhibits bipolar staining; ie, it resembles a safety pin, with a central clear area. Freshly isolated organisms possess a capsule, which can be lost with passage in the laboratory; loss of the capsule is accompanied by a loss of virulence. It is one of the **most virulent** bacteria known and has a strikingly low ID_{50}; ie, 1 to 10 organisms are capable of causing disease.

Pathogenesis & Epidemiology   The plague bacillus has been endemic in the wild rodents of Europe and Asia for thousands of years but entered North America in the early 1900s, probably carried by a rat that jumped ship at a California port. It is now endemic in the wild rodents in the western United States, although 99% of cases of plague occur in Southeast Asia.

The enzootic (sylvatic) cycle consists of transmission among **wild rodents by fleas.** In the United States, prairie dogs are the main reservoir. Rodents are relatively resistant to disease; most are asymptomatic. Humans are accidental hosts, and cases of plague in this country occur as a result of being bitten by a flea that is part of the sylvatic cycle.

The urban cycle, which does not occur in the United States, consists of transmission of the bacteria among urban rats, with the **rat flea** as vector. This cycle predominates during times of poor sanitation, eg, wartime, when rats proliferate and come in contact with the fleas in the sylvatic cycle.

The events within the flea are fascinating as well as essential. The flea ingests the bacteria while taking a blood meal from a bacteremic rodent. The blood clots in the flea's stomach owing to the action of the enzyme coagulase, which is made by the bacteria. The bacteria are trapped in the fibrin and proliferate to large numbers. The mass of organisms and fibrin block the proventriculus of the flea's intestinal tract, and during its next blood meal the flea regurgitates the organisms into the next animal. Because the proventriculus is blocked, the flea gets no nutrition, becomes hungrier, loses its natural host selectivity for rodents, and more readily bites a human.

The organisms inoculated at the time of the bite spread to the regional lymph nodes, which become swollen and tender. These swollen lymph nodes are the **buboes** that have led to the name **bubonic plague.** The organisms can reach high concentrations in the blood and disseminate to form abscesses in many organs. The endotoxin-related symptoms, including disseminated intravascular coagulation and cutaneous hemorrhages, probably were the genesis of the term "black death."

In addition to the sylvatic and urban cycles of transmission, respiratory droplet transmission of the organism from patients with pneumonic plague can occur.

The organism has five factors that contribute to its virulence: (1) the envelope antigen, called F-1, which protects against phagocytosis; (2) endotoxin; (3) an exotoxin; and two proteins known as (4) V antigen and (5) W antigen. The action of these last 3 proteins is unknown. Two additional correlates of virulence are the formation of pigmented colonies on certain media and the ability to synthesize purines.

Clinical Findings   Bubonic plague, which is the most frequent form, begins with pain and swelling of the lymph nodes draining the site of the flea bite and systemic symptoms such as high fever, myalgias, and prostration. The affected nodes enlarge and become exquisitely tender. These buboes are an early characteristic finding. Septic shock and pneumonia are the main life-threatening subsequent events. Pneumonic plague can arise either from inhalation of an aerosol or from septic emboli that reach the lungs. Untreated bubonic plague is fatal in approximately half of the cases, and untreated pneumonic plague is invariably fatal.

Laboratory Diagnosis   Smear and culture of blood or pus from the bubo is the best diagnostic procedure. Great care must be taken by the physician during aspiration of the pus and by laboratory workers doing the culture not to create an aerosol that might transmit the infection. Giemsa's or Wayson's stain reveals the typical safety-pin appearance of the organism better than does Gram's stain. Fluorescent-antibody staining can be used to identify the organism in tissues. A rise in antibody titer to the envelope antigen can be useful retrospectively.

Treatment   The treatment of choice is a combination of streptomycin and tetracycline, although streptomycin alone can be used. There is no significant antibiotic resistance. In view of the rapid progression of the disease, treatment should not wait for the results of the bacteriologic culture. Incision and drainage of the buboes are not usually necessary.

Prevention   Prevention of plague involves controlling the spread of rats in urban areas, preventing rats from entering the country by ship or airplane, and avoiding both flea bites and contact with dead wild rodents. A patient with plague must be placed in strict isolation (quarantine) for 72 hours after antibiotic therapy is started. Only close contacts need receive prophylactic tetracycline, but all contacts should be observed for fever. Reporting a case of plague to the public health authorities is mandatory.

A vaccine consisting of formalin-killed organisms provides partial protection against bubonic but not pneumonic plague. It was used in the armed forces during the Vietnam war but is not recommended for tourists traveling to Southeast Asia.

PASTEURELLA

Disease   *Pasteurella multocida* causes wound infections associated with cat and dog bites.

Important Properties   *P multocida* is a short, encapsulated gram-negative rod that exhibits bipolar staining.

Pathogenesis & Epidemiology   The organism is part of the normal flora in the mouths of many animals, particularly **domestic cats and dogs,** and is transmitted by **biting.** About 25% of animal bites become infected with the organism, with sutures acting as a predisposing factor to infection. Most bite infections are polymicrobial, with a variety of facultative anaerobes and anaerobic organisms present in addition to *P multocida*. Pathogenesis is not well understood, except that the capsule is a virulence factor and endotoxin is present in the cell wall. No exotoxins are made.

Clinical Findings   The rapid onset of cellulitis at the site of an animal bite is indicative of *P multocida* infection. Osteomyelitis can complicate cat bites in particular, because cats' sharp, pointed teeth can implant the organism under the periosteum.

Laboratory Diagnosis   The diagnosis is made by finding the organism in a culture of a sample from the wound site.

Treatment   Penicillin G is the treatment of choice. There is no significant antibiotic resistance.

Prevention   People who have been bitten by a cat should be given ampicillin to prevent *P multo-cida* infection. Animal bites, especially cat bites, should not be sutured.

Review Questions

1. How is brucellosis acquired?
2. In brucellosis, the organism is located primarily in which organ system and cells?
3. How can brucellosis be prevented?
4. How is tularemia acquired? How can it be prevented?
5. Infections caused by cat bites are associated with what organism?
6. What is the epidemiology of plague; ie, what is the reservoir, how is it transmitted, and where in the United States does it occur?
7. What is the pathogenesis of plague?

21

Mycobacteria

Mycobacteria are aerobic, **acid-fast** bacilli (rods). They are neither gram-positive nor gram-negative; ie, they are stained poorly by the dyes used in Gram's stain. They are virtually the only bacteria that are acid-fast. (One exception is *Nocardia asteroides,* the major cause of nocardiosis, which is also acid-fast.) The term "acid-fast" refers to an organism's ability to retain the carbolfuchsin stain despite subsequent treatment with an ethanol-hydrochloric acid mixture. The high lipid content (approximately 60%) of their cell wall makes mycobacteria acid-fast.

The major pathogens are *Mycobacterium tuberculosis,* the cause of tuberculosis, and *Mycobacterium leprae,* the cause of leprosy. Atypical mycobacteria, such as *Mycobacterium avium-intracellulare* complex and *Mycobacterium kansasii,* can cause tuberculosislike disease but are less frequent pathogens. Rapidly growing mycobacteria, such as *Mycobacterium chelonei,* are saprophytes that occasionally cause human disease in immunocompromised hosts (Table 21–1).

MYCOBACTERIUM TUBERCULOSIS

Disease   This organism causes tuberculosis.

Important Properties   *M tuberculosis* **grows slowly** (ie, it has a doubling time of 18 hours, in contrast to most bacteria, which can double in number in 1 hour or less). Because growth is so slow, cultures of clinical specimens must be held for 6–8 weeks before being recorded as negative. *M tuberculosis* can be cultured on bacteriologic media, whereas *M leprae* cannot. Media used for its growth (eg, Löwenstein-Jensen medium) contain complex nutrients (eg, egg yolk) and dyes (eg, malachite green). The dyes inhibit the unwanted normal flora present in sputum samples.

M tuberculosis is an **obligate aerobe;** this explains its predilection for causing disease in highly oxygenated tissue such as the upper lobe of the lung and the kidney. Its cell wall contains several complex lipids: (1) long-chain (C_{78}– C_{90}) fatty acids called **mycolic acids,** which contribute to the organism's acid-fastness; (2) wax D, one of the active components in Freund's adjuvant, which is used to enhance the immune response to many antigens in experimental animals; and (3) phosphatides, which play a role in caseation necrosis.

Table 21–1. Medically important mycobacteria.

Species	Growth on Bacteriologic Media	Preferred Temperature in Vivo (°C)	Source or Mode of Transmission
M tuberculosis	Slow (weeks)	37	Respiratory droplets
M bovis	Slow (weeks)	37	Milk from infected animals
M leprae	None	32	Prolonged close contact
Atypical mycobacteria[1] M kansasii	Slow (weeks)	37	Soil and water
M marinum	Slow (weeks)	32	Water
M avium-intracellulare complex	Slow (weeks)	37	Soil and water
M fortuitum-chelonei complex	Rapid (days)	37	Soil and water

[1]Only representative examples are given.

Cord factor (trehalose dimycolate) is correlated with virulence of the organism. Virulent strains grow in a characteristic "serpentine" cordlike pattern, whereas avirulent strains do not. The organism also contains several proteins, which, when combined with waxes, elicit delayed hypersensitivity. These proteins are the antigens in the **PPD (purified protein derivative)** skin test.

M tuberculosis is relatively resistant to acids and alkalis. NaOH is used to concentrate clinical specimens; it destroys unwanted bacteria, human cells, and mucus but not the organism. *M tuberculosis* is resistant to dehydration and so survives in dried expectorated sputum; this property may be important in its transmission by aerosol.

Strains of *M tuberculosis* resistant to the main antimycobacterial drug, isoniazid, as well as strains resistant to multiple antibiotics (called **multiple-drug-resistant or MDR** strains), have become a worldwide problem. This resistance is attributed to one or more chromosomal mutations, because no plasmids have been found in this organism. One of these mutations is in a gene for mycolic acid synthesis, and another is in a gene for catalase-peroxidase, an enzyme required to activate isoniazid within the bacterium.

Transmission & Epidemiology   *M tuberculosis* is transmitted from person to person by **respiratory aerosol,** and its initial site of infection is the lung. In the body, it resides chiefly within reticuloendothelial cells, eg, **macrophages. Humans are the natural reservoir** of *M tuberculosis;* there is no animal reservoir.

In the United States, tuberculosis is almost exclusively a human disease. In developing countries, *Mycobacterium bovis* also causes tuberculosis in humans. *M bovis* is found in cow's milk, which, unless pasteurized, can cause gastrointestinal tuberculosis in humans. The disease tuberculosis occurs in only a small proportion of infected individuals. In the United States, most tuberculosis is due to reactivation in elderly, malnourished men. The risk of infection and disease is highest among socioeconomically disadvantaged people, who have poor housing and poor nutrition. These factors, rather than genetic ones, probably account for the high rate of infection among Native Americans, blacks, and Eskimos.

Pathogenesis   *M tuberculosis* produces no exotoxins and does not contain endotoxin in its cell wall. In fact, no mycobacteria produce toxins. Lesions are dependent on the presence of the organism and the host response. There are two types of lesions:

(1) exudative lesions, which consist of an acute inflammatory response and occur chiefly in the lungs at the initial site of infection; and

(2) granulomatous lesions, which consist of a central area of giant cells containing tubercle bacilli surrounded by a zone of epithelioid cells. A **tubercle** is a granuloma surrounded by fibrous tissue that has undergone central caseation necrosis. Tubercles heal by fibrosis and calcification.

The primary lesion of tuberculosis usually occurs in the lungs. The parenchymal exudative lesion and the draining lymph nodes together are called a **Ghon complex.** Primary lesions usually occur in the lower lobes, whereas reactivation lesions usually occur in the apices. Reactivation lesions also occur in other well-oxygenated sites such as the kidneys, brain, and bone. Reactivation is seen primarily in immunocompromised or debilitated patients.

Spread of the organism within the body occurs by two mechanisms:

(1) A tubercle can erode into a brochus, empty its caseous contents, and thereby spread the organism to other parts of the lungs, to the gastrointestinal tract if swallowed, and to other persons if expectorated.

(2) It can disseminate via the bloodstream to many internal organs. Dissemination can occur at an early stage if cell-mediated immunity fails to contain the initial infection or at a late stage if a person becomes immunocompromised.

Immunity & Hypersensitivity   After recovery from the primary infection, resistance to the organism is mediated by **cellular immunity,** ie, by CD4-positive T cells and macrophages. Circulating antibodies also form, but they play no role in resistance and are not used for diagnostic purposes.

Prior infection can be detected by a positive **tuberculin skin test,** which is due to a delayed hypersensitivity reaction. **PPD** is used as the antigen in the tuberculin skin test. The intermediate-strength preparation of PPD, which contains 5 tuberculin units, is usually used. The test is positive if 10 mm of induration occurs 48–72 hours after intradermal injection of the PPD. **Induration** (thickening), not simply erythema (reddening), must be observed. Reactions of 5 to 9 mm in people known to be exposed and who have not received the BCG vaccine indicate that the person is probably infected. In AIDS patients, a 5-mm reaction is considered positive.

A positive skin test indicates previous infection by the organism but not necessarily active disease. The tuberculin test becomes positive 4–6 weeks after infection. Immunization with BCG vaccine can cause a positive test but the reactions are usually only 5 to 10 mm and tend to decrease with the passage of time. PPD reactions of 15 mm or more are assumed to be infected with *M tuberculosis* even if they have received the BCG vaccine. The skin test itself does *not* induce a positive response. Tuberculin reactivity is mediated by the cellular arm of the immune system; it can be transferred by CD4-positive T cells but not by serum. Infection with measles virus can suppress cell-mediated immunity, resulting in a loss of tuberculin skin test reactivity and, in some instances, reactivation of dormant organisms and clinical disease.

Clinical Findings   Clinical findings are protean; many organs can be involved. Fever, fatigue, night sweats, and weight loss are common. Pulmonary tuberculosis causes cough and hemoptysis. Scrofula is mycobacterial cervical adenitis that presents as swollen nontender lymph nodes, usually unilaterally. Both *M tuberculosis* and *M scrofulaceum* cause scrofula. Miliary tuberculosis is characterized by multiple disseminated lesions that resemble millet seeds. Tuberculous meningitis and tuberculous osteomyelitis, especially vertebral osteomyelitis (Pott's disease), are important disseminated forms.

Laboratory Diagnosis   **Acid-fast staining** of sputum or other specimens is the usual initial test. For rapid screening purposes, auramine stain, which can be visualized by fluorescence microscopy, can be used.

After digestion of the specimen by treatment with NaOH and concentration by centrifugation, the material is cultured on special media, such as Löwenstein-Jensen agar, for up to 8 weeks. It will *not* grow on a blood agar plate. In liquid BACTEC medium, radioactive metabolites are present and growth can be detected by the production of radioactive carbon dioxide in about 2 weeks. A liquid medium is preferred for isolation because the organism grows more rapidly and reliably than it does on agar. If growth in the culture occurs, the organism can be identified by biochemical tests. For example, *M tuberculosis* produces **niacin,** whereas almost no other mycobacteria do. More rapid identification tests using DNA probes are also available.

Because drug resistance, especially to isoniazid (see below), is a problem, susceptibility tests should be performed. However, the organism grows very slowly and susceptibility tests usually take several weeks, which is too long to guide the initial choice of drugs. A recently devised test called the **luciferase assay,** which can detect drug-resistant organisms in a few days, is a distinct improvement. Luciferase is an enzyme isolated from fireflies that produces flashes of light in the presence of ATP. If the organism isolated from the patient is resistant, it will not be damaged by the drug; ie, it will make a normal amount of ATP, and the luciferase will produce the normal amount of light. If the organism is sensitive to the drug, less ATP will be made and less light produced.

Treatment & Resistance   **Multiple-drug** therapy is used to prevent the emergence of drug-resistant mutants during the long (6–9-month) duration of treatment. (Organisms that become resistant to one drug will be inhibited by the other.) **Isoniazid** (isonicotinic acid hydrazide, INH), a bactericidal drug, is the mainstay of treatment. Treatment for most patients with pulmonary tuberculosis is with three drugs: INH, rifampin, and pyrazinamide. INH and rifampin are given for 6 months, but pyrazinamide treatment is stopped after 2 months. In patients who are immunocompromised (eg, AIDS patients), who have disseminated disease, or who are likely to have INH-resistant organisms, a fourth drug, ethambutol, is added and all four drugs are given for 9–12 months. Although therapy is usually given for months, the patient's sputum becomes noninfectious within 2–3 weeks. The necessity for protracted therapy is attributed to (1) the intracellular location of the organism; (2) caseous material, which blocks penetration by the drug; (3) the slow growth of the organism; and (4) metabolically inactive "persisters" within the lesion. Because metabolically inactive organisms may not be killed by antitubercular drugs, treatment may not eradicate the infection and reactivation of the disease may occur in the future.

Resistance to INH and other antituberculosis drugs is being seen with increasing frequency in the United States, especially in immigrants from Southeast Asia and Latin America. Strains of *M tuberculosis* resistant to multiple drugs have emerged, primarily in AIDS patients. The most common pattern is resistance to both INH and rifampin, but some isolates are resistant to three or more drugs. The treatment of multidrug-resistant organisms usually involves the use of four or five drugs, including such drugs as ciprofloxacin, amikacin, ethionamide, and cycloserine. The precise recommendations depend on the resistance pattern of the isolate and are beyond the scope of this book.

Previous treatment for tuberculosis predisposes to the selection of these multidrug-resistant organisms. **Noncompliance,** ie, the failure of patients to complete the full course of therapy, is a major factor in allowing the resistant organisms to survive. One approach to the problem of noncompliance is directly observed therapy (DOT), in which health care workers observe the patient taking the medication.

Prevention   The incidence of tuberculosis began to decrease markedly even before the advent of drug therapy in the 1940s. This is attributed to better housing and nutrition, which have improved host resistance.

The risk of progression to active tuberculosis is reduced by **chemoprophylaxis with INH** for 6–9 months. It is prescribed for (1) asymptomatic patients whose PPD skin test has recently converted to positive, (2) children exposed to patients with symptomatic pulmonary tuberculosis, and (3) patients with a positive PPD skin test who undergo immunosuppression. Patients receiving INH prophylaxis should be evaluated for drug-induced hepatitis, especially those over age 35 years, in view of the hepatotoxicity of the drug.

A vaccine containing a strain of live, attenuated *M bovis* (bacillus Calmette-Guérin or **BCG**) can be used to induce partial resistance to tuberculosis. Although in use in Europe and other areas of the world, it is *not* given in the United States because vaccinees become skin test-positive; hence, an important diagnostic tool is lost. Pasteurization of milk and destruction of infected cattle are important in preventing intestinal tuberculosis.

ATYPICAL MYCOBACTERIA

Several species of mycobacteria are characterized as atypical, because they differ in certain respects from the prototype, *M tuberculosis*. For example, atypical mycobacteria are widespread in the **environment** and are not pathogenic for guinea pigs, whereas *M tuberculosis* is found only in humans and is highly pathogenic for guinea pigs.

The atypical mycobacteria are classified into four groups according to their rate of growth and whether they produce pigment under certain conditions (Table 21–2). Group I organisms produce a yellow-orange-pigmented colony only when exposed to light (**photochromogens**), whereas group II organisms produce the pigment chiefly in the dark (**scotochromogens**). Group III mycobacteria produce little or no yellow-orange pigment, irrespective of the presence or absence of light (**nonchromogens**). In contrast to the organisms in the previous three groups, which grow slowly, group IV organisms grow rapidly, producing colonies in less than 7 days.

Group I (Photochromogens)   *M kansasii* causes lung disease clinically resembling tuberculosis. It is antigenically similar to *M tuberculosis,* and so patients are frequently tuberculin skin test-positive. Its habitat in the environment is unknown, but infections by this organism are localized to the midwestern states and Texas. It is susceptible to the standard antituberculosis drugs.

Mycobacterium marinum causes "swimming pool granuloma." These granulomatous, ulcerating lesions occur in the skin at the site of abrasions incurred at swimming pools and aquariums. The natural habitat of the organism is both fresh and salt water. Treatment with a tetracycline such as minocycline is effective.

Table 21–2. Runyon's classification of atypical mycobacteria.

Group	Growth Rate	Pigment Formation In:		Typical Species
		Light	Dark	
I	Slow	+	–	M kansasii, M marinum
II	Slow	+	+	M scrofulaceum
III	Slow	–	–	M avium-intracellulare complex
IV	Rapid	–	–	M fortuitum-chelonei complex

Group II (Scotochromogens) *Mycobacterium scrofulaceum* causes scrofula, a granulomatous cervical adenitis, usually in children. (*M tuberculosis* also causes scrofula.) The organism enters through the oropharynx and infects the draining lymph nodes. Its natural habitat is environmental water sources, but it has also been isolated as a saprophyte from the human respiratory tract. Scrofula can often be cured by surgical excision of the affected lymph nodes.

Group III (Nonchromogens) *M avium-intracellulare* complex (MAI, MAC) is composed of two species, *M avium* and *M intracellulare,* that are very difficult to distinguish from each other by standard laboratory tests. They cause pulmonary disease clinically indistinguishable from tuberculosis, primarily in immunocompromised patients such as those with AIDS who have CD4 cell counts of less than 200/mm³. MAI is the most common bacterial cause of disease in AIDS patients. The organisms are widespread in the environment, including water and soil, particularly in the southeastern United States. They are highly resistant to antituberculosis drugs, and as many as six drugs in combination are frequently required for adequate treatment. Current drugs of choice are clarithromycin plus one or more of the following: ethambutol, rifabutin, or ciprofloxacin. Clarithromycin is currently recommended for preventing disease in AIDS patients.

Group IV (Rapidly Growing Mycobacteria) *Mycobacterium fortuitum-chelonei* complex is composed of two similar species, *M fortuitum* and *M chelonei.* They are saprophytes, found chiefly in soil and water, which rarely cause human disease. Infections occur chiefly in two populations: (1) immunocompromised patients and (2) individuals with prosthetic heart valves and hip joints. They are frequently resistant to antituberculosis therapy, and therapy with multiple drugs in combination plus surgical excision may be required for effective treatment. Current drugs of choice are amikacin plus doxycycline.

    Mycobacterium smegmatis is a rapidly growing mycobacterium that is not associated with human disease. It is part of the normal flora of smegma, the material that collects under the foreskin of the penis.

MYCOBACTERIUM LEPRAE

Disease This organism causes leprosy.

Important Properties *M leprae* has **not been grown** in the laboratory, either on artificial media or in cell culture. It can be grown in the mouse footpad or in the armadillo. Humans are the natural hosts. The optimal temperature for growth (30 °C) is **lower** than body temperature; it therefore grows preferentially in the skin and superficial nerves.

Transmission Infection is acquired by **prolonged contact with patients** with lepromatous leprosy, who discharge *M leprae* in large numbers in nasal secretions and from skin lesions. In the United States, leprosy occurs primarily in Texas, Louisiana, California, and Hawaii. Most cases are found in immigrants from Mexico, the Philippines, southeast Asia, and India. The disease occurs worldwide, with most cases in the tropical areas of Asia and Africa.

Pathogenesis The organism replicates intracellularly, typically within skin histiocytes, endothelial cells, and the Schwann cells of nerves. There are two distinct forms of leprosy—**tuberculoid** and **lepromatous**—with several intermediate forms between the two extremes (Table 21–3).

Immunity to syphilis is incomplete. Antibodies to the organism are produced but do not stop the progression of the disease. Patients with early syphilis who have been treated can contract syphilis again. Patients with late syphilis are relatively resistant to reinfection.

Laboratory Diagnosis   There are three important approaches.

A.   Microscopy: Spirochetes are demonstrated in early lesions by **darkfield** or immunofluorescence microscopy. They are *not* seen on a Gram-stained smear.

B.   Nonspecific Serologic Tests: These tests involve the use of **nontreponemal** antigens. Extracts of normal mammalian tissues (eg, **cardiolipin** from beef heart) react with antibodies in serum samples from patients with syphilis. These antibodies, which are a mixture of IgG and IgM, are called "reagin" antibodies (see above). Flocculation tests, eg, VDRL (Venereal Disease Research Laboratory) and RPR (rapid plasma reagin) tests, detect the presence of these antibodies. These tests are positive in most cases of primary syphilis and are almost always positive in secondary syphilis. The titer of these nonspecific antibodies **decreases with effective treatment,** in contrast to the specific antibodies, which are positive for life (see below).

False-positive reactions occur in infections such as leprosy, hepatitis B, and infectious mononucleosis and in various autoimmune diseases. Therefore, positive results have to be confirmed by specific tests (see below). Results of nonspecific tests usually **become negative after treatment** and should be used to determine the response to treatment. These tests can also be falsely negative as a result of the prozone phenomenon. In the prozone phenomenon, the titer of antibody is too high (antibody excess) and no flocculation will occur. On dilution of the serum, however, the test becomes positive (see Chapter 64). These tests are inexpensive and easy to perform and therefore are used as a method of screening the population for infection. The nonspecific tests and the specific tests (see below) are described in more detail in Chapter 9.

The laboratory diagnosis of congenital syphilis is based on the finding that the infant has a higher titer of antibody in the VDRL test than has the mother. Furthermore, if a positive VDRL test on the infant is a false-positive result because maternal antibody has crossed the placenta, the titer will decline with time. If the infant is truly infected, the titer will remain high. However, irrespective of the VDRL results, any infant whose mother has syphilis should be treated.

C.   Specific Serologic Tests: These tests involve the use of treponemal antigens and therefore are more specific than those described above. In these tests, *T pallidum* reacts in immunofluorescence (FTA-ABS)* or hemagglutination (TPHA, MHA-TP)† assays with specific treponemal antibodies in the patient's serum. These antibodies arise within 2–3 weeks of infection, and so the tests are positive in most patients with primary syphilis. These **tests remain positive for life** after effective treatment and *cannot* be used to determine the response to treatment or reinfection. They are more expensive and more difficult to perform than the nonspecific tests and therefore are not used as screening procedures.

Treatment   Penicillin is effective in the treatment of all stages of syphilis. A single injection of benzathine penicillin G (2.4 million units) can eradicate *T pallidum* and cure early syphilis. If the patient is allergic to penicillin, tetracycline or erythromycin can be used but must be given for prolonged periods to effect a cure. In neurosyphilis, high doses of aqueous penicillin G are administered. No resistance to penicillin has been observed.

More than half of patients with secondary syphilis who are treated with penicillin experience fever, chills, myalgias, and other influenzalike symptoms a few hours after receiving the antibiotic. This response, called the **Jarisch-Herxheimer reaction,** is attributed to the lysis of the treponemes and the release of endotoxinlike substances. Patients should be alerted to this possibility, advised that it may last for up to 24 hours, and told that symptomatic relief can be obtained with aspirin. The Jarisch-Herxheimer reaction also occurs after treatment of other spirochetal diseases such as Lyme disease, leptospirosis, and relapsing fever.

Prevention   Prevention depends on early diagnosis and adequate treatment, use of condoms, administration of antibiotic after suspected exposure, and serologic follow-up of infected individuals

---

*FTA-ABS is the fluorescent treponemal antibody-absorbed test. The patient's serum is absorbed with nonpathogenic treponemes to remove cross-reacting antibodies prior to reacting with *T pallidum.*
†TPHA is the *T pallidum* hemagglutination assay. MHA-TP is a hemagglutination assay done in a microtiter plate.

and their contacts. The presence of any sexually transmitted disease makes testing for syphilis mandatory, because several different infections are often transmitted simultaneously. There is no vaccine against syphilis.

2. Nonvenereal Treponematoses

These are infections caused by spirochetes that are virtually indistinguishable from *T pallidum.* They are endemic in populations and are transmitted by direct contact. All of these infections result in positive (nontreponemal and treponemal) serologic tests for syphilis. None of these spirochetes have been grown on bacteriologic media. The diseases include bejel in Africa, yaws (caused by *T pallidum* subspecies *pertenue*) in many humid tropical countries, and pinta (caused by *T carateum*) in Central and South America. All can be cured by penicillin.

BORRELIA

Borrelia species are irregular, loosely coiled spirochetes which stain readily with Giemsa's and other stains. They can be cultured in bacteriologic media containing serum or tissue extracts. They are transmitted by **arthropods.** They cause two major diseases, Lyme disease and relapsing fever.

1. *Borrelia burgdorferi*

Disease   *Borrelia burgdorferi* causes Lyme disease (named after a town in Connecticut). Lyme disease is also known as Lyme borreliosis.

Important Properties   *B burgdorferi* is a flexible, motile spirochete that can be visualized by darkfield microscopy and by Giemsa's and silver stains. It can be grown in certain bacteriologic media, but routine cultures obtained from patients (eg, blood, spinal fluid) are typically negative. In contrast, culture of the organism from the tick vector is usually positive.

Transmission & Epidemiology   *B burgdorferi* is transmitted by tick bite. The tick *Ixodes dammini* (renamed *I scapularis*) is the vector on the East Coast and in the Midwest; *Ixodes pacificus* is involved on the West Coast. The organism is found in a much higher percentage of *I dammini* (35–50%) than *I pacificus* (ca 2%) ticks. This explains the lower incidence of disease on the West Coast. The main reservoir of the organism consists of small mammals, especially the white-footed mouse, upon which the nymphs feed.* Large mammals, especially deer, are an obligatory host in the tick's life cycle but are not an important reservoir of the organism.

The nymphal stage of the tick transmits the disease more often than the adult and larval stages do. Nymphs feed primarily in the summer, which accounts for the high incidence of disease at that time. The tick must feed for 24–48 hours to transmit an infectious dose. This implies that inspecting the skin after being exposed can prevent the disease. However, the nymphs are quite small and can easily be missed. There is no human-to-human spread.

The disease occurs worldwide. In the United States, three regions are primarily affected: the states along the North Atlantic seaboard; the northern Midwestern states, eg, Wisconsin; and the West Coast, especially California. In 1996, approximately 80% of the reported cases occurred in four states, New York, Connecticut, Pennsylvania, and New Jersey. Lyme disease is the most common vector-borne disease in the United States. The major bacterial diseases transmitted by ticks in the United States are Lyme disease, Rocky Mountain spotted fever, ehrlichiosis, relapsing fever, and tularemia.

Pathogenesis & Clinical Findings   Pathogenesis is associated with spread of the organism from the bite site through the surrounding skin followed by dissemination via the blood to various organs, especially the heart, joints, and central nervous system. No exotoxins, enzymes, or other important virulence factors have been identified.

---

*In California, the woodrat is the main reservoir and a second tick, *Ixodes neotomae,* perpetuates the infection in the woodrat but does not transmit the infection to humans.

The clinical findings have been divided into three stages; however, this is a progressive disease, and the stages are not discrete. In stage 1, **erythema chronicum migrans,** a spreading, nonpruritic, circular red rash with a clear center at the bite site is the most common finding. Both the tick bite and the rash are painless. The rash can, but need not, be accompanied by nonspecific "flulike" symptoms such as fever, chills, fatigue, and headache. Secondary skin lesions frequently occur. Arthralgias, but not arthritis, are another common finding in the early stage.

In stage 2, which occurs weeks to months later, cardiac and neurologic involvement predominates. Myocarditis or pericarditis, accompanied by various forms of heart block, occurs. Acute (aseptic) meningitis and cranial neuropathies, such as seventh-nerve palsy (Bell's palsy), are prominent during this stage. Peripheral neuropathies also occur. A latent phase lasting weeks to months typically ensues. In stage 3, arthritis, usually of the large joints, eg, knees, is a characteristic finding. Chronic progressive central nervous system disease also occurs.

Laboratory Diagnosis   Although the organism can be grown in the laboratory, cultures are rarely positive and so are usually not done. The diagnosis is typically made serologically by detecting either IgM antibody or a rising titer of IgG antibody with ELISA or an indirect immunofluorescence test. Unfortunately, there are problems with the specificity and sensitivity of these tests because of the presence of cross-reacting antibodies against spirochetes in the normal flora. A positive test should be confirmed with a Western blot analysis. In addition, patients treated early in the disease may not develop detectable antibodies. A PCR (polymerase chain reaction) test that detects the organism's DNA is also available.

Treatment & Prevention   The treatment of choice for stage 1 disease or other mild manifestations is either doxycycline or amoxicillin. For more severe forms or late-stage disease, penicillin G or ceftriaxone is more effective. There is no significant antibiotic resistance. Prevention centers on wearing protective clothing and using insect repellents. Examining the skin carefully for ticks is also very important, because the tick must feed for 24–48 hours to transmit an infective dose. If the risk of infection in a specific area is high, ie, *B burgdorferi* is found in a significant fraction of ixodid ticks, then either doxycycline or amoxicillin is a cost-effective preventive measure.

2.   *Borrelia recurrentis* & *Borrelia hermsii*

Borrelia recurrentis, Borrelia hermsii, and several other borreliae cause relapsing fever. During infection, the **antigens** of these organisms **undergo variation.** As antibodies develop against one antigen, variants emerge and produce relapses of the illness. This can be repeated 3–10 times.

B recurrentis is transmitted from person to person by the **human body louse.** Humans are the only hosts. *B hermsii* and many other *Borrelia* species are transmitted to humans by soft **ticks** (*Ornithodorus*). Rodents and other small animals are the main reservoirs. These species of *Borrelia* are passed transovarially in the ticks, a phenomenon that plays an important role in maintaining the organism in nature.

During infection, the arthropod bite introduces spirochetes, which then multiply in many tissues, producing fever, chills, headaches, and multiple-organ dysfunction. Each attack is terminated as antibodies arise.

Diagnosis is usually made by seeing the large spirochetes in stained smears of peripheral blood. They can be cultured in special media. Serologic tests are rarely useful. Tetracycline may be beneficial early in the illness and may prevent relapses. Avoidance of arthropod vectors is the best means of prevention.

LEPTOSPIRA

Leptospiras are tightly coiled, fine spirochetes that are not stained with dyes but are seen by dark-field microscopy. They grow in bacteriologic media containing serum.

Leptospira interrogans is the cause of leptospirosis. It is divided into serogroups that occur in different animals and geographic locations. Each serogroup is subdivided into serovars by the response to agglutination tests.

Leptospiras infect various animals including **rats** and other rodents, domestic livestock, and household pets. In the United States, dogs are the most important reservoir. Animals excrete leptospiras in **urine,** which contaminates water and soil. Swimming in contaminated water or consuming contaminated food or drink can result in human infection. Miners, farmers, and people who work in sewers are at high risk. Person-to-person transmission is rare.

Human infection results when leptospiras are ingested or pass through mucous membranes or skin. They circulate in the blood and multiply in various organs, producing fever and dysfunction of the liver (jaundice, hemorrhage), kidneys (uremia), and central nervous system (aseptic meningitis). The illness is typically **"biphasic,"** with fever, chills, and intense headache appearing early in the disease followed by a short period of resolution of these symptoms as the organisms are cleared from the blood. The second, "immune," phase is most often characterized by the findings of aseptic meningitis and, in severe cases, liver damage (jaundice) and impaired kidney function. Serovar-specific immunity develops with infection.

Diagnosis is based on history of possible exposure, suggestive clinical signs, and a marked rise in agglutinating-antibody titers. Occasionally, leptospiras are isolated from blood and urine cultures.

The treatment of choice is penicillin G. There is no significant antibiotic resistance. Prevention primarily involves avoiding contact with the contaminated environment. Doxycycline is effective in preventing the disease in exposed persons.

OTHER SPIROCHETES

Anaerobic saprophytic spirochetes are prominent in the normal flora of the human mouth. Such spirochetes participate in mixed anaerobic infections, infected human bites, stasis ulcers, etc.

Spirillum minor causes one type of rat bite fever in humans.

Review Questions

1. *Treponema pallidum* cannot be seen on Gram's stain. Why?
2. How is syphilis transmitted to an adult? to a fetus?
3. What are the number and distribution of the organisms in (a) primary, (b) secondary, and (c) late syphilis?
4. What are the differences between the treponemal and nontreponemal antibody tests?
5. How can syphilis be prevented?
6. What is the mode of transmission of (a) Lyme disease, (b) relapsing fever, and (c) leptospirosis?
7. What is the main reservoir for (a) *Treponema pallidum,* (b) *Borrelia burgdorferi?*
8. How is Lyme disease diagnosed in the laboratory?

25

Chlamydiae

Chlamydiae are obligate intracellular parasites. They are the agents of psittacosis, trachoma, lymphogranuloma venereum, and other infections.

Diseases   *Chlamydia psittaci* causes psittacosis; *Chlamydia trachomatis* causes eye, respiratory, and genital tract infections. *C trachomatis* is the **most common cause of sexually transmitted disease** in the United States. *Chlamydia pneumoniae* (formerly called the TWAR strain) causes atypical pneumonia (Table 25–1).

Table 25–1. Chlamydiae.

Medically Important Species	Disease	Natural Hosts	Mode of Transmission to Humans	Number of Immunologic Types	Diagnosis	Treatment
C psittaci	Psittacosis (pneumonia)	Birds	Inhalation of dried bird feces.	1	Serologic test (cell culture rarely done).	Tetracycline
C trachomatis	Urethritis, pneumonia, conjunctivitis, lymphogranuloma venereum, trachoma	Humans	Sexual contact; perinatal transmission.	More than 15	Inclusions in epithelial cells seen with Giemsa's stain or by immunofluorescence; also cell culture.	Tetracycline, erythromycin
C pneumoniae	Atypical pneumonia	Humans	Respiratory droplets.	1	Serologic test.	Tetracycline

Important Properties   Chlamydiae are **obligate intracellular** bacteria. They lack the ability to produce sufficient energy to grow independently and therefore can grow only inside host cells. They have a rigid cell wall but do not have a typical peptidoglycan layer. Their cell walls resemble those of gram-negative bacteria but lack muramic acid.

Chlamydiae have a replicative cycle different from that of all other bacteria. The cycle begins when the extracellular, metabolically inert, "sporelike," **elementary body** enters the cell and reorganizes into a larger, metabolically active **reticulate body** (Figure 25–1). The latter undergoes repeated binary fission to form daughter elementary bodies, which are released from the cell. Within cells, the site of replication appears as an inclusion body, which can be stained and visualized microscopically. These inclusions are useful in the diagnosis of these organisms in the clinical laboratory.

All chlamydiae share a group-specific lipopolysaccharide antigen, which is detected by complement fixation tests. They also possess species-specific and immunotype-specific antigens (proteins), which are detected by immunofluorescence. *C psittaci* and *C pneumoniae* each have one immunotype, whereas *C trachomatis* has at least 15.

Transmission & Epidemiology   *C psittaci* infects **birds** and many mammals. Humans are infected primarily by **inhaling** organisms in dry bird feces. *C trachomatis* infects **only humans** and is usually transmitted by close personal contact, eg, **sexually** or by **passage through the birth canal.** Individuals with **asymptomatic genital tract infections** are an important reservoir of infection for others. In trachoma, *C trachomatis* is transmitted by finger-to-eye or fomite-to-eye contact. *C pneumoniae* infects only humans and is transmitted from person to person by aerosol.

Disease caused by these organisms occurs worldwide, but trachoma is most frequently found in developing countries in dry, hot regions. Nongonococcal urethritis caused by *C trachomatis* is said to occur more frequently in higher socioeconomic groups, in contrast to gonorrhea, which is found predominantly in lower socioeconomic groups. However, the two diseases commonly occur simultaneously in the same individual.

Pathogenesis & Clinical Findings   Chlamydiae infect primarily **epithelial cells** of the mucous membranes or the lungs. They rarely cause invasive, disseminated infections. *C psittaci* infects the lungs primarily. The infection may be asymptomatic (detected only by a rising antibody titer) or may produce high fever and pneumonia. Human psittacosis is not generally communicable. *C pneumoniae* causes upper and lower respiratory tract infections, especially bronchitis and pneumonia, in young adults.

C trachomatis exists in more than 15 immunotypes (A–L). Types A, B, and C cause **trachoma,** a chronic conjunctivitis endemic in Africa and Asia. Trachoma may recur over many years and may lead to blindness but causes no systemic illness. Types D–K cause **genital tract infections,** which are occasionally transmitted to the eyes or the respiratory tract. In men, it is a common cause of nongonococcal urethritis, which may progress to epididymitis, prostatitis, or proctitis. In women, cervicitis develops and may progress to salpingitis and pelvic inflammatory disease (PID). Repeated

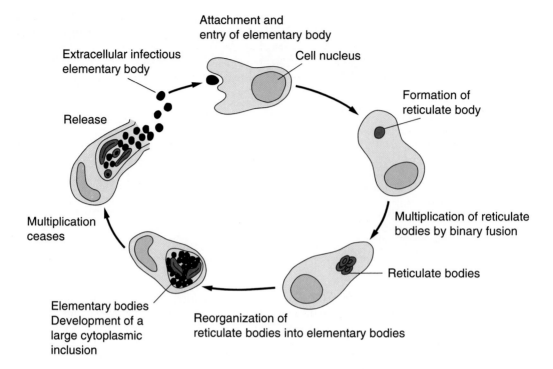

Figure 25–1. Life cycle of *Chlamydia*. The extracellular, inert elementary body enters an epithelial cell and changes into a reticulate body that divides many times by binary fission. The daughter reticulate bodies change into elementary bodies and are released from the epithelial cell. The cytoplasmic inclusion body, which is characteristic of chlamydial infections, consists of many daughter reticulate and elementary bodies. (Modified and reproduced, with permission, from Ryan K et al: *Sherris Medical Microbiology,* 3rd ed. Appleton & Lange, 1994.)

episodes of salpingitis or PID can result in infertility or ectopic pregnancy. Infants born to infected mothers often develop mucopurulent eye infections (neonatal inclusion conjunctivitis) 7–12 days after delivery, and some develop chlamydial pneumonitis 2–12 weeks after birth. Patients with genital tract infections caused by *C trachomatis* have a high incidence of **Reiter's syndrome,** which is characterized by urethritis, arthritis, and uveitis. Reiter's syndrome is an autoimmune disease caused by antibodies formed against *C trachomatis* cross-reacting with antigens on the cells of the urethra, joints, and uveal tract (see Chapter 66).

C trachomatis L1–L3 immunotypes cause **lymphogranuloma venereum,** a sexually transmitted disease with lesions on genitalia and in lymph nodes.

Infection by *C trachomatis* leads to formation of antibodies and cell-mediated reactions but not to resistance to reinfection or elimination of organisms.

Laboratory Diagnosis   Chlamydiae form **cytoplasmic inclusions,** which can be seen with special stains (eg, Giemsa's stain) or by immunofluorescence. The Gram stain is not useful. In exudates, the organism can be identified within epithelial cells by fluorescent antibody staining or hybridization with a DNA probe. Chlamydial antigens can also be detected in exudates or urine by ELISA. Tests not involving culture are now more commonly used than culture-based tests.

Chlamydiae can be grown in cell cultures treated with cycloheximide, which inhibits host cell but not chlamydial protein synthesis, thereby enhancing chlamydial replication. In culture, *C trachomatis* forms inclusions containing glycogen whereas *C psittaci* and *C pneumoniae* form inclusions that do not contain glycogen. The glycogen-filled inclusions are visualized by staining with iodine. Exudates from eyes, respiratory tract, or genital tract give positive cultures in about half of cases.

Serologic tests are used to diagnose infections by *C psittaci* and *C pneumoniae,* but are rarely helpful in diagnosing disease caused by *C trachomatis* because the frequency of infection is so high that many people already have antibodies.

Treatment   All chlamydiae are susceptible to tetracyclines and erythromycin. Treatment suppresses signs and symptoms but does not regularly eradicate the organisms. *C trachomatis* is susceptible to either tetracycline or erythromycin. The treatment of choice for *C psittaci* and *C pneumoniae* infections is tetracycline. The drug of choice for lymphogranuloma venereum is a tetracycline. The treatment of choice for *C trachomatis* sexually transmitted diseases is azithromycin.

Prevention   Psittacosis in humans is controlled by restricting the importation of psittacine birds, destroying sick birds, and adding tetracycline to bird feed. Domestic flocks of turkeys and ducks are surveyed for the presence of *C psittaci.*

   C trachomatis infection in humans should be diagnosed and treated early both in clinically manifest cases and in asymptomatic sexual contacts. Several types of sexually transmitted diseases are often present simultaneously. Thus, diagnosis of one requires a search for other etiologic agents. Erythromycin given to newborn infants of infected mothers can prevent inclusion conjunctivitis and pneumonitis.

   There is no vaccine available against any chlamydial disease.

Review Questions

   1. Why are chlamydiae obligate intracellular parasites?
   2. Describe the life cycle of chlamydiae.
   3. Contrast the natural reservoirs of *Chlamydia psittaci* and *Chlamydia trachomatis.*
   4. What is the relationship of serotype to disease with (a) *C psittaci* and (b) *C trachomatis?*
   5. How are chlamydial infections diagnosed in the clinical laboratory?

Rickettsiae

26

Rickettsiae are obligate intracellular parasites. They are the agents of typhus, spotted fevers, and Q fever.

Diseases   In the United States, there are two rickettsial diseases of significance: Rocky Mountain spotted fever, caused by *Rickettsia rickettsii,* and Q fever, caused by *Coxiella burnetii.* Several other rickettsial diseases such as epidemic, endemic, and scrub typhus are important in developing countries. Rickettsialpox, caused by *Rickettsia akari,* is a rare disease found in certain densely populated cities in the United States. *Ehrlichia chafeensis* is described in Chapter 27.

Important Properties   Rickettsiae are very short rods that are barely visible in the light microscope. Structurally, their cell wall resembles that of gram-negative rods, but they stain poorly with the standard Gram stain.

   Rickettsiae are **obligate intracellular parasites** because they are unable to produce sufficient energy to replicate extracellularly. Therefore, rickettsiae must be grown in cell culture, embryonated eggs, or experimental animals. Rickettsiae divide by binary fission within the host cell, in contrast to chlamydiae, which are also obligate intracellular parasites but replicate by a distinctive intracellular cycle.

   Several rickettsiae, such as *Rickettsia prowazekii, Rickettsia tsutsugamushi,* and *R rickettsii,* possess antigens that cross-react with antigens of the OX strains of *Proteus vulgaris.* The **Weil-Felix** test, which detects antirickettsial antibodies in a patient's serum by agglutination of the *Proteus* organisms, is based on this cross-reaction.

Transmission   The most striking aspect of the life cycle of the rickettsiae is that they are maintained in nature in certain arthropods such as ticks, lice, fleas, and mites and, with one exception, are transmitted to humans by the **bite of the arthropod.** The exception to arthropod transmission is *C burnetii,* the cause of Q fever, which is transmitted by aerosol and inhaled into the lungs. Virtually all rickettsial diseases are zoonoses (ie, they have an animal reservoir), with the prominent exception of **epidemic typhus, which occurs only in humans.** A summary of the vectors and reservoirs for selected rickettsial diseases is presented in Table 26–1.

The incidence of the disease depends on the geographic distribution of the arthropod vector and on the risk of exposure, which is enhanced by such things as poor hygienic conditions and camping in wooded areas. These factors are discussed below with the individual diseases.

Pathogenesis   The typical lesion caused by the rickettsiae is a **vasculitis,** particularly in the endothelial lining of the vessel wall where the organism is found. Damage to the vessels of the skin results in the characteristic rash and in edema and hemorrhage due to increased capillary permeability. The basis for pathogenesis by these organisms is unclear. There is some evidence that endotoxin is involved, which is in accord with the nature of some of the lesions such as fever and petechiae, but its role has not been confirmed. No exotoxins or cytolytic enzymes have been found.

Clinical Findings & Epidemiology   This section is limited to the two rickettsial diseases that are most common in the United States, ie, Rocky Mountain spotted fever and Q fever, and to the other major rickettsial disease, typhus.

A. Rocky Mountain Spotted Fever: This disease is characterized by the acute onset of nonspecific symptoms, eg, fever, severe headache, myalgias, and prostration. The typical rash, which appears 2–6 days later, begins with macules that frequently progress to petechiae. The rash usually appears first on the hands and feet and then moves inward to the trunk. In addition to headache, other profound central nervous system changes such as delirium and coma can occur. Disseminated intravascular coagulation, edema, and circulatory collapse may ensue in severe cases. The diagnosis must be made on clinical grounds and therapy started promptly, because the laboratory diagnosis is delayed until a rise in antibody titer can be observed.

The name of the disease is misleading, because it occurs primarily along the **East Coast** of the United States, where the dog tick, *Dermacentor variabilis,* is located. The name "Rocky Mountain spotted fever" is derived from the region in which the disease was first found.* The **tick** is an important reservoir of *R rickettsii* as well as the vector; the organism is passed by the transovarian route from tick to tick, and a lifetime infection results. Certain mammals, such as dogs and rodents, are also reservoirs of the organism. Humans are accidental hosts and are not required for the perpetuation of the organism in nature; there is no person-to-person transmission. Most cases occur in children during spring and early summer, when the ticks are active. Rocky Mountain spotted fever accounts for 95% of the rickettsial disease in the United States; there are about 1000 cases per year. It can be fatal if untreated, but if it is diagnosed and treated, a prompt cure results.

B. Q Fever†:   Unlike the other rickettsial diseases, the main focus of disease in Q fever is in the lungs. It begins suddenly with fever, severe headache, and influenzalike symptoms. This is all that occurs in many patients, but pneumonia ensues in about half. Hepatitis is frequent enough that the combination of pneumonia and hepatitis should suggest Q fever. A rash is rare, unlike in the other rickettsial diseases. In general, Q fever is an acute disease and recovery is expected even in the absence of antibiotic therapy. Rarely, chronic Q fever characterized by a life-threatening endocarditis occurs.

Q fever is the one rickettsial disease that is *not* transmitted to humans by the bite of an arthropod. The important reservoirs for human infection are cattle, sheep, and goats. The agent, *C burnetii,* which causes an inapparent infection in these reservoir hosts, is found in high concentrations in the urine, feces, placental tissue, and amniotic fluid of the animals. It is transmitted to humans by **inhalation of aerosols** of these materials. The disease occurs worldwide, chiefly in individuals whose occupations expose them to livestock, such as shepherds, abattoir employees, and farm workers.

---

*In the western United States, it is transmitted by the wood tick, *Dermacentor andersoni.*
†Q stands for "Query"; the cause of this disease was a question mark, ie, was unknown, when the disease was first described in Australia in 1937.

Table 26–1. Summary of selected rickettsial diseases.

Disease	Organism	Arthropod Vector	Mammalian Reservoir	Important in the United States
Spotted fevers Rocky Mountain spotted fever	R rickettsii	Ticks	Dogs, rodents	Yes (especially on the East Coast)
Rickettsialpox	R akari	Mites	Mice	No
Typhus group Epidemic	R prowazekii	Lice	Humans	No
Endemic	R typhi	Fleas	Rodents	No
Scrub	R tsutsugamushi	Mites	Rodents	No
Others Q fever	C burnetii	None	Cattle, sheep, goats	Yes

Cows' milk is usually responsible for subclinical infections rather than disease in humans. Pasteurization of milk kills the organism.

C. Typhus: There are several different forms of typhus, namely louse-borne epidemic typhus caused by *R prowazekii,* flea-borne endemic typhus caused by *Rickettsia typhi,* chigger-borne scrub typhus caused by *R tsutsugamushi,* and several other quite rare forms. The following description is limited to epidemic typhus, the most important of the typhus group of diseases.

Typhus begins with the sudden onset of chills, fever, headache, and other influenzalike symptoms approximately 1–3 weeks after the louse bite occurs. Between the fifth and ninth days after the onset of symptoms, a maculopapular rash begins on the trunk and spreads peripherally. Signs of severe meningoencephalitis, including delirium and coma, begin with the rash and continue into the second and third weeks. In untreated cases, death occurs from peripheral vascular collapse or from the most frequent complication, bacterial pneumonia.

Epidemic typhus is transmitted from person to person by the **human body louse,** *Pediculus.* When a bacteremic patient is bitten, the organism is ingested by the louse and multiplies in the gut epithelium. It is excreted in the feces of the louse during the act of biting the next person and autoinoculated by the person while scratching the bite. The infected louse dies after a few weeks, and there is no louse-to-louse transmission, so that human infection is an obligatory stage in the cycle. Epidemic typhus is associated with wars and poverty; at present it is found in developing countries in Africa and South America but not in the United States.

A recurrent form of epidemic typhus is called Brill-Zinsser disease. The signs and symptoms are similar to those of epidemic typhus but are less severe, of shorter duration, and rarely fatal. Recurrences can appear as long as 50 years later and can be precipitated by another intercurrent disease. In the United States, the disease is seen in older people who had epidemic typhus during World War II in Europe. Brill-Zinsser disease is epidemiologically interesting; persistently infected patients can serve as a source of the organism should a louse bite occur.

Laboratory Diagnosis Laboratory diagnosis of rickettsial diseases is based on serologic analysis rather than isolation of the organism. Although rickettsiae can be grown in cell culture or embryonated eggs, this is a hazardous procedure that is not available in the standard clinical laboratory.

Of the two serologic tests, complement fixation is more frequently used and provides more specific data than the Weil-Felix reaction. (A microagglutination test is used by public health laboratories but is not widely available.) As usual, a 4-fold rise in antibody titer found in a convalescent-phase serum sample is significant. However, in the presence of the clinical picture of Rocky Mountain spotted fever, a single acute-phase serum titer of 1:16 or greater is diagnostic.

The Weil-Felix test is based on the cross-reaction of an antigen present in many rickettsiae with the O antigen polysaccharide found in *P vulgaris* OX-2, OX-19, and OX-K. The test measures the presence of antirickettsial antibodies in the patient's serum by their ability to agglutinate *Proteus* bacteria. The specific rickettsial organism can be identified by the agglutination observed with one or another of these three different strains of *P vulgaris.* However, since there can be false-positive reactions following *Proteus* urinary tract infections and false-negative reactions due to variable antibody responses, and since no Weil-Felix agglutinins are made in Q fever, the test is of limited value.

Treatment   The treatment of choice for all rickettsial diseases is tetracycline, with chloramphenicol as the second choice.

Prevention   Prevention of many of these diseases is based on reducing exposure to the arthropod vector by wearing protective clothing and using insect repellent. Frequent examination of the skin for ticks is important in preventing Rocky Mountain spotted fever; the tick must be attached for several hours to transmit the disease. Prevention of typhus is based on personal hygiene and "delousing" with DDT. A typhus vaccine containing formalin-killed *R prowazekii* organisms is effective and useful in the military during wartime but is not available to civilians in the United States. Persons at high risk of contracting Q fever, such as veterinarians, shepherds, abattoir workers, and laboratory personnel exposed to *C burnetii,* should receive the vaccine that consists of the killed organism.

Review Questions

1. Why are most rickettsiae obligate intracellular parasites?
2. What is the common mode of transmission for all rickettsiae except *Coxiella burnetii?* How is *C burnetii* transmitted?
3. What is the pathogenesis of most rickettsial diseases (except Q fever)? Why do they cause a rash?
4. Contrast Rocky Mountain spotted fever and Q fever from the following points of view: (a) geographical distribution, (b) major symptoms, (c) Weil-Felix test reaction, and (d) possible mode of prevention.
5. Why is epidemic typhus not a zoonotic disease?
6. What is the Weil-Felix test, and what is its role in diagnosis?

27

Minor Bacterial Pathogens

The bacterial pathogens of lesser medical importance are briefly described in this chapter. Experts may differ on their choice of which organisms to put in this category. Nevertheless, separating the minor from the major pathogens should allow the reader to focus on the more important pathogens while providing at least some information about the less important ones.

These organisms are presented in alphabetical order. Table 27–1 lists the organisms according to their appearance on Gram's stain.

Achromobacter   *Achromobacter* species are gram-negative coccobacillary rods found chiefly in water supplies. They are opportunistic pathogens and are involved in sepsis, pneumonia, and urinary tract infections.

Acinetobacter   *Acinetobacter* species are gram-negative coccobacillary rods found commonly in soil and water, but they can be part of the normal flora. They are opportunistic pathogens that readily colonize patients with compromised host defenses. *Acinetobacter calcoaceticus,* the species usually involved in human infection, causes disease chiefly in a hospital setting usually associated with respiratory therapy equipment and indwelling catheters. Sepsis, pneumonia, and urinary tract infections are the most frequent manifestations. Previous names for this organism include *Herellea* and *Mima.*

Actinobacillus   *Actinobacillus* species are gram-negative coccobacillary rods. *Actinobacillus actinomycetemcomitans* is found as part of the normal flora in the upper respiratory tract. It is a rare opportunistic pathogen, causing endocarditis on damaged heart valves and sepsis.

Table 27–1. Minor bacterial pathogens.

Type of Bacterium	Genus or Species
Gram-positive cocci	*Micrococcus, Peptococcus, Peptostreptococcus, Sarcina*
Gram-positive rods	*Arachnia, Arcanobacterium, Bifidobacterium, Erysipelothrix, Eubacterium, Gardnerella, Lactobacillus, Mobiluncus, Propionibacterium, Rhodococcus*
Gram-negative cocci	*Veillonella*
Gram-negative rods	*Achromobacter, Acinetobacter, Actinobacillus, Aeromonas, Alcaligenes, Arizona, Bartonella, Calymmatobacterium, Capnocytophaga, Cardiobacterium, Chromobacterium, Citrobacter, Edwardsiella, Eikenella, Erwinia, Flavobacterium, Fusobacterium, HACEK group, Haemophilus ducreyi, Hafnia, Kingella, Moraxella, Pleisomonas, Porphyromonas, Pseudomonas pseudomallei, Spirillum, Streptobacillus, Vibrio vulnificus, Yersinia enterocolitica, Yersinia pseudotuberculosis*
Rickettsia	*Ehrlichia*
Unclassified	*Tropheryma*

Aeromonas   *Aeromonas* species are gram-negative rods found in water, soil, food, and animal and human feces. *Aeromonas hydrophila* causes wound infections, diarrhea, and sepsis, especially in immunocompromised patients.

Alcaligenes   *Alcaligenes* species are gram-negative coccobacillary rods that are found in soil and water and are associated with water-containing materials such as respirators in hospitals. *Alcaligenes faecalis* is an opportunistic pathogen, causing sepsis and pneumonia.

Arachnia   *Arachnia* species are anaerobic gram-positive rods that form long, branching filaments similar to those of *Actinomyces*. They are found primarily in the mouth (associated with dental plaque) and in the tonsillar crypts. *Arachnia propionica,* the major species, causes abscesses similar to those of *Actinomyces israelii,* including the presence of "sulfur granules" in the lesions.

Arcanobacterium   *Arcanobacterium haemolyticum* is a club-shaped gram-positive rod that closely resembles corynebacteria. It is a rare cause of pharyngitis and chronic skin ulcers. The pharyngitis can be accompanied by a rash resembling the rash of scarlet fever.

Arizona   *Arizona* species are gram-negative rods in the family *Enterobacteriaceae;* they ferment lactose slowly. *Arizona hinshawii* is found in the feces of chickens and other domestic animals and causes diseases similar to those caused by *Salmonella,* such as enterocolitis and enteric fevers. The organism is usually transmitted by contaminated food, eg, dried eggs.

Bartonella   *Bartonella* species are pleomorphic gram-negative rods. *Bartonella henselae* (formerly called *Rochalimaea henselae*) is the cause of **bacillary angiomatosis.** This disease occurs in immunocompromised individuals, especially AIDS patients. It is characterized by proliferative, vascular lesions resembling Kaposi's sarcoma in the skin and visceral organs. Treatment with doxycycline can be effective.

In immunocompetent people, *Bartonella henselae* causes **cat-scratch fever.** This disease is characterized by localized lymphadenopathy in a person who has had contact with a cat. The organism is a member of the oral flora of many cats. The diagnosis is supported by characteristic histopathology on a biopsied lymph node and a positive skin test. The disease is mild and self-limited, and no antibiotic therapy is recommended.

Bartonella quintana (formerly called *Rochalimaea quintana*) is the cause of trench fever. Trench fever is transmitted by body lice, and humans are the reservoir for the organism. *Bartonella bacilliformis* causes two rare diseases: Oroya fever and verruga peruana, both of which are stages of Carrión's disease. The disease occurs only in certain areas of the Andes Mountains, and an animal reservoir is suspected.

Bifidobacterium   *Bifidobacterium eriksonii* is a gram-positive, filamentous, anaerobic rod found as part of the normal flora in the mouth and gastrointestinal tract. It occurs in mixed anaerobic infections.

Branhamella   *Branhamella catarrhalis* has been renamed *Moraxella catarrhalis* (see *Moraxella,* below).

Calymmatobacterium   *Calymmatobacterium granulomatis* is a gram-negative rod that causes granuloma inguinale, a sexually transmitted disease characterized by genital ulceration and soft-tissue and bone destruction. The diagnosis is made by visualizing the stained organisms (Donovan bodies) within large macrophages from the lesion. Tetracycline is the treatment of choice for this disease, which is rare in the United States but endemic in many developing countries.

Capnocytophaga   *Capnocytophaga gingivalis* is a gram-negative fusiform rod that is associated with periodontal disease, but it can also be an opportunistic pathogen, causing sepsis.

Cardiobacterium   *Cardiobacterium hominis* is a gram-negative pleomorphic rod. It is a member of the normal flora of the human colon, but it can be an opportunistic pathogen, causing mainly endocarditis.

Chromobacterium   *Chromobacterium violaceum* is a gram-negative rod that produces a violet pigment. It is found in soil and water and can cause wound infections, especially in subtropical parts of the world.

Citrobacter   *Citrobacter* species are gram-negative rods (members of the *Enterobacteriaceae*) related to *Salmonella* and *Arizona*. They occur in the environment and in the human colon and can cause sepsis in immunocompromised patients.

Edwardsiella   *Edwardsiella* species are gram-negative rods (members of the *Enterobacteriaceae*) resembling *Salmonella*. They can cause enterocolitis, sepsis, and wound infections.

Eikenella   *Eikenella corrodens* is a gram-negative rod that is a member of the normal flora in the human mouth and causes skin and bone infections associated with **human bites** and "clenched fist" injuries. It also causes sepsis and soft tissue infections of the head and neck, especially in immunocompromised patients and in drug abusers who lick needles prior to injection.

Ehrlichia   *Ehrlichia chaffeensis* is a member of the rickettsia family and causes human monocytic ehrlichiosis (HME). This disease resembles Rocky Mountain spotted fever, except that the typical rash usually does not occur. High fever, severe headache, and myalgias are prominent symptoms. The organism is endemic in dogs and is transmitted to humans by ticks, especially the dog tick, *Dermacentor* and the Lone star tick, *Amblyomma*. *E chaffeensis* primarily infects mononuclear leukocytes and forms characteristic **"morulae"** in the cytoplasm. (A morula is an inclusion body that resembles a mulberry.) Lymphopenia, thrombocytopenia, and elevated liver enzyme values are seen. In the United States, the disease occurs primarily in the southern states, especially Arkansas. The diagnosis is usually made serologically. Doxycycline is the treatment of choice.

Another form of ehrlichiosis, called human granulocytic ehrlichiosis (HGE), is caused by an organism closely resembling *E equi*. Either *Dermacentor* or *Ixodes* ticks are the vectors. In HGE, granulocytes are infected rather than mononuclear cells, but the disease is clinically indistinguishable from that caused by *E chaffeensis*. The diagnostic approach and the treatment are the same for both forms of ehrlichiosis.

Erwinia   *Erwinia* species are gram-negative rods (members of the *Enterobacteriaceae*) found in soil and water and are rarely involved in human disease.

Erysipelothrix   *Erysipelothrix rhusiopathiae* is a gram-positive rod that causes erysipeloid, a skin infection that resembles erysipelas (caused by streptococci). Erysipeloid usually occurs on the hands of meat and **fish handlers.**

Eubacterium   *Eubacterium* species are gram-positive, anaerobic, non-spore-forming rods that are present in large numbers as part of the normal flora of the human colon. They rarely cause human disease.

Flavobacterium   *Flavobacterium* species are gram-negative rods found in soil and water. They can be opportunistic pathogens, causing meningitis and sepsis especially in premature infants.

Fusobacterium   *Fusobacterium* species are anaerobic gram-negative rods with pointed ends. They are part of the human normal flora of the mouth, colon, and female genital tract and are sometimes isolated from pulmonary, intra-abdominal, and pelvic abscesses. They are frequently found in mixed infections with other anaerobes and facultative anaerobes. *Fusobacterium nucleatum* occurs in cases of Vincent's angina (trench mouth), along with various spirochetes.

Gardnerella *Gardnerella vaginalis* is a facultative gram-variable rod associated with **bacterial vaginosis,** characterized by a malodorous vaginal discharge and **"clue cells,"** which are vaginal epithelial cells covered with bacteria. The drug of choice is metronidazole. *Mobiluncus* (see below), an anaerobic rod, is often found in this disease as well.

HACEK Group This is a group of small gram-negative rods that have in common the following: slow growth in culture, the requirement for high CO_2 levels to grow in culture, and the ability to cause endocarditis. The name "HACEK" is an acronym of the first letters of the genera of the following bacteria: *Haemophilus aphrophilus* and *H paraphrophilus, Actinobacillus actinomycetemcomitans, Cardiobacterium hominus, Eikenella corrodens,* and *Kingella kingae.*

Haemophilus aegyptius *Haemophilus aegyptius* (Koch-Weeks bacillus) is a small gram-negative rod that is an important cause of conjunctivitis in children. Certain strains of *H aegyptius* cause Brazilian purpuric fever, a life-threatening childhood infection characterized by purpura and shock.

Haemophilus ducreyi This small gram-negative rod causes the sexually transmitted disease **chancroid** (soft chancre), which is common in tropical countries but uncommon in the United States. The disease begins with penile lesions, which are painful; nonindurated (soft) ulcers; and local lymphadenitis (bubo). The diagnosis is made by isolating *Haemophilus ducreyi* from the ulcer or from pus aspirated from a lymph node. The organism requires heated (chocolate) blood agar supplemented with X factor (heme) but, unlike *Haemophilus influenzae,* does not require V factor (NAD). Chancroid can be treated with erythromycin, azithromycin, or ceftriaxone.

Hafnia *Hafnia* species are gram-negative rods (members of the *Enterobacteriaceae*) found in soil and water and are rare opportunistic pathogens.

Kingella *Kingella kingae* is a gram-negative rod in the normal flora of the human oropharynx. It is a rare cause of opportunistic infection and endocarditis.

Lactobacillus Lactobacilli are gram-positive non-spore-forming rods found as members of the normal flora in the mouth, colon, and female genital tract. In the mouth, they may play a role in the production of dental caries. In the vagina, they are the main source of lactic acid, which keeps the pH low. Lactobacilli are rare causes of opportunistic infection.

Micrococcus Micrococci are gram-positive cocci that are part of the normal flora of the skin. They are rare human pathogens.

Mobiluncus *Mobiluncus* species are anaerobic gram-positive curved rods that often stain gram-variable. They are associated with **bacterial vaginosis** in women. *Gardnerella* (see above), a facultative rod, is often found in this disease as well.

Moraxella *Moraxella* species are gram-negative coccobacillary rods resembling neisseriae. *Moraxella catarrhalis* is the major pathogen in this genus. Although considered to be a member of the normal flora of the upper respiratory tract, it can cause sinusitis, otitis, bronchitis, and pneumonia, especially in immunocompromised patients. Trimethoprim-sulfamethoxazole or amoxicillin-clavulanate can be used to treat these infections. Most clinical isolates produce β-lactamase. *Moraxella nonliquefaciens* is one of the two common causes of blepharitis (infection of the eyelid); *Staphylococcus aureus* is the other. The usual treatment is local application of antibiotic ointment, such as erythromycin.

Peptococcus Peptococci are anaerobic gram-positive cocci, resembling staphylococci, found as members of the normal flora of the mouth and colon. They are also isolated from abscesses of various organs, usually from mixed anaerobic infections.

Peptostreptococcus Peptostreptococci are anaerobic gram-positive cocci found as members of the normal flora of the mouth and colon. They are also isolated from abscesses of various organs, usually from mixed anaerobic infections.

Pleisomonas *Pleisomonas shigelloides* is a gram-negative rod associated with water sources. It causes self-limited gastroenteritis, primarily in tropical areas, and can cause invasive disease in immunocompromised individuals.

Porphyromonas *Porphyromonas gingivalis* and *P endodontalis* are anaerobic gram-negative rods found in the mouth. They cause periodontal infections, such as gingivitis and dental abscesses.

Propionibacterium Propionibacteria are pleomorphic, anaerobic gram-positive rods found on the skin and in the gastrointestinal tract. *Propionibacterium acnes* is part of the normal flora of the skin and can cause opportunistic infections. Its lipase contributes to the genesis of acne.

Pseudomonas pseudomallei *Pseudomonas pseudomallei* is a gram-negative rod that causes melioidosis, a rare disease found primarily in Southeast Asia. The organism is found in soil and is transmitted most often when soil contaminates skin abrasions. This disease has been seen in the United States since infections acquired by members of the armed forces during the Vietnam War have reactivated many years later. The acute disease is characterized by high fever and bloody, purulent sputum. Untreated cases can proceed to sepsis and death. In the chronic form, the disease can appear as pneumonia or lung abscess or may resemble tuberculosis. Diagnosis is made by culturing the organism from blood or sputum. The treatment of choice is ceftazidime, which is administered for several weeks.

Rhodococcus *Rhodococcus equi* is a gram-positive bacterium whose shape varies from a coccus to a club-shaped rod. It is a rare cause of pneumonia and cavitary lung disease in patients whose cell-mediated immunity is compromised. The diagnosis is made by isolating the organism on laboratory agar and observing salmon-pink colonies that do not ferment most carbohydrates. The treatment of choice is a combination of rifampin and erythromycin.

Sarcina *Sarcina* species are anaerobic gram-positive cocci grouped in clusters of four or eight. They are minor members of the normal flora of the colon and are rarely pathogens.

Spirillum *Spirillum minor* is a gram-negative, spiral-shaped rod that causes rat-bite fever ("sodoku"). The disease is characterized by a reddish brown rash spreading from the bite, accompanied by fever and local lymphadenopathy. The diagnosis is made by a combination of microscopy and animal inoculation.

Streptobacillus *Streptobacillus moniliformis* is a gram-negative rod that causes another type of rat-bite fever (see *Spirillum,* above).

Tropheryma *Tropheryma whippelii* is the putative cause of Whipple's disease. Bacilli seen in duodenal lesions were identified as an actinomycete on the basis of amplification of the bacterial 16S ribosomal RNA and comparison with known related organisms. This identification is tentative because the organism has not been reproducibly grown in culture.

Veillonella *Veillonella parvula* is an anaerobic gram-negative diplococcus that is part of the normal flora of the mouth, colon, and vagina. It is a rare opportunistic pathogen that causes abscesses of the sinuses, tonsils, and brain, usually in mixed anaerobic infections.

Vibrio vulnificus *Vibrio vulnificus* is a comma-shaped gram-negative rod that is found in seawater. It is a "halophilic" organism; ie, it grows preferentially in water, such as seawater, that contains a high concentration of NaCl. It causes severe skin and soft tissue infections **(cellulitis), especially in shellfish handlers,** who often sustain skin wounds. It can also cause a rapidly fatal **septicemia in immunocompromised people who have eaten raw shellfish** containing the organism. Chronic liver disease, eg, cirrhosis, predisposes to severe infections. The recommended treatment is doxycycline.

Yersinia enterocolitica & Yersinia pseudotuberculosis *Yersinia enterocolitica* and *Yersinia pseudotuberculosis* are gram-negative oval rods that are larger than *Yersinia pestis.* The virulence factors produced by *Y pestis* are not made by these species. These organisms are transmitted to humans by contamination of food with the excreta of domestic animals such as dogs, cats, and cattle. *Yersinia* infections are relatively infrequent in the United States, but the number of documented cases has increased during the past few years, perhaps as a result of improved laboratory procedures.

Y enterocolitica causes enterocolitis that is clinically indistinguishable from that caused by *Salmonella* or *Shigella*. Both *Y enterocolitica* and *Y pseudotuberculosis* can cause **mesenteric adenitis** that clinically resembles acute appendicitis. Rarely, these organisms are involved in bacteremia or abscesses of the liver or spleen, mainly in persons with underlying diseases.

Y enterocolitica is usually isolated from stool specimens and forms a lactose-negative colony on MacConkey's agar. It grows better at 25 °C than at 37 °C; most biochemical tests are positive at 25 °C and negative at 37 °C. Incubation of a stool sample at 4 °C for 1 week, a technique called "cold enrichment," increases the frequency of recovery of the organism. *Y enterocolitica* can be distinguished from *Y pseudotuberculosis* by biochemical reactions.

The laboratory is usually not involved in the diagnosis of *Y pseudotuberculosis;* cultures are rarely performed in cases of mesenteric adenitis, and the organism is rarely recovered from stool specimens. Serologic tests are not available in most hospital clinical laboratories.

Enterocolitis and mesenteric adenitis caused by the organisms do not require treatment. In cases of bacteremia or abscess, either trimethoprim-sulfamethoxazole or ciprofloxacin is usually effective. There are no preventive measures except to guard against contamination of food by the excreta of domestic animals.

Part III: Basic Virology

In contrast to bacteria, fungi, and parasites, viruses are *not* cells, ie, they are not capable of reproducing independently, do not have a nucleus, and do not have organelles such as ribosomes, mitochondria, and lysosomes. Viruses are smaller than cells and cannot be seen in the light microscope.

(1) Viruses are particles composed of an internal core containing *either* DNA *or* RNA (but not both) covered by a protective protein coat. Some viruses have an outer lipoprotein membrane, called an envelope, external to the coat.

(2) Viruses must reproduce (replicate) within cells, because they cannot generate energy or synthesize proteins. Because they can reproduce only within cells, viruses are **"obligate intracellular parasites."**

(3) Viruses replicate in a manner different from that of cells; ie, viruses do not undergo binary fission or mitosis.

Table 1 compares some of the attributes of viruses and cells.

Table 1. Comparison of viruses and cells.

Property	Viruses	Cells
Type of nucleic acid	DNA or RNA but not both	DNA and RNA
Proteins	Few	Many
Lipoprotein membrane	Envelope present in some viruses	Cell membrane present in all cells
Ribosomes	Absent[1]	Present
Mitochondria	Absent	Present in eukaryotic cells
Enzymes	None or few	Many
Multiplication by binary fission or mitosis	No	Yes

[1] Arenaviruses have a few nonfunctional ribosomes.

28

Structure

SIZE & SHAPE

Viruses range from 20 to 300 nm in diameter; this corresponds roughly to a range of sizes from that of the largest protein to that of the smallest cell (see Fig 2–2). Their shapes are frequently referred to in colloquial terms, eg, spheres, rods, bullets, or bricks, but in reality they are complex structures of precise geometric symmetry (see below). The shape of virus particles is determined by the arrangement of the **repeating subunits** that form the protein coat (**capsid**) of the virus. The shapes and sizes of some important viruses are depicted in Fig 28–1.

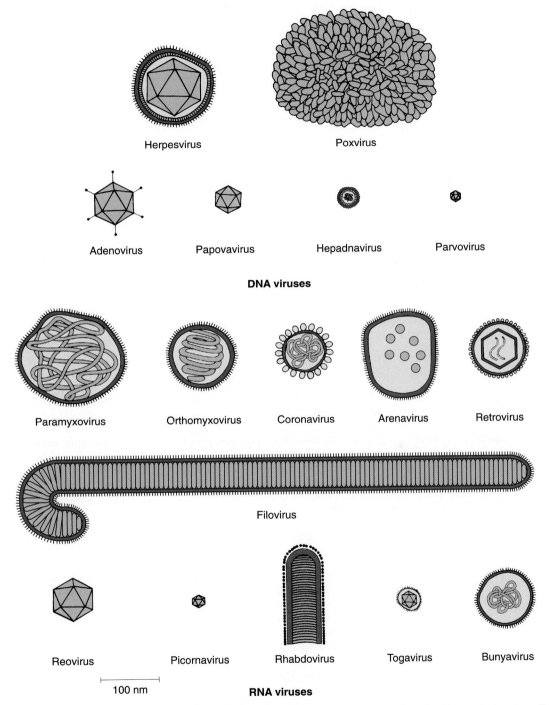

Figure 28–1. Shapes and sizes of medically important viruses. (Modified and reproduced, with permission, from Fenner F, White DO: *Medical Virology,* 4th ed. Academic Press, 1994.)

VIRAL NUCLEIC ACIDS

The anatomy of two representative types of virus particles is shown in Fig 28–2. The viral nucleic acid (genome) is located internally and can be either single- or double-stranded DNA or single- or double-stranded RNA.* Only viruses have genetic material composed of single-stranded DNA or of single-stranded or double-stranded RNA. The nucleic acid can be either linear or circular. The DNA is always a single molecule; the RNA can exist either as a single molecule or in several pieces. Almost all viruses contain only a single copy of their genome; ie, they are haploid. The exception is the retrovirus family, whose members have two copies of their RNA genome; ie, they are diploid.

CAPSID & SYMMETRY

The nucleic acid is surrounded by a protein coat called a **capsid,** made up of subunits called capsomers. Each capsomer, consisting of one or several proteins, can be seen in the electron microscope as a spherical particle, sometimes with a central hole. The arrangement of capsomers gives the virus structure its geometric symmetry. There are two forms of symmetry in virus capsids: (1) **icosahedral,** in which the capsomers are arranged in 20 triangles that form a symmetric figure (an icosahedron) with the approximate outline of a sphere; and (2) **helical,** in which the capsomers are arranged in a hollow coil that appears rod-shaped. The helix can be either rigid or flexible. Both the icosahedral and the helical forms can exist either as a "naked" **nucleocapsid** or with an outer **envelope** layer (Fig 28–2).

The advantage of building the virus particle from identical protein subunits is 2-fold: (1) it reduces the need for genetic information, and (2) it promotes self-assembly; ie, no enzyme or energy is required. In fact, functional virus particles have been assembled in the test tube by combining the purified nucleic acid with the purified proteins in the absence of cells, energy source, and enzymes.

VIRAL PROTEINS

Viral proteins serve several important functions. The outer capsid proteins **protect** the genetic material and **mediate the attachment** of the virus to specific receptors on the host cell surface. This interaction of the viral proteins with the cell receptor is the major determinant of species and organ **specificity.** Outer viral proteins are also **important antigens** that induce neutralizing antibody and activate cytotoxic T cells to kill virus-infected cells. The outer proteins induce these immune responses following both the natural infection and immunization (see below). Some of the internal proteins are associated with the nucleic acid, eg, nucleic acid polymerases, which are essential for replication. Histonelike proteins, which may have a regulatory function or may neutralize the negative charge on the nucleic acid during assembly of the virus particle, are also located internally.

ENVELOPE

In addition to the capsid and internal proteins, there are two other types of proteins, both of which are associated with the envelope. The **envelope** is a **lipoprotein** membrane composed of lipid derived from the host cell membrane and protein that is virus-specific. Furthermore, there are frequently glycoproteins in the form of spikelike projections on the surface, which attach to host cell receptors during the entry of the virus into the cell. Another protein, the **matrix** protein, mediates the interaction between the capsid proteins and the envelope.

In general, the presence of an envelope confers **instability** on the virus. Enveloped viruses are more sensitive to heat, detergents, and lipid solvents such as alcohol and ether than are nonenveloped (nucleocapsid) viruses, which are composed only of nucleic acid and capsid proteins.

The surface proteins of the virus, whether they are the capsid proteins or the envelope glycoproteins, are the principal **antigens** against which the host mounts its immune response to viruses. They are also the determinants of type specificity. For example, poliovirus types 1, 2, and 3 are distinguished by the antigenicity of their capsid proteins. It is important to know the number of serotypes of a virus, since vaccines should contain the prevalent serotypes. There is often little cross protection between different serotypes.

---

*The nature of the nucleic acid of each virus is listed in Tables 31–1 and 31–2.

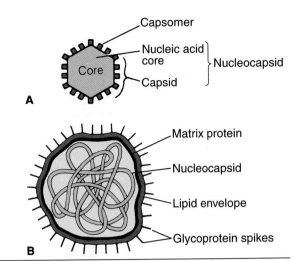

Figure 28–2. Cross section of two types of virus particles. **A:** Nonenveloped virus with an icosahedral nucleocapsid. **B:** Enveloped virus with a helical nucleocapsid. (Modified and reproduced, with permission, from Brooks GF et al: *Medical Microbiology,* 20th ed. Appleton & Lange, 1995.)

ATYPICAL VIRUSLIKE AGENTS

There are four exceptions to the typical virus as described above:

(1) Defective viruses are composed of viral nucleic acid and proteins but cannot replicate without a "helper" virus, which provides the missing function. Defective viruses usually have a mutation or a deletion of part of their genetic material. During the growth of most human viruses, many more defective than infectious virus particles are produced. The ratio of defective to infectious particles can be as high as 100:1. Because these defective particles can interfere with the growth of the infectious particles, it has been hypothesized that the defective viruses may aid in recovery from an infection by limiting the ability of the infectious particles to grow.

(2) Pseudovirions contain host cell DNA instead of viral DNA within the capsid. They are formed during infection with certain viruses when the host cell DNA is fragmented and pieces of it are incorporated within the capsid protein. Pseudovirions can infect cells, but they do not replicate.

(3) Viroids consist solely of a single molecule of circular RNA without a protein coat or envelope. There is extensive homology between bases in the viroid RNA, leading to large double-stranded regions. The RNA is quite small (MW 1×10^5) and apparently does not code for any protein. Nevertheless, viroids replicate but the mechanism is unclear. They cause several plant diseases but are not implicated in any human disease.

(4) Prions are infectious protein particles that are composed **solely of protein;** ie, they contain no detectable nucleic acid. They are implicated as the cause of certain "slow" diseases such as Creutzfeldt-Jakob disease in humans and scrapie in sheep (see Chapter 44). Since neither DNA nor RNA has been detected in prions, they are clearly different from viruses (Table 28–1). Furthermore, electron microscopy reveals filaments rather than virus particles. Prions are much **more resistant** to inactivation by ultraviolet light and heat than are viruses. They are remarkably resistant to formaldehyde and nucle-

Table 28–1. Comparison of prions and conventional viruses.

Feature	Prions	Conventional Viruses
Particle contains nucleic acid	No	Yes
Particle contains protein	Yes, encoded by cellular genes	Yes, encoded by viral genes
Inactivated rapidly by UV light or heat	No	Yes
Appearance in electron microscope	Filamentous rods (amyloid-like)	Icosahedral or helical symmetry
Infection induces antibody	No	Yes
Infection induces inflammation	No	Yes

ases. However, they are inactivated by hypochlorite, NaOH, and autoclaving. Hypochlorite is used to sterilize surgical instruments and other medical supplies that cannot be autoclaved.

Prions are composed of a single glycoprotein with a molecular weight of 27,000–30,000. With scrapie prions as the model, it was found that this protein is encoded by a single **cellular** gene. This gene is found in equal numbers in the cells of both infected and uninfected animals. Furthermore, the amount of prion protein mRNA is the same in uninfected as in infected cells. In view of these findings, **post-translational** modifications of the prion protein are hypothesized to be the important distinction between the protein found in infected and uninfected cells. There is evidence that a change in the conformation from the normal alpha-helical form to the **abnormal beta-pleated sheet** form is the important modification. The abnormal form then recruits additional normal forms to change their configuration, and the number of abnormal pathogenic particles increases. The prion protein in normal cells is protease-sensitive, whereas the prion protein in infected cells is protease-resistant, probably because of the change in configuration.

The function of the normal prion protein is unknown. "Knockout" mice in which the gene encoding the prion protein is inactive appear normal. There is some evidence that it is a copper-binding protein.

The observation that the prion protein is the product of a normal cellular gene may explain why **no immune response** is formed against this protein; ie, tolerance occurs. Similarly, there is **no inflammatory response** in infected brain tissue. A vacuolated **(spongiform)** appearance is found, without inflammatory cells. Prion proteins in infected brain tissue form rod-shaped particles that are morphologically and histochemically indistinguishable from **amyloid,** a substance found in the brain tissue of individuals with various central nervous system diseases (as well as diseases of other organs).

The role of prions in the pathogenesis of "slow" diseases such as Creutzfeldt-Jakob disease remains unclear. The central question is: are prions the cause of these diseases or a pathologic byproduct? At present, prions are the most plausible causative agents and no alternative explanation has gathered much support.

Review Questions

1. What are the two types of symmetry of viral capsids?
2. What are the functions of viral proteins?
3. What is the composition of the viral envelope, and how is it formed?
4. Which proteins of the virus induce protective antibody?
5. What are the differences between viroids and prions?

29

Replication

The viral replication cycle is described below in two different ways. The first approach is a growth curve, which shows the amount of virus produced at different times after infection. The second is a stepwise description of the specific events within the cell during virus growth.

VIRAL GROWTH CURVE

A typical growth curve is depicted in Fig 29–1. The amount of virus produced is plotted on a logarithmic scale as a function of time after infection. Note that the time required for the growth cycle varies; it is minutes for some bacterial viruses and hours for some human viruses.

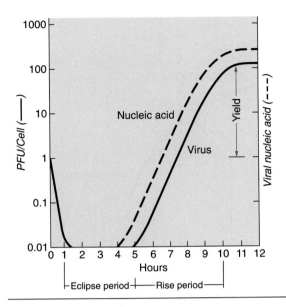

Figure 29–1. Viral growth curve. Note the eclipse period during which no infectious virus is detectable within the infected cells. PFU, plaque-forming units. Plaque-forming units are a measure of the number of infectious units of virus. In this growth curve, the amount of infecting virus is 1 PFU/cell, ie, 1 infectious unit/cell. (Modified and reproduced, with permission, from Joklik WK et al: *Zinsser Microbiology,* 20th ed. Appleton & Lange, 1992.)

The first event is quite striking: the virus disappears, as represented by the solid line dropping to the *X* axis. Although the virus particle, as such, is no longer present, the viral nucleic acid continues to function and begins to accumulate within the cell, as indicated by the dotted line. The time during which no virus is found inside the cell is known as the **eclipse period.** The eclipse period ends with the appearance of virus (solid line). The **latent period,** in contrast, is defined as the time from the onset of infection to the appearance of virus extracellularly. Note that infection begins with one virus particle and ends with several hundred virus particles having been produced; this type of reproduction is unique to viruses. Alterations of cell morphology accompanied by marked derangement of cell function begin toward the end of the latent period. This **cytopathic effect** (CPE) culminates in the lysis and death of cells. Not all viruses cause CPE; some can replicate while causing little morphologic or functional change in the cell.

Table 29–1. Stages of the viral growth cycle.

Attachment and penetration by parental virion
↓
Uncoating of the viral genome
↓
Early[1] viral mRNA synthesis[2]
↓
Early viral protein synthesis
↓
Viral genome replication
↓
Late viral mRNA synthesis
↓
Late viral protein synthesis
↓
Progeny virion assembly
↓
Virion release from cell

[1] "Early" is defined as the period before genome replication. Not all viruses exhibit a distinction between early and late functions. In general, early proteins are enzymes, whereas late proteins are structural components of the virus.
[2] In some cases, the viral genome is functionally equivalent to mRNA; thus, early mRNA need not be synthesized.

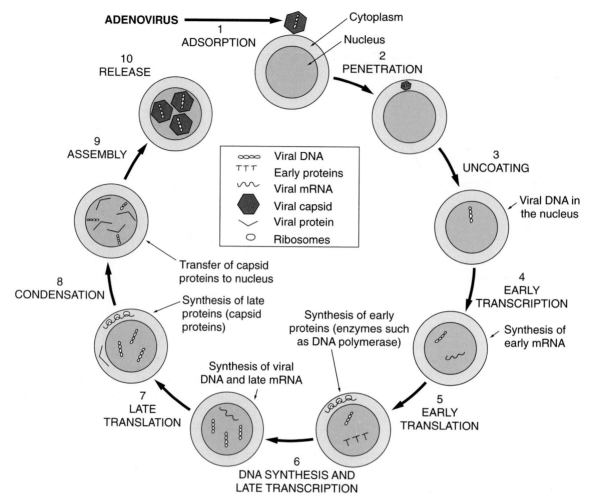

Figure 29–2. Viral growth cycle. The growth cycle of adenovirus, a nonenveloped DNA virus, is shown. (Modified and reproduced, with permission, from Jawetz E, Melnick JL, Adelberg EA: *Review of Medical Microbiology,* 16th ed. Appleton & Lange, 1984.)

SPECIFIC EVENTS DURING THE GROWTH CYCLE

An overview of the events is described in Table 29–1 and presented in diagrammatic fashion in Fig 29–2. The infecting parental virus particle attaches to the cell membrane and then penetrates the host cell. The viral genome is "uncoated" by removing the capsid proteins, and the genome is free to function. Early mRNA and proteins are synthesized; the **early proteins are enzymes** used to replicate the viral genome. Late mRNA and proteins are then synthesized. These **late proteins are the structural, capsid proteins.** The progeny virions are assembled from the replicated genetic material and newly made capsid proteins and are then released from the cell.

Another, more general way to describe the growth cycle is as follows: (1) early events, ie, **attachment, penetration,** and **uncoating;** (2) middle events, ie, **gene expression** and **genome replication;** and (3) late events, ie, **assembly** and **release.** With this sequence in mind, each stage will be described in more detail.

Attachment, Penetration, & Uncoating   The proteins on the surface of the virion attach to specific receptor proteins on the cell surface through weak, noncovalent bonding. The **specificity** of attachment determines the **host range** of the virus. Some viruses have a narrow range, whereas others have quite a broad range. For example, poliovirus can enter the cells of only humans and other primates, whereas rabies virus can enter all mammalian cells. The organ specificity of viruses is governed by receptor interaction as well. Those cellular receptors that have been identified are surface proteins that serve various other functions. For example, herpes simplex virus type 1 attaches to the fibroblast growth factor receptor, rabies virus to the acetylcholine receptor, and human immunodeficiency virus to the CD4 protein on helper T lymphocytes.

The virus particle penetrates by being engulfed in a pinocytotic vesicle, within which the process of uncoating begins. A low pH within the vesicle favors uncoating. Rupture of the vesicle or fusion of the outer layer of virus with the vesicle membrane deposits the inner core of the virus into the cytoplasm.

Certain bacterial viruses (bacteriophages) have a special mechanism for entering bacteria that has no counterpart in either human viruses or those of animals or plants. Some of the T group of bacteriophages infect *Escherichia coli* by attaching several tail fibers to the cell surface and then using lysozyme from the tail to degrade a portion of the cell wall. At this point, the tail sheath contracts, driving the tip of the core through the cell wall. The viral DNA then enters the cell through the tail core, while the capsid proteins remain outside.

It is appropriate at this point to describe the phenomenon of **infectious nucleic acid,** since it provides a transition between the concepts of host specificity described above and early genome functioning, which is discussed below. Note that we are discussing whether the purified genome is infectious. All viruses are "infectious" in a person or in cell culture, but not all purified genomes are infectious.

Infectious nucleic acid is purified viral DNA or RNA (without any protein) that can carry out the entire viral growth cycle and result in the production of complete virus particles. This is interesting from three points of view:

(1) The observation that purified nucleic acid is infectious is the definitive proof that nucleic acid, not protein, is the genetic material.

(2) Infectious nucleic acid can bypass the host range specificity provided by the viral protein-cell receptor interaction. For example, although intact poliovirus can grow only in primate cells, purified poliovirus RNA can enter nonprimate cells, go through its usual growth cycle, and produce normal poliovirus. The poliovirus produced in the nonprimate cells can infect only primate cells, since it now has its capsid proteins. These observations indicate that the internal functions of the nonprimate cells are capable of supporting viral growth once entry has occurred.

(3) Only certain viruses yield infectious nucleic acid. The reason for this is discussed below. Note that all viruses are infectious but not all purified viral DNA's or RNA's (genomes) are infectious.

Gene Expression & Genome Replication   The first step in viral gene expression is **mRNA synthesis.** It is at this point that viruses follow different pathways depending on the nature of their nucleic acid and the part of the cell in which they replicate (Fig 29–3).

DNA viruses, with one exception, **replicate in the nucleus** and use the host cell DNA-dependent RNA polymerase to synthesize their mRNA. The poxviruses are the exception because they replicate in the cytoplasm, where they do not have access to the host cell RNA polymerase. They therefore carry their own polymerase within the virus particle. **The genome of all DNA viruses consists of double-stranded DNA, except for the parvoviruses, which have a single-stranded DNA genome** (Table 29–2).

Most RNA viruses undergo their entire replicative cycle in the cytoplasm. The two principal exceptions are retroviruses and influenza viruses, both of which have an important replicative step in the nucleus. Retroviruses integrate a DNA copy of their genome into the host cell DNA, and influenza viruses synthesize their progeny genomes in the nucleus.

RNA viruses fall into four groups with quite different strategies for synthesizing mRNA (Table 29–3).

(1) The simplest strategy is illustrated by poliovirus, which has **single-stranded RNA** of **positive polarity*** as its genetic material. These viruses use their RNA genome directly as mRNA.

---

*Positive polarity is defined as an RNA with the same base sequence as the mRNA. RNA with negative polarity has a base sequence that is complementary to the mRNA. For example, if the mRNA sequence is a A-C-U-G, an RNA with negative polarity would be U-G-A-C and an RNA with positive polarity would be A-C-U-G.

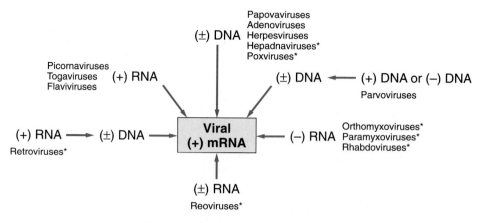

Legend: (+) = Strand with same polarity as mRNA   (±) = Double-stranded
           (−) = Strand complementary to mRNA   *   = These viruses contain a polymerase in the virion.

Figure 29–3. Synthesis of viral mRNA by medically important viruses. The following information starts at the top of the figure and moves clockwise. Viruses with a double-stranded DNA genome, eg, papovaviruses such as human papillomavirus, use host cell RNA polymerase to synthesize viral mRNA. Note that hepadnaviruses, eg, hepatitis B virus, contain a virion DNA polymerase that synthesizes the missing portion of the DNA genome but the viral mRNA is synthesized by host cell RNA polymerase. Parvoviruses use host cell DNA polymerase to synthesize viral double-stranded DNA and host cell RNA polymerase to synthesize viral mRNA. Viruses with a single-stranded, negative-polarity RNA genome, eg, orthomyxoviruses such as influenza virus, use a virion RNA polymerase to synthesize viral mRNA. Viruses with a double-stranded RNA genome, eg, reoviruses, use a virion RNA polymerase to synthesize viral mRNA. Some viruses with a single-stranded, positive-polarity RNA genome, eg, retroviruses, use a virion DNA polymerase to synthesize a DNA copy of the RNA genome but a host cell RNA polymerase to synthesize the viral mRNA. Some viruses with a single-stranded, positive-polarity RNA genome, eg, picornaviruses, use the virion genome RNA itself as their mRNA. (Modified and reproduced, with permission, from Ryan K et al: *Sherris Medical Microbiology,* 3rd ed. Appleton & Lange, 1994.)

(2) The second group has **single-stranded RNA** of **negative polarity** as its genetic material. An mRNA must be transcribed by using the negative strand as a template. Because the cell does not have an RNA polymerase capable of using RNA as a template, the virus carries its own **RNA-dependent RNA polymerase.** There are two subcategories of negative-polarity RNA viruses: those that have a single piece of RNA, eg, measles virus (a paramyxovirus) or rabies virus (a rhabdovirus), and those that have multiple pieces of RNA, eg, influenza virus (a myxovirus).

Table 29–2. Important features of DNA viruses.

DNA Genome	Location of Replication	Virion Polymerase	Infectivity of Genome	Prototype Human Virus
Single strand	Nucleus	No[1,2]	Yes	Parvovirus B19
Double strand				
Circular	Nucleus	No[1]	Yes	Papillomavirus
Circular; partially single strand	Nucleus	Yes[3]	No	Hepatitis B virus
Linear	Nucleus	No[1]	Yes	Herpesvirus, adenovirus
Linear	Cytoplasm	Yes	No	Smallpox virus, vaccinia virus

[1] mRNA is synthesized by host cell RNA polymerase in the nucleus.
[2] Single-stranded genome DNA is converted to double-stranded DNA by host cell polymerase. A virus-encoded DNA polymerase then synthesizes progeny DNA.
[3] Hepatitis B virus uses a virion-encoded RNA-dependent DNA polymerase to synthesize its progeny DNA with full-length mRNA as the template. This enzyme is a type of "reverse transcriptase" but functions at a different stage in the replicative cycle than does the reverse transcriptase of retroviruses.
Note: All DNA viruses encode their own DNA polymerase that replicates the genome. They do not use the host cell DNA polymerase (with the minor exception of the parvoviruses as mentioned above).

Table 29–3. Important features of RNA viruses.

RNA Genome	Polarity	Virion Polymerase	Source of mRNA	Infectivity of Genome	Prototype Human Virus
Single strand, nonsegmented	+	No	Genome	Yes	Poliovirus
Single strand,					
Nonsegmented	–	Yes	Transcription	No	Measles virus, rabies virus
Segmented	–	Yes	Transcription	No	Influenza virus
Double strand, segmented	±	Yes	Transcription	No	Rotavirus
Single strand, diploid	+	Yes[1]	Transcription[2]	No[3]	HTLV, HIV[4]

[1] Retroviruses contain an RNA-dependent DNA polymerase.
[2] mRNA transcribed from DNA intermediate.
[3] Although the retroviral genome RNA is not infectious, the DNA intermediate is.
[4] HTLV, human T cell leukemia virus; HIV, human immunodeficiency virus.

(3) The third group has **double-stranded RNA** as its genetic material. Because the cell has no enzyme capable of transcribing this RNA into mRNA, the virus carries its own polymerase. Reovirus, the best-studied member of this group, has 10 segments of double-stranded RNA.

(4) The fourth group, exemplified by retroviruses, has single-stranded RNA of positive polarity that is transcribed into double-stranded DNA by the RNA-dependent DNA polymerase (**reverse transcriptase**) carried by the virus. This DNA copy is then transcribed into viral mRNA by the regular host cell RNA polymerase (polymerase II). Retroviruses are the only family of viruses that are **"diploid,"** ie, that have two copies of their genome RNA.

These differences explain why some viruses yield infectious nucleic acid and others do not. Viruses that do not require a polymerase in the virion can produce infectious DNA or RNA. By contrast, viruses such as the poxviruses, the negative-stranded RNA viruses, the double-stranded RNA viruses, and the retroviruses, which require a virion polymerase, cannot yield infectious nucleic acid. Several additional features of viral mRNA are described in the box.

Once the viral mRNA of either DNA or RNA viruses is synthesized, it is translated by host cell ribosomes into viral proteins, some of which are **"early"** proteins, ie, **enzymes** required for replication of the viral genome, and others are **"late proteins,"** ie, **structural proteins** of the progeny viruses. (The term "early" is defined as occurring before the replication of the genome, and "late" is defined as occurring after genome replication.) The most important of the early proteins for many RNA viruses is the polymerase that will synthesize many copies of viral genetic material for the progeny virus particles. No matter how a virus makes its mRNA, virtually all viruses make a virus-encoded polymerase (a **replicase**) that replicates the genome, ie, that makes many copies of the parental genome that will become the genome of the progeny virions.

Some viral mRNAs are translated into **precursor polypeptides that must be cleaved by proteases** to produce the functional structural proteins (Fig 29–4), whereas other viral mRNAs are translated directly into structural proteins. A striking example of the former occurs during the replication of picornaviruses (eg, poliovirus, rhinovirus, and hepatitis A virus), in which the genome RNA, acting as mRNA, is translated into a **single polypeptide,** which is then cleaved by a virus-coded protease into various proteins. This protease is one of the proteins in the single polypeptide, an interesting example of a protease acting upon its own polypeptide.

Another important family of viruses in which precursor polypeptides are synthesized is the retrovirus family. For example, the *gag, pol,* and *env* genes of human immunodeficiency virus are translated into precursor polypeptides, which are then cleaved by a virus-encoded protease. It is this protease that is inhibited by the drugs classified as **protease inhibitors.** Flaviviruses, such as hepatitis C virus and yellow fever virus, also synthesize precursor polypeptides that must be cleaved to form functional proteins. In contrast, other viruses, such as influenza virus and rotavirus, have segmented genomes, and each segment encodes a specific functional polypeptide rather than a precursor polypeptide.

Replication of the viral genome is governed by the principle of **complementarity,** which requires that a strand with a complementary base sequence be synthesized; this strand then serves as the template for the synthesis of the actual viral genome. The following examples from Table 29–4 should

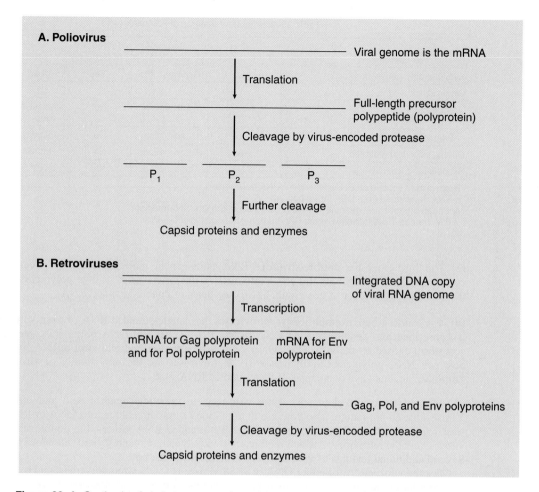

Figure 29–4. Synthesis of viral precursor polypeptides. **A:** Poliovirus mRNA is translated into a full-length precursor polypeptide, which is cleaved by the virus-encoded protease into the functional viral proteins. **B:** Retroviral mRNAs are translated into several precursor polypeptides, which are then cleaved by the virus-encoded protease into the functional viral proteins. Inhibitors of the protease are effective drugs against human immunodeficiency virus.

Table 29–4. Complementarity in viral genome replication.

Prototype Virus	Parental Genome[1]	Intermediate Form	Progeny Genome
Poliovirus	+ ssRNA	− ssRNA	+ ssRNA
Influenza virus, measles virus, rabies virus	− ssRNA	+ ssRNA	− ssRNA
Rotavirus	dsRNA	+ ssRNA	dsRNA
Retrovirus	+ ssRNA	dsDNA	+ ssRNA
Parvovirus B19	ssDNA	dsDNA	ssDNA
Hepatitis B virus	dsDNA	+ ssRNA	dsDNA
Papovavirus, adenovirus, herpesvirus, poxvirus	dsDNA	dsDNA	dsDNA

[1] Code: ss, single-stranded; ds, double-stranded; +, positive polarity; −, negative polarity.

Viral mRNA

There are four interesting aspects of viral mRNA and its expression in eukaryotic cells. (1) Viral mRNAs have three attributes in common with cellular mRNAs: on the 5′ end there is a methylated GTP "cap," which is linked by an "inverted" (3′-to-5′) bond instead of the usual 5′-to-3′ bond; on the 3′ end there is a tail of 100–200 adenosine residues [poly(A)]; and the mRNA is generated by splicing from a larger transcript of the genome. In fact, these three modifications were first observed in studies on viral mRNAs and then extended to cellular mRNAs. (2) Some viruses use their genetic material to the fullest extent by making more than one type of mRNA from the same piece of DNA by "shifting the reading frame." This is done by starting transcription 1 or 2 bases downstream from the original initiation site. (3) With some DNA viruses, there is temporal control over the region of the genome that is transcribed into mRNA. During the beginning stages of the growth cycle, before DNA replication begins, only the early region of the genome is transcribed and, therefore, only certain early proteins are made. One of the early proteins is a repressor of the late genes; this prevents transcription until the appropriate time. (4) Three different processes are used to generate the monocistronic mRNAs that will code for a single protein from the polycistronic viral genome:

(1) Individual mRNAs are transcribed by starting at many specific initiation points along the genome, which is the same mechanism used by eukaryotic cells and by herpesviruses, adenoviruses, and the DNA and RNA tumor viruses;

(2) in the reoviruses and influenza viruses, the genome is segmented into multiple pieces, each of which codes for a single mRNA; and

(3) in polioviruses, the entire RNA genome is translated into one long polypeptide, which is then cleaved into specific proteins by a protease.

---

make this clear: (1) poliovirus makes a negative-strand intermediate, which is the template for the positive-strand genome; (2) influenza, measles, and rabies viruses make a positive-strand intermediate, which is the template for the negative-strand genome; (3) reovirus makes a positive strand that acts both as mRNA and as the template for the negative strand in the double-stranded genome RNA; (4) retroviruses use the negative strand of the DNA intermediate to make positive-strand progeny RNA; (5) hepatitis B virus uses its mRNA as a template to make progeny double-stranded DNA; and (6) the other double-stranded DNA viruses replicate their DNA by the same semiconservative process by which cell DNA is synthesized.

As the replication of the viral genome proceeds, the structural capsid proteins to be used in the progeny virus particles are synthesized. In some cases, the newly replicated viral genomes can serve as templates for the late mRNA to make these capsid proteins.

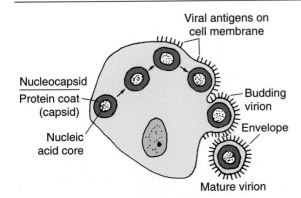

Figure 29–5. Budding. Most enveloped viruses derive their lipoprotein envelope from the cell membrane. The matrix protein mediates the interaction between the viral nucleocapsid and the viral envelope. (Reproduced, with permission, from Mims CA: *The Pathogenesis of Infectious Disease,* 3rd ed. Academic Press, 1987.)

Assembly & Release   The progeny particles are assembled by packaging the viral nucleic acid within the capsid proteins. Little is known about the precise steps in the assembly process. Surprisingly, certain viruses can be assembled in the test tube by using only purified RNA and purified protein. This indicates that the specificity of the interaction resides within the RNA and protein and that the action of enzymes and expenditure of energy are not required.

Virus particles are released from the cell by either of two processes. One is rupture of the cell membrane and release of the mature particles; this usually occurs with unenveloped viruses. The other, which occurs with enveloped viruses, is release of viruses by **"budding"** through the outer cell membrane (Fig 29–5). (An exception is the **herpesvirus** family, whose members acquire their envelopes from the **nuclear membrane** rather than from the outer cell membrane.) The budding process begins when virus-specific proteins enter the cell membrane at specific sites. The viral nucleocapsid then interacts with the specific membrane site mediated by the **matrix protein.** The cell

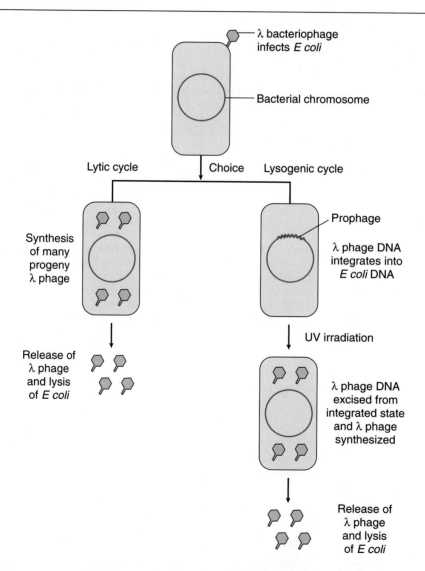

Figure 29–6. Comparison of the lytic and lysogenic cycles of bacteriophage (phage) replication. In the lytic cycle, replication of the phage is completed without interruption. In the lysogenic cycle, replication of the phage is interrupted and the phage DNA integrates into the bacterial DNA. The integrated DNA is called a prophage and can remain in the integrated state for long periods. If the bacteria are exposed to UV light, the prophage DNA is excised from the bacterial DNA and the phage enters the lytic cycle, which ends with the production of progeny phage.

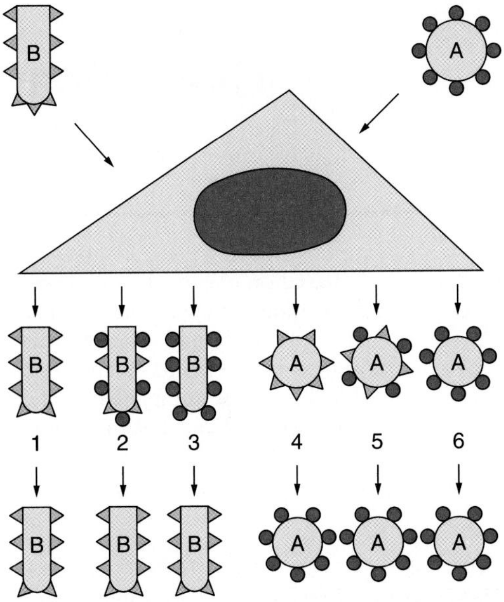

Figure 30–2. Phenotypic mixing. A retrovirus (A) and a rhabdovirus (B) infect the same cell. The progeny viruses include phenotypically mixed particles (2, 3, 4, and 5) and normal progeny virions (1 and 6). Assume that virus A can infect human cells but not chicken cells (a property determined by the circular surface proteins) and that virus B can infect chicken cells but not human cells (a property determined by the triangular surface proteins). However both virus A and virus B can infect a mouse cell. As shown in the figure, six types of progeny viruses can arise when both virus A and virus B infect a mouse cell. Progeny virus #1 is not phenotypically mixed and can infect chicken cells but not human cells because it has the triangular surface proteins. If progeny virus #1 infects chicken cells, the progeny virus from that infection is determined by the B genome and will be identical to the parental B virus. Progeny virus #2 is phenotypically mixed and can infect both chicken cells and human cells because it has both the triangular and the circular surface proteins. Note that when progeny virus #2 infects in either chicken cells or human cells, the progeny of that infection is determined by the B genome and will be identical to the parental B virus. Progeny virus #3 is phenotypically mixed and can infect human cells but not chicken cells because it has the circular surface proteins. Note that when progeny virus #3 infects human cells, the progeny of that infection is determined by the B genome and will be identical to the parental B virus. The reader should use the interpretation of progeny viruses 1, 2, and 3 to understand the properties of progeny viruses 4, 5, and 6. (Modified and reproduced, with permission, from Boettiger D: Animal virus pseudotypes. *Prog Med Virol* 1979;**25**:37.)

gene that is not essential for viral replication is deleted and the gene from the other virus that encodes the antigen which elicits neutralizing antibody is introduced. For example, the gene for the surface antigen of hepatitis B virus has been introduced into vaccinia virus and is expressed in infected cells. Recombinant vaccines are not yet clinically available, but vaccines of this type promise to greatly improve the efficiency of our immunization programs.

Review Questions

1. What are temperature-sensitive conditional-lethal mutants?
2. What are defective interfering particles?
3. Distinguish between complementation and phenotypic mixing.
4. Why are retroviruses excellent vectors for gene therapy?
5. Describe the process by which a retroviral vector for a human gene is produced.

31

Classification of Medically Important Viruses

The classification of viruses is based on chemical and morphologic criteria. The two major components of the virus used in classification are (1) the nucleic acid (its molecular weight and structure); and (2) the capsid (its size and symmetry and whether it is enveloped). A classification scheme based on these factors is presented in Tables 31–1 and 31–2 for DNA and RNA viruses, respectively. This scheme was simplified from the complete classification to emphasize organisms of medical importance. Only the virus families are listed; subfamilies are described in the chapter on the specific virus.

DNA VIRUSES

The families of DNA viruses are described in Table 31–1. The three **naked** (ie, nonenveloped) icosahedral virus families—the parvoviruses, papovaviruses, and adenoviruses—are presented in order of increasing particle size, as are the three **enveloped** families. The hepadnavirus family, which includes hepatitis B virus, and the herpesviruses are enveloped icosahedral viruses. The largest viruses, the poxviruses, have a complex internal symmetry.

Parvoviruses   These are very small (22 nm in diameter), naked icosahedral viruses with single-stranded linear DNA. There are two types of parvoviruses: defective and nondefective. The defective parvoviruses, eg, adeno-associated virus, require a helper virus for replication. The DNA of defective parvoviruses is unusual, because plus-strand DNA and minus-strand DNA are carried in separate particles. The nondefective parvoviruses are best illustrated by B19 virus, which is associated with aplastic crises in sickle cell anemia patients and with erythema infectiosum, an innocuous childhood disease characterized by a "slapped-cheeks" rash.

Papovaviruses   These are naked icosahedral viruses (55 nm in diameter) with double-stranded circular supercoiled DNA. The name "papova" is an acronym of *pa*pilloma, *po*lyoma, and simian *va*cuolating viruses. Three human papovaviruses are JC virus, isolated from patients with progressive multifocal leukoencephalopathy; BK virus, isolated from the urine of immunosuppressed kidney

Table 31–1. Classification of DNA viruses.

Virus Family	Envelope Present	Capsid Symmetry	Particle Size (nm)	DNA MW ($\times 10^6$)	DNA Structure[1]	Medically Important Viruses
Parvovirus	No	Icosahedral	22	2	SS, linear	B19 virus
Papovavirus	No	Icosahedral	55	3–5	DS, circular, supercoiled	Papillomavirus
Adenovirus	No	Icosahedral	75	23	DS, linear	Adenovirus
Hepadnavirus	Yes	Icosahedral	42	1.5	DS, incomplete circular	Hepatitis B virus
Herpesvirus	Yes	Icosahedral	100[2]	100–150	DS, linear	Herpes simplex virus, varicella-zoster virus, cytomegalovirus, Epstein-Barr virus
Poxvirus	Yes	Complex	250 × 400	125–185	DS, linear	Smallpox virus, vaccinia virus

[1]SS, single-stranded; DS, double-stranded.
[2]The herpesvirus nucleocapsid is 100 nm, but the envelope varies in size. The entire virus can be as large as 200 nm in diameter.

transplant patients; and human papillomavirus. Polyomavirus and simian vacuolating virus 40 (SV40 virus) are papovaviruses of mice and monkeys, respectively, that induce malignant tumors in a variety of species.

Adenoviruses   These are naked icosahedral viruses (75 nm in diameter) with double-stranded linear DNA. They cause pharyngitis, upper and lower respiratory tract disease, and a variety of other less common infections. There are at least 40 antigenic types, some of which cause sarcomas in animals but no tumors in humans.

Hepadnaviruses   These are double-shelled viruses (42 nm in diameter) with an icosahedral capsid covered by an envelope. The DNA is a double-stranded circle that is unusual because the complete strand is not a covalently closed circle and the other strand is missing approximately 25% of its length. Hepatitis B virus is the human pathogen in this family.

Herpesviruses   These are enveloped viruses (100 nm in diameter) with an icosahedral nucleocapsid and double-stranded linear DNA. They are noted for causing latent infections. The five important human pathogens are herpes simplex virus types 1 and 2, varicella-zoster virus, cytomegalovirus, and Epstein-Barr virus (the cause of infectious mononucleosis).

Poxviruses   These are the largest viruses, with a bricklike shape, an envelope with an unusual appearance, and a complex capsid symmetry. They are named for the skin lesions, or "pocks," that they cause. Smallpox virus and vaccinia virus are the two important members. The latter virus is used in the smallpox vaccine.

RNA VIRUSES

The 14 families of RNA viruses are described in Table 31–2. The three **naked icosahedral** virus families are listed first and are followed by the three **enveloped icosahedral** viruses. The remaining eight families are **enveloped helical** viruses; the first five have single-stranded linear RNA as their genome, whereas the last three have single-stranded circular RNA.

Picornaviruses   These are the smallest (28 nm in diameter) RNA viruses. They have single-stranded, linear, nonsegmented, positive-polarity RNA within a naked icosahedral capsid. The name "picorna" is derived from *pico* (small), *RNA*-containing. There are two groups of human pathogens: (1) enteroviruses such as poliovirus, coxsackievirus, echovirus, and hepatitis A virus; and (2) rhinoviruses.

Caliciviruses   These are naked viruses (38 nm in diameter) with an icosahedral capsid. They have single-stranded, linear, nonsegmented, positive-polarity RNA. There are two human pathogens: Norwalk virus and hepatitis E virus.

Reoviruses   These are naked viruses (75 nm in diameter) with two icosahedral capsid coats. They have 10 segments of double-stranded linear RNA. The name is an acronym of *r*espiratory *e*nteric *o*rphan, because they were originally found in the respiratory and enteric tracts and were not associated with any human disease. The main human pathogen is rotavirus, which causes diarrhea, mainly in infants.

Flaviviruses   These are enveloped viruses with an icosahedral capsid and single-stranded, linear, nonsegmented, positive-polarity RNA. The flaviviruses include hepatitis C virus, yellow fever virus, dengue virus, and St. Louis and Japanese encephalitis viruses.

Togaviruses   These are enveloped viruses with an icosahedral capsid and single-stranded, linear, nonsegmented, positive-polarity RNA. There are two major groups of human pathogens: the alphaviruses and rubiviruses. The alphavirus group includes eastern and western encephalitis viruses; the rubivirus group consists only of rubella virus.

Retroviruses   These are enveloped viruses with an icosahedral capsid and two identical strands of single-stranded, linear, positive-polarity RNA. The term "retro" pertains to the reverse transcription

Table 31–2. Classification of RNA viruses.

Virus Family	Envelope Present	Capsid Symmetry	Particle Size (nm)	RNA MW ($\times 10^6$)	RNA Structure[1]	Medically Important Viruses
Picornavirus	No	Icosahedral	28	2.5	SS linear, nonsegmented, positive polarity	Poliovirus, rhinovirus, hepatitis A virus
Calicivirus	No	Icosahedral	38	2.7	SS linear, nonsegmented, positive polarity	Norwalk virus, hepatitis E virus
Reovirus	No	Icosahedral	75	15	DS linear, 10 segments	Reovirus, rotavirus
Flavivirus	Yes	Icosahedral	45	4	SS linear, nonsegmented, positive polarity	Yellow fever virus, dengue virus, hepatitis C virus
Togavirus	Yes	Icosahedral	60	4	SS linear, nonsegmented, positive polarity	Rubella virus
Retrovirus	Yes	Icosahedral	100	7[2]	SS linear, 2 segments, positive polarity	HIV, human T-cell leukemia virus
Orthomyxovirus	Yes	Helical	80–120	4	SS linear, 8 segments, negative polarity	Influenza virus
Paramyxovirus	Yes	Helical	150	6	SS linear, nonsegmented, negative polarity	Measles virus, mumps virus, respiratory syncytial virus
Rhabdovirus	Yes	Helical	75 × 180	4	SS linear, nonsegmented, negative polarity	Rabies virus
Filovirus	Yes	Helical	80[3]	4	SS linear, nonsegmented, negative polarity	Ebola virus, Marburg virus
Coronavirus	Yes	Helical	100	5	SS linear, nonsegmented, positive polarity	Coronavirus
Arenavirus	Yes	Helical	80–130	5	SS circular, 2 segments with cohesive ends, negative polarity	Lymphocytic choriomeningitis virus
Bunyavirus	Yes	Helical	100	5	SS circular, 3 segments with cohesive ends, negative polarity	California encephalitis virus, hantavirus
Deltavirus	Yes	Helical	37	0.5	SS circular, closed circle, negative polarity	Hepatitis delta virus

[1]SS, single-stranded; DS, double-stranded.
[2]Retrovirus RNA contains 2 identical molecules of MW 3.5×10^6.
[3]Particles are 80 nm wide but can be thousands of nanometers long.

of the RNA genome into DNA. There are two medically important groups: (1) the oncovirus group, which contains the sarcoma and leukemia viruses, eg, human T cell leukemia virus (HTLV); and (2) the lentivirus ("slow virus") group, which includes human immunodeficiency virus (HIV) and certain animal pathogens, eg, visna virus. A third group, spumaviruses, is described in Chapter 46.

Orthomyxoviruses These viruses (myxoviruses) are enveloped, with a helical nucleocapsid and eight segments of linear, single-stranded, negative-polarity RNA. The term "myxo" refers to the affinity of these viruses for mucins, and "ortho" is added to distinguish them from the paramyxoviruses. Influenza virus is the main human pathogen.

Paramyxoviruses   These are enveloped viruses with a helical nucleocapsid and single-stranded, linear, nonsegmented, negative-polarity RNA. The important human pathogens are measles, mumps, parainfluenza, and respiratory syncytial viruses.

Rhabdoviruses   These are bullet-shaped enveloped viruses with a helical nucleocapsid and a single-stranded, linear, nonsegmented, negative-polarity RNA. The term "rhabdo" refers to the bullet shape. Rabies virus is the only important human pathogen.

Filoviruses   These are enveloped viruses with a helical nucleocapsid and single-stranded, linear, nonsegmented, negative-polarity RNA. They are highly pleomorphic, long filaments that are 80 nm in diameter but can be thousands of nanometers long. The term "filo" means "thread" and refers to the long filaments. The two human pathogens are Ebola virus and Marburg virus.

Coronaviruses   These are enveloped viruses with a helical nucleocapsid and a single-stranded, linear, nonsegmented, positive-polarity RNA. The term "corona" refers to the prominent halo of spikes protruding from the envelope. Coronaviruses cause respiratory tract infections (eg, the common cold) in humans.

Arenaviruses   These are enveloped viruses with a helical nucleocapsid and a single-stranded, circular, negative-polarity RNA in two segments. The term "arena" means "sand" and refers to granules on the virion surface that are nonfunctional ribosomes. Two human pathogens are lymphocytic choriomeningitis virus and Lassa fever virus.

Bunyaviruses   These are enveloped viruses with a helical nucleocapsid and a single-stranded, circular, negative-polarity RNA in three segments. The term "bunya" refers to the prototype, Bunyamwera virus, which is named for the place in Africa where it was isolated. These viruses cause encephalitis and various fevers such as Korean hemorrhagic fever. Hantaviruses, such as Sin Nombre virus (see Chapter 46), are members of this family.

Deltavirus   Hepatitis delta virus (HDV) is the only member of this genus. It is an enveloped virus with a helical nucleocapsid and an RNA genome that is a single-stranded, negative-polarity, covalently closed circle. It is a defective virus because it cannot replicate unless hepatitis B virus (HBV) is present within the same cell. HBV is required because it encodes hepatitis B surface antigen (HBsAg), which serves as the outer protein coat of HDV. The RNA genome of HDV encodes only one protein, the internal core protein called delta antigen.

Pathogenesis 32

The ability of viruses to cause disease can be viewed on two distinct levels: (1) the changes that occur within individual cells and (2) the process that takes place in the infected patient.

THE INFECTED CELL

There are four main effects of virus infection on the cell: (1) death, (2) fusion of cells to form multinucleated cells, (3) malignant transformation, and (4) no apparent morphologic or functional change.

Death of the cell is probably due to inhibition of macromolecular synthesis. Inhibition of host cell protein synthesis frequently occurs first and is probably the most important. Inhibition of DNA and RNA synthesis may be a secondary effect. It is important to note that synthesis of **cellular** proteins is inhibited but **viral** protein synthesis still occurs. For example, poliovirus inactivates an initiation factor (IF) required for cellular mRNA to be translated into cellular proteins, but poliovirus mRNA has a special ribosome-initiating site that allows it to bypass the IF so that viral proteins can be synthesized.

Infected cells frequently contain **inclusion bodies,** which are discrete areas containing viral proteins or viral particles. They have a characteristic intranuclear or intracytoplasmic location and appearance depending on the virus. One of the best examples of inclusion bodies that can assist in clinical diagnosis is that of **Negri bodies,** which are eosinophilic cytoplasmic inclusions found in rabies virus-infected brain neurons. Electron micrographs of inclusion bodies can also aid in the diagnosis when virus particles of typical morphology are visualized.

Fusion of virus-infected cells produces **multinucleated giant cells,** which characteristically form after infection with **herpesviruses and paramyxoviruses.** Fusion occurs as a result of cell membrane changes, which are probably due to the insertion of viral proteins into the membrane. The clinical diagnosis of herpesvirus skin infections is aided by the finding of multinucleated giant cells with eosinophilic intranuclear inclusions in skin scrapings.

A hallmark of viral infection of the cell is the **cytopathic effect** (CPE). This change in the appearance of the infected cell usually begins with a rounding and darkening of the cell and culminates in either lysis (disintegration) or giant cell formation. Detection of virus in a clinical specimen frequently is based on the appearance of CPE in cell culture. In addition, CPE is the basis for the plaque assay, an important method for quantifying the amount of virus in a sample.

Infection with certain viruses causes **malignant transformation,** which is characterized by unrestrained growth, prolonged survival, and morphologic changes such as focal areas of rounded, piled-up cells. These changes are described in more detail in Chapter 43.

Infection of the cell accompanied by virus production can occur **without** morphologic or gross functional changes. This observation highlights the wide variations in the nature of the interaction between the virus and the cell, ranging from rapid destruction of the cell to a symbiotic relationship in which the cell survives and multiplies despite the replication of the virus.

THE INFECTED PATIENT

Pathogenesis in the infected patient involves (1) transmission of the virus and its entry into the host; (2) replication of the virus and damage to cells; (3) spread of the virus to other cells and organs; (4) the immune response, both as a host defense and as a contributing cause of certain diseases; and (5) persistence of the virus in some instances.

The stages of a typical viral infection are the same as those described for a bacterial infection in Chapter 7, namely, an **incubation period** during which the patient is asymptomatic, a **prodromal period** during which nonspecific symptoms occur, a **specific-illness period** during which the characteristic symptoms and signs occur, and a **recovery period** during which the illness wanes and the patient regains good health. In some patients, the infection persists and a chronic carrier state or a latent infection occurs (see below).

Transmission & Portal of Entry   Viruses are transmitted to the individual by many different routes, and their portals of entry are varied (Table 32–1). For example, person-to-person spread occurs by transfer of respiratory secretions, saliva, blood, or semen and by fecal contamination of water or food. Transmission can occur also between mother and offspring in utero across the placenta, at the time of delivery, or during breast feeding. Animal-to-human transmission can take place either directly from a bite of a reservoir host as in rabies or indirectly through the bite of an insect vector, such as a mosquito, which transfers the virus from an animal reservoir to the person. The zoonotic diseases caused by viruses are described in Table 32–2. In addition, activation of a latent, nonreplicating virus to form an active, replicating virus can occur within the individual, with no transmission from an external source.

Localized or Disseminated Infections   Viral infections are either **localized** to the portal of entry or spread **systemically** through the body. The best example of the localized infection is the common cold, which involves only the upper respiratory tract. Influenza is localized primarily to the upper and lower respiratory tracts. One of the best-understood systemic viral infections is paralytic poliomyelitis (Fig 32–1). After poliovirus is ingested, it infects and multiplies within the cells of the small intestine and then spreads to the mesenteric lymph nodes, where it multiplies again. It then enters the bloodstream and is transmitted to certain internal organs, where it multiplies again. The virus

Table 32–1. Main portal of entry of important viral pathogens.

Portal of Entry	Virus	Disease
Respiratory tract[1]	Influenza virus Rhinovirus Respiratory syncytial virus Epstein-Barr virus Varicella-zoster virus Herpes simplex virus type 1 Cytomegalovirus Measles virus Mumps virus Rubella virus Hantavirus Adenovirus	Influenza Common cold Bronchiolitis Infectious mononucleosis Chickenpox Herpes labialis Mononucleosis syndrome Measles Mumps Rubella Pneumonia Pneumonia
Gastrointestinal tract[2]	Hepatitis A virus Poliovirus Rotavirus	Hepatitis A Poliomyelitis Diarrhea
Skin	Rabies virus[3] Yellow fever virus[3] Dengue virus[3] Human papillomavirus	Rabies Yellow fever Dengue Papillomas (warts)
Genital tract	Human papillomavirus Hepatitis B virus Human immunodeficiency virus Herpes simplex virus type 2	Papillomas (warts) Hepatitis B AIDS Herpes genitalis and neonatal herpes
Blood	Hepatits B virus Hepatits C virus Human immunodeficiency virus Cytomegalovirus	Hepatitis B Hepatitis C AIDS Mononucleosis syndrome or pneumonia
Transplacental	Cytomegalovirus Rubella	Congenital abnormalities Congenital abnormalities

[1] Transmission of these viruses is typically by respiratory aerosols or saliva.
[2] Transmission of these viruses is typically by the fecal-oral route in contaminated food or water.
[3] Transmission of these viruses is typically by the bite of an infected animal.

reenters the bloodstream and is transmitted to the central nervous system, where damage to the anterior horn cells occurs, resulting in the characteristic muscle paralysis. It is during this obligatory viremia that circulating IgG antibodies induced by the polio vaccine can prevent the virus from infecting the central nervous system. Viral replication in the gastrointestinal tract results in the presence of poliovirus in the feces, thus perpetuating its transmission to others.

Some of the molecular determinants of pathogenesis have been determined by using reovirus infection in mice as a model system. This virus has three different outer capsid proteins, each of which has a distinct function in determining the course of the infection. One of the proteins binds to specific receptors on the cell surface and thereby determines tissue tropism. A second protein conveys resistance to proteolytic enzymes in the gastrointestinal tract and acts as the antigen that stimulates

Table 32–2. Viruses that cause important zoonotic diseases.

Virus	Animal Reservoir	Mode of Transmission	Disease
Rabies virus	In United States, skunks, raccoons, and bats; in developing countries, dogs.	Usually bite of infected animal; also aerosol of bat saliva.	Rabies
Hantavirus[1]	Deer mice.	Aerosol of dried excreta.	Hantavirus pulmonary syndrome (pneumonia)
Yellow fever virus	Monkeys.	Bite of *Aedes* mosquito.	Yellow fever
Dengue virus	Monkeys.	Bite of *Aedes* mosquito.	Dengue
Encephalitis viruses[2]	Wild birds, eg, sparrows.	Bite of various mosquitoes.	Encephalitis

[1] Sin Nombre virus is the most important hantavirus in the United States.
[2] Important encephalitis viruses in the United States include eastern and western equine encephalitis viruses and St. Louis encephalitis virus.

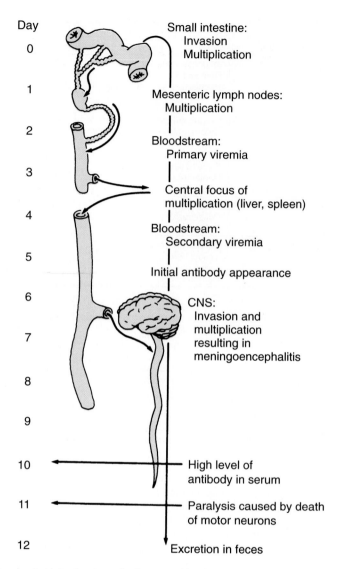

Figure 32–1. Systemic viral infection by poliovirus, resulting in paralytic poliomyelitis. (Modified and reproduced, with permission, from Brooks GF et al: *Medical Microbiology,* 20th ed. Appleton & Lange, 1995.)

the cellular immune response. The third protein inhibits cellular RNA and protein synthesis, leading to death of the cell. Alternatively, this third protein can play a role in the initiation of persistent viral infection.

Pathogenesis & Immunopathogenesis   The signs and symptoms of most viral diseases undoubtedly are the result of cell killing by virus-induced inhibition of macromolecular synthesis. Death of the virus-infected cells results in a loss of function and in the symptoms of disease. For example, when poliovirus kills motor neurons, paralysis of the muscles innervated by those neurons results.

However, there are certain diseases in which cell killing by **immunologic attack** plays an important role in pathogenesis. Both cytotoxic T cells and antibodies play a role in immunopathogenesis.

(1) The best-studied system is lymphocytic choriomeningitis (LCM) in mice; LCM occurs in humans also but is quite rare. When LCM virus is inoculated into the brain of an adult mouse, virus replication occurs and death follows. However, when LCM virus is inoculated into the brain of an immunosuppressed adult mouse or a newborn mouse, the animal remains well despite extensive virus replication. When immune lymphocytes are inoculated into these infected, healthy mice, death ensues. It appears that death of the cells is caused by immune attack by cytotoxic T cells on the new viral antigens in the cell membrane rather than by virus-induced inhibition of cell functions.

(2) Cytotoxic T cells are involved in the pathogenesis of hepatitis caused by hepatitis A, B, and C viruses. These viruses do not cause a cytopathic effect, and the damage to the hepatocytes is the result of the recognition of viral antigens on the hepatocyte surface by cytotoxic T cells. The rash of measles is similarly caused by these cells attacking the infected vascular endothelium in the skin.

(3) Immune-mediated pathogenesis also occurs when virus-antibody-complement complexes form and are deposited in various tissues. This occurs in hepatitis B virus infection, in which immune complexes play a role in producing the arthritis characteristic of the early stage of hepatitis B. The pathogenesis of pneumonia caused by respiratory syncytial virus in infants is attributed to immune complexes formed by maternal IgG and viral antigens.

Virulence   Strains of viruses differ greatly in their ability to cause disease. For example, there are strains of poliovirus which have mutated sufficiently that they have lost the ability to cause polio in immunocompetent individuals; ie, they are **attenuated.** These strains are used in vaccines. The viral genes that control the virulence of the virus are poorly characterized, and the process of virulence is poorly understood.

In the early 1990s, some insight was gained with the finding that some viruses encode the receptors for various mediators of immunity such as interleukin-1 (IL-1) and tumor necrosis factor (TNF). For example, vaccinia virus encodes a protein that binds to IL-1 and fibroma virus encodes a protein that binds to TNF. When released from virus-infected cells, these proteins bind to the immune mediators and block their ability to interact with receptors on their intended targets, our immune cells that mediate host defenses against the viral infection. By reducing our host defenses, the virulence of the virus is enhanced. In addition, some viruses (eg, HIV) can reduce the expression of class I MHC proteins, thereby reducing the ability of cytotoxic T cells to kill the virus-infected cells, and others (eg, herpes simplex virus) inhibit complement. Several viruses (HIV, Epstein-Barr virus, and adenovirus) synthesize RNAs that block the phosphorylation of an initiation factor (eIF-2), which reduces the ability of interferon to block viral replication (see Chapter 33). Collectively, these viral virulence factors are called **virokines.**

Persistent Viral Infections   In most viral infections, the virus does not remain in the body for a significant period after clinical recovery. However, in certain instances, the virus persists for long periods either intact or in the form of a subviral component, eg, the genome. The mechanisms that may play a role in the persistence of viruses include (1) integration of a DNA provirus into host cell DNA, as occurs with retroviruses; (2) immune tolerance, because neutralizing antibodies are not formed; (3) formation of virus-antibody complexes, which remain infectious; (4) location within an immunologically sheltered "sanctuary," eg, the brain; (5) rapid antigenic variation; (6) spread from cell to cell without an extracellular phase, so that virus is not exposed to antibody; and (7) immunosuppression, as in AIDS.

There are three types of persistent viral infections of clinical importance. They are distinguished primarily by whether virus is usually produced by the infected cells and by the timing of the appearance both of the virus and of the symptoms of disease.

A. Chronic-Carrier Infections: Some patients who have been infected with certain viruses continue to produce significant amounts of the virus for long periods. This **carrier state** can follow an asymptomatic infection as well as the actual disease and can itself either be asymptomatic or result in chronic illness. Important clinical examples are chronic hepatitis, which occurs in hepatitis B and hepatitis C virus carriers, and neonatal rubella virus and cytomegalovirus infections, in which carriers can produce virus for years.

B. Latent Infections: In these infections, best illustrated by the herpesvirus group, the patient recovers from the initial infection and virus production stops. Subsequently, the symptoms may **recur,** accompanied by the production of virus. In herpes simplex virus infections, the virus enters the latent state in the cells of the sensory ganglia. The molecular nature of the latent state is unknown. Herpes simplex virus type 1, which causes infections primarily of the eyes and face, is latent in the trigeminal ganglion, whereas herpes simplex virus type 2, which causes infections primarily of the genitals, is latent in the lumbar and sacral ganglia. Varicella-zoster virus, another member of the herpesvirus family, causes varicella (chickenpox) as its initial manifestation and then remains latent, primarily in the trigeminal or thoracic ganglion cells. It can recur in the form of the painful vesicles of zoster (shingles), usually on the face or trunk.

C. Slow Virus Infections: The term "slow virus" refers to the **prolonged period** between the initial infection and the onset of disease, which is usually measured in years. In instances in which the cause has been identified, the virus has been shown to have a normal, not prolonged, growth cycle. It is not, therefore, that virus growth is slow; rather, the incubation period and the progression of the disease are prolonged. Two of these diseases are caused by conventional viruses, namely, subacute sclerosing panencephalitis, which follows several years after measles virus infections, and progressive multifocal leukoencephalopathy (PML), which is caused by JC virus, a papovavirus. PML occurs primarily in patients who have lymphomas or are immunosuppressed. Other slow infections in humans, eg, Creutzfeldt-Jakob disease and kuru, may be caused by unconventional agents called **prions** (see Chapter 28). Slow virus infections are described in Chapter 44.

Review Questions

1. What are inclusion bodies? Why are they important in viral diagnosis?
2. How are giant cells formed in viral infection? What is their importance in viral diagnosis?
3. What is the cytopathic effect? How is it used in viral diagnosis?
4. Describe immunopathogenesis.
5. Distinguish between chronic carrier infections and latent infections.
6. What are slow virus infections?

33

Host Defenses

Host defenses against viruses fall into two major categories: (1) **nonspecific,** of which the most important are interferons; and (2) **specific,** including both humoral and cell-mediated immunity. Interferons are an early, first-line defense, whereas humoral immunity and cell-mediated immunity are effective only later since it takes several days to induce an immune response.

NONSPECIFIC DEFENSES

1. Interferons

Interferons are a heterogeneous group of glycoproteins produced by human and other animal cells after viral infection (or after exposure to other inducers). They inhibit the growth of viruses by **blocking the translation of viral proteins.** Interferons are divided into three groups based on the cell of origin, namely, leukocyte, fibroblast, and lymphocyte. They are also known as alpha, beta, and gamma interferons, respectively. Alpha and beta interferons are induced by viruses, whereas gamma (T cell, immune) interferon is induced by antigens and is one of the effectors of cell-mediated immunity (see Chapter 58). Interferons are cytokines that inhibit the growth of certain cancer

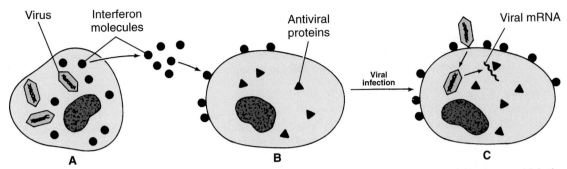

Figure 33–1. Induction and action of interferon. **A:** Virus infection induces the synthesis of interferon, which then leaves the infected cell. **B:** Interferon binds to the surface receptor of an uninfected cell and induces the synthesis of 3 new enzymes (antiviral proteins). **C:** A new virion enters the cell, but the translation of viral mRNA is inhibited by the interferon-induced antiviral proteins. One of these antiviral proteins is a ribonuclease that degrades viral, but not cellular, mRNA. (Modified and reproduced, with permission, from Tortora G, Funk B, Case C: *Microbiology: An Introduction,* 5th ed. Benjamin/Cummings, 1995.)

cells, bacteria, and protozoa, but the focus here will be on their inhibitory effect on viral growth. The following discussion of alpha and beta interferons focuses on two aspects of their antiviral effect: induction and action (Fig 33–1).

Induction of Alpha & Beta Interferons The strong inducers of these interferons are **viruses** and **double-stranded RNAs.** Induction is not specific for a particular virus; many DNA and RNA viruses of humans, other animals, plants, and bacteria are competent, although they differ in effectiveness. The finding that double-stranded RNA, but not single-stranded RNA or DNA, is a good inducer has led to the hypothesis that a double-stranded RNA is synthesized as part of the replicative cycle of all inducing viruses. The double-stranded RNA poly(rI-rC) is one of the strongest inducers and was under consideration as an antiviral agent, but toxic side effects prevented its clinical use. The weak inducers of microbiologic interest include a variety of intracellular bacteria and protozoa, as well as certain bacterial substances such as endotoxin.

This extensive list of inducers makes it clear that **induction** of these interferons is **not specific.** Similarly, their inhibitory **action** is **not specific** for any particular virus. However, they are typically **specific** in regard to the **host species** in which they act; ie, interferons produced by human cells are active in human cells but are much less effective in cells of other species. It is clear, therefore, that other animals cannot be used as a source of interferons for human therapy. Rather, the genes for human interferons have been cloned and material for medical trials is now produced by genetic engineering techniques.

Action of Alpha & Beta Interferons Interferons inhibit the intracellular replication of a **wide variety** of viruses but have little effect on the metabolism of normal cells; ie, they exhibit a remarkable degree of **selective inhibition.** They act by inducing the synthesis of three proteins that **inhibit the translation of viral mRNA** without affecting the translation of cellular mRNA. The three proteins are (1) a 2,5-oligonucleotide synthetase that synthesizes an adenine trinucleotide [2,5-oligo(A)]; (2) a **ribonuclease** that is activated by 2,5-oligo(A) and that degrades viral but not cellular mRNAs; and (3) a protein kinase that phosphorylates an initiation factor for protein synthesis (eIF-2), thereby inactivating it. The endonuclease selectively degrades viral mRNAs by recognizing a nucleotide sequence on viral mRNAs that is not present on cellular mRNAs. Interferons have **no direct effect** on extracellular virus particles.

Because interferons are produced within a few hours of the initiation of viral replication, they may act in the early phase of viral diseases to limit the spread of virus. In contrast, antibody begins to appear in the blood several days after infection.

Alpha interferon has been approved for use in patients with condyloma acuminatum and chronic active hepatitis caused by hepatitis C virus. Gamma interferon reduces recurrent infections in patients with chronic granulomatous disease (see Chapter 68). Interferons are also used clinically in patients with cancers such as Kaposi's sarcoma and hairy cell leukemia.

2. Phagocytosis

Macrophages, particularly fixed macrophages of the reticuloendothelial system and alveolar macrophages, are the important cell types in limiting virus infection. In contrast, polymorphonuclear leukocytes are the predominant cellular defense in bacterial infections.

3. Fever

Elevated body temperature may play a role in host defenses, but its importance is uncertain. Fever may act in two ways. (1) The higher body temperature may directly inactivate the virus particles, particularly enveloped viruses, which are more heat-sensitive than nonenveloped viruses. (2) Replication of some viruses is reduced at higher temperatures, and so fever may inhibit replication.

4. Mucociliary Clearance

The mucociliary clearance mechanism of the respiratory tract may protect the host. Its damage, eg, from smoking, results in an increased frequency of viral respiratory tract infections, especially influenza.

5. Factors that Modify Host Defenses

Several factors influence host defenses in a nonspecific or multifactorial way.

(1) Age is a significant variable in the outcome of viral infections. In general, infections are more severe in neonates and in the elderly than in older children and young adults. For example, influenza is typically more severe in older people than in younger adults and herpes simplex virus infections are more severe in neonates than in adults.

(2) Increased corticosteroid levels predispose to more severe infections with some viruses, such as varicella-zoster virus; the use of topical cortisone in herpetic keratitis can exacerbate eye damage. It is not clear how these effects are mediated, because corticosteroids can cause a variety of pertinent effects, namely, lysis of lymphocytes, decreased recruitment of monocytes, inhibition of interferon production, and stabilization of lysosomes.

(3) Malnutrition leads to more severe viral infections; eg, there is a much higher death rate from measles in developing countries than in developed ones. Poor nutrition causes decreased immunoglobulin production and phagocyte activity as well as reduced skin and mucous membrane integrity.

SPECIFIC DEFENSES

There is evidence for natural resistance to some viruses in certain species, which is probably based on the absence of receptors on the cells of the resistant species. However, by far the most important type of defense is **acquired immunity,** either actively acquired by exposure to the virus or passively acquired by the transfer of immune serum. Active immunity can be elicited by contracting the actual disease, by having an inapparent infection, or by being vaccinated.

1. Active Immunity

Active immunity is important in the **prevention** of disease, but its ability to enhance the patient's **recovery** from a viral disease is limited. Disease prevention is chiefly due to the presence of immunoglobulins; eg, passive transfer of serum containing specific antibodies is typically protective. Cell-mediated immunity is also important, because when it is suppressed, severe viral infections commonly occur, eg, in AIDS patients.

The duration of protection varies; disseminated viral infections such as measles and mumps confer lifelong immunity against recurrences, but localized infections such as the common cold usually impart only a brief immunity of several months. IgA confers protection against viruses that enter through the respiratory and gastrointestinal mucosa, and IgM and IgG protect against viruses that en-

Antiviral Drugs

35

Compared with the number of drugs available to treat bacterial infections, the number of antiviral drugs is **very small.** The major reason for this difference is the **difficulty in obtaining selective toxicity** against viruses; their replication is intimately involved with the normal synthetic processes of the cell. Despite the difficulty, several virus-specific replication steps have been identified that are potentially useful (Table 35–1).

Another limitation of antiviral drugs is that they are relatively ineffective, because many cycles of viral replication occur during the incubation period when the patient is well. By the time the patient has a recognizable systemic viral disease, the virus has spread throughout the body and it is too late to interdict it. Furthermore, some viruses, eg, herpesviruses, become latent within cells, and no current antiviral drug can eradicate them.

Another potential limiting factor is the emergence of drug-resistant viral mutants. At present, this is not of major clinical significance. Mutants of herpesvirus resistant to acyclovir have been recovered from patients, but they do not interfere with recovery.

INHIBITION OF EARLY EVENTS

Amantadine (α-adamantanamine, Symmetrel) is a tricyclic compound (Fig 35–1) that is used to prevent influenza A infections. It **inhibits uncoating of the virus** by binding to the matrix protein in the virion. Absorption and penetration occur normally, but transcription by the virion RNA polymerase does not. This drug specifically inhibits influenza A virus; influenza B and C viruses are not affected. Despite its efficacy in preventing influenza, it is not widely used in the United States because the vaccine is preferred for the high-risk population. The main side effects of amantadine are central nervous system alterations such as dizziness, ataxia, and insomnia. Rimantadine (Flumadine) is a derivative of amantadine and has the same mode of action but fewer side effects.

INHIBITION OF VIRAL NUCLEIC ACID SYNTHESIS

Inhibitors of Herpesviruses

A. Acyclovir: Acyclovir (acycloguanosine, Zovirax) is a nucleoside analogue with a three-carbon fragment in place of the normal sugar, ribose (Fig 35–1). Acyclovir is active primarily against herpes simplex virus types 1 and 2 (HSV-1 and -2) and varicella-zoster virus (VZV). It is relatively nontoxic, because it is incorporated preferentially into virus-infected cells. This is due to the **virus-encoded thymidine kinase,** which phosphorylates acyclovir much more effectively than

Table 35–1. Potential sites for antiviral chemotherapy.

Site of Action	Effective Drugs
Early events (entry or uncoating of the virus)	Amantadine, rimantadine
Nucleic acid synthesis by viral DNA and RNA polymerases	Acyclovir, ganciclovir, vidarabine, idoxuridine, trifluridine, foscarnet, zidovudine (azidothymidine), didanosine (dideoxyinosine), zalcitabine (dideoxycytidine), stavudine (d4T), lamivudine (3TC), nevirapine, ribavirin
Cleavage of precursor polypeptides	Saquinavir, indinavir, ritonavir
Protein synthesis directed by viral mRNA	Interferon, methisazone
Action of viral regulatory proteins	
Assembly of the particle, including the matrix protein	
Release of the particle by budding	

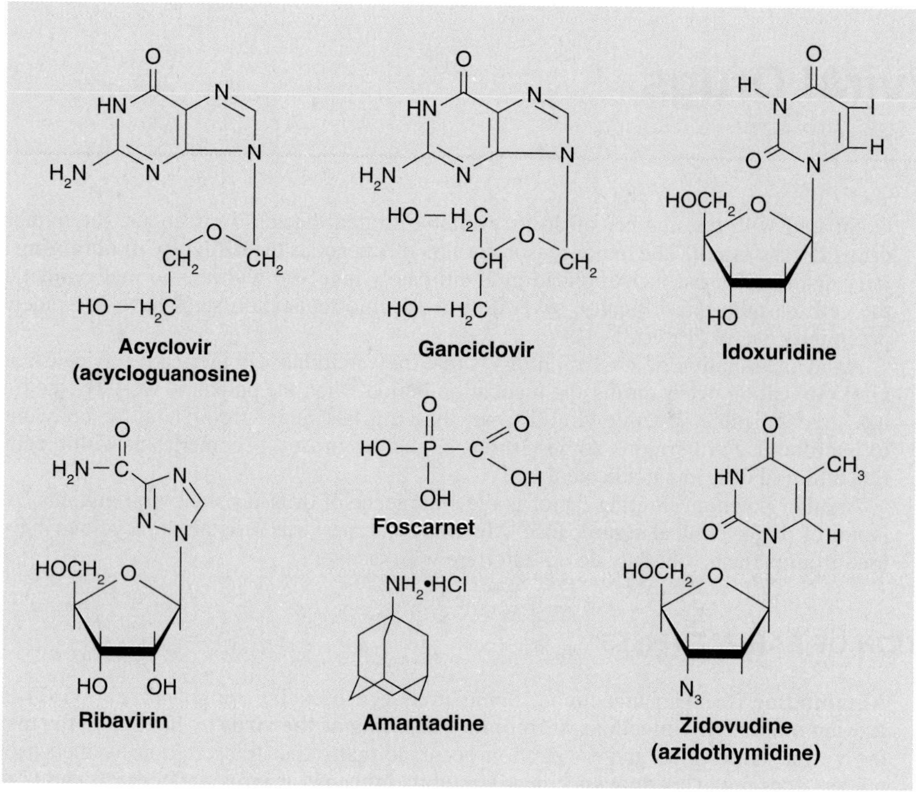

Figure 35–1. Structures of some medically important antiviral drugs.

does the cellular thymidine kinase. Because only HSV and VZV encode a kinase that efficiently phosphorylates the drug, it is active primarily against these viruses. It has no activity against cytomegalovirus (CMV). Once the drug is phosphorylated to acyclovir monophosphate by the viral thymidine kinase, cellular kinases synthesize acyclovir triphosphate, which **inhibits viral DNA polymerase** much more effectively than it inhibits cellular DNA polymerase. Acyclovir and ganciclovir (see below) cause chain termination because they lack a hydroxyl group in the 3′ position.

To recap, the selective action of acyclovir is based on two features of the drug. (1) Acyclovir is phosphorylated to acyclovir monophosphate much more effectively by herpesvirus-encoded thymidine kinase than by cellular thymidine kinase. It is therefore preferentially activated in herpesvirus-infected cells and much less so in uninfected cells, which accounts for its relatively few side effects. (2) Acyclovir triphosphate inhibits herpesvirus-encoded DNA polymerase much more effectively than it does cellular DNA polymerase. It therefore inhibits viral DNA synthesis to a much greater extent than cellular DNA synthesis.

Topical acyclovir is effective in the treatment of primary genital herpes and reduces the frequency of recurrences while it is being taken. However, it has **no effect on latency** or on the rate of recurrences after treatment is stopped. Acyclovir is the treatment of choice for HSV-1 encephalitis and is effective in preventing systemic infection by HSV-1 or VZV in immunocompromised patients. It is not effective treatment for HSV-1 recurrent lesions in immunocompetent hosts. Acyclovir-resistant mutants have been isolated from HSV-1- and VZV-infected patients.

B. Ganciclovir: Ganciclovir (dihydroxypropoxymethylguanine, DHPG) is a nucleoside analogue of guanosine with a four-carbon fragment in place of the normal sugar, ribose (Fig 35–1). It is structurally similar to acyclovir but is more active against cytomegalovirus than is acyclovir. It is effective in the treatment of retinitis caused by CMV in AIDS patients and may be useful in other disseminated infections caused by this virus. The main side effects of ganciclovir are leukopenia and thrombocytopenia as a result of bone marrow suppression.

C. Vidarabine: Vidarabine (adenine arabinoside, ara-A) is a nucleoside analogue with arabinose in place of the normal sugar, ribose. On entering the cell, the drug is phosphorylated by cellular kinases to the triphosphate, which inhibits the herpesvirus-encoded DNA polymerase more effectively than the cellular DNA polymerase. Vidarabine is effective against HSV-1 infections such as encephalitis and keratitis but is less effective and more toxic than acyclovir.

D. Iododeoxyuridine: Iododeoxyuridine (idoxuridine, IDU, IUDR) is a nucleoside analogue in which the methyl group of thymidine is replaced by an iodine atom (Fig 35–1). The drug is phosphorylated to the triphosphate by cellular kinases and incorporated into DNA. Because IDU has a high frequency of mismatched pairing to guanine, it causes the formation of faulty progeny DNA and mRNA. However, because IDU is incorporated into normal cell DNA as well as viral DNA, it is too toxic to be used systemically. It is clinically useful in the topical treatment of herpes simplex virus keratoconjunctivitis.

E. Trifluorothymidine: Trifluorothymidine (trifluridine, Viroptic) is a nucleoside analogue in which the methyl group of thymidine contains 3 fluorine atoms instead of 3 hydrogen atoms. Its mechanism of action is probably similar to that of IDU. Like IDU, it is too toxic for systemic use but is clinically useful in the topical treatment of herpes simplex virus keratoconjunctivitis.

F. Foscarnet: Foscarnet (trisodium phosphonoformate, Foscavir), unlike the previous drugs which are nucleoside analogues, is a pyrophosphate analogue. It inhibits the DNA polymerases of all herpesviruses, especially HSV and CMV. Unlike acyclovir, it does not require activation by thymidine kinase. Foscarnet also inhibits the reverse transcriptase of HIV. It is approved for use in patients with CMV retinitis but ganciclovir is the treatment of first choice. Foscarnet is also used to treat patients infected with acyclovir-resistant mutants of HSV-1 and VZV.

Inhibitors of Retroviruses

A. Nucleoside inhibitors: The selective toxicity of azidothymidine, dideoxyinosine, dideoxycytidine, d4T, and 3TC is based on their ability to **inhibit DNA synthesis by the reverse transcriptase** of human immunodeficiency virus (HIV) to a much greater extent that they inhibit DNA synthesis by the DNA polymerase in human cells. The effect of these drugs on the replication of HIV is depicted in Fig 45–3.

1. Azidothymidine—Azidothymidine (zidovudine, Retrovir, AZT) is a nucleoside analogue that causes **chain termination** during DNA synthesis; it has an azido group in place of the hydroxyl group on the ribose (Fig 35–1). It is particularly effective against DNA synthesis by the reverse transcriptase of HIV and inhibits growth of the virus in cell culture. It is currently the drug of choice in patients with AIDS. The main side effects of AZT are bone marrow suppression and myopathy.

2. Dideoxyinosine—Dideoxyinosine (didanosine, Videx, ddI) is a nucleoside analogue that causes chain termination during DNA synthesis; it is missing hydroxyl groups on the ribose. The administered drug ddI is metabolized to ddATP, which is the active compound. It is effective against DNA synthesis by the reverse transcriptase of HIV and is used to treat patients with AIDS who are intolerant of or resistant to AZT. The main side effects of ddI are pancreatitis and peripheral neuropathy.

3. Dideoxycytidine—Dideoxycytidine (zalcitabine, Hivid, ddC) is a nucleoside analogue that causes chain termination during DNA synthesis; it is missing hydroxyl groups on the ribose. The administered drug ddC is metabolized to ddCTP, which is the active compound. It is effective against DNA synthesis by the reverse transcriptase of HIV and is used to treat patients who are intolerant of or resistant to AZT. The main side effects of ddC are the same as those of ddI but occur less often.

4. d4T—d4T (stavudine, Zerit) is a nucleoside analogue that causes chain termination during DNA synthesis. It inhibits DNA synthesis by the reverse transcriptase of HIV and is used to treat patients with advanced AIDS who are intolerant of or resistant to other approved therapies. The molecular name of d4T is didehydro-dideoxythymidine. The main side effect is peripheral neuropathy.

5. 3TC—3TC (lamivudine, Epivir) is a nucleoside analogue that causes chain termination during DNA synthesis by the reverse transcriptase of HIV. When used in combination with AZT, it is very effective both in reducing the viral load and in elevating the CD4 cell count. The molecular name of

3TC is dideoxythiacytidine. It is one of the best-tolerated of the nucleoside inhibitors, but side effects such as neutropenia, pancreatitis, and peripheral neuropathy do occur.

B. Non-nucleoside inhibitors: Unlike the drugs described above, the drugs in this group are not nucleoside analogues and do not cause chain termination. The non-nucleoside inhibitors act by binding near the active site of the enzyme and inducing a conformational change that inhibits the synthesis of viral DNA.

1. Nevirapine—Nevirapine (Viramune) is the non-nucleoside inhibitor currently approved for use in the treatment of HIV infection. It is usually used in combination with AZT and ddI. There is no cross-resistance with AZT, ddI, ddC, d4T, or 3TC. The main side effect of nevirapine is a severe skin rash (Stevens-Johnson syndrome). Nevirapine is a member of a class of drugs called the dipyridodiazepinones; its precise name is beyond the scope of this book.

Inhibitors of Other Viruses
A. Ribavirin: Ribavirin (Virazole) is a nucleoside analogue in which a triazole-carboxamide moiety is substituted in place of the normal purine precursor aminoimidazole-carboxamide (Fig 35–1). The drug inhibits the synthesis of guanine nucleotides, which are essential for both DNA and RNA viruses. Ribavirin aerosol is used clinically to treat pneumonitis caused by respiratory syncytial virus in infants and to treat severe influenza B infections.

INHIBITION OF CLEAVAGE OF PRECURSOR POLYPEPTIDES

Saquinavir, ritonavir, and indinavir are inhibitors of the protease encoded by human immunodeficiency virus (Fig 35–2). The protease cleaves the *gag* and *pol* precursor polypeptides to produce several nucleocapsid proteins, eg, p24, and enzymatic proteins, eg, reverse transcriptase, required for viral replication. The effect of protease inhibitors on the replication of HIV is depicted in Fig 45–3.

INHIBITION OF VIRAL PROTEIN SYNTHESIS

A. Interferon: The mode of action of interferon is described in Chapter 33. Recombinant alpha interferon is effective in the treatment of some patients with chronic hepatitis B and chronic hepatitis C infections. It also causes regression of condylomata acuminata lesions.

B. Methisazone: Methisazone (*N*-methylisatin-β-thiosemicarbazone) specifically inhibits the protein synthesis of poxviruses, such as smallpox and vaccinia viruses, by blocking the translation of late mRNA. The drug can be used to treat certain rare, severe side effects of the smallpox vaccine, eg, disseminated vaccinia. However, it is rarely (if ever) used, because the smallpox vaccine is no longer administered except to military personnel.

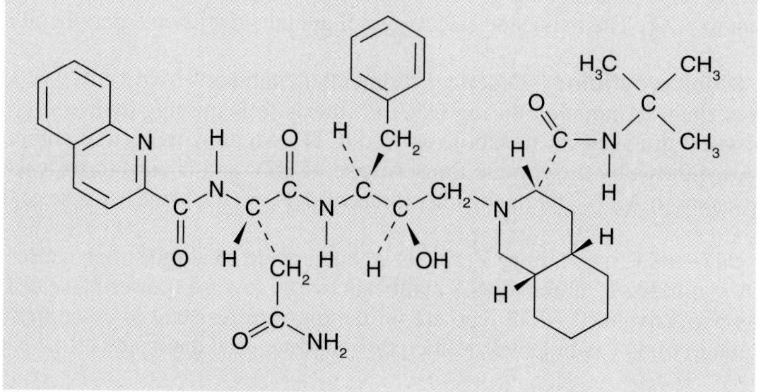

Figure 35–2. Structure of the protease inhibitor saquinavir. Note the presence of several peptide bonds, which interact with the active site of the protease.

Table 35–2. Chemoprophylactic use of drugs described in this chapter.

Drug	Use	Number of Chapter for Additional Information
Amantadine	Prevention of influenza during outbreaks caused by influenza A virus	39
Acyclovir	Prevention of disseminated HSV or VZV disease in immunocompromised patients	37
Ganciclovir	Prevention of disseminated CMV disease in immunocompromised patients, especially retinitis in AIDS patients	37
Azidothymidine	Possible prevention of HIV infection in needle-stick injuries	45

CHEMOPROPHYLAXIS

In most instances, the antiviral agents described in this chapter are used to *treat* infectious diseases. However, there are times when they are used to *prevent* diseases from occurring, a process called **chemoprophylaxis.** Table 35–2 describes the drugs used for this purpose and the situations in which they are used. For more information, see the chapters on the individual viruses.

Review Questions

1. Why are there fewer antiviral drugs than antibacterial drugs?
2. What is the basis of the selective action of acyclovir against herpes simplex viruses?
3. Describe amantadine, azidothymidine, and ganciclovir from two points of view: (a) mechanism of action and (b) spectrum of activity.

Viral Vaccines

36

Because few drugs are useful against viral infections, prevention of infection by the use of vaccines is very important. Prevention of viral diseases can be achieved by the use of vaccines that induce active immunity or by the administration of preformed antibody that provides passive immunity.

ACTIVE IMMUNITY

There are two types of vaccines that induce **active** immunity: those that contain **live virus** whose pathogenicity has been **attenuated*** and those that contain **killed virus.** The attributes of the two

---

*An attenuated virus is one that is unable to cause disease but retains its antigenicity and can induce protection.

Table 36–1. Characteristics of live and killed viral vaccines.

Characteristic	Live Vaccine	Killed Vaccine
Duration of immunity	Longer	Shorter
Effectiveness of protection	Greater	Lower
Immunoglobulins produced	IgA[1] and IgG	IgG
Cell-mediated immunity produced	Yes	Weakly or none
Interruption of transmission of virulent virus	More effective	Less effective
Reversion to virulence	Possible	No
Stability at room temperature	Low	High
Excretion of vaccine virus and transmission to nonimmune contacts	Possible	No

[1] If the vaccine is given by the natural route.

types of vaccines are listed in Table 36–1. In general, live vaccines are preferred to vaccines containing killed virus because their protection is **greater** and **longer-lasting.** With live vaccines, the virus multiplies in the host, producing a prolonged antigenic stimulus, and both IgA and IgG are elicited when the vaccine is administered by the natural route of infection, eg, when polio vaccine is given orally. Killed vaccines, which are usually given intramuscularly, do not stimulate a major IgA response. Killed vaccines typically do not stimulate a cytotoxic T cell response, because the virus in the vaccine does not replicate. In the absence of replication, no viral epitopes are presented in association with class I MHC proteins and the cytotoxic T cell response is not activated (see Chapter 58). Although live vaccines stimulate a long-lasting response, booster doses are now recommended with measles and polio vaccines.

There are three concerns about the use of live vaccines:

(1) They are composed of attenuated viral mutants, which can **revert to virulence** either during vaccine production or in the immunized person. Reversion to virulence during production can be detected by quality control testing, but there is no test to predict whether reversion will occur in the immunized individual.

(2) The live vaccine can be **excreted** by the immunized person. This is a double-edged sword. It is advantageous if the spread of the virus successfully immunizes others, as occurs with the live polio vaccine. However, it could be a problem if, eg, a virulent poliovirus revertant spreads to a susceptible person. Rare cases of paralytic polio occur in the USA each year by this route of infection.

(3) A second virus could **contaminate** the vaccine if it was present in the cell cultures used to prepare the vaccine. This concern exists for both live and killed vaccines, although, clearly, the live vaccine presents a greater problem, because the process that inactivates the virus in the killed vaccine could inactivate the contaminant as well. It is interesting, therefore, that the most striking incidence of contamination of a vaccine occurred with the *killed* polio vaccine. In 1960, it was reported that live simian vacuolating virus 40 (SV40 virus), an inapparent "passenger" virus in monkey kidney cells, had contaminated some lots of polio vaccine and was resistant to the formaldehyde used to inactivate the poliovirus. There was great concern when it was found that SV40 virus causes sarcomas in a variety of rodents. Fortunately, it has not caused cancer in the individuals inoculated with the contaminated polio vaccine.

Certain viral vaccines, namely, influenza, measles, mumps and yellow fever vaccines, are grown in chick embryos. These vaccines should *not* be given to those who have had an **anaphalactic reaction to eggs.** People with allergies to chicken feathers can be immunized.

In addition to the disadvantages of the killed vaccines already mentioned—namely, that they induce a **shorter duration** of protection, are **less protective,** and **induce fewer IgA antibodies**—there is the potential problem that the inactivation process might be inadequate. Although this is rare, it happened in the early days of the manufacture of the killed polio vaccine. However, killed vaccines do have two advantages: they **cannot revert to virulence** and they are **more heat-stable,** so they can be used more easily in tropical climates.

Table 2. The 10 most common notifiable viral diseases in the United States in 1995.[1]

Disease	Number of Cases
Chickenpox (varicella)	120,624
AIDS	71,547
Hepatitis A	31,582
Hepatitis B	10,805
Hepatitis C (non-A, non-B)	4,576
Mumps	906
Measles	281
Rubella	128
Rabies	5
Poliomyelitis	2

[1]The latest year for which complete data are available.

Table 2 lists the frequency of the 10 most common notifiable viral diseases in the United States for 1995 (the latest year for which complete data are available). Chickenpox (varicella) is by far the most frequent, with AIDS in second place. Hepatitis A and hepatitis B are in third and fourth places, respectively. Note that the common cold, which is probably the most frequent disease, is not listed because it is not a notifiable disease.

DNA Enveloped Viruses

37

Herpesviruses

The herpesvirus family contains five important human pathogens: herpes simplex virus types 1 and 2, varicella-zoster virus, cytomegalovirus, and Epstein-Barr virus.

All herpesviruses are structurally similar. Each has an **icosahedral** core surrounded by a lipoprotein **envelope.** The genome is linear double-stranded DNA. The virion does not contain a polymerase. They are large (120–200 nm in diameter), second in size only to poxviruses. They replicate in the nucleus, form intranuclear inclusions, and are the only viruses that obtain their envelopes by budding from the nuclear membrane.

Herpesviruses are noted for their ability to cause **latent infections.** In these infections, the acute disease is followed by an asymptomatic period during which the virus remains in a quiescent (latent) state. When the patient is exposed to an inciting agent or immunosuppression occurs, reactivation of virus replication and disease can occur. With some herpesviruses, eg, herpes simplex virus, the symptoms of the subsequent episodes are similar to those of the initial one; however, with others, eg, varicella-zoster virus, they are different (Table 37–1).

Three of the herpesviruses, herpes simplex virus types 1 and 2, and varicella-zoster virus, cause a **vesicular rash,** both in primary infections and in reactivations. Primary infections are usually more severe than reactivations. The other two herpesviruses, cytomegalovirus and Epstein-Barr virus, do not cause a vesicular rash.

Certain herpesviruses are suspected of causing cancer in humans; eg, Epstein-Barr virus is associated with Burkitt's lymphoma and nasopharyngeal carcinoma, and human herpesvirus 8 (described in Chapter 46) is associated with Kaposi's sarcoma. Several herpesviruses cause cancer in animals, eg, leukemia in monkeys and lymphomatosis in chickens (see tumor viruses, Chapter 43).

Table 37–1. Important features of common herpesvirus infections.

Virus	Primary Infection	Usual Site of Latency	Recurrent Infection	Route of Transmission
HSV-1	Gingivostomatitis[1]	Cranial sensory ganglia	Herpes labialis,[2] encephalitis, keratitis	Via respiratory secretions and saliva
HSV-2	Herpes genitalis, perinatal disseminated disease	Lumbar or sacral sensory ganglia	Herpes genitalis	Sexual contact, perinatal infection
VZV	Varicella	Cranial or thoracic sensory ganglia	Zoster[2]	Via respiratory secretions
EBV	Infectious mononucleosis[1]	B lymphocytes	None[3]	Via respiratory secretions and saliva
CMV	Congenital infection (in utero), mononucleosis	Uncertain[4]	Asymptomatic shedding[2]	Intrauterine infection, transfusions, sexual contact, via secretions (eg, saliva and urine)

[1] Primary infection is often asymptomatic.
[2] In immunocompromised patients, dissemination is common.
[3] The relationship of EBV infection to "chronic fatigue syndrome" and B cell neoplasms is unclear.
[4] CMV may be latent within circulating lymphoid cells or epithelial cells.

HERPES SIMPLEX VIRUSES (HSV)

Herpes simplex virus type 1 (HSV-1) and type 2 (HSV-2) are distinguished by two main criteria: antigenicity and location of lesions. Lesions caused by HSV-1 are, in general, above the waist, whereas those caused by HSV-2 are below the waist.

Diseases   HSV-1 causes acute gingivostomatitis, recurrent herpes labialis (cold sores), keratoconjunctivitis, and encephalitis. HSV-2 causes genital herpes, neonatal herpes, and aseptic meningitis.

Important Properties   HSV-1 and HSV-2 are structurally and morphologically indistinguishable. They can, however, be differentiated by the restriction endonuclease patterns of their genome DNA and by type-specific monoclonal antisera. Humans are the natural hosts of both HSV-1 and HSV-2.

Summary of Replicative Cycle   HSV-1 attaches to the cell surface at the site of the receptor for fibroblast growth factor. After entry into the cell, the virion is uncoated and the genome DNA enters the nucleus. Early virus messenger RNA (mRNA) is transcribed by host cell RNA polymerase and then translated into early, nonstructural proteins in the cytoplasm. Two of these early proteins, thymidine kinase and DNA polymerase, are important because they are sufficiently different from the corresponding cellular enzymes to be involved in the action of antiviral drugs, eg, acyclovir.

The viral DNA polymerase replicates the genome DNA, at which time early protein synthesis is shut off and late protein synthesis begins. These late, structural proteins are transported to the nucleus, where virion assembly occurs. The virion obtains its envelope by budding through the nuclear membrane and exits the cell via tubules or vacuoles that communicate with the exterior. In latently infected cells, multiple copies of HSV-1 DNA are found in the cytoplasm of infected neurons. Only a few genes are transcribed, and none are translated into protein.

Transmission & Epidemiology   HSV-1 is transmitted primarily in **saliva,** whereas HSV-2 is transmitted by **sexual contact.** As a result, HSV-1 infections occur mainly on the face whereas HSV-2 lesions occur in the genital area. However, oral-genital sexual practices can result in HSV-1 infections of the genitals and HSV-2 lesions in the oral cavity (this occurs in about 10–20% of cases). Although transmission occurs most often when active lesions are present, asymptomatic shedding of both HSV-1 and HSV-2 does occur and plays an important role in transmission.

The number of HSV-2 infections has markedly increased in recent years, whereas that of HSV-1 infections has not. Roughly 80% of people in the United States are infected with HSV-1, and 40% have recurrent herpes labialis. Most primary infections by HSV-1 occur in childhood, as evidenced by the early appearance of antibody. In contrast, antibody to HSV-2 does not appear until the age of sexual activity.

Pathogenesis & Immunity The virus replicates in the skin or mucous membrane at the initial site of infection, then migrates up the neuron and becomes latent in the sensory ganglion cells. In general, HSV-1 becomes latent in the **trigeminal ganglia** whereas HSV-2 becomes latent in the **lumbar and sacral ganglia.** The precise nature of the virus during latency is unknown, but lysogeny in bacterial viruses can be used as a model. The virus can be reactivated from the latent state by a variety of inducers, eg, sunlight, hormonal changes, trauma, stress, and fever, at which time it migrates down the neuron and replicates in the skin, causing lesions.

The typical skin lesion is a **vesicle** that contains serous fluid filled with virus particles and cell debris. When the vesicle ruptures, virus is liberated and can be transmitted to other individuals. **Multinucleated giant cells** are typically found at the base of herpesvirus lesions.

Immunity is type-specific, but some cross-protection exists. However, immunity is incomplete, and both reinfection and reactivation occur in the presence of circulating IgG. **Cell-mediated immunity** is important in limiting herpesviruses, since its suppression often results in reactivation, spread, and severe disease.

Clinical Findings HSV-1 causes several forms of primary and recurrent disease:

(1) Gingivostomatitis occurs primarily in children and is characterized by fever, irritability, and vesicular lesions in the mouth. The primary disease is more severe and lasts longer than recurrences. The lesions heal spontaneously in 2–3 weeks. Many children have asymptomatic primary infections.

(2) Herpes labialis (fever blisters or cold sores) is the milder, recurrent form and is characterized by crops of vesicles, usually at the mucocutaneous junction of the lips or nose. Recurrences frequently reappear at the same site.

(3) Keratoconjunctivitis is characterized by corneal ulcers and lesions of the conjunctival epithelium. Recurrences can lead to scarring and blindness.

(4) Encephalitis, which usually involves the temporal lobe, has a high mortality rate and causes severe neurologic sequelae in those who survive.

(5) Herpetic whitlow is a pustular lesion of the skin of the finger or hand. It can occur in medical personnel as a result of contact with patient's lesions.

(6) Disseminated infections, such as esophagitis and pneumonia, occur in immunocompromised patients with depressed T cell function.

HSV-2 causes several diseases, both primary and recurrent:

(1) Genital herpes is characterized by painful vesicular lesions of the male and female genitals and anal area. The lesions are more severe and protracted in primary disease than in recurrences. Primary infections are associated with fever and inguinal adenopathy. Asymptomatic infections occur in both men (in the prostate or urethra) and women (in the cervix) and can be a source of infection of other individuals. Many infections are asymptomatic; ie, many people have antibody to HSV-2 but have no history of disease.

(2) Neonatal herpes originates chiefly from contact with vesicular lesions within the birth canal. In some cases, there are no visible lesions; nevertheless, HSV-2 is being shed (asymptomatic shedding) and can infect the child during birth. Neonatal herpes varies from a severe generalized disease or encephalitis through milder local lesions to asymptomatic infection. Neonatal disease may be prevented by performing cesarean section on women with either active lesions or positive viral cultures. Both HSV-1 and HSV-2 can cause severe neonatal infections that are acquired after birth from carriers handling the child. Despite their association with neonatal infections, neither HSV-1 nor HSV-2 causes congenital abnormalities to any significant degree.

(3) Aseptic meningitis caused by HSV-2 is usually a mild, self-limited disease with few sequelae.

Laboratory Diagnosis The most important diagnostic procedure is isolation of the virus from the lesion by growth in cell culture. The typical cytopathic effect occurs in 1–3 days, after which the virus is identified by fluorescent-antibody staining of the infected cells or by detecting virus-specific glycoproteins in ELISAs. A rapid diagnosis from skin lesions can be made by using the **Tzanck smear,** in which cells from the base of the vesicle are stained with Giemsa's stain. The presence of multinucleated giant cells suggests herpesvirus infection. A rapid diagnosis of encephalitis can be made by fluorescent-antibody staining of a brain biopsy, but virus is rarely recovered from the cerebrospinal fluid.

Serologic tests such as the neutralization test can be used in the diagnosis of primary infections, since a significant rise in antibody titer is readily observed. However, they are of no use in the diagnosis of recurrent infections, because many adults already have circulating antibodies and recurrences rarely cause a rise in antibody titer.

Treatment   **Acyclovir** (acycloguanosine, Zovirax) is the treatment of choice for encephalitis and systemic disease caused by HSV-1. It is also the treatment for primary and recurrent genital herpes; it **shortens the duration** of the lesions and **reduces the extent of shedding** of the virus. Acyclovir is also used to treat neonatal infections caused by HSV-2. Mutants of HSV-1 resistant to acyclovir have been isolated from patients; foscarnet can be used in these cases. For HSV-1 eye infections, other nucleoside analogues, eg, trifluridine (Viroptic), are used topically. Penciclovir can be used to treat recurrences of orolabial HSV-1 infections in immunocompetent adults. Note that no drug treatment of the primary infection prevents recurrences; drugs have **no effect on the latent state,** but prophylactic long-term acyclovir administration can suppress clinical recurrences.

Prevention   Prevention involves avoiding contact with the vesicular lesion or ulcer. Cesarean section is recommended for women who are at term and who have genital lesions or positive viral cultures.

VARICELLA-ZOSTER VIRUS (VZV)

Disease   Varicella (chickenpox) is the primary disease; zoster (shingles) is the recurrent form.

Important Properties   VZV is structurally and morphologically identical to other herpesviruses but is antigenically different. It has a single serotype. The same virus causes both varicella and zoster. Humans are the natural hosts.

Summary of Replicative Cycle   The cycle is similar to that of HSV (see p 194).

Transmission & Epidemiology   The virus is transmitted by **respiratory droplets** and by direct contact with the lesions. Varicella is a highly contagious disease of childhood; over 90% of people in the United States have antibody by age 10 years. Varicella occurs worldwide.

Pathogenesis & Immunity   VZV infects the mucosa of the upper respiratory tract, then spreads via the blood to the skin, where the typical **vesicular rash** occurs. **Multinucleated giant cells** with intranuclear inclusions are seen in the base of the lesions. After the host has recovered, the virus becomes **latent,** probably in the **dorsal root ganglia.** Later in life, frequently at times of reduced cell-mediated immunity or local trauma, the virus is activated and causes the vesicular skin lesions and **nerve pain** of zoster.

Immunity following varicella is lifelong: a person gets varicella only once, but zoster can occur despite this immunity to varicella. Zoster usually occurs only once. The frequency of zoster increases with advancing age, perhaps as a consequence of waning immunity.

Clinical Findings

A.   Varicella: After an incubation period of 14–21 days, brief prodromal symptoms of fever and malaise occur. A papulovesicular rash then appears in crops on the trunk and spreads to the head and extremities. The rash evolves from papules to vesicles, pustules, and, finally, crusts. Itching is marked. Varicella is mild in children but more severe in adults. Varicella pneumonia and encephalitis are the major rare complications. **Reye's syndrome,** characterized by encephalopathy and liver degeneration, is associated with VZV and influenza B virus infection, especially in children given aspirin. Its pathogenesis is unknown.

B. Zoster: The occurrence of painful vesicles along the course of a sensory nerve of the head or trunk is the usual picture. The pain can last for weeks, and postzoster neuralgia can be debilitating. In immunocompromised patients, life-threatening disseminated infections such as pneumonia can occur.

Laboratory Diagnosis Although most diagnoses are made clinically, laboratory tests are available. A presumptive diagnosis can be made by using the Tzanck smear. Multinucleated giant cells are seen in VZV as well as HSV lesions. The definitive diagnosis is made by isolation of the virus in cell culture and identification with specific antiserum. A rise in antibody titer can be used to diagnose varicella but is less useful in the diagnosis of zoster, since antibody is already present.

Treatment No antiviral therapy is necessary for chickenpox or shingles in normal patients. Systemic disease in immunocompromised patients can be treated with acyclovir. Systemic disease caused by acyclovir-resistant strains of VZV can be treated with foscarnet. Acyclovir and two similar drugs, famciclovir (Famvir) and valacyclovir (Valtrex), can be used in patients with zoster to accelerate healing of the lesions, but these drugs do not cure the latent state and have little effect on postzoster neuralgia.

Prevention **Acyclovir** is useful in preventing varicella and disseminated zoster in immunocompromised people exposed to the virus. **Varicella-zoster immune globulin** (VZIG), which contains a high titer of antibody to the virus, is also used for such prophylaxis. A **vaccine containing live, attenuated VZV** (Varivax) was approved by the FDA in 1995. The vaccine is very effective in preventing varicella, but zoster can still occur in those previously infected because the vaccine does not eliminate the latent state. One dose is recommended for children ages 1 to 12 years. Teenagers and adults who have not had the disease should receive two doses.

CYTOMEGALOVIRUS (CMV)

Diseases CMV causes cytomegalic inclusion disease (especially congenital abnormalities) in neonates. It is the **most common cause of congenital abnormalities** in the United States. It also causes pneumonia and other diseases in immunocompromised patients and heterophil-negative mononucleosis in immunocompetent individuals.

Important Properties CMV is structurally and morphologically identical to other herpesviruses but is antigenically different. It has a single serotype. Humans are the natural hosts; animal CMV strains do not infect humans. Giant cells are formed, hence the name "cytomegalo."

Summary of Replicative Cycle The cycle is similar to that of HSV (see p 194).

Transmission & Epidemiology CMV is transmitted by a **variety of modes.** Early in life it is transmitted across the placenta, within the birth canal, and quite commonly in mother's milk. Its most common mode of transmission is via saliva in young children. Later in life it is transmitted sexually; it is present in both semen and cervical secretions. It can also be transmitted during blood transfusions and organ transplants. CMV infection occurs worldwide, and over 80% of adults have antibody.

Pathogenesis & Immunity Infection of the fetus can cause **cytomegalic inclusion disease,** characterized by multinucleated giant cells with prominent intranuclear inclusions. Many organs are affected, and widespread congenital abnormalities result. Infection of the fetus occurs mainly when a **primary infection** occurs in the pregnant woman, ie, when she has no antibodies that will neutralize the virus before it can infect the fetus. The fetus usually will not be infected if the pregnant woman has antibodies against the virus. Congenital abnormalities are **more common when a fetus is infected during the first trimester** than later in gestation because the first trimester is the time when development of organs occurs and the death of any precursor cells can result in congenital defects.

Infections of children and adults are usually asymptomatic, except in immunocompromised individuals. CMV enters a **latent** state in leukocytes and can be reactivated when cell-mediated immunity is decreased. CMV can also persist in kidneys for years. Reactivation of CMV from the latent state in cervical cells can result in infection of the newborn during passage through the birth canal.

CMV infection causes an immunosuppressive effect by inhibiting T cells. Host defenses against CMV infection include both circulating antibody and cell-mediated immunity. Cellular immunity is more important, because its suppression can lead to systemic disease.

Clinical Findings   Approximately 20% of infants infected with CMV during gestation show clinically apparent manifestations of cytomegalic inclusion disease such as microcephaly, seizures, deafness, jaundice, and purpura. Hepatosplenomegaly is very common. Cytomegalic inclusion disease is one of the leading causes of mental retardation in the United States. Infected infants can continue to excrete CMV, especially in the urine, for several years.

In immunocompetent adults, CMV can cause **"heterophil-negative" mononucleosis,** which is characterized by fever, lethargy, and the presence of abnormal lymphoctyes in peripheral blood smears. Systemic CMV infections, especially pneumonitis and hepatitis, occur in a high proportion of immunosuppressed patients, eg, those with renal and bone marrow transplants. In AIDS patients, CMV commonly infects the intestinal tract and causes intractable diarrhea. CMV also causes retinitis in AIDS patients which can lead to blindness.

Laboratory Diagnosis   The virus can be recovered in cell culture, but the appearance of cytopathic effect is slow, usually taking 1–2 weeks. Most of the virus produced remains cell-associated. The virus is identified by immunofluorescence. Other diagnostic methods include fluorescent-antibody and histologic staining of inclusion bodies in giant cells in urine and in tissue. The inclusion bodies are intranuclear and have an oval **"owl's-eye"** shape. A 4-fold or greater rise in antibody titer is also diagnostic.

Treatment   Ganciclovir (Cytovene) is moderately effective in the treatment of CMV retinitis and pneumonia in patients with AIDS. Foscarnet (Foscavir) is also effective but causes more side effects. Unlike HSV and VZV, CMV is largely resistant to acyclovir.

Prevention   There is no vaccine. Ganciclovir can suppress progressive retinitis in AIDS patients. Infants with cytomegalic inclusion disease who are shedding virus in their urine should be kept isolated from other infants. Blood for transfusion to newborns should be CMV antibody-negative. If possible, only organs from CMV antibody-negative donors should be transplanted to antibody-negative recipients.

EPSTEIN-BARR VIRUS (EBV)

Diseases   EBV causes infectious mononucleosis. It is associated with Burkitt's lymphoma, other B cell lymphomas, and nasopharyngeal carcinoma. EBV is also associated with hairy leukoplakia, a whitish, nonmalignant lesion on the tongue seen especially in AIDS patients.

Important Properties   EBV is structurally and morphologically identical to other herpesviruses but is antigenically different. The most important antigen is the **viral capsid antigen** (VCA), because it is used most often in diagnostic tests. The early antigens (EA), which are produced prior to viral DNA synthesis, and nuclear antigen (EBNA), which is located in the nucleus bound to chromosomes, are sometimes diagnostically helpful as well. Two other antigens, lymphocyte-determined membrane antigen and viral membrane antigen, have been detected also. Neutralizing activity is directed against the viral membrane antigen.

Humans are the natural hosts. EBV infects mainly lymphoid cells, primarily **B lymphocytes.** In latently infected cells, multiple copies of EBV DNA are found in the cytoplasm of infected B lymphocytes. Some, but not all, genes are transcribed, and only a subset of those are translated into protein.

Summary of Replicative Cycle   The cycle is similar to that of HSV (see p 194). EBV enters B lymphocytes at the site of the C3 receptor.

Transmission & Epidemiology   EBV is transmitted primarily by the exchange of **saliva,** eg, during kissing. EBV infection is one of the most common infections worldwide; over 90% of adults in the United States have antibody. Infection in the first few years of life is usually asymptomatic. Early infection tends to occur in individuals in lower socioeconomic groups. The frequency of clinically apparent infectious mononucleosis, however, is highest in those who are exposed to the virus later in life, eg, college students.

Pathogenesis & Immunity   The infection first occurs in the oropharynx (?epithelium, ?lymphoid tissue) and then spreads to the blood, where it infects B lymphocytes. Cytotoxic T lymphocytes react against the infected B cells. The T cells are the "atypical lymphs" seen in the blood smear. EBV remains **latent within B lymphocytes.** A few copies of EBV DNA are integrated into the cell genome; many copies of circular EBV DNA are found in the cytoplasm.

The immune response to EBV infection consists first of IgM antibody to the VCA. IgG antibody to the VCA follows and persists for life. The IgM response is therefore useful for diagnosing acute infection, whereas the IgG response is best for revealing prior infection. Lifetime immunity against second episodes of infectious mononucleosis is based on antibody to the viral membrane antigen.

In addition to the EBV-specific antibodies, nonspecific **heterophil antibodies** are found. The term "heterophil" refers to antibodies that are detected by tests using antigens different from the antigens that induced them. The heterophil antibodies formed in infectious mononucleosis agglutinate sheep or horse red blood cells in the laboratory. (Cross-reacting Forssman antibodies in human serum are removed by adsorption with guinea pig kidney extract prior to agglutination.) Note that these antibodies do not react with any component of EBV. It seems likely that EBV infection modifies a cell membrane constituent so that it becomes antigenic and induces the heterophil antibody. Heterophil antibodies usually disappear within 6 months after recovery. These antibodies are not specific for EBV infection and are also seen in individuals with hepatitis B and serum sickness.

Clinical Findings   Infectious mononucleosis is characterized primarily by fever, sore throat, lymphadenopathy, and splenomegaly. Anorexia and lethargy are prominent. Hepatitis is frequent; encephalitis occurs in some patients. Spontaneous recovery usually occurs in 2–3 weeks. Splenic rupture, associated with contact sports such as football, is a feared but rare complication of the splenomegaly. In certain immunosuppressed patients, a severe, often fatal EBV infection called X-linked immunoproliferative syndrome occurs.

Laboratory Diagnosis   The diagnosis of infectious mononucleosis in the clinical laboratory is based primarily on two approaches:

(1) In the **hematologic** approach, an absolute lymphocytosis occurs and as many as 30% abnormal lymphocytes are seen on a smear. These **"atypical lymphs"** are large and have a lobulated nucleus and a vacuolated, basophilic cytoplasm. They are cytotoxic T cells.

(2) In the **immunologic** approach, there are two types of serologic tests. (a) The **heterophil antibody** test is useful for the early diagnosis of infectious mononucleosis because it is usually positive by week 2 of illness. However, the antibody titer declines after recovery and so is not useful for detection of prior infection. The Monospot test is often used to detect the heterophil antibody; it is more sensitive, more specific, and cheaper than the tube agglutination test. (b) The **EBV-specific antibody** tests are used primarily in diagnostically difficult cases. The IgM VCA antibody response can be used to detect early illness; the IgG VCA antibody response can be used to detect prior infection. In certain instances, antibodies to EA and EBNA can be useful diagnostically.

Although EBV can be isolated from clinical samples such as saliva by morphologic transformation of cord blood lymphocytes, it is a technically difficult procedure and is not readily available. No virus is synthesized in the cord lymphocytes; its presence is detected by fluorescent-antibody staining of the nuclear antigen.

Treatment   No antiviral therapy is necessary for uncomplicated infectious mononucleosis. Acyclovir has little activity against EBV, but administration of high doses may be useful in life-threatening EBV infections.

Prevention   There is no EBV vaccine.

Association With Cancer   EBV infection is associated with cancers of lymphoid origin: **Burkitt's lymphoma** in African children, other B cell lymphomas, nasopharyngeal carcinoma in the Chinese population, and thymic carcinoma in the United States. The initial evidence of an association of EBV infection with Burkitt's lymphoma was the production of EBV by the lymphoma cells in culture. In fact, this was how EBV was discovered by Epstein and Barr in 1964. Additional evidence includes the finding of EBV DNA and EBNA in the tumor cells. EBV DNA and antigens are found in nasopharyngeal and thymic carcinoma cells also. The role of EBV in carcinogenesis is unclear.

Poxviruses

The poxvirus family includes three viruses of medical importance: smallpox virus, vaccinia virus, and molluscum contagiosum virus. Poxviruses are the **largest and most complex** viruses.

SMALLPOX VIRUS

Disease   Smallpox virus, also called variola virus, is the agent of smallpox, the only disease that has been eradicated from the face of the Earth. **Eradication** is due to the vaccine.

Important Properties   Poxviruses are brick-shaped particles containing linear double-stranded DNA, a disk-shaped core within a double membrane, and a lipoprotein envelope. The virion contains a DNA-dependent RNA polymerase. This enzyme is required because the virus replicates in the cytoplasm and does not have access to the cellular RNA polymerase, which is located in the nucleus.

Smallpox virus has a single, stable serotype, which is the key to the success of the vaccine. If the antigenicity varied as it does in influenza virus, eradication would not have succeeded.

Summary of Replicative Cycle   Vaccinia virus, a poxvirus virtually nonpathogenic for humans, is used for studies on poxvirus replication and as a vector in certain gene therapy experiments. After penetration of the cell and uncoating, the virion DNA-dependent RNA polymerase synthesizes early mRNA, which is translated into early, nonstructural proteins, mainly enzymes required for subsequent steps in viral replication. The viral DNA is replicated in typical semiconservative fashion, after which late, structural proteins are synthesized that will form the progeny virions. The virions are assembled and acquire their envelopes by budding from the cell membrane as they are released from the cell. Note that all steps in replication occur in the cytoplasm, which is unusual for a DNA virus.

Transmission & Epidemiology   Before the disease was eradicated, smallpox virus was transmitted via respiratory aerosol or by direct contact with virus either in the skin lesions or on fomites such as bedding.

Prior to the 1960s, smallpox was widespread throughout large areas of Africa, Asia, and South America, and millions of people were affected. In 1967, the World Health Organization embarked on a vaccination campaign that led to the eradication of smallpox. The last naturally occurring case was in Somalia in 1977.

Pathogenesis & Immunity   Smallpox begins when the virus infects the upper respiratory tract and local lymph nodes and then enters the blood (primary viremia). Internal organs are infected; then the virus reenters the blood (secondary viremia) and spreads to the skin. These events occur during the incubation period, when the patient is still well. The rash is the result of virus replication in the skin, but there may be an immune component as well.

Immunity following smallpox disease is lifelong; immunity following vaccination lasts about 10 years.

Clinical Findings   After an incubation period of 7–14 days, there is a sudden onset of prodromal symptoms such as fever and malaise. This is followed by the rash, which begins on the face and spreads over the body to include the extremities. The rash evolves through stages from macules to papules, vesicles, pustules, and, finally, crusts in 2–3 weeks.

Laboratory Diagnosis   In the past when the disease occurred, the diagnosis was made either by growing the virus in cell culture or chick embryos or by detecting viral antigens in vesicular fluid by immunofluorescence.

Prevention   The disease was eradicated by global use of the **vaccine,** which contains live, attenuated **vaccinia virus.** The success of the vaccine is dependent upon five critical factors: (1) smallpox virus has a single, stable serotype; (2) there is no animal reservoir, and humans are the only hosts; (3) the antibody response is prompt, so that exposed persons can be protected; (4) the disease is easily recognized clinically, so that exposed persons can be immunized promptly; and (5) there is no carrier state or subclinical infection.

The vaccine is inoculated intradermally, where virus replication occurs. The formation of a vesicle is indicative of a "take" (success). Although the vaccine was relatively safe, it became apparent in the 1970s that the incidence of side effects such as encephalitis, generalized vaccinia, and vaccinia gangrenosa exceeded the incidence of smallpox. Routine vaccination of civilians was discontinued, and it is no longer a prerequisite for international travel. Military personnel are still vaccinated.

Methisazone was used to treat the complications of vaccination. Rifampin inhibits viral DNA-dependent RNA polymerase but was not used clinically against smallpox.

MOLLUSCUM CONTAGIOSUM VIRUS

Molluscum contagiosum virus (MCV) is a member of the poxvirus family but is quite distinct from smallpox and vaccinia viruses. It causes small, pink, papular, wartlike benign tumors of the skin or mucous membranes. The lesions have a characteristic cup-shaped crater with a white core. Note that these lesions are different from warts, which are caused by papillomavirus, a member of the papovavirus family.

MCV is transmitted by close personal contact, including sexually. The disease is quite common in children, and the lesions can be widespread in patients with reduced cellular immunity. In immunocompetent patients, the lesions are self-limited but may last for months. The diagnosis is typically made clinically; the virus is not isolated in the clinical laboratory, and antibody titers are not helpful. There is no specific antiviral treatment and no vaccine. Removal of the lesions by curettage or with liquid nitrogen is often effective.

Hepatitis B Virus

Hepatitis B virus, a DNA-enveloped virus, is described in Chapter 41 with the other hepatitis viruses.

Review Questions

1. Herpesviruses cause latent infections. In which cells are the five important human herpesviruses typically latent?
2. What are the main differences between HSV-1 and HSV-2?
3. Describe the important steps in the replication of HSV.
4. What is the best way to make the diagnosis of HSV infection in the laboratory?
5. What is the characteristic appearance of HSV-infected cells?
6. Acyclovir is effective treatment for infections by certain herpesviruses. Which ones? What accounts for the selective antiviral effect of acyclovir?
7. What is the relationship between varicella (chickenpox) and zoster (shingles)?
8. You can get varicella only once. Why?
9. What is the predisposing factor to disseminated disease from VZV? How can the likelihood of dissemination be reduced?
10. What are the modes of transmission of CMV? To fetuses? In infants? In young children? In adults?
11. Describe the effects of CMV on fetuses and newborn infants.
12. What disease does EBV cause?
13. How is EBV transmitted, and which cells are initially infected?
14. Describe the heterophil antibody test.
15. Antibodies against which antigen indicate prior, rather than current, EBV infection?
16. What are the laboratory findings in a typical case of infectious mononucleosis?
17. What is the relationship of EBV and cancer?

18. What attributes of smallpox virus have led to the successful eradication of the disease?

19. Smallpox and vaccinia viruses are DNA viruses that contain a virion RNA polymerase. Why do they require this enzyme in the virion?

20. In the 1970s before smallpox was eradicated, the vaccine was no longer required in the United States. Why?

38 DNA Nonenveloped Viruses

ADENOVIRUSES

Diseases   Adenoviruses cause a variety of upper and lower respiratory tract diseases such as pharyngitis, conjunctivitis, and pneumonia. Keratoconjunctivitis, hemorrhagic cystitis, and gastroenteritis also occur. Some adenoviruses cause sarcomas in rodents.

Important Properties   Adenoviruses are **nonenveloped** viruses with double-stranded linear DNA and an **icosahedral** nucleocapsid. They are the only viruses with a **fiber** protruding from each of the 12 vertices of the capsid. The fiber is the organ of attachment and is a hemagglutinin. When purified free of virions, the fiber is toxic to human cells.

There are 41 known antigenic types; the fiber protein is the main type-specific antigen. All adenoviruses have a common group-specific antigen located on the hexon protein.

Certain serotypes of human adenoviruses (especially 12, 18, and 31) cause **sarcomas** at the site of injection in laboratory rodents such as newborn hamsters. There is no evidence that adenoviruses cause tumors in humans.

Summary of Replicative Cycle   After attachment to the cell surface via its fiber, the virus penetrates and uncoats and the viral DNA moves to the nucleus. Host cell DNA-dependent RNA polymerase transcribes the early genes, and splicing enzymes remove the RNA representing the introns, resulting in functional mRNA (note that introns and exons, which are common in eukaryotic DNA, were first described for adenovirus DNA). Early mRNA is translated into nonstructural proteins in the cytoplasm. After viral DNA replication in the nucleus, late mRNA is transcribed and then translated into structural virion proteins. Viral assembly occurs in the nucleus, and the virus is released by lysis of the cell, not by budding.

Transmission & Epidemiology   Adenoviruses are transmitted by several mechanisms: **aerosol** droplet, the **fecal-oral** route, and **direct inoculation** of conjunctivas by tonometers or fingers. The fecal-oral route is the most common mode of transmission among young children and their families. Many species of animals are infected by strains of adenovirus, but these strains are not pathogenic for humans.

Adenovirus infections are endemic worldwide, but outbreaks occur among military recruits, apparently as a result of the close living conditions that facilitate transmission. Certain serotypes are associated with specific syndromes; eg, types 3, 4, 7, and 21 cause respiratory disease, especially in military recruits; types 8 and 19 cause epidemic keratoconjunctivitis; types 11 and 21 cause hemorrhagic cystitis; and types 40 and 41 cause infantile gastroenteritis.

Pathogenesis & Immunity   Adenoviruses infect the mucosal epithelium of several organs, eg, the **respiratory tract** (both upper and lower), the **gastrointestinal tract,** and the **conjunctivas.** Immunity based on neutralizing antibody is type-specific and lifelong.

In addition to acute infection leading to death of the cells, adenoviruses cause a latent infection, particularly in the adenoidal and tonsillar tissues of the throat. In fact, these viruses were named for the adenoids, from which they were first isolated in 1953.

Clinical Findings   In the upper respiratory tract, adenoviruses cause infections such as pharyngitis, pharyngoconjunctival fever, and acute respiratory disease, characterized by fever, sore throat, coryza, and conjunctivitis. In the lower respiratory tract, they cause bronchitis and atypical pneumonia. Hematuria and dysuria are prominent in hemorrhagic cystitis. Gastroenteritis with nonbloody diarrhea occurs mainly in children under 2 years of age. Most adenovirus infections resolve spontaneously. Approximately half of all adenovirus infections are asymptomatic.

Laboratory Diagnosis   The most frequent methods of diagnosis are isolation of the virus in cell culture and detection of a 4-fold or greater rise in antibody titer. Complement fixation and hemagglutination inhibition are the most important serologic tests.

Treatment   There is no antiviral therapy.

Prevention   Three **live, nonattenuated** vaccines against serotypes 4, 7, and 21 are available but are used only by the military. Each of the three vaccines is monovalent; ie, it contains only one serotype. The viruses are administered separately because they interfere with each other when given together. The vaccines are delivered in an enteric-coated capsule, which protects the live virus from inactivation by stomach acid. The virus infects the gastrointestinal tract, where it causes an asymptomatic infection and induces immunity to respiratory disease. This vaccine is not available for civilian use.

Epidemic keratoconjunctivitis is an iatrogenic disease, preventable by strict asepsis and hand washing by those who examine eyes.

PAPILLOMAVIRUSES

Diseases   Papillomaviruses cause papillomas, which are benign tumors of squamous cells, eg, warts on the skin. Several types of human papillomaviruses, eg, HPV-16, are implicated as the cause of carcinomas, especially **carcinoma of the cervix.**

Important Properties   Papillomaviruses are nonenveloped viruses with double-stranded circular DNA and an icosahedral nucleocapsid. They are members of the papovavirus family. They are similar to polyomavirus and SV40 virus (see Chapter 43) but are larger, have a larger genome, and are antigenically distinct. Two of the early genes, **E6 and E7,** are implicated in carcinogenesis. They encode proteins that inactivate proteins encoded by tumor suppressor genes in human cells, eg, the p53 gene and the retinoblastoma (RB) gene, respectively. Inactivation of the p53 and RB proteins is an important step in the process by which a normal cell becomes a cancer cell.

There are at least 100 types of papillomaviruses, classified primarily on the basis of DNA restriction fragment analysis. There is a pronounced **predilection of certain types to infect certain tissues.** For example, skin warts are caused primarily by HPV-1 through HPV-4 whereas genital warts are usually caused by HPV-6 and HPV-11.

Summary of Replicative Cycle   Little is known of the specifics of viral replication because the virus grows poorly, if at all, in cell culture. In human tissue, infectious virus particles are found in the terminally differentiated squamous cells rather than in the basal cells. In malignant cells, viral DNA is integrated into host cell DNA in the vicinity of cellular proto-oncogenes and E6 and E7 are overexpressed. However, in latently infected, nonmalignant cells, the viral DNA is episomal and E6 and E7 are not overexpressed. This difference occurs because another early gene E2 controls E6 and E7 expression. The E2 gene is functional when the viral DNA is episomal but is inactivated when it is integrated.

Transmission & Epidemiology   Papillomaviruses are transmitted primarily by skin-to-skin contact and by genital contact. Genital warts are one of the **most common sexually transmitted diseases.** Skin warts are more common in children and young adults and tend to regress in older adults. Many species of animals are infected with their own types of papillomaviruses, but these viruses are not an important source of human infection.

Pathogenesis & Immunity   Papillomaviruses infect squamous epithelial cells and produce a characteristic cytoplasmic vacuole, a process called **koilocytosis.** Koilocytes are a hallmark of infection by these viruses. Most warts are benign and do not progress to malignancy. However, HPV infection is associated with carcinoma of the uterine cervix and penis. The proteins encoded by viral genes E6 and E7 interfere with the growth-inhibitory activity of the proteins encoded by the p53 and RB tumor suppressor genes and thereby contribute to oncogenesis by these viruses.

Both cell-mediated immunity and antibody are induced by viral infection and are involved in the spontaneous regression of warts. Immunosuppressed patients, eg, AIDS patients, have more extensive warts.

Clinical Findings   Papillomas of various organs are the predominant finding. These papillomas are caused by specific HPV types. For example, skin and plantar warts are caused primarily by HPV-1 through HPV-4, whereas genital warts (**condylomata acuminata**) are caused primarily by HPV-6 and HPV-11. Carcinoma of the uterine cervix, the penis, and the anus, as well as premalignant lesions called intraepithelial neoplasia, are associated with infection by HPV-16 and HPV-18. Occult premalignant lesions of the cervix and penis can be revealed by applying acetic acid to the tissue.

Laboratory Diagnosis   Infections are usually diagnosed clinically. The presence of koilocytes in the lesions indicates HPV infection. DNA hybridization tests to detect the presence of viral DNA are commercially available. Serologic tests are rarely done, and the virus has not been isolated in cell culture.

Treatment & Prevention   The usual treatment for genital warts is podophyllin; alpha interferon is also effective and is better at preventing recurrences than are non-antiviral treatments. Liquid nitrogen is commonly used for skin warts. Plantar warts can be removed surgically or treated with salicylic acid topically. There are no preventive measures (no vaccine is available).

PARVOVIRUSES

Diseases   Parvovirus B19 causes erythema infectiosum (slapped-cheeks syndrome, fifth disease), aplastic crisis (especially in patients with sickle cell anemia), and fetal infections, including hydrops fetalis. It is the most important human parvovirus.

Important Properties   Parvovirus B19 is a very small (22-nm) nonenveloped virus with a **single-stranded DNA genome.** The genome is negative-strand DNA, but there is no virion polymerase. The capsid has icosahedral symmetry. There is one serotype.

Summary of Replicative Cycle   After adsorption to host cell receptors, the virion penetrates and moves to the nucleus, where replication occurs. The single-stranded genome DNA has "hairpin" loops at both of its ends that provide double-stranded areas for the cellular DNA polymerase to initiate the synthesis of the progeny genomes. The viral mRNA is synthesized by cellular RNA polymerase from the double-stranded DNA intermediate. The progeny virions are assembled in the nucleus. B19 virus replicates only when a cell is in S phase, which explains why the virus replicates in red cell precursors but not in mature red cells.

Transmission & Epidemiology   B19 virus is transmitted primarily by the respiratory route; transplacental transmission also occurs. Blood donated for transfusions also is a source of infection because a high-titer viremia occurs in the infected patient. B19 virus infection occurs worldwide, and about half the people in the United States over the age of 18 years have antibodies to the virus. Humans are the natural reservoir; animals are not a source of human infection.

Pathogenesis & Immunity   B19 virus infects primarily two types of cells: **red blood cell precursors** in the bone marrow, which accounts for the aplastic crisis, and endothelial cells in the blood vessels, which accounts, in part, for the rash associated with erythema infectiosum. Immune complexes composed of virus and IgM or IgG also contribute to the pathogenesis of the rash and to the arthritis that is seen in some adults infected with B19 virus. Infection provides lifelong immunity against reinfection.

Clinical Findings   There are four main clinical presentations.

A. Erythema Infectiosum (slapped-cheeks syndrome, fifth disease): This is a mild disease, primarily of childhood, characterized by a bright red rash that is most prominent on the cheeks, accompanied by low-grade fever, runny nose (coryza), and sore throat. A "lacy" less intense, erythematous rash appears on the body. The symptoms resolve in about a week. The main complication of B19 infection is arthritis, which is more common in adults, mostly women, than in children.

B. Aplastic Crisis: Children with chronic anemia, such as sickle cell anemia, thalassemia, and spherocytosis, can have a transient but severe aplastic anemia (aplastic crisis) when infected with B19 virus. People with normal red cells do not have a clinically apparent anemia, although their red cell precursors are infected.

C. Fetal Infections: If a woman is infected with B19 virus during the first or second trimester of pregnancy, the virus may cross the placenta and infect the fetus. Infection during the first trimester is associated with fetal death, whereas infection during the second trimester leads to hydrops fetalis. Third-trimester infections do not result in important clinical findings. B19 virus is not a common cause of congenital abnormalities.

D. Chronic B19 Infection: People with immunodeficiencies, especially HIV-infected, chemotherapy, or transplant patients, can have chronic anemia, leukopenia, or thrombocytopenia as a result of chronic B19 infection.

Laboratory Diagnosis Fifth disease and aplastic crisis are usually diagnosed by detecting IgM antibodies. B19 virus can be isolated from throat swabs, but this is not commonly done. In immunocompromised patients, antibodies may not be detectable; therefore, viral DNA in the blood can be assayed by PCR methods. Fetal infection can be determined by PCR analysis of amniotic fluid.

Treatment & Prevention There is no specific treatment of B19 infection. Pooled immune globulins may have a beneficial effect on chronic B19 infection in patients with immunodeficiencies. There is no vaccine or chemoprophylaxis.

Review Questions

1. What are the important sites of infection for the various types of adenoviruses?
2. What is the importance of the fibers on the surface of adenoviruses?
3. What measures are available for prevention of adenovirus infection?
4. Which human cancer is associated with human papillomavirus (HPV) types 16 and 18?
5. What is the proposed relationship of HPV genes E6 and E7 to cancer in humans?
6. What is the significance of finding koilocytes in a skin biopsy specimen?
7. How does the genome of the parvoviruses differ from those of the papillomaviruses and the adenoviruses?
8. What is the pathogenesis of the following clinical features of parvovirus B19 infection: (a) anemia, (b) rash, (c) arthritis?
9. Is there an antiviral drug effective against parvovirus B19 infection? Is there an effective vaccine?

39

RNA Enveloped Viruses

Orthomyxoviruses

INFLUENZA VIRUSES

Influenza viruses are the only members of the orthomyxovirus family. The term "myxo" refers to the observation that these viruses interact with mucins (glycoproteins). The orthomyxoviruses differ from the paramyxoviruses primarily in that the former have a segmented RNA genome (usually eight pieces), whereas the RNA genome of the latter consists of a single piece.* In addition, the orthomyxoviruses are smaller (110 nm in diameter) than the paramyxoviruses (150 nm in diameter). See Table 39–1 for additional differences.

Table 39–2 shows a comparison of influenza A virus with several other viruses that infect the respiratory tract.

Disease   Influenza A virus causes worldwide epidemics (pandemics) of influenza; influenza B virus causes major outbreaks of influenza; and influenza C virus causes mild respiratory tract infections but does not cause outbreaks of influenza. The pandemics caused by influenza A virus occur approximately every 10–20 years, but major outbreaks caused by this virus occur virtually every year in various countries. Influenza B virus does not cause pandemics, and the major outbreaks caused by this virus do not occur as often as those caused by influenza A virus.

Important Properties   Influenza virus is composed of a **segmented** single-stranded RNA genome, a **helical** nucleocapsid, and an outer lipoprotein **envelope.** The virion contains an RNA-dependent **RNA polymerase,** which transcribes the **negative-polarity** genome into mRNA. The genome is therefore not infectious. The envelope is covered with two different types of spikes, a **hemagglutinin** and a **neuraminidase.**†

The function of the hemagglutinin is to bind to the cell surface receptor (neuraminic acid, sialic acid) to initiate infection. In the clinical laboratory, the hemagglutinin agglutinates red blood cells, which is the basis of a diagnostic test called the hemagglutination inhibition test. The hemagglutinin is also the target of neutralizing antibody.

The neuraminidase cleaves neuraminic acid (sialic acid) to release progeny virus from the infected cell. The hemagglutinin functions at the beginning of infection, whereas the neuraminidase functions at the end. Neuraminidase also degrades the protective layer of mucus in the respiratory tract. This enhances the ability of the virus to infect the respiratory epithelium.

Influenza viruses, especially influenza A virus, show **changes in the antigenicity** of their hemagglutinin and neuraminidase proteins; this property contributes to their capacity to cause devastating **worldwide epidemics.** These changes are attributed to the **reassortment** (high-frequency recombination) of the segments of the genome RNA. Note that in reassortment, entire segments of RNA are exchanged, each one of which codes for a single protein, eg, the hemagglutinin (Fig 39–1).

Influenza viruses have both **group-specific** and **type-specific** antigens.

(1) The internal ribonucleoprotein is the group-specific antigen that distinguishes influenza A, B, and C viruses.

(2) The hemagglutinin and the neuraminidase are the type-specific antigens located on the surface. Antibody against the hemagglutinin neutralizes the infectivity of the virus (and prevents disease), whereas antibody against the group-specific antigen (which is located internally) does not. Antibody

---

*The total molecular weight of influenza virus RNA is approximately $2-4 \times 10^6$, whereas the molecular weight of paramyxovirus RNA is higher, approximately $5-8 \times 10^6$.

†Paramyxoviruses also have a hemagglutinin and a neuraminidase, but the two proteins are located on the same spike.

Table 39–1. Properties of orthomyxoviruses and paramyxoviruses.

Property	Orthomyxoviruses	Paramyxoviruses
Viruses	Influenza A, B, and C viruses	Measles, mumps, respiratory syncytial, and parainfluenza viruses
Genome	Segmented (eight pieces) single-stranded RNA of negative polarity	Nonsegmented single-stranded RNA of negative polarity
Virion RNA polymerase	Yes	Yes
Capsid	Helical	Helical
Envelope	Yes	Yes
Size	Smaller (110 nm)	Larger (150 nm)
Surface spikes	Hemagglutinin and neuraminidase on different spikes	Hemagglutinin and neuraminidase on the same spike[1]
Giant cell formation	No	Yes

[1] Individual viruses differ in detail. See Table 39–3.

against the neuraminidase does not neutralize infectivity but does reduce disease, perhaps by decreasing the amount of virus released from the infected cell and thus reducing spread.

Many species of animals (eg, aquatic birds, chickens, swine, and horses) have their own influenza A viruses. These **animal viruses are the source of the new antigenic types** that cause epidemics among humans. For example, if an equine and a human A influenza virus infect the same cell (eg, in a farmer's respiratory tract), reassortment could occur and a new variant of the human A virus, bearing the equine virus hemagglutinin, may appear.

A/Philippines/82 (H3N2) illustrates the nomenclature of influenza viruses. "A" refers to the group antigen. Next are the location and year the virus was isolated. H3N2 is the designation of the hemagglutinin (H) and neuraminidase (N) types. The H1N1 and H3N2 strains of influenza A virus are the most common at this time and are the strains included in the current vaccine. The H2N2 strain

Table 39–2. Features of viruses that infect the respiratory tract.

Virus	Disease	Number of Serotypes	Lifelong Immunity to Disease	Vaccine Available	Viral Latency	Treatment
RNA viruses Influenza A virus	Influenza	Many	No	+	−	Amantadine
Parainfluenza virus	Croup	Many	No	−	−	None
Respiratory syncytial virus	Bronchiolitis	One	Incomplete	−	−	Ribavirin
Rubella virus	Rubella	One	Yes	+	−	None
Measles virus	Measles	One	Yes	+	−	None
Mumps virus	Parotitis, meningitis	One	Yes	+	−	None
Rhinovirus	Common cold	Many	No	−	−	None
Coronavirus	Common cold	Many	No	−	−	None
Coxsackievirus	Herpangina, pleurodynia	Many	No	−	−	None
DNA viruses Herpes simplex virus type 1	Gingivostomatitis	One	No	−	+	Acyclovir in immunodeficient patients
Epstein-Barr virus	Infectious mononucleosis	One	Yes	−	+	None
Varicella-zoster virus	Chickenpox, shingles	One	Yes[1]	−	+	Acyclovir in immunodeficient patients
Adenovirus	Pharyngitis, pneumonia	Many	No	+[2]	+	None

[1]Lifelong immunity to varicella (chickenpox) but not to zoster (shingles).
[2]For military recruits only.

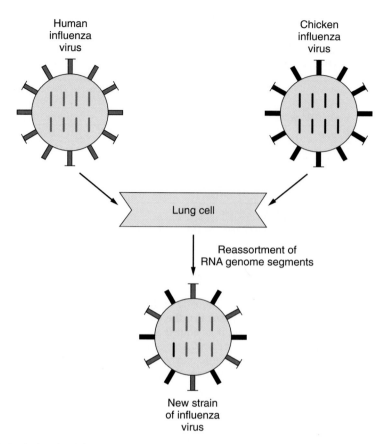

Figure 39–1. Antigenic shift in influenza virus. A human strain of influenza virus containing the gene encoding one antigenic type of hemagglutinin (colored orange) infects the same lung cell as a chicken strain of influenza virus containing the gene encoding a different antigenic type of hemagglutinin (colored black). Reassortment of the genome RNA segments that encode the hemagglutinin occurs, and a new strain of influenza virus is produced containing the chicken type of hemagglutinin (colored black).

caused a pandemic in 1968. In 1997, a new strain, H5N1, that previously was limited to chickens, caused human disease in Hong Kong.

Summary of Replicative Cycle   The virus adsorbs to the cell as the viral hemagglutinin interacts with sialic acid receptors on the cell surface. The virus then enters the cell in vesicles and uncoats. The virion RNA polymerase transcribes the eight genome segments into eight mRNAs, which are translated into virion proteins in the cytoplasm. Progeny RNA genomes are synthesized in the nucleus. The helical ribonucleoprotein assembles in the cytoplasm; matrix protein mediates the interaction of the nucleocapsid with the envelope; and the virion is released from the cell by budding from the outer cell membrane at the site where the hemagglutinin and neuraminidase are located. The neuraminidase may play a role in release of the virus by cleaving neuraminic acid on the cell surface. Influenza virus and retroviruses are the **only RNA viruses** that have an important stage of their replication take place in the **nucleus.**

Transmission & Epidemiology   The virus is transmitted by **airborne respiratory droplets.** The ability of influenza A virus to cause epidemics is dependent on antigenic changes in the hemagglutinin and neuraminidase. There are two types of changes: **antigenic shifts,** which are major changes based on the **reassortment** of genome pieces, and **antigenic drifts,** which are minor changes based on **mutation.** Antigenic shifts appear less frequently, about every 10 or 11 years, whereas drift variants appear virtually every year. Epidemics and pandemics (worldwide epidemics) occur when the antigenicity of the virus has changed sufficiently that the preexisting immunity of many people is no longer effective. The antigenicity of influenza B virus also varies but not as dramatically or as often.

Influenza occurs primarily in the winter months, when it and secondary bacterial pneumonia cause a significant number of deaths, especially in older people.

Pathogenesis & Immunity   After the virus has been inhaled, the neuraminidase degrades the protective mucus layer, allowing the virus to gain access to the cells of the upper and lower respiratory tract. The infection is limited primarily to this area, and, despite systemic symptoms, viremia rarely occurs. The systemic symptoms, such as the severe myalgias, are due to cytokines circulating in the blood. There is necrosis of the superficial layers of the respiratory epithelium. Influenza virus pneumonia, which can complicate influenza, is interstitial in location.

Immunity rests mainly upon secretory IgA in the respiratory tract. IgG is also produced but is less protective. Cytotoxic T cells also play a protective role.

Clinical Findings   After an incubation period of 24–48 hours, fever, myalgias, headache, and cough develop suddenly. Vomiting and diarrhea are rare. The symptoms usually resolve spontaneously in 4–7 days, but influenzal or bacterial pneumonia may complicate the course.

Reye's syndrome, characterized by encephalopathy and liver degeneration, is a rare, life-threatening complication in children following some viral infections, particularly influenza B and chickenpox. Aspirin given to reduce fever in viral infections has been implicated in the pathogenesis of Reye's syndrome.

Laboratory Diagnosis   Although most diagnoses of influenza are made on clinical grounds, two laboratory diagnostic approaches are available. (1) The virus can be grown in cell culture from throat washings and identified by fluorescent-antibody staining of the infected cells by using antisera to influenza A and B. This process takes several days. (2) A rise in antibody titer of at least 4-fold in paired serum samples taken early in the illness and 10 days later is sufficient for diagnosis. Either the hemagglutination inhibition or complement fixation (CF) test can be used to assay the antibody titer.

Treatment   **Amantadine** (Symmetrel) is approved for use as both treatment for and prevention of influenza A. Its main indication is in the prevention of influenza in a confined, elderly, unimmunized population, such as in a retirement home, where influenza can be life-threatening. Note that amantadine is effective only against influenza A, not against influenza B. A derivative of amantadine, **rimantadine** (Flumadine), can also be used for treatment and prevention and has fewer side effects than amantadine.

Prevention   The main mode of prevention is the **vaccine,** which consists of killed influenza A and B viruses, typically two A strains and one B strain. The vaccine is usually reformulated each year to contain the current antigenic strains. Because the virus in the vaccine is killed, there is no replication in the respiratory tract and, consequently, little secretory IgA appears on the respiratory mucosa. The vaccine does induce IgG, which offers some protection.

The vaccine is not a good immunogen, because little IgA is made and the titer of IgG is relatively low. Protection lasts only 6 months. Yearly boosters are recommended and should be given shortly before the flu season, eg, in October. These boosters also provide an opportunity to immunize against the latest antigenic changes. The vaccine should be given to people over age 65 years and to those with chronic diseases, particularly respiratory and cardiovascular conditions. In 1994, the recommendations were expanded to include all those who want to reduce their risk of acquiring influenza.

In addition to the vaccine containing whole, killed virus, two other forms of the vaccine are available. One contains "split" (disrupted) virus and, the other contains purified surface antigen. They are used particularly in children because they cause fewer side effects. An experimental vaccine containing a live, temperature-sensitive mutant is effective and may become available. This virus can replicate in the cooler (33 °C) nasal passages, where it induces IgA, but not in the warmer (37 °C) lower respiratory tract. It therefore immunizes but does not cause disease.

Paramyxoviruses

The paramyxovirus family contains four important human pathogens: measles virus, mumps virus, respiratory syncytial virus (RSV), and parainfluenza viruses. They differ from orthomyxoviruses in that their **genomes are not segmented,** they have a larger diameter, and their surface spikes are different (Table 39–1).

Paramyxoviruses are composed of **one piece** of single-stranded RNA, a **helical** nucleocapsid, and an outer lipoprotein envelope. The virion contains an RNA-dependent **RNA polymerase,** which transcribes the **negative-polarity** genome into mRNA. The genome is therefore not infectious. The envelope is covered with spikes, which contain either hemagglutinin, neuraminidase, or a fusion protein that causes cell fusion and, in some cases, hemolysis (Table 39–3).

MEASLES VIRUS

Disease   This virus causes measles.

Important Properties   The genome RNA and nucleocapsid of measles virus are those of a typical paramyxovirus (see above). The virion has two types of envelope spikes, one with hemagglutinating activity and the other with cell-fusing and hemolytic activities (Table 39–3). It has a single serotype, and the hemagglutinin is the antigen against which neutralizing antibody is directed. Humans are the natural host.

Summary of Replicative Cycle   After adsorption to the cell surface via its hemagglutinin, the virus penetrates and uncoats and the virion RNA polymerase transcribes the negative-strand genome into mRNA. Multiple mRNAs are synthesized, each of which is translated into the specific viral proteins; no polyprotein analogous to that synthesized by poliovirus is made. The helical nucleocapsid is assembled, the matrix protein mediates the interaction with the envelope, and the virus is released by budding from the cell membrane.

Transmission & Epidemiology   Measles virus is transmitted via **respiratory droplets** produced by coughing and sneezing both during the prodromal period and for a few days after the rash appears. Measles occurs worldwide, usually in outbreaks every 2–3 years, when the number of susceptible children reaches a high level. The attack rate is one of the highest of viral diseases; most children contract the clinical disease on exposure. When this virus is introduced into a population that has not experienced measles, such as the inhabitants of the Hawaiian Islands in the 1800s, devastating epidemics occur. In malnourished children, especially those in developing countries, measles is a much more serious disease than in well-nourished children. Patients with deficient cell-mediated immunity, eg, AIDS patients, have a severe, life-threatening disease when they contract measles.

In the United States a marked increase in the number of measles cases has occurred in the last few years. This increase is caused primarily by three factors: (1) failure to immunize many preschool children, (2) inadequate immunity in children immunized before 15 months of age, and (3) waning immunity in those who received only one dose of the vaccine.

Pathogenesis & Immunity   After infecting the cells lining the upper respiratory tract, the virus enters the blood and infects reticuloendothelial cells, where it replicates again. It then spreads via the blood to the skin. The **rash** is caused primarily by cytotoxic T cells attacking the measles virus-infected vascular endothelial cells in the skin. An antibody-mediated vasculitis may also play a role. Shortly after the rash appears, the virus can no longer be recovered and the patient can no longer spread the virus to others. **Multinucleated giant cells,** which form as a result of the fusion protein in the spikes, are characteristic of the lesions.

Table 39–3. Envelope spikes of paramyxoviruses.

Virus	Hemagglutinin	Neuraminidase	Fusion Protein[1]
Measles virus	+	–	+
Mumps virus[2]	+	+	+
Respiratory syncytial virus	–	–	+
Parainfluenza virus[2]	+	+	+

[1] The measles and mumps fusion proteins are hemolysins also.
[2] In mumps and parainfluenza viruses, the hemagglutinin and neuraminidase are on the same spike and the fusion protein is on a different spike.

Lifelong immunity occurs in individuals who have had the disease. Although IgG antibody may play a role in neutralizing the virus during the viremic stage, cell-mediated immunity is more important; agammaglobulinemic children have a normal course of disease, are subsequently immune, and are protected by immunization. Maternal antibody passes the placenta, and infants are protected during the first 6 months of life.

Infection with measles virus can **transiently depress cell-mediated immunity** against other intracellular microorganisms, such as *M tuberculosis,* leading to a loss of PPD skin test reactivity, reactivation of dormant organisms, and clinical disease. The proposed mechanism for this unusual finding is that when measles virus binds to its receptor (called CD46) on the surface of human macrophages, the production of IL-12, which is necessary for cell-mediated immunity to occur, is suppressed.

Clinical Findings   After an incubation period of 10–14 days, a prodromal phase characterized by fever, conjunctivitis (causing photophobia), running nose, and coughing occurs. **Koplik's spots** are bright red lesions with a white, central dot that are located on the buccal mucosa and are virtually diagnostic. A few days later, a maculopapular rash appears on the face and proceeds gradually down the body to the lower extremities. The rash develops a brownish hue several days later.

The complications of measles can be quite severe. Encephalitis occurs at a rate of 1 per 1000 cases of measles. The mortality rate of encephalitis is 10%, and there are permanent sequelae in 40% of cases. In addition, both primary measles (giant-cell) pneumonia and secondary bacterial pneumonia occur. Bacterial otitis media is quite common. Although very rare, subacute sclerosing panencephalitis (SSPE) is a fatal disease of the central nervous system that occurs several years after measles (see Chapter 44).

Atypical measles occurs in some people who were given the killed vaccine and were subsequently infected with measles virus. It is characterized by an atypical rash without Koplik's spots. Because the killed vaccine has not been used for many years, atypical measles occurs only in adults and is infrequent.

Laboratory Diagnosis   Most diagnoses are made on clinical grounds, but the virus can be isolated in cell culture; a rise in antibody titer of greater than 4-fold can be used to diagnose difficult cases.

Treatment   There is no antiviral therapy available.

Prevention   Prevention rests on immunization with the **live, attenuated vaccine.** The vaccine is effective and causes few side effects. It is given subcutaneously to children at 15 months of age, usually in combination with rubella and mumps vaccines. The vaccine should not be given to children prior to **15 months of age, because maternal antibody in the child can neutralize the virus** and reduce the immune response. Since immunity can wane, a **booster dose** is recommended. Because it is a live vaccine, it should not be given to immunocompromised persons or pregnant women. The vaccine has decreased the number of cases of measles markedly in the United States. However, outbreaks still occur among unimmunized individuals, eg, children in the inner cities and in developing countries.

The killed vaccine should not be used. Immune globulin can be used to modify the disease if given to unimmunized individuals early in the incubation period.

MUMPS VIRUS

Disease   This virus causes mumps.

Important Properties   The genome RNA and nucleocapsid are those of a typical paramyxovirus. The virion has two types of envelope spikes, one with both hemagglutinin and neuraminidase activities and the other with cell-fusing and hemolytic activities (Table 39–3).

The virus has a single serotype. Neutralizing antibody is directed against the hemagglutinin. The internal nucleocapsid protein is the S (soluble) antigen detected in the complement fixation test used for diagnosis. Humans are the natural host.

Summary of Replicative Cycle   Replication is similar to that of measles virus (see p 210).

Transmission & Epidemiology   Mumps virus is transmitted via **respiratory droplets.** Mumps occurs worldwide, with a peak incidence in the winter. About 30% of children have a subclinical (inapparent) infection, which confers immunity.

Pathogenesis & Immunity   The virus infects the upper respiratory tract and then spreads through the blood to infect the parotid glands, testes, ovaries, pancreas, and, in some cases, meninges. Alternatively, the virus may ascend from the buccal mucosa up Stensen's duct to the parotid gland.

    Lifelong immunity occurs in persons who have had the disease. There is a popular misconception that unilateral mumps can be followed by mumps on the other side. Mumps occurs only once; subsequent cases of parotitis can be caused by other viruses such as parainfluenza viruses, by bacteria, and by duct stones. Maternal antibody passes the placenta and provides protection during the first 6 months of life.

Clinical Findings   After an incubation period of 18–21 days, a prodromal stage of fever, malaise, and anorexia is followed by tender swelling of the parotid glands, either unilateral or bilateral. There is a characteristic increase in parotid pain when drinking citrus juices. The disease is typically benign and resolves spontaneously within a week.

    Two complications are of significance. One is orchitis in postpubertal males, which, if bilateral, can result in sterility. Postpubertal males have a fibrous tunica albuginea, which resists expansion, thereby causing pressure necrosis of the spermatocytes. Unilateral orchitis, although quite painful, does not lead to sterility. The other complication is meningitis, which is usually benign, self-limited, and without sequelae. Mumps virus, coxsackievirus, and echovirus are the three most frequent causes of viral (aseptic) meningitis. The widespread use of the vaccine in the United States has led to a marked decrease in the incidence of mumps meningitis.

Laboratory Diagnosis   The diagnosis of mumps is usually made clinically, but laboratory tests are available for confirmation. The virus can be isolated in cell culture from saliva, spinal fluid, or urine. In addition, a 4-fold rise in antibody titer in either the hemagglutination inhibition or the CF test is diagnostic. A single CF test that assays both the S and the V (viral) antigens can also be used. Because antibody to S antigen appears early and is short-lived, it indicates current infection. If only V antibody is found, the patient has had mumps in the past.

    A mumps skin test based on delayed hypersensitivity can be used to detect previous infection, but serologic tests are preferred. The mumps skin test is widely used to determine whether a patient's cell-mediated immunity is competent.

Treatment   There is no antiviral therapy for mumps.

Prevention   Prevention consists of immunization with the **live, attenuated vaccine.** The vaccine is effective and long-lasting (at least 10 years) and causes few side effects. It is given subcutaneously to children at 15 months of age, usually in combination with measles and rubella vaccines. Because it is a live vaccine, it should not be given to immunocompromised persons or pregnant women. Immune globulin is not useful for preventing or mitigating mumps orchitis.

RESPIRATORY SYNCYTIAL VIRUS (RSV)

Diseases   This virus is the most important cause of pneumonia and bronchiolitis in infants.

Important Properties   The genome RNA and nucleocapsid are those of a typical paramyxovirus (Table 39–1). Its surface spikes are **fusion proteins,** not hemagglutinins or neuraminidases (Table 39–3). The fusion protein causes cells to fuse, forming **multinucleated giant cells (syncytia),** which give rise to the name of the virus.

    Humans and chimpanzees are the natural hosts of RSV. For many years, RSV was thought to have one serotype; however, two serotypes, designated subgroup A and subgroup B, have been detected by monoclonal antibody tests. Antibody against the fusion protein neutralizes infectivity.

Summary of Replicative Cycle   Replication is similar to that of measles virus (see p 210).

Transmission & Epidemiology   Transmission occurs via **respiratory droplets** and by direct contact of contaminated hands with the nose or mouth. RSV causes **outbreaks** of respiratory infections **every winter,** in contrast to many other "cold" viruses, which reenter the community every few years. It occurs worldwide, and virtually everyone has been infected by the age of 3 years. RSV also causes **outbreaks** of respiratory infections in **hospitalized infants;** these outbreaks can be controlled by hand-washing and use of gloves, which interrupt transmission by hospital personnel.

Pathogenesis & Immunity   RSV infection in **infants is more severe** and more often involves the lower respiratory tract than in older children and adults, in whom it causes mild upper respiratory infections. The infection is localized to the respiratory tract; viremia does not occur.

The severe disease in infants may have an **immunopathogenetic** mechanism. Maternal antibody passed to the infant may react with the virus and damage the respiratory tract cells. Immune complexes (IgG plus virus), as well as IgE antibody and histamine, may be involved. Trials with a killed vaccine resulted in more severe disease, an unexpected finding that supports such a mechanism.

Most individuals have multiple infections due to RSV, indicating that immunity is incomplete. The reason for this is unknown, but it is not due to antigenic variation of the virus. IgA respiratory antibody reduces the frequency of RSV infection as a person ages.

Clinical Findings   In infants, lower respiratory tract disease such as bronchiolitis and pneumonia predominates. Surprisingly, secondary bacterial pneumonia is rare. In older children and adults, upper respiratory tract infections resemble the common cold.

Laboratory Diagnosis   The presence of the virus can be detected rapidly by immunofluorescence on smears of respiratory epithelium or by isolation in cell culture. The cytopathic effect in cell culture is characterized by the formation of multinucleated giant cells. A rise in antibody titer of at least 4-fold is also diagnostic.

Treatment   Aerosolized ribavirin (Virazole) is recommended for severely ill hospitalized infants, but there is uncertainty regarding its effectiveness. A combination of ribavirin and hyperimmune globulins against RSV may be more effective.

Prevention   There is **no vaccine.** Previous attempts to protect with a killed vaccine resulted in an increase in severity of symptoms. Hyperimmune globulins against RSV are used for prophylaxis in premature or immunocompromised infants. Nosocomial outbreaks can be limited by hand-washing and use of gloves.

PARAINFLUENZA VIRUSES

Diseases   These viruses cause croup (acute laryngotracheobronchitis) and pneumonia in children and a disease resembling the common cold in adults.

Important Properties   The genome RNA and nucleocapsid are those of a typical paramyxovirus (Table 39–1). The surface spikes consist of hemagglutinin (H), neuraminidase (N), and fusion (F) proteins (Table 39–3). The fusion protein mediates the formation of multinucleated giant cells. The H and N proteins are on the same spike; the F protein is on a separate spike. Both humans and animals are infected by parainfluenza viruses, but the animal strains do not infect humans. There are four types, which are distinguished by antigenicity, cytopathic effect, and pathogenicity (see below). Antibody to either the H or the F protein neutralizes infectivity.

Summary of Replicative Cycle   Replication is similar to that of measles virus (see p 210).

Transmission & Epidemiology   These viruses are transmitted via **respiratory droplets.** They cause disease worldwide, primarily in the winter months.

Pathogenesis & Immunity   These viruses cause upper and lower respiratory tract disease without viremia. A large proportion of infections are subclinical. Parainfluenza viruses 1 and 2 are **major causes of croup** but cause pharyngitis as well. Parainfluenza virus 3 causes disease less frequently, and parainfluenza virus 4 rarely causes disease, except for the common cold.

Clinical Findings   Parainfluenza viruses are best known as the main cause of croup in children under 5 years of age. Croup is characterized by a harsh cough and hoarseness. In addition to croup, these viruses cause a variety of respiratory diseases such as the common cold, pharyngitis, bronchitis, and pneumonia.

Laboratory Diagnosis   Most infections are diagnosed clinically. The diagnosis can be made in the laboratory either by isolating the virus in cell culture or by observing a 4-fold or greater rise in antibody titer.

Treatment & Prevention   There is neither antiviral therapy nor a vaccine available.

Togaviruses

RUBELLA VIRUS

Diseases   This virus causes rubella (German measles) and congenital rubella syndrome.

Important Properties   Rubella virus is a member of the togavirus family. It is composed of one piece of **single-stranded** RNA, an **icosahedral** nucleocapsid, and a lipoprotein **envelope.** However, unlike the paramyxoviruses, such as measles and mumps viruses, it has a **positive-strand** RNA and therefore has no virion polymerase. Its surface spikes contain hemagglutinin. The virus has a single antigenic type. Antibody against hemagglutinin neutralizes infectivity. Humans are the natural host.

Summary of Replicative Cycle   Because knowledge of rubella virus replication is incomplete, the following cycle is based on the replication of other togaviruses. After penetration of the cell and uncoating, the plus-strand RNA genome is translated into several nonstructural and structural proteins. Note the difference between togaviruses and poliovirus, which also has a plus-strand RNA genome but translates its RNA into a single large polyprotein, which is subsequently cleaved. One of the nonstructural rubella proteins is an RNA-dependent RNA polymerase, which replicates the genome first by making a minus-strand template and then, from that, plus-strand progeny. Both replication and assembly occur in the cytoplasm, and the envelope is acquired from the outer membrane as the virion exits the cell.

Transmission & Epidemiology   The virus is transmitted via **respiratory droplets.** The disease occurs worldwide. In areas where the vaccine is not used, epidemics occur every 6–9 years. In the United States, approximately 10% of young adult women are susceptible and are therefore at risk of giving birth to children with congenital malformations.

Pathogenesis & Immunity   Initial replication of the virus occurs in the nasopharynx and local lymph nodes. From there it spreads via the blood to the internal organs and skin. The origin of the rash is unclear; it may be due to an antigen–antibody-mediated vasculitis.

Natural infection leads to **lifelong immunity.** Second cases of rubella do not occur; similar rashes are caused by other viruses, such as coxsackieviruses and echoviruses. Antibody crosses the placenta and protects the newborn.

Clinical Findings

A.   Rubella: Rubella is a milder, shorter disease than measles. After an incubation period of 14–21 days, a brief prodromal period with fever and malaise is followed by a maculopapular rash, which starts on the face and progresses downward to involve the extremities. Posterior auricular lymphadenopathy is characteristic. The rash typically lasts for 3 days. When rubella occurs in adults, especially women, polyarthritis due to immune complexes often occurs.

B.   Congenital Rubella Syndrome: The significance of rubella virus is not as a cause of mild childhood disease but as a **teratogen.** When a nonimmune pregnant woman is **infected during the first trimester,** especially the first month, significant congenital malformations can occur as a result of maternal viremia and fetal infection. The increased rate of abnormalities during the early weeks of pregnancy is attributed to the very sensitive organ development that occurs at that time. The malformations are widespread and involve primarily the heart (eg, patent ductus arteriosus), the eyes (eg, cataracts), and the brain (eg, deafness and mental retardation).

In addition, some children infected in utero can **continue to excrete** rubella virus for months following birth, which is a significant public health hazard because the virus can be transmitted to pregnant women. Some congenital shedders are asymptomatic and without malformations and hence can be diagnosed only if the virus is isolated. Congenitally infected infants also have significant IgM titers and persistent IgG titers long after maternal antibody has disappeared.

Laboratory Diagnosis   Rubella virus can be grown in cell culture, but it produces little cytopathic effect (CPE). It is therefore usually identified by its ability to interfere with echovirus CPE. If rubella virus is present in the patient's specimen and has grown in the cell culture, no CPE will appear when the culture is superinfected with an echovirus. The diagnosis can also be made by observing a 4-fold or greater rise in antibody titer between acute-phase and convalescent-phase sera in the hemagglutination inhibition test or ELISA or by observing the presence of IgM antibody in a single acute-phase serum sample. In a pregnant woman exposed to rubella virus, the presence of **IgM antibody indicates recent infection,** whereas a 1:8 or greater titer of IgG antibody indicates immunity and consequent protection of the fetus. If recent infection has occurred, an **amniocentesis** can reveal whether there is rubella virus in the amniotic fluid, which indicates definite fetal infection.

Treatment   There is no antiviral therapy.

Prevention   Prevention involves immunization with the **live, attenuated vaccine.** The vaccine is effective and long-lasting (at least 10 years) and causes few side effects, except for transient arthralgias in some women. It is given subcutaneously to children at 15 months of age (usually in combination with measles and mumps vaccine) and to unimmunized young adult women if they are not pregnant and will use contraception for the next 3 months. There is no evidence that the vaccine virus causes malformations. Because it is a live vaccine, it should not be given to immunocompromised patients.

The vaccine has caused a marked reduction in the incidence of both rubella and congenital rubella syndrome. It induces some respiratory IgA, thereby interrupting the spread of virulent virus by nasal carriage. Administration of immune globulin does not prevent fetal infection in pregnant women who have been exposed to rubella virus.

To protect pregnant women from exposure to rubella virus, many hospitals require their personnel to demonstrate immunity, either by serologic testing or by proof of immunization.

OTHER TOGAVIRUSES

Several other medically important togaviruses are described in the chapter on arboviruses (see Chapter 42).

Rhabdoviruses

RABIES VIRUS

Disease   This virus causes rabies.

Important Properties   Rabies virus is the only medically important member of the rhabdovirus family. It has a **single-stranded RNA** enclosed within a **bullet-shaped** capsid surrounded by a lipoprotein **envelope.** Because the genome RNA has **negative polarity,** the virion contains an RNA-dependent **RNA polymerase.** Rabies virus has a single antigenic type. The antigenicity resides in the envelope glycoprotein spikes.

Rabies virus has a **broad host range:** it can infect all mammals, but only certain mammals are important sources of infection for humans (see below).

Summary of Replicative Cycle   Rabies virus attaches to the **acetylcholine receptor** on the cell surface. After entry into the cell, the virion RNA polymerase synthesizes five mRNAs that code for viral proteins. After replication of the genome viral RNA by a virus-encoded RNA polymerase, progeny RNA is assembled with virion proteins to form the nucleocapsid, and the envelope is acquired as the virion buds through the cell membrane.

Transmission & Epidemiology   The virus is transmitted by the **bite** of a rabid animal. In the United States, this is usually due to the bite of **wild animals** such as skunks, raccoons, and bats; dogs and cats are frequently immunized and therefore are rarely sources of human infection. Bats are remarkable for their ability to transmit the virus while remaining healthy, whereas in other animals the ability to transmit is associated with aberrant behavior caused by viral encephalitis. Rodents and rabbits do not transmit rabies. In the United States, fewer than 10 cases of rabies occur each year (mostly imported), whereas in developing countries there are hundreds of cases, mostly due to rabid dogs.

Pathogenesis & Immunity   The virus multiplies locally at the bite site and then infects the sensory neurons and **moves by axonal transport to the central nervous system.** During its transport within the nerve, the virus is sheltered from the immune system and little, if any, immune response occurs. The virus multiplies in the central nervous system and then travels down the peripheral nerves to the salivary glands and other organs. From the salivary glands, it enters the saliva to be transmitted by the bite. There is no viremic stage.

Within the central nervous system, an **encephalitis** develops, with the death of neurons and demyelination. Infected neurons contain an eosinophilic cytoplasmic inclusion called a **Negri body,** which is important in laboratory diagnosis of rabies. Because so few individuals have survived rabies, there is no information regarding immunity to disease upon being bitten again.

Clinical Findings   The incubation period varies, according to the location of the bite, from as short as 2 weeks to 16 weeks or longer. It is shorter when bites are sustained on the head rather than on the leg, because the virus has a shorter distance to travel to reach the central nervous system.

Clinically, the patient exhibits a prodrome of nonspecific symptoms such as fever, anorexia, and changes in sensation at the bite site. Within a few days, signs such as confusion, lethargy, and increased salivation develop. Most notable is the painful spasm of the throat muscles on swallowing. This results in **hydrophobia,** an aversion to swallowing water because it is so painful. Within several days, the disease progresses to seizures, paralysis, and coma. Death almost invariably ensues, but with the advent of life support systems a few individuals have survived.

Laboratory Diagnosis   Rapid diagnosis of rabies infection in the animal is usually made by examination of brain tissue by using either fluorescent antibody to rabies virus or histologic staining of Negri bodies in the cytoplasm of hippocampal neurons. The virus can be isolated from the animal brain by growth in cell culture, but this takes too long to be useful in the decision of whether to give the vaccine.

Rabies in humans can be diagnosed by fluorescent-antibody staining of a biopsy specimen, usually taken from the skin of the neck at the hairline; by isolation of the virus from sources such as saliva, spinal fluid, and brain tissue; or by a rise in titer of antibody to the virus. Negri bodies can be demonstrated in corneal scrapings and in autopsy specimens of the brain.

Treatment   There is no antiviral therapy for a patient with rabies. Only supportive treatment is available.

Prevention   There are two approaches to prevention of rabies in humans: **preexposure** and **postexposure.** Preexposure immunization with rabies vaccine should be given to individuals in high-risk groups, such as veterinarians, zoo keepers, and travelers to areas of hyperendemic infection, eg, Peace Corps members. The rabies vaccine is the only vaccine that is routinely used postexposure, ie, after the person has been exposed to the virus via animal bite. The long incubation period of the disease allows the virus in the vaccine sufficient time to induce protective immunity.

In the United States, the **rabies vaccine** contains inactivated virus grown in human diploid cells. In other countries, the duck embryo vaccine or various nerve tissue vaccines are available as well. Duck embryo vaccine has low immunogenicity, and the nerve tissue vaccines can cause an allergic encephalomyelitis as a result of a cross-reaction with human myelin; for these reasons, the human diploid cell vaccine (HDCV) is preferred.

Postexposure immunization involves the use of both the **vaccine and human rabies immune globulin** (RIG, obtained from hyperimmunized persons) plus immediate cleaning of the wound. This is an example of passive-active immunization. Tetanus immunization should also be considered.

The decision to give postexposure immunization depends on a variety of factors, such as (1) the type of animal (all wild-animal attacks demand immunization); (2) whether an attack by a domestic animal was provoked, whether the animal was immunized adequately, and whether the animal is available to be observed; and (3) whether rabies is endemic in the area. The advice of local public health officials should be sought. Hospital personnel exposed to a patient with rabies need not be immunized unless a significant exposure has occurred, eg, a traumatic wound to the health care worker.

If the decision is to immunize, both HDCV and RIG are recommended. Five doses of HDCV are given, but RIG is given only once with the first dose of HDCV (at a different site). HDCV and RIG are given at different sites to prevent neutralization of the virus in the vaccine by the antibody in the RIG. As much as possible of the RIG is given into the bite site, and the remainder is given intramuscularly. If the animal has been captured, it should be observed for 10 days and sacrificed if symptoms develop. The brain of the animal should be examined by immunofluorescence.

The vaccine for immunization of dogs and cats consists of live, attenuated rabies virus grown in chick embryos. Vaccination must be repeated at intervals.

Review Questions

1. Describe the genome and proteins of influenza virus.
2. What is the origin of the changing antigenicity of the influenza virus surface proteins?
3. What is the basis on which influenza virus is divided into A, B, and C viruses?
4. Antibody against which proteins protects against influenza virus infection?
5. What is the function of the influenza virion polymerase?
6. Distinguish between antigenic shift and antigenic drift. What is the impact of each on disease occurrence?
7. What is the mode of action of amantadine? What is its clinical use?
8. Describe influenza vaccine (the nature of the antigen, the number of virus types, its effectiveness, and its target population).
9. What are the main differences between orthomyxoviruses and paramyxoviruses?
10. Why do paramyxoviruses have a virion RNA polymerase?
11. You get measles only once. What factors contribute to this?
12. What is the pathogenesis of measles?
13. What is the relationship between measles and subacute sclerosing panencephalitis?
14. What is the nature of the measles vaccine? How effective is it?
15. What is the pathogenesis of mumps?
16. What is the nature of the mumps vaccine? How effective is it?
17. Why is mumps of concern in a man but less so in a young boy?
18. Respiratory syncytial virus is a major cause of which disease in which age group?
19. Why is the term "syncytial" in the name "respiratory syncytial virus"? What causes syncytia?
20. What is the major disease caused by parainfluenza viruses in children?
21. How does the rubella virus genome differ from the orthomyxovirus and paramyxovirus genomes?
22. What is the most important complication of rubella infection in young women?
23. What is congenital rubella syndrome?
24. What is the nature of rubella vaccine? How effective is it?
25. What is the host range of rabies virus?
26. What are the main reservoirs of rabies virus in the United States and in developing countries?
27. What is the pathogenesis of rabies?
28. Trace the path of rabies virus from its entry into the normal animal to its appearance in the saliva of the rabid animal.
29. What are the laboratory procedures for the diagnosis of rabies in animals and in humans?
30. Discuss the criteria that determine whether postexposure rabies prophylaxis should be given.
31. What is the nature of the rabies vaccine? In which cells is it made? Why?

40

RNA Nonenveloped Viruses

Picornaviruses

Picornaviruses are small (20–30-nm) **nonenveloped** viruses composed of an **icosahedral nucleo-capsid** and a **single-stranded** RNA genome. The genome RNA has **positive polarity;** ie, on entering the cell, it functions as the viral mRNA. The genome RNA is unusual because it has a protein on the 5′ end that serves as a primer for transcription by RNA polymerase. Picornaviruses replicate in the cytoplasm of cells. They are not inactivated by lipid solvents, such as ether, because they do not have an envelope.

The picornavirus family includes two groups of medical importance: the **enteroviruses** and the **rhinoviruses.** Among the major enteroviruses are poliovirus, coxsackieviruses, echoviruses, and hepatitis A virus (which is described in Chapter 41). Enteroviruses infect primarily the enteric tract, whereas rhinoviruses are found in the nose and throat (hence their name). Important features of viruses that commonly infect the intestinal tract are summarized in Table 40–1. Enteroviruses replicate optimally at 37 °C, whereas rhinoviruses grow better at 33 °C, in accordance with the lower temperature of the nose. Enteroviruses are stable under acid conditions (pH 3–5), which enables them to survive exposure to gastric acid, whereas rhinoviruses are acid-labile. This may explain why rhinoviruses are restricted to the nose and throat.

ENTEROVIRUSES

1. Poliovirus

Disease   This virus causes poliomyelitis.

Important Properties   The host range is limited to **primates,** ie, humans and nonhuman primates such as apes and monkeys. This limitation is due to the binding of the viral capsid protein to a receptor found only on primate cell membranes. However, note that purified viral RNA (without the capsid protein) can enter and replicate in many nonprimate cells; the RNA can bypass the cell membrane receptor; ie, it is "infectious RNA."

There are **three serologic (antigenic) types** based on different antigenic determinants on the outer capsid proteins. Because there is little cross reaction, protection from disease requires the presence of antibody against each of the three types.

Summary of Replicative Cycle   The virion interacts with specific cell receptors on the cell membrane and then enters the cell. The capsid proteins are then removed. After uncoating, the genome RNA functions as mRNA and is translated into **one very large polypeptide** called noncapsid viral protein 00. This polypeptide is cleaved by proteases in multiple steps to form both the capsid proteins of the progeny virions and several noncapsid proteins including the RNA polymerase that synthesizes the progeny RNA genomes. Replication of the genome occurs by synthesis of a complementary negative strand, which then serves as the template for the positive strands. Some of these positive strands function as mRNA to make more viral proteins, and the remainder become progeny virion genome RNA. Assembly of the progeny virions occurs by coating of the genome RNA with capsid proteins. Virions accumulate in the cell cytoplasm and are released upon death of the cell. They do not bud from the cell membrane.

Transmission & Epidemiology   Poliovirus is transmitted by the **fecal-oral** route. It replicates in the oropharynx and intestinal tract. Humans are the only natural hosts.

As a result of the success of the vaccine, poliomyelitis caused by naturally occurring "wild-type" virus has been **eradicated** from the United States and, indeed, **from the entire Western hemisphere.** The rare cases in the United States occur mainly in (1) people exposed to virulent revertants of the at-

Table 40–1. Features of viruses commonly infecting the intestinal tract.

Virus	Nucleic Acid	Disease	Number of Serotypes	Lifelong Immunity to Disease	Vaccine Available	Antiviral Therapy
Poliovirus	RNA	Poliomyelitis	3	Yes (type-specific)	+	–
Echoviruses	RNA	Meningitis, etc	Many	No	–	–
Coxsackieviruses	RNA	Meningitis, carditis, etc	Many	No	–	–
Hepatitis A virus (enterovirus 72)	RNA	Hepatitis	1	Yes	–	–
Rotavirus	RNA	Diarrhea	Several[1]	No	–	–
Norwalk virus	RNA	Diarrhea	Unknown	Unknown	–	–
Adenovirus	DNA	Diarrhea	2 of 41[2]	Unknown	–	–

[1]Exact number uncertain.
[2]Two of the 41 serotypes of adenovirus are known to cause diarrhea.

tenuated virus in the live vaccine and (2) unimmunized people exposed to "wild-type" poliovirus while traveling abroad. Before the vaccine was available, epidemics occurred in the summer and fall.

Poliomyelitis occurs worldwide with varying frequency. In developing countries, particularly in areas where hygiene and sanitation are poor, children are exposed at an early age and experience mostly asymptomatic infections. In more developed countries, exposure is frequently delayed, with a consequent increase in the frequency of symptomatic infection among the unimmunized.

Pathogenesis & Immunity   After replicating in the oropharynx and small intestine, especially in lymphoid tissue, the virus spreads through the bloodstream to the central nervous system. It can also spread retrograde along nerve axons.

In the central nervous system, poliovirus preferentially replicates in the **motor neurons** located in the **anterior horn** of the spinal cord. Death of these cells results in paralysis of the muscles innervated by those neurons. Paralysis is not due to virus infection of muscle cells. The virus also affects the brain stem, leading to "bulbar" poliomyelitis (with respiratory paralysis), but rarely damages the cerebral cortex.

In infected individuals, the immune response consists of both intestinal IgA and humoral IgG to the specific serotype. Infection provides lifelong type-specific immunity.

Clinical Findings   The range of responses to poliovirus infection includes (1) inapparent, asymptomatic infection; (2) abortive poliomyelitis; (3) nonparalytic poliomyelitis; and (4) paralytic poliomyelitis. Asymptomatic infection is quite common. Roughly 1% of infections are clinically apparent. The incubation period is usually 10–14 days.

The most common clinical form is abortive poliomyelitis, which is a mild, febrile illness characterized by headache, sore throat, nausea, and vomiting. Most patients recover spontaneously. Nonparalytic poliomyelitis manifests as an aseptic meningitis with fever, headache, and a stiff neck. This also usually resolves spontaneously. In paralytic poliomyelitis, flaccid paralysis is the predominant finding but brain stem involvement can lead to life-threatening respiratory paralysis. Painful muscle spasms also occur. The motor nerve damage is permanent, but some recovery of muscle function occurs as other nerve cells take over.

A post-polio syndrome that occurs many years after the acute illness has been described. Marked deterioration of the residual function of the affected muscles occurs many years after the acute phase. The cause of this deterioration is unknown.

No permanent carrier state occurs following infection by poliovirus, but virus excretion in the feces can occur for several months.

Laboratory Diagnosis   The diagnosis is made either by isolation of the virus or by a rise in antibody titer. Virus can be recovered from the throat, stool, or spinal fluid by inoculation of cell cultures. The virus causes a cytopathic effect (CPE) and can be identified by neutralization of the CPE with specific antisera.

Treatment   There is no antiviral therapy. Treatment is limited to symptomatic relief and respiratory support, if needed. Physiotherapy for the affected muscles is important.

Prevention   Poliomyelitis can be prevented by both the **killed** vaccine (Salk vaccine, inactivated vaccine, IPV) and the **live, attenuated** vaccine (Sabin vaccine, oral vaccine, OPV) (Table 40–2). Both vaccines induce humoral antibodies, which neutralize virus entering the blood and hence prevent central nervous system infection and disease. The **live vaccine is currently preferred** in the United States for two main reasons. (1) It interrupts fecal-oral transmission by inducing secretory IgA in the gastrointestinal tract. IgA is induced by the live virus because it replicates in the gastrointestinal tract, whereas the killed vaccine does not. (2) It is given orally and so is more readily accepted than the killed vaccine, which must be injected.

The live vaccine has four disadvantages: (1) Rarely, **reversion** of the attenuated virus to virulence will occur, and disease may ensue (especially for the type 3 virus); (2) it can cause disease in immunodeficient persons and therefore should not be given to them; (3) infection of the gastrointestinal tract by other enteroviruses can limit replication of the vaccine virus and reduce protection; and (4) it must be kept refrigerated to prevent heat inactivation of the live virus.

The duration of immunity is thought to be longer with the live than with the killed vaccine, but booster doses are recommended with both.

The killed vaccine is used in the United States in two special instances: (1) initial vaccination of unimmunized adults, because the risk of disease from the live vaccine is higher in adults than in children; and (2) vaccination of immunodeficient individuals. The enhanced-potency inactivated vaccine (eIPV) is recommended for these purposes.

Both the killed and the live vaccines contain all three serologic types. The live vaccine should be given at 2, 4, 6, and 18 months of age, with a booster when the child enters school. In 1996, an alternative vaccine schedule consisting of two doses of inactivated vaccine followed by two doses of live vaccine was approved. This approach should prevent some of the approximately 10 cases per year of paralytic polio that arise from reversion of the attenuated virus in the vaccine.

In the past, some lots of poliovirus vaccines were contaminated with a papovavirus, SV40 virus, which causes sarcomas in rodents. SV40 virus was a "passenger" virus in the monkey kidney cells used to grow the poliovirus for the vaccine. Fortunately, no increase in cancer occurred in persons inoculated with the SV40 virus-containing polio vaccine. At present, cell cultures used for vaccine purposes are carefully screened to exclude the presence of adventitious viruses.

Passive immunization with immune serum globulin is available for protection of unimmunized individuals known to have been exposed. Passive immunization of newborns as a result of passage of maternal IgG antibodies across the placenta also occurs.

Quarantine of patients with disease is not effective, because fecal excretion of the virus occurs in infected individuals prior to the onset of symptoms and in those who remain asymptomatic.

Table 40–2. Important features of poliovirus vaccines.

Attribute	Killed (Salk)	Live (Sabin)
Prevents disease	Yes	Yes
Interrupts transmission	No	Yes
Induces humoral IgG	Yes	Yes
Induces intestinal IgA	No	Yes
Affords secondary protection by spread to others	No	Yes
Interferes with replication of virulent virus in gut	No	Yes
Reverts to virulence	No	Yes (rarely)
Coinfection with other enteroviruses may impair immunization	No	Yes
Can cause disease in the immuno-compromised	No	Yes
Route of administration	Injection	Oral
Requires refrigeration	No	Yes
Duration of immunity	Shorter	Longer

2. Coxsackieviruses

Coxsackieviruses are named for the town of Coxsackie, NY, where they were first isolated.

Diseases   Coxsackieviruses cause a variety of diseases. Group A viruses cause, for example, herpangina and hand-foot-and-mouth disease, whereas group B viruses cause pleurodynia, myocarditis, and pericarditis. Both types cause nonspecific upper respiratory tract disease, febrile rashes, and aseptic meningitis.

Important Properties   Group classification is based on pathogenicity in mice. Group A viruses cause widespread myositis and flaccid paralysis, which is rapidly fatal, whereas group B viruses cause generalized, less severe lesions of the heart, pancreas, and central nervous system and a focal myositis. At least 24 serotypes of coxsackievirus A and 6 serotypes of coxsackievirus B are recognized.

The size and structure of the virion and the nature of the genome RNA are similar to those of poliovirus. Unlike poliovirus, they can infect mammals other than primates.

Summary of Replicative Cycle   Replication is similar to that of poliovirus.

Transmission & Epidemiology   Coxsackieviruses are transmitted primarily by the **fecal-oral** route, but respiratory **aerosols** also play a role. They replicate in the oropharynx and the intestinal tract. Humans are the only natural hosts. Coxsackievirus infections occur worldwide, primarily in the summer and fall.

Pathogenesis & Immunity   Group A viruses have a predilection for skin and mucous membranes, whereas group B viruses cause disease in various organs such as the heart, pleura, pancreas, and liver. Both group A and B viruses can affect the meninges and the motor neurons (anterior horn cells) to cause paralysis. From their original site of replication in the oropharynx and gastrointestinal tract, they disseminate via the bloodstream.

Immunity following infection is provided by type-specific IgG antibody.

Clinical Findings

A.   Group A-Specific Diseases: **Herpangina** is characterized by fever, sore throat, and tender vesicles in the oropharynx. Hand-foot-and-mouth disease is characterized by a vesicular rash on the hands and feet and ulcerations in the mouth, mainly in children.

B.   Group B-Specific Diseases: **Pleurodynia** (Bornholm disease, epidemic myalgia, "devil's grip") is characterized by fever and severe pleuritic-type chest pain. **Myocarditis** and pericarditis are characterized by fever, chest pain, and signs of congestive failure. **Diabetes** in mice can be caused by pancreatic damage as a result of infection with coxsackievirus B4. This virus is suspected to have a similar role in juvenile diabetes in humans.

C.   Diseases Caused by Both Groups: Both groups of viruses can cause **aseptic meningitis,** mild paresis, and transient paralysis. Upper respiratory infections and minor febrile illnesses with or without rash can occur also.

Laboratory Diagnosis   The diagnosis is made either by isolating the virus in cell culture or suckling mice or by observing a rise in titer of neutralizing antibodies.

Treatment & Prevention   There is neither antiviral drug therapy nor a vaccine available against these viruses. No passive immunization is recommended.

3. Echoviruses

The prefix ECHO is an acronym for *e*nteric *c*ytopathic *h*uman *o*rphan. Although called "orphans" because they were not initially associated with any disease, they are now known to cause a variety of diseases such as aseptic meningitis, upper respiratory infection, febrile illness with and without rash, infantile diarrhea, and hemorrhagic conjunctivitis.

The structure of echoviruses is similar to that of other enteroviruses. More than 30 serotypes have been isolated. In contrast to coxsackieviruses, they are not pathogenic for mice. Unlike polioviruses, they do not cause disease in monkeys. They are transmitted by the **fecal-oral** route and occur world-wide. Pathogenesis is similar to that of the other enteroviruses.

Along with coxsackieviruses, echoviruses are one of the **leading causes of aseptic (viral) meningitis.** The diagnosis is made by isolation of the virus in cell culture. Serologic tests are of little value, because there are a large number of serotypes and no common antigen. There is no antiviral therapy or vaccine available.

4. Other Enteroviruses

In view of the difficulty in classifying many enteroviruses, all new isolates have been given a simple numerical designation since 1969.

Enterovirus 70 is the main cause of acute hemorrhagic conjunctivitis, characterized by petechial hemorrhages on the bulbar conjunctivas. Complete recovery usually occurs, and there is no therapy. Enterovirus 71 is one of the leading causes of viral central nervous system disease, including meningitis, encephalitis, and paralysis. Enterovirus 72 is hepatitis A virus, which is described in Chapter 41.

RHINOVIRUSES

Disease   These viruses are the main cause of the common cold.

Important Properties   There are **more than 100 serologic types.** They **replicate better at 33 °C** than at 37 °C, which explains why they affect primarily the nose and conjunctiva rather than the lower respiratory tract. They are **acid-labile** and so are killed by gastric acid when swallowed. This explains why they do not infect the gastrointestinal tract, unlike the enteroviruses. The host range is limited to humans and chimpanzees.

Summary of Replicative Cycle   Replication is similar to that of poliovirus. The cell surface receptor for rhinoviruses is ICAM-1, an adhesion protein located on the surface of many types of cells.

Transmission & Epidemiology   There are **two modes** of transmission for these viruses. In the past, it was accepted that they were transmitted directly from person to person via aerosols of respiratory droplets. However, now it appears that an indirect mode, in which respiratory droplets are deposited on the hands or on a surface such as a table and then transported by fingers to the nose or eyes, is also important.

The common cold is reputed to be the most common human infection, although data are difficult to obtain because it is not a well-defined or notifiable disease. Millions of days of work and school are lost each year as a result of "colds." Rhinoviruses occur worldwide, causing disease particularly in the fall and winter. The reason for this seasonal variation is unclear. Low temperatures per se do not predispose to the common cold, but the crowding that occurs at schools, for example, may enhance transmission during fall and winter. The frequency of colds is high in childhood and tapers off during adulthood, presumably owing to the acquisition of immunity.

A few serotypes of rhinoviruses are prevalent during one season, only to be replaced by other serotypes during the following season. It appears that the population builds up immunity to the prevalent serotypes but remains susceptible to the others.

Pathogenesis & Immunity   The portal of entry is the upper respiratory tract, and the infection is limited to that region. Rhinoviruses rarely cause lower respiratory tract disease, probably because they grow poorly at 37 °C.

Immunity is serotype-specific and is a function of nasal secretory antibody rather than humoral antibody.

Clinical Findings   After an incubation period of 2–4 days, sneezing, nasal discharge, sore throat, cough, and headache are common. A chilly sensation may occur, but there are few other systemic symptoms. The illness lasts about 1 week. Note that other viruses such as coronaviruses, adenoviruses, influenza C virus, and coxsackieviruses also cause the common cold syndrome.

Laboratory Diagnosis Diagnosis can be made by isolation of the virus from nasal secretions in cell culture, but this is rarely attempted. Serologic tests are not done.

Treatment & Prevention No specific antiviral therapy is available. Vaccines appear impractical because of the large number of serotypes. Paper tissues impregnated with disinfectants, such as iodine, limit transmission when used to remove rhinoviruses from fingers contaminated with respiratory secretions. High doses of vitamin C have little ability to prevent rhinovirus-induced colds. Lozenges containing zinc gluconate are available for the treatment of the common cold, but their efficacy remains unproven.

Reoviruses

REO is an acronym for *r*espiratory *e*nteric *o*rphan; when the virus was discovered, it was isolated from the respiratory and enteric tracts and was not associated with any disease. Rotaviruses are the most important human pathogens in the reovirus family.

ROTAVIRUS

Disease Rotavirus is the most common cause of gastroenteritis in young children.

Important Properties Reoviruses, including rotavirus, are composed of a **segmented,* double-stranded RNA genome** surrounded by a double-layered icosahedral capsid without an envelope. The virion contains an **RNA-dependent RNA polymerase.** A virion polymerase is required because human cells do not have an RNA polymerase that can synthesize mRNA from a double-stranded RNA template.

Many domestic animals are infected with their own strains of rotaviruses, but these are not a source of human disease. There are at least six serotypes of human rotavirus. The viral hemagglutinin is the type-specific antigen.

Summary of Replicative Cycle Reoviruses attach to the cell surface at the site of the beta-adrenergic receptor. After entry of the virion into the cell, the RNA-dependent RNA polymerase synthesizes mRNA from each of the 10 or 11 segments within the cytoplasm. The 10 or 11 mRNAs are translated into the corresponding number of structural and nonstructural proteins. One of these, an RNA polymerase, synthesizes minus strands that will become part of the genome of the progeny virus. Capsid proteins form an incomplete capsid around the minus strands, and then the plus strands of the progeny genome segments are synthesized. The virus is released from the cytoplasm by lysis of the cell, not by budding.

Transmission & Epidemiology Rotavirus is transmitted by the **fecal-oral** route. Infection occurs worldwide, and by age 6 years the majority of children have antibodies to at least one serotype.

Pathogenesis & Immunity Rotavirus replicates in the mucosal cells of the small intestine, damaging the transport mechanisms. The consequent loss of salt, glucose, and water leads to diarrhea. No inflammation occurs, and the diarrhea is nonbloody.

The virulence of certain reoviruses in mice has been localized to the proteins encoded by several specific genome segments. For example, one gene governs tissue tropism, whereas another controls the inhibition of cell RNA and protein synthesis.

Immunity to rotavirus infection is unclear. It is likely that intestinal IgA directed against specific serotypes protects against reinfection and that colostrum IgA protects newborns up to the age of 6 months.

---

*Rotaviruses have 11 segments; other reoviruses have 10.

Clinical Findings   Rotavirus infection is characterized by nausea, vomiting, and watery, non-bloody diarrhea. **Gastroenteritis** is most serious in **young children,** in whom dehydration and electrolyte imbalance are a major concern. Adults usually have minor symptoms.

Laboratory Diagnosis   Although the diagnosis of most cases of viral gastroenteritis does not involve the laboratory, a diagnosis can be made by **detection of rotavirus in the stool** by using radioimmunoassay or ELISA. This approach is feasible because there are large numbers of virus particles in the stool. The original demonstration of rotavirus in the stool was done by immunoelectron microscopy, in which antibody aggregated the virions, allowing them to be visualized in the electron microscope. This technique is not feasible for routine clinical use. In addition to antigen detection, the diagnosis can be made by observation of a 4-fold or greater rise in antibody titer. Although the virus can be cultured, this procedure is not routinely done.

Treatment & Prevention   There is neither antiviral therapy nor a vaccine available. A vaccine containing four serotypes of live, attenuated rotavirus is likely to be approved by the FDA soon. Prevention rests on sanitation.

Review Questions

1. What are the differences between enteroviruses and rhinoviruses?
2. What is the nature of the picornavirus genome?
3. Why does poliovirus infect only primate cells?
4. Poliovirus has three serotypes. What is the importance of this for the prevention of poliomyelitis?
5. What is the nature of the translation product of the poliovirus RNA? How are viral capsid proteins formed?
6. How is poliovirus transmitted?
7. What is the pathogenesis of paralytic poliomyelitis?
8. Compare the advantages and disadvantages of the killed and live poliovirus vaccines.
9. How did SV40 virus get into some lots of poliovirus vaccine? Why is this of concern?
10. On what basis are coxsackievirus groups A and B distinguished?
11. What clinical entities do coxsackievirus groups A and B specifically cause? What disease do both groups A and B cause?
12. What is the significance of the fact that there are more than 100 serotypes of rhinoviruses?
13. What are two modes of transmission of rhinoviruses?
14. What is the nature of the reovirus genome? Why is there a virion polymerase?
15. Rotaviruses are clinically important reoviruses. What disease do they cause? In what population?
16. How is rotavirus infection diagnosed in the laboratory?

41

Hepatitis Viruses

Many viruses cause hepatitis. Of these, five medically important viruses are commonly described as "hepatitis viruses": hepatitis A virus (HAV); hepatitis B virus (HBV); non-A, non-B viruses, of which hepatitis C virus (HCV) is the most common; hepatitis D virus (HDV, delta agent); and hepatitis E virus (HEV) (Tables 41–1 and 41–2). Other viruses, such as Epstein-Barr virus (the cause of infectious mononucleosis), cytomegalovirus, and yellow fever virus, cause inflammation of the liver but are not called hepatitis viruses per se. They are discussed elsewhere.

Table 41–1. Glossary of hepatitis viruses and their serologic markers.

Abbreviation	Name and Description
HAV	Hepatitis A virus (enterovirus 72), a picornavirus (nonenveloped RNA virus).
IgM HAVAb	IgM antibody to HAV; best test to detect acute hepatitis A.
HBV	Hepatitis B virus, a hepadnavirus (enveloped, partially double-stranded DNA virus); also known as Dane particle.
HBsAg	Antigen found on surface of HBV, also found on noninfectious particles in patient's blood; positive during acute disease; continued presence indicates carrier state.
HBsAb	Antibody to HBsAg; provides immunity to hepatitis B.
HBcAg	Antigen associated with core of HBV.
HBcAb	Antibody to HBcAg; positive during window phase. IgM HBcAb is an indicator of recent disease.
HBeAg	A second, different antigenic determinant in the HBV core. Important indicator of transmissibility.
HBeAb	Antibody to e antigen; indicates low transmissibility.
Non-A, non-B	Hepatitis viruses that are neither HAV nor HBV.
HCV	Enveloped RNA virus; one of the non-A, non-B viruses.
HEV	Nonenveloped RNA virus; one of the non-A, non-B viruses.
HDV (delta agent)	Small RNA virus with HBsAg envelope; defective virus that replicates only in HBV-infected cells.

HEPATITIS A VIRUS

Disease HAV causes hepatitis A.

Important Properties HAV is a typical **enterovirus** classified in the picornavirus family. It has a single-stranded RNA genome and a nonenveloped icosahedral nucleocapsid and replicates in the cytoplasm of the cell. It is also known as enterovirus 72. It has one serotype, and there is no antigenic relationship to HBV or other hepatitis viruses.

Summary of Replicative Cycle HAV has a replicative cycle similar to that of other enteroviruses (the replicative cycle of poliovirus is discussed in Chapter 40).

Transmission & Epidemiology HAV is transmitted by the **fecal-oral** route. Humans are the reservoir for HAV. Virus appears in the feces roughly 2 weeks before the appearance of symptoms, so quarantine of patients is ineffective. **Children are the most frequently infected** group, and outbreaks occur in special living situations such as summer camps and boarding schools. Common-source outbreaks arise from fecally contaminated water or food such as oysters grown in polluted water and eaten raw. Unlike HBV, HAV is **rarely transmitted via the blood,** because the level of viremia is low and chronic infection does not occur. About 50–75% of adults in the United States have been infected, as evidenced by IgG antibody.

Pathogenesis & Immunity The pathogenesis of HAV infection is not completely understood. The virus probably replicates in the gastrointestinal tract and spreads to the liver via the blood. He-

Table 41–2. Important properties of hepatitis viruses.

Virus	Genome	Replication Defective	DNA Polymerase in Virion	HBsAg in Envelope	Virus Family
HAV	ssRNA	No	No	No	Picornavirus
HBV	dsDNA[1]	No	Yes	Yes	Hepadnavirus
HCV	ssRNA	No	No	No	Flavivirus
HDV	ssRNA[2]	Yes	No	Yes	Deltavirus
HEV	ssRNA	No	No	No	Calicivirus

[1] Interrupted, circular dsDNA.
[2] Circular, negative-stranded ssRNA.

Table 41–3. Clinical features of hepatitis viruses.

Virus	Mode of Transmission	Chronic Carriers	Laboratory Test Usually Used for Diagnosis	Vaccine Available	Immune Globulins Useful
HAV	Fecal-oral	No	IgM HAV	Yes	Yes
HBV	Blood, sexual, at birth	Yes	HBsAg, HBsAb, IgM HBcAb	Yes	Yes
HCV	Blood, sexual[1]	Yes	HCV Ab	No	No
HDV	Blood, sexual[1]	Yes	Ab to delta Ag	No	No
HEV	Fecal-oral	No	None	No	No

[1] Sexual transmission seems likely but is poorly documented.

patocytes are infected, but the mechanism by which cell damage occurs is unclear. HAV infection of cultured cells produces no cytopathic effect. It is likely that attack by cytotoxic T cells causes the damage to the hepatocytes. The infection is cleared, the damage is repaired, and no chronic infection ensues. Hepatitis caused by the different viruses cannot be distinguished pathologically.

The immune response consists initially of IgM antibody, which is detectable at the time jaundice appears. It is therefore important in the laboratory diagnosis of hepatitis A. The appearance of IgM is followed 1–3 weeks later by the production of IgG antibody, which provides lifelong protection.

Clinical Findings   The clinical manifestations of hepatitis are virtually the same, regardless of which hepatitis virus is the cause (Table 41–3). Fever, anorexia, nausea, vomiting, and jaundice are typical. Dark urine, pale feces, and elevated transaminase levels are seen. Most cases resolve spontaneously in 2–4 weeks. Hepatitis A has a short incubation period (3–4 weeks), in contrast to that of hepatitis B, which is 10–12 weeks. Most HAV infections are asymptomatic and are detected solely by the presence of IgG antibody. No chronic hepatitis or chronic carrier state occurs, and there is no predisposition to hepatocellular carcinoma.

Laboratory Diagnosis   The detection of **IgM antibody** is the most important test. A 4-fold rise in IgG antibody titer can also be used. Isolation of the virus in cell culture is possible but not available in the clinical laboratory.

Treatment & Prevention   No antiviral therapy is available. **Active immunization** with a vaccine containing inactivated HAV is available. The virus is grown in human cell culture and inactivated with formalin. An initial dose followed by a booster 6 to 12 months later should be given to adults. The vaccine is recommended for travelers to developing countries. However, because many people have antibodies to HAV, it may be cost-effective to determine whether antibodies are present before giving the vaccine. **Passive immunization** with immune serum globulin prior to infection or early in the incubation period can prevent or mitigate the disease. Observation of proper hygiene, eg, sewage disposal and hand washing after bowel movements, is of prime importance.

HEPATITIS B VIRUS

Disease   HBV causes hepatitis B.

Important Properties   HBV is a member of the hepadnavirus family. It is a 42-nm **enveloped virion,*** with an icosahedral nucleocapsid core containing a **partially double-stranded circular DNA genome** (Fig 41–1 and Table 41–1). The envelope contains a protein called the **surface antigen** (HBsAg), which is important for laboratory diagnosis and immunization.† Within the core is a **DNA-dependent DNA polymerase.** The genome encodes only five proteins: surface antigen, core antigen, DNA polymerase, and two regulatory proteins that activate transcription of RNA.

Electron microscopy of a patient's serum reveals three different types of particles: a few 42-nm virions and many 22-nm **spheres** and long **filaments** 22 nm wide, which are composed of surface antigen. HBV is the only human virus that produces these spheres and filaments in such large numbers in the patient's blood.

---

*Also known as a Dane particle (named for the scientist who first published electron micrographs of the virion).
†HBsAg was known as Australia antigen, because it was first found in the serum of an Australian aborigine.

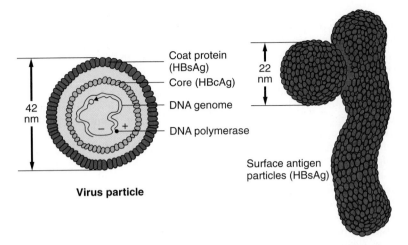

Figure 41–1. Hepatitis B virus. **Left:** Cross-section of the HBV virion. **Right:** The 22-nm spheres and filaments composed only of hepatitis B surface antigen. There is no viral DNA in the spheres and filaments, and so they are not infectious. (Modified and reproduced, with permission from Ryan K et al: *Sherris Medical Microbiology,* 3rd ed. Appleton & Lange, 1994.)

In addition to HBsAg, there are two other important antigens: the **core antigen** (HBcAg) and the **e antigen** (HBeAg), both of which are located in the core but have different antigenicities. HBeAg is an important indicator of **transmissibility.**

For vaccine purposes, HBV has one serotype based on HBsAg. However, for epidemiologic purposes, there are four serologic subtypes of HBsAg based on a group-specific antigen, "a," and two sets of mutually exclusive epitopes, d or y and w or r. This leads to four serotypes—adw, adr, ayw, and ayr—which are useful in epidemiologic studies because they are concentrated in certain geographic areas.

Humans are the only natural hosts of HBV.

Summary of Replicative Cycle   After entry of the virion into the cell and its uncoating, the virion DNA polymerase synthesizes the missing portion of DNA and a double-stranded closed-circular DNA is formed in the nucleus. This DNA serves as a template for mRNA synthesis by cellular RNA polymerase. mRNA not only functions in protein synthesis but also is the template for the minus strand of the progeny DNA. The minus strand then serves as the template for the plus strand of the genome DNA. This **RNA-dependent DNA synthesis** takes place within the newly assembled virion core in the cytoplasm. Hepadnaviruses are the *only* viruses that produce genome DNA by reverse transcription with mRNA as the template. (Note that this type of RNA-dependent DNA synthesis is similar to but different from the process in retroviruses, in which the genome RNA is transcribed into a DNA intermediate.) Some of the progeny DNA integrates into the host cell genome, and this seems likely to be the DNA that maintains the carrier state. Progeny HBV with its HBsAg-containing envelope is released from the cell by budding through the cell membrane.

Transmission & Epidemiology   The three main modes of transmission are via blood, during sexual intercourse, and perinatally from mother to newborn. The observation that needle-stick injuries can transmit the virus indicates that only very small amounts of blood are necessary. HBV infection is especially prevalent in addicts who use intravenous drugs. Screening of blood for the presence of HBsAg has greatly decreased the number of transfusion-associated cases of hepatitis B.* However, because blood transfusion is a modern procedure, there must be another, natural route of transmission. It is likely that **sexual** transmission and transmission from **mother to child** during birth or breast-feeding are the natural routes. Note that enveloped viruses, such as HBV, are more sensitive to the environment than nonenveloped viruses and hence are more efficiently transmitted by intimate contact, eg, sexual contact. Nonenveloped viruses, such as HAV, are quite stable and are transmitted well via the environment, eg, fecal-oral transmission.

---

*In the United States, donated blood is screened for HBsAg and antibodies to HBcAg, HCV, HIV-1, HIV-2, and HTLV-I. Two other tests are also performed: a VDRL test for syphilis and a transaminase assay, which, if elevated, indicates liver damage and is a surrogate marker of viral infection.

Hepatitis B is found worldwide but is particularly prevalent in the Orient. In that region, there is a high incidence of **hepatocellular carcinoma (hepatoma),** a finding which indicates that HBV may be a human tumor virus (see Chapter 43). Immunization against HBV in Taiwan has significantly reduced the incidence of hepatoma in children. It appears that the HBV vaccine is the **first vaccine to prevent a human cancer.**

Pathogenesis & Immunity   After entering the blood, the virus infects hepatocytes, and viral antigens are displayed on the surface of the cells. Cytotoxic T cells mediate an immune attack against the viral antigens, and inflammation and necrosis occur. **Immune attack** against viral antigens on infected hepatocytes is mediated by cytotoxic T cells. The pathogenesis of hepatitis B is probably the result of this cell-mediated immune injury, because HBV itself does not cause a cytopathic effect. Antigen-antibody complexes cause some of the early symptoms, eg, arthralgias, and some of the complications in chronic hepatitis, eg, immune-complex glomerulonephritis and vasculitis.

Unlike hepatitis A patients, about 5% of patients with hepatitis B become **chronic carriers** of HBV. A chronic carrier is someone who has **HBsAg persisting in their blood for at least 6 months.** The chronic carrier state is attributed to a persistent infection of the hepatocytes which results in the prolonged presence of HBV and HBsAg in the blood. The main determinant of whether a person clears the infection or becomes a chronic carrier is the adequacy of the cytotoxic T cell response. HBV DNA exists primarily as an episome in the cytoplasm of persistently infected cells; a small number of copies of HBV DNA are integrated into cell DNA. A high rate of **hepatocellular carcinoma occurs in chronic carriers.** The HBV genome has no oncogene, and hepatocellular carcinoma appears to be the result of persistent cellular regeneration that attempts to replace the dead hepatocytes. Chronic carriage is more likely to occur when infection occurs in a newborn than in an adult, probably because a newborn's immune system is less competent than an adult's. Approximately 90% of those infected as neonates become chronic carriers.

Lifelong immunity occurs after the natural infection and is mediated by humoral antibody against HBsAg. Antibody against HBcAg is not protective.

Clinical Findings   Many HBV infections are asymptomatic and are detected only by the presence of antibody to HBsAg. The mean incubation period for hepatitis B is 10–12 weeks, which is much longer than that of hepatitis A (3–4 weeks). The clinical appearance of acute hepatitis B is similar to that of hepatitis A. However, with hepatitis B, symptoms tend to be more severe and life-threatening hepatitis can occur. Most chronic carriers are asymptomatic, but some have chronic active hepatitis, which can lead to cirrhosis and death.

Laboratory Diagnosis   The most important laboratory test for the detection of early HBV infection is the immunoassay for **HBsAg.** HBsAg appears during the incubation period and is detectable in most patients during the prodrome and acute disease (Fig 41–2). It falls to undetectable levels during convalescence in most cases; its **prolonged presence** (at least 6 months) indicates the carrier state and the risk of chronic hepatitis and hepatic carcinoma. As described in Table 41–4, HBsAb is not detectable in the chronic carrier state. Note that HBsAb is, in fact, being made but is not detectable in the laboratory tests because it is bound to the large amount of HBsAg present in the blood. HBsAb is also being made during the acute dsease but is similarly undetectable because it is bound in immune complexes.

Note that there is a period of several weeks when HBsAg has disappeared but HBsAb is not yet detectable. This is the **"window phase."** At this time, the HBcAb is always positive and can be used to make the diagnosis. HBcAb is present in those with acute infection and chronic infection, as well as those who have recovered from acute infection. Therefore, it cannot be used to distinguish between acute and chronic infection. The IgM form of HBcAb is present during acute infection and disappears approximately 6 months after infection. The test for HBcAg is not readily available. Table 41–4 describes the serologic test results that characterize the four important stages of HBV infection.

HBeAg arises during the incubation period and is present during the prodrome and early acute disease, and in certain chronic carriers. Its presence is an important **indicator of transmissibility,** and, conversely, the finding of HBeAb indicates low transmissibility. DNA polymerase activity is detectable during the incubation period and early in the disease, but the assay is not available in most clinical laboratories. The detection of viral DNA in the serum is strong evidence that infectious virions are present.

Treatment & Prevention   Alpha interferon is clinically useful for the treatment of chronic hepatitis B infections. Some nucleoside analogues, such as lamivudine (thiacytidine), that inhibit the reverse transcriptase of HIV, also are effective against HBV. These drugs reduce hepatic inflammation and lower the levels of HBV in chronic carriers.

Prevention involves the use of either the **vaccine** or **hyperimmune globulin,** or both.

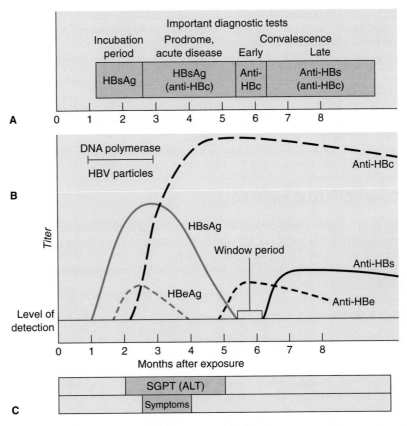

Figure 41–2. *A:* Important diagnostic tests during various stages of hepatitis B. *B:* Serologic findings in a patient with acute hepatitis B. *C:* Duration of increased liver enzyme activity and of symptoms in a patient with acute hepatitis B. (Modified and reproduced, with permission, from Hollinger FB, Dienstag JL: Hepatitis viruses. Chapter 81 in: *Manual of Clinical Microbiology,* 4th ed. Lennette EH et al [editors]. American Society for Microbiology, 1985.)

(1) The vaccine contains HBsAg produced in yeasts by genetic engineering techniques. The vaccine is highly effective in preventing hepatitis B and has few side effects. It is indicated for people who are frequently exposed to blood or blood products, such as certain health care personnel (eg, medical students, surgeons, and dentists), patients receiving multiple transfusions or dialysis, patients with frequent sexually transmitted disease, and abusers of illicit intravenous drugs. The U.S. Public Health Service recommends that all newborns and adolescents receive the vaccine. At present, booster doses after the initial three-dose regimen are not recommended.

Table 41–4. Serologic test results in four stages of HBV infection.

Test	Acute Disease	Window Phase	Complete Recovery	Chronic Carrier State
HBsAg	Positive	Negative	Negative	Positive
HbsAb	Negative	Negative	Positive	Negative
HBcAb	Positive[1]	Positive	Positive	Positive

[1] IgM is found in the acute stage; IgG is found in subsequent stages.
Note: People immunized with HBV vaccine have HBsAb but not HBcAb because the immunogen in the vaccine is purified HbsAg.

(2) Hepatitis B immune globulin (HBIG) contains a high titer of HBsAb, because it is prepared from sera of patients who have recovered from hepatitis B. It is used to provide immediate, passive protection to individuals known to be exposed to HBsAg-positive blood, eg, after an accidental needle stick.

Precise recommendations for use of the vaccine and HBIG are beyond the scope of this book. However, the recommendation regarding one common concern of medical students, the needle-stick injury from a patient with HBsAg-positive blood, is that both the vaccine and HBIG be given (at separate sites). Both the vaccine and HBIG should also be given to a newborn whose mother is infected with HBV. These are good examples of **"passive-active"** immunization, in which both immediate and long-term protection are provided.

All blood for transfusion should be screened for HBsAg. No one with a history of hepatitis (of any type) should donate blood, because non-A, non-B viruses may be present.

NON-A, NON-B HEPATITIS VIRUSES

The term "non-A, non-B hepatitis" was coined to describe the cases of hepatitis for which existing serologic tests had ruled out all known viral causes. The term is not often used because the main cause of non-A, non-B hepatitis, namely hepatitis C virus, has been identified. In addition, hepatitis D virus and hepatitis E virus have been described. Cross-protection experiments indicate additional hepatitis viruses exist.

HEPATITIS C VIRUS

Disease   HCV causes hepatitis C.

Important Properties   HCV is a member of the flavivirus family. It is an enveloped virion containing a genome of single-stranded, positive-polarity RNA. It has no virion polymerase. Multiple serotypes exist; the gene encoding the envelope glycoprotein has hypervariable regions similar to those of HIV.

Summary of Replicative Cycle   The replication of HCV is uncertain, because it has not been grown in cell culture. Other flaviviruses replicate in the cytoplasm and translate their genome RNA into large polyproteins, from which functional viral proteins are cleaved. It is likely that HCV replication follows this model.

Transmission & Epidemiology   Humans are the reservoir for HCV. It is transmitted via blood, sexually, and from mother to child. It is uncertain whether maternal transmission is across the placenta or during birth. Unlike yellow fever virus, another flavivirus that infects the liver and is transmitted by mosquitoes, there is no evidence for an insect vector for HCV.

In the United States, about 1% of blood donors have antibody to HCV. People who abuse intravenous drugs are very commonly infected. Commercially prepared immune globulin preparations are generally very safe, but several instances of the transmission of HCV have occurred. This is the only example of an infectious disease transmitted by immune globulins.

Pathogenesis & Immunity   HCV infects hepatocytes primarily, but there is no evidence for a virus-induced cytopathic effect on the liver cells. Rather, death of the hepatocytes is probably caused by immune attack by cytotoxic T cells. HCV infection strongly predisposes to hepatocellular carcinoma, but there is no evidence for an oncogene in the viral genome or for insertion of a copy of the viral genome into the DNA of the cancer cells.

Antibodies against HCV are made, but approximately 75% of patients are chronically infected and continue to produce virus for at least a year. (Note that the rate of **chronic carriage of HCV is much higher** than the rate of chronic carriage of HBV.) Chronic active hepatitis and cirrhosis occur in approximately 10% of these patients. For patients who clear the infection, it is not known whether reinfection can occur or whether there is lifelong immunity.

Clinical Findings   Clinically, the acute infection with HCV is milder than infection with HBV. Fever, anorexia, nausea, vomiting, and jaundice are common. Dark urine, pale feces, and elevated transaminase levels are seen. Hepatitis C resembles hepatitis B as far as the ensuing chronic liver disease and the predisposition to hepatocellular carcinoma are concerned. Similar to HBV, a chronic carrier state occurs with HCV. Many infections with HCV are asymptomatic and are detected only by the presence of antibody. The mean incubation period is 8 weeks.

Laboratory Diagnosis   HCV infection is diagnosed by detecting antibodies to HCV in an ELISA. The antigen in the assay is a recombinant protein formed from three immunologically stable HCV proteins and does not include the highly variable envelope proteins. The test does not distinguish between IgM and IgG. Because false-positive results can occur in the ELISA, a RIBA (recombinant immunoblot assay) should be performed as a confirmatory test. If the RIBA is positive, a PCR-based test that detects the presence of viral RNA in the serum should be used to determine whether active disease exists. Isolation of the virus from patient specimens is not done.

Treatment & Prevention   Alpha interferon is used for the treatment of chronic hepatitis C. It can mitigate the symptoms but does not eliminate the carrier state. Blood for transfusion is screened for the presence of HCV antibody, which has prevented many cases of hepatitis C. There is no vaccine, and hyperimmune globulins are not available.

HEPATITIS D VIRUS (DELTA AGENT)

Disease   Hepatitis D virus (HDV) causes hepatitis D (hepatitis delta).

Important Properties & Replicative Cycle   HDV is unusual in that it is a **defective** virus; ie, it cannot replicate by itself, because it does not have the genes for its envelope protein. HDV can replicate only in cells also infected with HBV, because HDV uses the surface antigen of HBV (HBsAg) as its envelope protein. HBV is therefore the helper virus for HDV (Fig 41–3).

HDV is an enveloped virus with an RNA genome that is a single-stranded, negative polarity, covalently closed circle. The RNA genome of HDV is very small and encodes only one protein, the internal core protein called **delta antigen.** HDV genome RNA has no sequence homology to HBV genome DNA. HDV has no virion polymerase; the genome RNA is replicated and transcribed by the host cell RNA polymerase. HDV genome RNA is a "ribozyme"; ie, it has the ability to self-cleave and self-ligate, properties that are employed during replication of the genome. HDV replicates in the nucleus, but the specifics of the replicative cycle are complex and beyond the scope of this book.

HDV has one serotype because HBsAg has only one serotype. There is no evidence for the existence of an animal reservoir for HDV.

Transmission & Epidemiology   HDV is transmitted by the same means as is HBV, ie, sexually, by blood, and perinatally. In the United States, most HDV infections occur in intravenous drug abusers who share needles. HDV infections occur worldwide with a similar distribution to that of HBV infections.

Pathogenesis & Immunity   It seems likely that the pathogenesis of hepatitis caused by HDV and HBV is the same; ie, the virus-infected hepatocytes are damaged by cytotoxic T cells. There is some evidence that delta antigen is cytopathic for hepatocytes.

IgG antibody against delta antigen is not detected for long periods after infection, so it is uncertain whether long-term immunity to HDV exists.

Clinical Findings   Because HDV can replicate only in cells also infected with HBV, hepatitis delta can occur only in a person infected with HBV. A person can either be infected with both HDV and HBV at the same time, ie, be "coinfected," or be previously infected with HBV and then "superinfected" with HDV.

Hepatitis in patients coinfected with HDV and HBV is more severe than in those infected with HBV alone, but the incidence of chronic hepatitis is about the same in patients infected with HBV alone. However, hepatitis in chronic carriers of HBV who become superinfected with HDV is much more severe, and the incidence of fulminant, life-threatening hepatitis, chronic hepatitis, and liver failure is significantly higher.

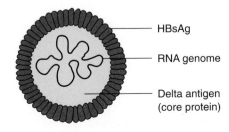

HBsAg

RNA genome

Delta antigen
(core protein)

Figure 41–3. Hepatitis D virus. Note that hepatitis B surface antigen forms the outer envelope and the genome consists of circular RNA. (Modified and reproduced, with permission, from Ryan K et al: *Sherris Medical Microbiology,* 3rd ed. Appleton & Lange, 1994.)

Laboratory Diagnosis   The diagnosis of HDV infection in the laboratory is made by detecting either delta antigen or IgM antibody to delta antigen in the patient's serum.

Treatment & Prevention   Alpha interferon can mitigate some of the effects of the chronic hepatitis caused by HDV but does not eradicate the chronic carrier state. There is no specific antiviral therapy against HDV. There is no vaccine against HDV, but a person immunized against HBV will not be infected by HDV.

HEPATITIS E VIRUS

Hepatitis E virus (HEV) is a major cause of enterically transmitted hepatitis. It is a common cause of water-borne epidemics of hepatitis in Asia, Africa, India, and Mexico but is uncommon in the United States. HEV is a nonenveloped, single-stranded RNA virus tentatively classified as a member of the calicivirus family. Clinically the disease resembles hepatitis A, with the exception of a high mortality rate in pregnant women. Chronic liver disease does not occur, and there is no prolonged carrier state.

   The test for HEV antibody is not readily available, so the diagnosis is typically made by excluding HAV and other causes. There is no antiviral treatment and no vaccine.

HEPATITIS G VIRUS

In 1996, hepatitis G virus (HGV) was isolated from patients with posttransfusion hepatitis. HGV is a member of the flavivirus family, as is HCV. However, unlike HCV, which is clearly the cause of both acute hepatitis and chronic active hepatitis and predisposes to hepatocellular carcinoma, HGV has not been documented to cause any of these clinical findings. The role of HGV in the causation of liver disease has yet to be established.

Review Questions

1. Compare HAV and HBV according to the following criteria: classification, genome, presence of envelope, number of serotypes, and existence of animal reservoir.
2. How is HAV transmitted?
3. How is the diagnosis of acute hepatitis A made in the laboratory?
4. How can hepatitis A be prevented?
5. What are the three important antigens in the HBV particle?
6. What is the function of the DNA polymerase in the virion?
7. In the replication of HBV, there is a step in which RNA is transcribed into DNA, analogous to reverse transcription in retroviruses. When does this step occur in HBV replication?
8. HBV is transmitted by blood transfusion. What are thought to be the natural modes of transmission?
9. What is the role of the immune response in the pathogenesis of hepatitis B?
10. HBV infection is associated with hepatoma. What step in HBV replication might explain this relationship?
11. HBV can cause a chronic carrier state. What step in HBV replication might explain the persistence of the virus?
12. Is there lifelong immunity against (a) HAV? (b) HBV?
13. What laboratory test is used (a) to detect acute infection with HBV? (b) as the best indicator of transmissibility? (c) to indicate immunity? (d) to indicate the chronic carrier state?
14. What are the two modes of prevention of hepatitis B?
15. What is the antigen in the HBV vaccine?
16. Why do we think there are non-A, non-B hepatitis viruses?
17. Which virus is the most common cause of non-A, non-B hepatitis?
18. How is HCV transmitted?
19. Which features of the clinical picture of hepatitis C resemble hepatitis B more than hepatitis A?
20. How is the diagnosis of hepatitis C made in the clinical laboratory?
21. What is the nature of the agent of delta hepatitis?
22. Why is the delta agent found only in persons infected with HBV?
23. How is delta agent transmitted?
24. Clinically, does delta hepatitis resemble hepatitis A or hepatitis B more closely?
25. What is the mode of transmission of HEV?
26. Does the clinical picture of hepatitis E resemble hepatitis A or hepatitis B?
27. How is the diagnosis of hepatitis E made?

Arboviruses

42

The term "arbovirus" is an acronym for *ar*thropod-*bo*rne virus and highlights the fact that these viruses are transmitted by **arthropods,** primarily mosquitoes and ticks. It is a collective name for a large group of diverse viruses, more than 400 at last count. In general, they are named either for the diseases they cause, eg, yellow fever virus, or for the place where they were first isolated, eg, St. Louis encephalitis virus.

IMPORTANT PROPERTIES

Most arboviruses are classified in three families,* namely, togaviruses, flaviviruses, and bunyaviruses (Table 42–1).

(1) Togaviruses† are characterized by an icosahedral nucleocapsid surrounded by an envelope and a single-stranded, positive-polarity RNA genome. They are 70 nm in diameter, in contrast to the flaviviruses, which are 40–50 nm in diameter (see below). Togaviruses are divided into two families, alphaviruses and rubiviruses. Only alphaviruses are considered here. The only rubivirus is rubella virus, which is discussed in Chapter 39.

(2) Flaviviruses‡ are similar to togaviruses in that they also have an icosahedral nucleocapsid surrounded by an envelope and a single-stranded, positive-polarity RNA genome but the flaviviruses are only 40–50 nm in diameter whereas the togaviruses have a diameter of 70 nm.

(3) Bunyaviruses§ have a helical nucleocapsid surrounded by an envelope and a genome consisting of three segments of negative-polarity RNA that are hydrogen-bonded together.

TRANSMISSION

The life cycle of the arboviruses is based on the ability of these viruses to multiply in **both** the vertebrate host and the bloodsucking vector. For effective transmission to occur, the virus must be present in the bloodstream of the vertebrate host (viremia) in sufficiently high titer to be taken up in the small volume of blood ingested during an insect bite. After ingestion, the virus replicates in the gut of the arthropod and then spreads to other organs, including the salivary glands. Only the female of the species serves as the vector of the virus, because only she requires a blood meal in order for progeny to be produced. An obligatory length of time, called the **extrinsic incubation period,#** must pass before the virus has replicated sufficiently for the saliva of the vector to contain enough virus to transmit an infectious dose. For most viruses, the extrinsic incubation period ranges from 7 to 14 days.

In addition to transmission through vertebrates, some arboviruses are transmitted by vertical "transovarian" passage from the mother tick to her offspring. Vertical transmission has important survival value for the virus if a vertebrate host is unavailable.

Humans are involved in the transmission cycle of arboviruses in two different ways. Usually, humans are **"dead-end" hosts,** because the concentration of virus in human blood is too low and the duration of viremia too brief for the next bite to transmit the virus. However, in some diseases, eg, yellow fever and dengue, humans have a high-level viremia and act as reservoirs of the virus.

---

*A few arboviruses belong to two other families. For example, Colorado tick virus is a reovirus; Kern Canyon virus and vesicular stomatitis virus are rhabdoviruses.

†Toga means cloak.

‡Flavi means yellow, as in yellow fever.

§"Bunya" is short for Bunyamwera, the town in Africa where the prototype virus was isolated.

#The intrinsic incubation period is the interval between the time of the bite and the appearance of symptoms in the human host.

Table 42–1. Classification of the major arboviruses.

Family	Genus	Viruses of Medical Interest in the Americas
Togavirus	Alphavirus[1]	Eastern equine encephalitis virus, western equine encephalitis virus
Flavivirus	Flavivirus[2]	St. Louis encephalitis virus, yellow fever virus, dengue virus
Bunyavirus	Bunyavirus[3]	California encephalitis virus
Reovirus	Orbivirus	Colorado tick fever virus

[1] Alphaviruses of other regions include Chikungunya, Mayaro, O'Nyong-Nyong, Ross River, and Semliki Forest viruses.
[2] Flaviviruses of other regions include Japanese encephalitis, Kyasanur Forest, Murray Valley encephalitis, Omsk hemorrhagic fever, Powassan encephalitis, and West Nile fever viruses.
[3] Bunyaviruses of other regions include the Bunyamwera complex of viruses and Oropouche virus.

Infection by arboviruses usually does not result in disease either in the arthropod vector or in the vertebrate animal that serves as the natural host. Disease occurs primarily when the virus infects dead-end hosts. For example, yellow fever virus cycles harmlessly among the jungle monkeys in South America, but when the virus infects a human, yellow fever can occur.

CLINICAL FINDINGS & EPIDEMIOLOGY

The diseases caused by arboviruses range in severity from mild to rapidly fatal. The clinical picture usually fits one of three categories: (1) **encephalitis;** (2) **hemorrhagic fever;** or (3) fever with myalgias, arthralgias, and nonhemorrhagic rash. The pathogenesis of these diseases involves not only the cytocidal effect of the virus but also, in some, a prominent immunopathologic component. Following recovery from the disease, immunity is usually lifelong.

The arboviral diseases occur primarily in the **tropics** but are also found in temperate zones such as the United States and as far north as Alaska and Siberia. They have a tendency to cause sudden outbreaks of disease, generally at the interface between human communities and jungle or forest areas.

Arboviruses That Cause Disease in the United States

EASTERN EQUINE ENCEPHALITIS VIRUS

Of the four encephalitis viruses listed in Table 42–2, eastern equine encephalitis (EEE) virus causes the **most severe** disease and is associated with the highest fatality rate (approximately 50%). In its natural habitat, the virus is transmitted primarily by the swamp **mosquito,** *Culiseta,* among the small wild birds of the Atlantic and Gulf Coast states. Species of *Aedes* mosquitoes are suspected of carrying the virus from its **wild-bird reservoir** to the principal **dead-end hosts, horses and humans.** The number of cases of human encephalitis caused by EEE virus in the United States usually ranges from zero to four per year, but outbreaks involving hundreds of cases also occur. Subclinical infections greatly exceed the number of overt cases.

The encephalitis is characterized by the sudden onset of severe headache, nausea, vomiting, and fever. Changes in mental status, such as confusion and stupor, ensue. A rapidly progressive downhill course with nuchal rigidity, seizures, and coma occurs. If the patient survives, the central nervous system sequelae are usually severe. Immunity following the infection is lifelong.

The diagnosis is made by either isolating the virus or demonstrating a rise in antibody titer. Clinicians should have a high index of suspicion in the summer months in the appropriate geographic areas. The disease does not occur in the winter, because mosquitoes are not active. It is not known how the virus survives the winter—in birds, mosquitoes, or perhaps some other animal.

No antiviral therapy is available. A killed vaccine is available to protect horses but not humans. The disease is too rare for production of a human vaccine to be economically feasible.

Table 42–2. Epidemiology of important arbovirus diseases in the United States.

Disease[1]	Vector	Animal Reservoir	Geographic Distribution	Approximate Incidence per Year[2]
EEE	Mosquito	Wild birds[3]	Atlantic and Gulf states	0–4
WEE	Mosquito	Wild birds[3]	West of Mississippi	5–20[4]
SLE	Mosquito	Wild birds	Widespread in southern, central, and western states	10–30[4]
CE	Mosquito	Small mammals	North-central states	40–80
CTF	Tick	Small mammals	Rocky Mountains	100–300

[1] Venezuelan equine encephalitis virus causes disease in the United States too rarely to be included.
[2] Human cases.
[3] Horses are dead-end hosts, not reservoirs.
[4] Hundreds of cases during an outbreak.

WESTERN EQUINE ENCEPHALITIS VIRUS

Western equine encephalitis (WEE) virus causes disease more frequently than does EEE virus, but the illness is less severe. Inapparent infections outnumber the apparent by at least 100:1. The number of cases in the United States usually ranges between 5 and 20 per year, and the fatality rate is roughly 2%.

The virus is transmitted primarily by *Culex* **mosquitoes** among the **wild-bird** population of the western states, especially in areas with irrigated farmland.

The clinical picture of WEE virus infection is similar to but less severe than that caused by EEE virus. Sequelae are less common. The diagnosis is made by isolating the virus or observing a rise in antibody titer. There is no antiviral therapy. There is a killed vaccine for horses but not for humans.

ST. LOUIS ENCEPHALITIS VIRUS

St. Louis encephalitis (SLE) virus causes disease over a wider geographic area than do EEE and WEE virus. It is found in the southern, central, and western states and causes 10–30 cases of encephalitis per year in the United States.

The virus is transmitted by several species of *Culex* **mosquitoes** that vary depending upon location. Again, small **wild birds,** especially English sparrows, are the reservoir and humans are dead-end hosts. Although EEE and WEE viruses are predominantly rural, SLE virus occurs in **urban areas** because these mosquitoes prefer to breed in stagnant wastewater.

SLE virus causes a moderately severe encephalitis with a fatality rate that approaches 10%. Most infections are inapparent. Sequelae are uncommon.

The diagnosis is usually made serologically, because the virus is difficult to isolate. No antiviral therapy or vaccine is available.

CALIFORNIA ENCEPHALITIS VIRUS

California encephalitis (CE) virus was first isolated from mosquitoes in California in 1952, but its name is something of a misnomer because most human disease occurs in the north-central states. The strain of the 11 CE viruses that causes encephalitis most frequently is called La Crosse for the city in Wisconsin where it was isolated. CE virus is the only one of the four major encephalitis viruses in the United States that is a member of the **bunyavirus** family.

The La Crosse strain of CE virus is transmitted by the **mosquito** *Aedes triseriatus* among forest **rodents.** The virus is passed transovarially in mosquitoes and thus survives the winter when mosquitoes are not active.

The clinical picture varies from mild to severe, but death is rare. Diagnosis is usually made serologically rather than by isolation of the virus. No antiviral therapy or vaccine is available.

COLORADO TICK FEVER VIRUS

Of the five diseases described in Table 42–2, Colorado tick fever (CTF) is the most easily distinguished from the others, both biologically and clinically. CTF virus is a **reovirus** transmitted by the wood **tick** *Dermacentor andersoni* among the small **rodents,** eg, chipmunks and squirrels, of the Rocky Mountains. There are approximately 100–300 cases per year in the United States.

The disease occurs primarily in people hiking or camping in the Rocky Mountains and is characterized by fever, headache, retro-orbital pain, and severe myalgia. The diagnosis is made either by isolating the virus from the blood or by detecting a rise in antibody titer. No antiviral therapy or vaccine is available. Prevention involves wearing protective clothing and inspecting the skin for ticks.

Important Arboviruses That Cause Disease Outside the United States

Although yellow fever and dengue are not endemic in the United States, extensive travel by Americans to tropical areas means that imported cases occur. It is reasonable, therefore, that physicians in the United States be acquainted with these two diseases. Both yellow fever virus and dengue virus are classified as flaviviruses. Japanese encephalitis virus, also a flavivirus and an important cause of epidemic encephalitis in Asia, is described in Chapter 46.

YELLOW FEVER VIRUS

As the name implies, yellow fever is characterized by jaundice and fever. It is a severe, life-threatening disease that begins with the sudden onset of fever, headache, myalgias, and photophobia. After this prodrome, the symptoms progress to involve the liver, kidneys, and heart. Prostration and shock, accompanied by upper gastrointestinal tract hemorrhage with hematemesis, follow. Diagnosis in the laboratory can be made either by isolating the virus or by detecting a rise in antibody titer. No antiviral therapy is available, and the mortality rate is high. If the patient recovers, no chronic infection ensues and lifelong immunity is conferred.

In the epidemiology of yellow fever, **two distinct cycles** exist in nature, with different reservoirs and vectors.

(1) Jungle yellow fever is a disease of **monkeys** in tropical Africa and South America; it is transmitted primarily by the treetop **mosquitoes** of the *Haemagogus* species. Monkeys are the permanent reservoir, whereas humans are accidental hosts. Humans (eg, tree cutters) are infected when they enter the jungle occupationally.

(2) In contrast, urban yellow fever is a disease of **humans** that is transmitted by the **mosquito** *Aedes aegypti,* which breeds in stagnant water. In the urban form of the disease, humans are the reservoir. For effective transmission to occur, the virus must replicate in the mosquito during the 12–14-day extrinsic incubation period. After the infected mosquito bites the person, the intrinsic incubation period is 3–6 days.

Prevention of yellow fever involves mosquito control and immunization with the **vaccine** containing live, attenuated yellow fever virus. Travelers to and residents of endemic areas should be immunized. Protection lasts up to 10 years, and boosters are required every 10 years for travelers entering certain countries. Epidemics still occur in parts of tropical Africa and South America.

DENGUE VIRUS

Although dengue is **not endemic** in the United States, some tourists to the Caribbean and other tropical areas return with this disease. In recent years, there were 100–200 cases per year in the United States, mostly in the southern and eastern states. No indigenous transmission occurred within the United States.

Classic dengue (**"breakbone fever"**) begins suddenly with an influenzalike syndrome consisting of fever, malaise, cough, and headache. Severe pains in muscles and joints (breakbone) occur. Enlarged lymph nodes, a maculopapular rash, and leukopenia are common. After a week or so, the symptoms regress but weakness may persist. Although unpleasant, this typical form of dengue is rarely fatal and has few sequelae.

In contrast, **dengue hemorrhagic fever** is a much more severe disease, with a fatality rate that approaches 10%. The initial picture is the same as classic dengue, but then shock and hemorrhage, especially into the gastrointestinal tract and skin, develop. Dengue hemorrhagic fever occurs particularly in southern Asia, whereas the classic form is found in tropical areas worldwide.

Hemorrhagic shock syndrome is due to the production of large amounts of **cross-reacting antibody** at the time of a second dengue infection. The pathogenesis is as follows: The patient recovers from classic dengue caused by one of the four serotypes, and antibody against that serotype is produced. When the patient is infected with another serotype of dengue virus, an anamnestic, heterotypic response occurs and large amounts of cross-reacting antibody to the first serotype are produced. Immune complexes composed of virus and antibody are formed that activate complement, causing increased vascular permeability and thrombocytopenia. Shock and hemorrhage result.

Dengue virus is transmitted by the *A aegypti* **mosquito,** which is also the vector of yellow fever virus. Humans are the reservoir for dengue virus, but a jungle cycle involving monkeys as the reservoir and other *Aedes* species as vectors is suspected.

No antiviral therapy or vaccine for dengue is available. Outbreaks are controlled by using insecticides and draining stagnant water that serves as the breeding place for the mosquitoes. Personal protection includes using mosquito repellent and wearing clothing that covers the entire body.

Review Questions

1. What does the term "arbovirus" mean?
2. Contrast the structure and genomes of togaviruses and bunyaviruses.
3. Distinguish between extrinsic and intrinsic incubation periods.
4. Humans are frequently dead-end hosts for arboviruses. What does this mean, and why does it occur?
5. Regarding EEE, WEE, and SLE, (a) what is the vector? (b) what is the reservoir? (c) which one is the most severe? (d) which one is most likely to occur in an urban setting?
6. Describe the two epidemiologic cycles of yellow fever.
7. How can yellow fever be prevented?
8. Cases of dengue seen in the United States occur primarily in travelers returning from which geographic region? How is the disease transmitted?
9. What is the pathogenesis of dengue hemorrhagic shock?

Tumor Viruses

43

OVERVIEW

Viruses can cause benign or malignant tumors in many species of animals, eg, frogs, fishes, birds, and mammals. Despite the common occurrence of tumor viruses in animals, only a few viruses are associated with **human** tumors and evidence that they are truly the causative agents exists for very few.

Tumor viruses have no characteristic size, shape, or chemical composition. Some are large, and some are small; some are enveloped, and others are naked (ie, nonenveloped); some have DNA as their genetic material, and others have RNA. The factor that unites all of them is their common ability to cause tumors.

Tumor viruses are at the forefront of cancer research for two main reasons:

(1) They are more rapid, reliable, and efficient tumor producers than either chemicals or radiation. For example, many of these viruses can cause tumors in all susceptible animals in 1 or 2 weeks and can produce malignant transformation in cultured cells in just a few days.

(2) They have a small number of genes compared with a human cell (only three, four, or five for many retroviruses), and hence their role in the production of cancer can be readily analyzed and understood. To date, the genomes of many tumor viruses have been cloned and sequenced and the number of genes and their functions have been determined; all of this has provided important information.

MALIGNANT TRANSFORMATION OF CELLS

The term "malignant transformation" refers to changes in the growth properties, shape, and other features of the tumor cell (Table 43–1). Malignant transformation can be induced by tumor viruses not only in animals but also in cultured cells. In culture, the following changes occur when cells become malignantly transformed.

Altered Morphology   Malignant cells lose their characteristic differentiated shape and appear rounded and more refractile when visualized under a microscope. The rounding may be due to the disaggregation of actin filaments, and the reduced adherence of the cell to the surface of the culture dish may be due to changes in the surface charge of the cell.

Altered Growth Control

(1) Malignant cells grow in a disorganized, piled-up pattern in contrast to normal cells, which have an organized, flat appearance. The term applied to this change in growth pattern in malignant cells is **loss of contact inhibition.** Contact inhibition is a property of normal cells that refers to their ability to stop their growth and movement upon contact with another cell. Malignant cells have lost this ability and consequently move on top of one another, continue to grow to large numbers, and form a random array of cells.

Table 43–1. Features of malignant transformation.

Feature	Description
Altered morphology	Loss of differentiated shape Rounded as a result of disaggregation of actin filaments and decreased adhesion to surface More refractile
Altered growth control	Loss of contact inhibition of growth Loss of contact inhibition of movement Reduced requirement for serum growth factors Increased ability to be cloned from a single cell Increased ability to grow in suspension Increased ability to continue growing ("immortalization")
Altered cellular properties	Induction of DNA synthesis Chromosomal changes Appearance of new antigens Increased agglutination by lectins
Altered biochemical properties	Reduced level of cyclic AMP Enhanced secretion of plasminogen activator Increased anaerobic glycolysis Loss of fibronectin Changes in glycoproteins and glycolipids

(2) Malignant cells are able to grow in vitro at a much lower concentration of serum than are normal cells.

(3) Malignant cells grow well in suspension, whereas normal cells grow well only when they are attached to a surface, eg, a culture dish.

(4) Malignant cells are easily cloned; ie, they can grow into a colony of cells starting with a single cell, whereas normal cells cannot do this effectively.

(5) Infection of a cell by a tumor virus "immortalizes" that cell by enabling it to continue growing long past the time when its normal counterpart would have died. Normal cells in culture have a lifetime of about 50 generations, but malignantly transformed cells grow indefinitely.

Altered Cellular Properties

(1) DNA synthesis is induced. If cells resting in the G1 phase are infected with a tumor virus, they will promptly enter the S phase, ie, synthesize DNA and go on to divide.

(2) The karyotype becomes altered; ie, there are changes in the number and shape of the chromosomes as a result of deletions, duplications, and translocations.

(3) Antigens different from those in normal cells appear. These new antigens can be either virus-encoded proteins, preexisting cellular proteins that have been modified, or previously repressed cellular proteins that are now being synthesized. Some new antigens are on the cell surface and elicit either circulating antibodies or a cell-mediated response that can kill the tumor cell. These new antigens are the recognition sites for immune surveillance against tumor cells.

(4) Agglutination by lectins is enhanced. Lectins are plant glycoproteins that bind specifically to certain sugars on the cell membrane surface, eg, wheat germ agglutinin. The increased agglutination of malignant cells may be due to the clustering of existing receptor sites rather than to the synthesis of new ones.

Altered Biochemical Properties

(1) Reduced levels of cyclic AMP (cAMP) occur in malignant cells. Addition of cAMP will cause the malignant cells to revert to the appearance and growth properties of normal cells.

(2) Malignant cells secrete more plasminogen activator than do normal cells. This activator is a protease that converts plasminogen to plasmin, the enzyme that dissolves the fibrin clot.

(3) Increased anaerobic glycolysis leads to increased lactic acid production (Warburg effect). The mechanism for this change is unknown.

(4) There is a loss of high-molecular-weight glycoprotein called fibronectin. The effect of this loss is unknown.

(5) There are changes in the sugar components of glycoproteins and glycolipids in the membranes of malignant cells.

ROLE OF TUMOR VIRUSES IN MALIGNANT TRANSFORMATION

Malignant transformation is a permanent change in the behavior of the cell. Must the viral genetic material be present and functioning at all times, or can it alter some cell component and not be required subsequently? The answer to this question was obtained by using a temperature-sensitive mutant of Rous sarcoma virus. This mutant has an altered transforming gene that is functional at the low, permissive temperature (35 °C) but not at the high, restrictive temperature (39 °C). When chicken cells were infected at 35 °C they transformed as expected, but when incubated at 39 °C they regained their normal morphology and behavior within a few hours. Days or weeks later, when these cells were returned to 35 °C, they recovered their transformed phenotype. Thus, continued production of some functional virus-encoded protein is required for the maintenance of the transformed state.

Although malignant transformation is a permanent change, revertants to normality do appear, albeit rarely. In the revertants studied, the viral genetic material remains integrated in cellular DNA but changes in the quality and quantity of the virus-specific RNA occur.

PROVIRUSES & ONCOGENES

The two major concepts of the way viral tumorigenesis occurs are expressed in the terms **"provirus"** and **"oncogene."** These contrasting ideas address the fundamental question of the source of the genes for malignancy.

(1) In the provirus model, the genes enter the cell at the time of infection by the tumor virus.

(2) In the oncogene model, the genes for malignancy are already present in all cells of the body by virtue of being present in the initial sperm and egg. These oncogenes encode proteins that encourage cell growth, eg, fibroblast growth factor. In the oncogene model, carcinogens such as chemicals, radiation, and tumor viruses activate cellular oncogenes to overproduce these growth factors. This initiates inappropriate cell growth and malignant transformation.

Both proviruses and oncogenes may play a role in malignant transformation. Evidence for the provirus mode consists of finding copies of viral DNA integrated into cell DNA only in cells that have been infected with the tumor virus. The corresponding uninfected cells have no copies of the viral DNA.

The first direct evidence that oncogenes exist in normal cells was based on results of experiments in which a DNA copy of the *onc* gene of the chicken retrovirus Rous sarcoma virus was used as a probe. DNA in normal embryonic cells hybridized to the probe, indicating that the cells contain a gene homologous to the viral gene. It is hypothesized that the **cellular oncogenes** (proto-oncogenes) may be the precursors of viral oncogenes. Although cellular oncogenes and viral oncogenes are similar, they are not identical. They differ in base sequence at various points; and cellular oncogenes have exons and introns, whereas viral oncogenes do not. It seems likely that viral oncogenes were acquired by incorporation of cellular oncogenes into retroviruses lacking these genes. Retroviruses can be thought of as **transducing agents,** carrying oncogenes from one cell to another.

Since this initial observation, **more than 20 cellular oncogenes** have been identified by using either the Rous sarcoma virus DNA probe or probes made from other viral oncogenes. Many cells contain several different cellular oncogenes. In addition, the same cellular oncogenes have been found in species as diverse as fruit flies, rodents, and humans. Such conservation through evolution suggests a normal physiologic function for these genes. Some are known to be expressed during normal embryonic development.

A marked **diversity** of viral oncogene function has been found. Some encode a **protein kinase** that specifically phosphorylates the amino acid tyrosine,* in contrast to the commonly found protein kinase of cells, which preferentially phosphorylates serine. Other oncogenes have a base sequence almost identical to that of the gene for certain cellular **growth factors,** eg, epidermal growth factor. Several proteins encoded by oncogenes have their effect at the cell membrane (eg, the *ras* oncogene encodes a G protein), whereas some act in the nucleus by binding to DNA (eg, the *myc* oncogene). These observations suggest that growth control is a multistep process and that carcinogenesis can be induced by affecting one or more of several steps.

Based on the known categories of oncogenes, the following model of growth control can be constructed. After a **growth factor** binds to its **receptor** on the cell membrane, membrane-associated **G proteins** and **tyrosine kinases** are activated. These, in turn, interact with **cytoplasmic proteins** or produce **second messengers,** which are transported to the nucleus and interact with **nuclear factors.** DNA synthesis is activated, and cell division occurs. Overproduction or inappropriate expression of any of the above factors **in boldface type** can result in malignant transformation. Not all tumor viruses of the retrovirus family contain *onc* genes. How do these viruses cause malignant transfor-

---

*The cellular protein(s) phosphorylated by this kinase are unknown.

mation? It appears that the DNA copy of the viral RNA integrates near a cellular oncogene, causing a marked increase in its expression. **Overexpression** of the cellular oncogene may play a key role in malignant transformation by these viruses.

Although it has been demonstrated that viral oncogenes can cause malignant transformation, it has not been directly shown that cellular oncogenes can do so. However, as described in Table 43–2, the following evidence suggests that they do:

(1) DNA containing cellular oncogenes isolated from certain tumor cells can transform normal cells in culture. When the base sequence of these "transforming" cellular oncogenes was analyzed, it was found to have a **single base change** from the normal cellular oncogene; ie, it had **mutated.** In several tumor cell isolates, the altered sites in the gene are the same.

(2) In certain tumors, characteristic **translocations** of chromosomal segments can be seen. In Burkitt's lymphoma cells, a translocation occurs that moves a cellular oncogene (c-*myc*) from its normal site on chromosome 8 to a new site adjacent to an immunoglobulin heavy-chain gene on chromosome 14. This shift enhances expression of the c-*myc* gene.

(3) Some tumors have multiple copies of the cellular oncogenes, either on the same chromosome or on multiple tiny chromosomes. The **amplification** of these genes results in overexpression of their mRNA and proteins.

(4) Insertion of the DNA copy of the retroviral RNA (proviral DNA) near a cellular oncogene stimulates expression of the c-*onc* gene.

(5) Certain cellular oncogenes isolated from normal cells can cause malignant transformation if they have been modified to be **overexpressed** within the recipient cell.

In summary, two different mechanisms—**mutation** and **increased expression**—appear to be able to activate the quiescent "proto-oncogene" into a functioning oncogene capable of transforming a cell. Cellular oncogenes provide a rationale for carcinogenesis by chemicals and radiation; eg, a chemical carcinogen might act by enhancing the expression of a cellular oncogene. Furthermore, DNA isolated from cells treated with a chemical carcinogen can malignantly transform other normal cells. The resulting tumor cells contain cellular oncogenes from the chemically treated cells, and these genes are expressed with high efficiency.

There is another mechanism of carcinogenesis involving cellular genes, namely, mutation of a **tumor suppressor** gene. A well-documented example is the retinoblastoma susceptibility gene, which normally acts as a suppressor of retinoblastoma formation. When both alleles of this **"antioncogene"** are mutated (made nonfunctional), retinoblastoma occurs. Human papillomavirus and SV40 virus produce a protein that binds to and inactivates the protein encoded by the retinoblastoma gene. Human papillomavirus also produces a protein that inactivates the protein encoded by the p53 gene, another tumor suppressor gene in human cells. The p53 gene encodes a transcription factor that activates the synthesis of a second protein, which blocks the cyclin-dependent kinases required for cell division to occur.

Inactivation of tumor suppressor genes appears likely to be an important general mechanism of viral oncogenesis. Tumor suppressor genes are involved in the formation of other cancers as well, eg,

Table 43–2. Evidence that cellular oncogenes (c-*onc*) can cause tumors.

Evidence	Description
Mutation of c-*onc* gene	DNA isolated from tumor cells can transform normal cells. This DNA has a c-*onc* gene with a mutation consisting of a single base change.
Translocation of c-*onc* gene	Movement of c-*onc* gene to a new site on a different chromosome results in malignancy accompanied by increased expression of the gene.
Amplification of c-*onc* gene	The number of copies of c-*onc* genes is increased, resulting in enhanced expression of their mRNA and proteins.
Insertion of retrovirus near c-*onc* gene	Proviral DNA inserts near c-*onc* gene, which alters its expression and causes tumors.
Overexpression of c-*onc* gene by modification in the laboratory	Addition of an active promoter site enhances expression of the c-*onc* gene, and malignant transformation occurs.

breast and colon carcinomas and various sarcomas. For example, in many colon carcinomas, two genes are inactivated, the p53 gene and the DCC (*d*eleted in *c*olon *c*arcinoma) gene. **Over half of human cancers have a mutated p53 gene** within the malignant cells.

OUTCOME OF TUMOR VIRUS INFECTION

The outcome of tumor virus infection is dependent on the virus and the type of cell. Some tumor viruses go through their entire replicative cycle with the production of progeny virus, whereas others undergo an interrupted cycle, analogous to lysogeny, in which the **proviral DNA is integrated** into cellular DNA and limited expression of proviral genes occurs. Therefore, malignant transformation does not require that progeny virus be produced. Rather, all that is required is the expression of one or, at most, a few viral genes. Note, however, that some tumor viruses transform by inserting their proviral DNA in a manner that activates a cellular oncogene.

In most cases, the DNA tumor viruses such as the papovaviruses transform only cells in which they do not replicate. These cells are called "nonpermissive" because they do not permit viral replication. Cells of the species from which the DNA tumor virus was initially isolated are "permissive"; ie, the virus replicates and usually kills the cells, and no tumors are formed. For example, SV40 virus replicates in the cells of the African green monkey (its species of origin) and causes a cytopathic effect but no tumors. However, in rodent cells the virus does not replicate, expresses only its early genes, and causes malignant transformation. In the "nonproductive" transformed cell, the viral DNA is integrated into the host chromosome and remains there through subsequent cell divisions. The underlying concept applicable to both DNA and RNA tumor viruses is that **only viral gene expression,** not replication of the viral genome or production of progeny virus, is required for transformation.

The essential step required for a DNA tumor virus, eg, SV40 virus, to cause malignant transformation is expression of the **"early" genes** of the virus (Table 43–3). (The early genes are those expressed prior to the replication of the viral genetic material.) These required early genes produce a set of proteins called **T antigens.*** The large T antigen, which is both necessary and sufficient to induce transformation, binds to SV40 virus DNA at the site of initiation of viral DNA synthesis. This is compatible with the finding that the large T antigen is required for the initiation of cellular DNA synthesis in the virus-infected cell. Biochemically, large T antigen has protein kinase and adenosine triphosphate (ATPase) activity. Almost all of the large T antigen is located in the cell nucleus, but some of it is in the outer cell membrane. In that location, it can be detected as a transplantation antigen called **tumor-specific transplantation antigen** (TSTA). TSTA is the antigen that induces the immune response against the transplantation of virally transformed cells. Relatively little is known about the SV40 virus small T antigen, except that if it is not synthesized the efficiency of transformation decreases. In polyomavirus-infected cells, the middle T antigen plays the same role as the SV40 virus large T antigen.

Table 43–3. Viral oncogenes.

Characteristic	DNA Virus	RNA Virus
Prototype virus	SV40 virus	Rous sarcoma virus
Name of gene	Early-region A gene	*src* gene
Name of protein	T antigen	*src* protein
Function of protein	Protein kinase, ATPase activity, binding to DNA, and stimulation of DNA synthesis	Protein kinase that phosphorylates tyrosine[1]
Location of protein	Primarily nuclear, but some in plasma membrane	Plasma membrane
Required for viral replication	Yes	No
Required for cell transformation	Yes	Yes
Gene has cellular homolog	No	Yes

[1] Some retroviruses have *onc* genes that code for other proteins such as platelet-derived growth factor and epidermal growth factor.

---

*In SV40 virus-infected cells, two T antigens, large (MW 100,000) and small (MW 17,000), are produced, whereas in polyomavirus-infected cells, three T antigens, large (MW 90,000), middle (MW 60,000), and small (MW 22,000), are made. Other tumor viruses such as adenoviruses also induce T antigens, which are immunologically distinct from those of the two papoviruses.

In RNA tumor virus-infected cells, this required gene has one of several different functions depending on the retrovirus. The oncogene of Rous sarcoma virus and several other viruses codes for a protein kinase that phosphorylates tyrosine. Some viruses have a gene for a factor that regulates cell growth (eg, epidermal growth factor or platelet-derived growth factor), and still others have a gene that codes for a protein that binds to DNA. The conclusion is that normal growth control is a multistep process that can be affected at any one of several levels. The addition of a viral oncogene perturbs the growth control process, and a tumor cell results.

The viral genetic material remains stably integrated in host cell DNA by a process similar to lysogeny. In the lysogenic cycle, bacteriophage DNA becomes stably integrated into the bacterial genome. The linear DNA genome of the temperate phage, lambda, forms a double-stranded circle within the infected cell and then covalently integrates into bacterial DNA (Table 43–4). A repressor is synthesized that prevents transcription of most of the other lambda genes. Similarly, the double-stranded circular DNA of the DNA tumor virus covalently integrates into eukaryotic-cell DNA and only early genes are transcribed. Thus far, no repressor has been identified in any DNA tumor virus-infected cell. With RNA tumor viruses (retroviruses), the single-stranded linear RNA genome is transcribed into a double-stranded linear DNA that integrates into cellular DNA. In summary, despite the differences in their genomes and in the nature of the host cells, these viruses go through the common pathway of a double-stranded DNA intermediate followed by covalent integration into cellular DNA and subsequent expression of certain genes.

Just as a lysogenic bacteriophage can be induced to enter the replicative cycle by ultraviolet radiation and certain chemicals, tumor viruses can be induced by several mechanisms. Induction is one of the approaches used to determine whether tumor viruses are present in human cancer cells; eg, human T cell leukemia virus was discovered by inducing the virus from leukemic cells with iododeoxyuridine.

Three techniques have been used to induce tumor viruses to replicate in the transformed cells.

(1) The most frequently used method is the addition of nucleoside analogues, eg, iododeoxyuridine. The mechanism of induction by these analogues is uncertain.

(2) The second method involves fusion with "helper" cells; ie, the transformed, nonpermissive cell is fused with a permissive cell, in which the virus undergoes a normal replicative cycle. Within the heterokaryon (a cell with two or more nuclei that is formed by the fusion of two different cell types), the tumor virus is induced and infectious virus is produced. The mechanism of induction is unknown.

(3) In the third method, helper viruses provide a missing function to complement the integrated tumor virus. Infection with the helper virus results in the production of both the integrated tumor virus and the helper virus.

The process of rescuing tumor viruses from cells revealed the existence of **"endogenous"** viruses. Treatment of *normal, uninfected* embryonic cells with nucleoside analogues resulted in the production of retroviruses. Retroviral DNA is integrated within the chromosomal DNA of all cells and serves as the template for viral replication. This proviral DNA probably arose by retrovirus infection of the germ cells of some prehistoric ancestor.

Endogenous retroviruses, which have been rescued from the cells of many species (including humans), differ depending upon the species of origin. Endogenous viruses are xenotropic (**xeno** means foreign; **tropism** means to be attracted to); ie, they infect cells of other species more efficiently than

Table 43–4. Lysogeny as a model for the integration of tumor viruses.

Type of Virus	Name	Genome[1]	Integration	Limited Transcription of Viral Genes
Temperate phage	Lambda phage	Linear dsDNA	+	+
DNA tumor virus	SV40 virus	Circular dsDNA	+	+
RNA tumor virus	Rous sarcoma virus	Linear ssRNA	+	+[2]

[1]Abbreviations: ds, double-stranded; ss, single-stranded.
[2]Limited transcription in some cells or under certain conditions but full transcription with viral replication in others.

they infect the cells of the species of origin. Entry of the endogenous virus into the cell of origin is limited as a result of defective viral envelope-cell receptor interaction. Although they are retroviruses, most endogenous viruses are not tumor viruses; ie, only a few cause leukemia.

TRANSMISSION OF TUMOR VIRUSES

Tumor virus transmission in experimental animals can occur by two processes, vertical and horizontal. **Vertical transmission** indicates movement of the virus from mother to newborn offspring, whereas **horizontal transmission** describes the passage of virus between animals that do not have a mother-offspring relationship. Vertical transmission occurs by three methods: (1) the viral genetic material is in the sperm and the egg; (2) the virus is passed across the placenta; and (3) the virus is transmitted in the breast milk.

When vertical transmission occurs, exposure to the virus early in life can result in tolerance to viral antigens and the immune system will not recognize the virus. Large amounts of virus are produced, and a high frequency of cancer occurs. In contrast, when horizontal transmission occurs, the immunocompetent animal produces antibody against the virus and the frequency of cancer is low. If an immunocompetent animal is experimentally made immunodeficient, the frequency of cancer increases markedly.

Horizontal transmission probably does not occur in humans; those in close contact with cancer patients, eg, family members and medical personnel, do not have an increased frequency of cancer. There have been "outbreaks" of leukemia in several children at the same school, but these have been interpreted statistically as random, rare events that happen to coincide.

EVIDENCE FOR HUMAN TUMOR VIRUSES

At present, only two viruses, human T cell leukemia virus and human papillomavirus, are considered to be human tumor viruses. However, several other candidate viruses are implicated by epidemiologic correlation, by serologic relationship, or by recovery of virus from tumor cells.

Human T Cell Leukemia Virus
There are two human T cell leukemia virus (HTLV) isolates so far, HTLV-I and HTLV-II, both of which are associated with leukemias and lymphomas. HTLV-I was isolated in 1980 from the cells of a patient with a cutaneous T cell lymphoma. It was induced from the tumor cells by exposure to iododeoxyuridine. Its RNA and proteins are different from those of all other retroviruses. In addition to cancer, HTLV is the cause of tropical spastic paraparesis, an autoimmune disease in which progressive weakness of the legs occurs.

HTLV-I may cause cancer by a mechanism different from that of other retroviruses. It has **no viral oncogene.** Rather, it has two special genes (in addition to the standard retroviral genes *gag, pol,* and *env*) called *tax* and *rex* that play a role in oncogenesis by regulating mRNA transcription and translation. The Tax protein has two activities: (1) it acts on the viral long terminal repeat (LTR) sequences to stimulate viral mRNA synthesis, and (2) it induces NF-κB, which stimulates the production of interleukin-2 (IL-2) and the IL-2 receptor. The increase in IL-2 and its receptor stimulates the T cells to continue growing, thus increasing the likelihood that the cells will become malignant. The Rex protein determines which viral mRNAs can exit the nucleus and enter the cytoplasm to be translated.

HTLV-I is not an endogenous virus; ie, proviral DNA corresponding to its RNA genome is not found in normal human cell DNA. It is an **exogenously acquired** virus, because its proviral DNA is found only in the DNA of the malignant lymphoma cells. It infects CD4-positive T cells preferentially and will induce malignant transformation in these cells in vitro. Some (but not all) patients with T cell lymphomas have antibodies against the virus, indicating that it may not be the cause of all T cell lymphomas. Antibodies against the virus are not found in the general population, indicating that infection is not widespread.

Transmission occurs primarily by sexual contact and by exchange of contaminated blood, eg, in transfusions and intravenous drug users. In the United States, blood for transfusions is screened for antibodies to HTLV-I and HTLV-II and discarded if positive. In recent years, HTLV-I and HTLV-II were found in equal frequency in donated blood. Serologic tests for HTLV do not cross-react with human immunodeficiency virus (HIV).

At about the same time that HTLV-I was found, a similar virus was isolated from malignant T cells in Japan. In that country, a clustering of cases in the rural areas of the west coast of Kyushu was found. Antibodies in the sera of leukemic individuals and in the sera of 25% of the normal population of Kyushu react with the Japanese isolate and with HTLV-I. (Only a small fraction of infected individuals contract leukemia, indicating that HTLV infection alone is insufficient to cause a cancer.) In addition, HTLV-I is endemic in some areas of Africa and on several Caribbean islands, as shown by the high frequency of antibodies. The number of people with positive antibody titers in the United States is quite small, except in certain parts of the southeastern states.

HTLV-II has 60% genetic homology with HTLV-I. Like HTLV-I, it is transmitted primarily by blood and semen and infects CD4-positive cells. Routine serologic tests do not distinguish between HTLV-I and HTLV-II; therefore, other techniques, eg, polymerase chain reaction, are required.

Human Papillomavirus Human papillomavirus (HPV) is one of the two viruses definitely known to cause tumors in humans (see Chapter 38). Papillomas (warts) are benign but can progress to form carcinomas, especially in an immunocompromised person. HPV primarily infects keratinizing or mucosal squamous epithelium.

Papillomaviruses are members of the family of papovaviruses, an acronym of *papilloma*, *polyoma*, and *va*cuolating (eg, SV40 virus) viruses. They are DNA nucleocapsid viruses with double-stranded, circular supercoiled DNA and an icosahedral nucleocapsid. The papillomaviruses have a somewhat larger genome and diameter than do polyomavirus and SV40 virus.* Carcinogenesis by HPV involves two proteins encoded by HPV genes E6 and E7 that interfere with the activity of the proteins encoded by two tumor suppressor genes, p53 and Rb (retinoblastoma), found in normal cells.

There are at least 60 different types of HPV, many of which cause distinct clinical entities. For example, HPV-1 through HPV-4 cause plantar warts on the soles of the feet whereas HPV-6 and HPV-11 cause anogenital warts (condylomata acuminata) and laryngeal papillomas. Certain types of HPV, especially types 16 and 18, are implicated as the cause of carcinoma of the cervix. Approximately 90% of anogenital cancers contain the DNA of these HPV types. In most of these tumor cells, the viral DNA is integrated into the cellular DNA and the E6 and E7 proteins are produced.

Epstein-Barr Virus Epstein-Barr virus (EBV; also discussed in Chapter 37) is a herpesvirus that was isolated from the cells of an East African individual with **Burkitt's lymphoma.** EBV, the cause of infectious mononucleosis, transforms B lymphocytes in culture and causes lymphomas in marmoset monkeys. It is also associated with **nasopharyngeal carcinoma,** a tumor that occurs primarily in China, and with thymic carcinoma and B cell lymphoma in the United States. However, cells from Burkitt's lymphoma patients in the United States show no evidence of EBV infection.

Cells isolated from East African individuals with Burkitt's lymphoma contain EBV DNA and EBV nuclear antigen. Only a small fraction of the many copies of EBV DNA is integrated; most viral DNA is in the form of closed circles in the cytoplasm.

The difficulty in proving that EBV is a human tumor virus is that infection by the virus is widespread but the tumor is rare. The current hypothesis is that EBV infection induces B cells to proliferate, thus increasing the likelihood that a second event (such as activation of a cellular oncogene) will occur. In Burkitt's lymphoma cells, a cellular oncogene, c-*myc*, which is normally located on chromosome 8, is **translocated** to chromosome 14 at the site of immunoglobulin heavy-chain genes. This translocation brings the c-*myc* gene in juxtaposition to an active promoter, and large amounts of c-*myc* RNA are synthesized.

Herpes Simplex Virus Type 2 Herpes simplex virus type 2 (HSV-2) is included as a possible human tumor virus on the basis of two main lines of evidence: (1) epidemiologic; ie, women with HSV-2 genital infections have a higher incidence of **carcinoma of the cervix** than do matched controls, and women with carcinoma of the cervix have antibody to HSV-2 more frequently than do matched controls; and (2) molecular; ie, HSV-2 DNA and proteins are located in cervical carcinoma cells, and HSV-2 can malignantly transform certain cells in vitro.

Despite this evidence, HSV-2 is not considered to be a human tumor virus; most of these findings can be explained by the alternative hypothesis that HSV-2 causes latent genital infections in patients who began sexual activity at an early age. Human papillomavirus is now considered more likely to be the cause of carcinoma of the cervix than is HSV-2 (see above).

---

*Papillomaviruses are 55 nm in diameter with a DNA molecular weight of 5×10^6, in contrast to the others, which have a diameter of 45 nm and a DNA molecular weight of 3×10^6.

Hepatitis B Virus Hepatitis B virus (HBV) infection is significantly more common in patients with primary hepatocellular carcinoma **(hepatoma)** than in controls. This relationship is striking in areas of Africa and Asia where the incidence of both HBV infection and hepatoma is high. Chronic HBV infection commonly causes cirrhosis of the liver; these two events are the main predisposing factors to hepatoma. Part of the HBV genome is integrated into cellular DNA in malignant cells. However, no HBV gene has been definitely implicated in oncogenesis. The integration of HBV DNA may cause insertional mutagenesis, resulting in the activation of a cellular oncogene.

Hepatitis C Virus Chronic infection with hepatitis C virus (HCV), like HBV, also predisposes to hepatocellular carcinoma. HCV is an RNA virus that has no oncogene and forms no DNA intermediate during replication. It does cause chronic hepatitis, which seems likely to be the main predisposing event.

Human Herpesvirus 8 HHV8, also known as Kaposi's sarcoma-associated herpesvirus (KSHV), may cause Kaposi's sarcoma. The DNA of the virus has been detected in the sarcoma cells, but the role of the virus in oncogenesis remains to be determined (see Chapter 46).

DO ANIMAL TUMOR VIRUSES CAUSE CANCER IN HUMANS?

There is no evidence that animal tumor viruses cause tumors in humans. In fact, the only available information suggests that they do not, because (1) people who were inoculated with poliovirus vaccine contaminated with SV40 virus have no greater incidence of cancers than do uninoculated controls, (2) soldiers inoculated with yellow fever vaccine contaminated with avian leukemia virus do not have a high incidence of tumors, and (3) members of families whose cats have died of leukemia caused by feline leukemia virus show no increase in the occurrence of leukemia over control families.

ANIMAL TUMOR VIRUSES

1. DNA Tumor Viruses

The important DNA tumor viruses are listed in Table 43–5.

Papovaviruses The two best-characterized oncogenic papovaviruses are **polyomavirus** and **SV40 virus.** Polyomavirus (*poly* means many; *oma* means tumor) causes a wide variety of histologically different tumors when inoculated into newborn rodents. Its natural host is the mouse. SV40 virus, which was isolated from normal rhesus monkey kidney cells, causes sarcomas in newborn hamsters.

Polyomavirus and SV40 virus share many chemical and biologic features, eg, double-stranded, circular, supercoiled DNA of molecular weight 3×10^6 and a 45-nm icosahedral nucleocapsid. However, the sequence of their DNA and the antigenicity of their proteins are quite distinct. Both undergo a lytic (permissive) cycle in the cells of their natural hosts, with the production of progeny virus. However, when they infect the cells of a heterologous species, the nonpermissive cycle ensues, no virus is produced, and the cell is malignantly transformed.* In the transformed cell, the viral DNA integrates into the cell DNA and only early proteins are synthesized. Some of these proteins, eg, the T antigens described on p 242, are required for induction and maintenance of the transformed state.

JC virus, a human papovavirus, is the cause of progressive multifocal leukoencephalopathy (see Chapter 44). It also causes brain tumors in monkeys and hamsters. There is no evidence that it causes human cancer.

Adenoviruses Some human adenoviruses, especially serotypes 12, 18, and 31, induce sarcomas in newborn hamsters and transform rodent cells in culture. There is no evidence that these viruses cause tumors in humans, and no adenoviral DNA has been detected in the DNA of any human tumor cells.

---

*The ability of polyomaviruses to transform mouse cells is an exception to the generalization that cells of the natural host do not become malignant. Polyomavirus not only causes a cytopathic effect in most mouse cells but also can induce a rare transformed cell.

Adenoviruses undergo both a permissive cycle in some cells and a nonpermissive, transforming cycle in others. The linear genome DNA (MW 23×10^6) circularizes within the infected cell, but—in contrast to the papovaviruses, whose entire genome integrates—only a small region (10%) of the adenovirus genome does so; yet transformation still occurs. This region codes for several proteins, one of which is the T (tumor) antigen. Adenovirus T antigen is required for transformation and is antigenically distinct from the polyomavirus and SV40 virus T antigens.

Herpesviruses   Several animal herpesviruses are known to cause tumors. Four species of herpesviruses cause **lymphomas** in nonhuman primates. Herpesviruses saimiri and ateles induce T cell lymphomas in New World monkeys, and herpesviruses pan and papio transform B lymphocytes in chimpanzees and baboons, respectively.

A herpesvirus of chickens causes Marek's disease, a contagious, rapidly fatal neurolymphomatosis. Immunization of chickens with a live, attenuated vaccine has resulted in a marked decrease in the number of cases. A herpesvirus is implicated as the cause of kidney carcinomas in frogs.

Poxviruses   Two poxviruses cause tumors in animals; these are the fibroma-myxoma virus, which causes fibromas or myxomas in rabbits and other animals, and Yaba monkey tumor virus, which causes benign histiocytomas in animals and human volunteers. Little is known about either of these viruses.

2. RNA Tumor Viruses (Retroviruses)

RNA tumor viruses have been isolated from a large number of species: snakes, birds, and mammals including nonhuman primates. The important RNA tumor viruses are listed in Table 43–5. They are important because of their ubiquity, their ability to cause tumors in the host of origin, their small number of genes, and the relationship of their genes to cellular oncogenes (see p 240).

These viruses belong to the retrovirus family (the prefix "retro" means reverse), so named because a **"reverse transcriptase"** is located in the virion. This enzyme transcribes the genome RNA into double-stranded proviral DNA and is essential to their replication. The viral genome consists of two identical molecules of positive-strand RNA. Each molecule has a molecular weight of approximately 2×10^6 (these are the only viruses that are diploid, ie, have two copies of their genome in the virion). The two molecules are hydrogen-bonded together by complementary bases located near the 5′ end of both RNA molecules. Also bound near the 5′ end of each RNA is a transfer RNA (tRNA) that serves as the primer* for the transcription of the RNA into DNA. The icosahedral capsid is surrounded by an envelope with glycoprotein spikes. Some internal capsid proteins are group-specific antigens, which are common to retroviruses within a species. There are three important morphologic types of retroviruses, labeled B, C, and D, depending primarily on the location of the capsid or core. Most of the retroviruses are C-type particles, but mouse mammary tumor virus is a B-type particle, and human immunodeficiency virus (HIV), the cause of AIDS, is a D-type particle.

The gene sequence of the RNA of a typical avian sarcoma virus is *gag, pol, env,* and *src.* The nontransforming retroviruses have three genes; they are missing *src.* The *gag* region codes for the group-specific antigens, the *pol* gene codes for the reverse transcriptase, the *env* gene codes for the two envelope spike proteins, and the *src* gene codes for the protein kinase. In other oncogenic retroviruses, such as HTLV-I, there is a fifth coding region (the *tax* gene) near the 3′ end, which encodes a protein that enhances viral transcription.

Table 43–5. Varieties of tumor viruses.

Nucleic Acid	Virus
DNA	Papovaviruses, eg, polyomavirus, SV40 virus; papillomaviruses; adenoviruses, especially types 12, 18 and 31; herpesviruses, eg, herpesvirus saimiri; poxviruses, eg, fibroma-myxoma virus.
RNA	Avian sarcoma viruses, eg, Rous sarcoma virus; avian leukemia viruses; murine sarcoma viruses; murine leukemia viruses; mouse mammary tumor virus; feline sarcoma virus; feline leukemia virus; simian sarcoma virus; human T cell leukemia virus.

*The purpose of the primer tRNA is to act as the point of attachment for the first deoxynucleotide at the start of DNA synthesis. The primers are normal-cell tRNAs that are characteristic for each retrovirus.

The sequences at the 5′ and 3′ ends function in the integration of the proviral DNA and in the transcription of mRNA from the integrated proviral DNA by host cell RNA polymerase II. At each end is a sequence* called a long terminal repeat (LTR) that is composed of several regions, one of which, near the 5′ end, is the binding site for the primer tRNA.

After infection of the cell by a retrovirus, the following events occur. Using the genome RNA as the template, the reverse transcriptase (RNA-dependent DNA polymerase) synthesizes double-stranded proviral DNA. The DNA then integrates into cellular DNA. Integration of the proviral DNA is an obligatory step, but there is no specific site of integration. Insertion of the viral LTR can enhance the transcription of adjacent host cell genes. If this host gene is a cellular oncogene, malignant transformation may result. This explains how retroviruses without viral oncogenes can cause transformation.

Review Questions

1. Describe some of the changes that occur when cells undergo malignant transformation.
2. Distinguish between a provirus and an oncogene.
3. What is the relationship between viral and cellular oncogenes?
4. What are some of the functions of oncogenes?
5. What is the fate of viral DNA when a DNA tumor virus infects a nonpermissive cell? What typically happens to the cell?
6. Describe the importance of the T antigen of papovaviruses.
7. Describe the similarities between the temperate bacteriophages, the papovaviruses, and the retroviruses.
8. What are three techniques to recover viruses from the integrated state?
9. What are endogenous viruses?
10. Describe the vertical transmission of viruses. What is its consequence for the immune system?
11. Describe HTLV-I: (a) the nature of the virus, (b) its *tax* gene, (c) how it was first isolated, (d) the locations where it is endemic.
12. What is the relationship of the following viruses to human cancers? (a) EBV, (b) HSV-2, (c) HBV, (d) HPV, (e) adenoviruses.
13. What is the nature of papovaviruses, eg, SV40 virus, and their relationship to cancer?
14. What is the nature of retroviruses and their relationship to cancer?

44

Slow Viruses

This is a heterogeneous group of agents containing both conventional viruses and unconventional agents, eg, prions. **Prions** are **protein-containing particles** with **no detectable nucleic acid** that are highly resistant to inactivation by heat, formaldehyde, and ultraviolet light but are killed by protein- and lipid-disrupting agents such as phenol, ether, NaOH, and hypochlorite (see Chapter 28).

In humans, the "slow" agents cause **central nervous system** diseases characterized by a long incubation period, a gradual onset, and a progressive, invariably fatal course. There is no antimicrobial therapy for these diseases. Note that the term "slow" refers to the disease, not to the rate of replication of the causative viruses. The replication rate of these viruses is similar to that of most other viruses.

---

*The length of the sequence varies from 250 to 1200 bases, depending on the virus.

DISEASES CAUSED BY CONVENTIONAL VIRUSES

Progressive Multifocal Leukoencephalopathy Progressive multifocal leukoencephalopathy (PML) is a fatal demyelinating disease of the white matter and involves multiple areas of the brain. It occurs primarily in individuals with compromised cell-mediated immunity, especially AIDS patients. PML is caused by JC virus, a papovavirus antigenically distinct from other papovaviruses such as human papillomavirus. Antibodies to JC virus are found in approximately 75% of normal human sera, showing that infection is widespread. Disease occurs when latent JC virus is activated in an immunocompromised patient. There is no antiviral treatment.

Subacute Sclerosing Panencephalitis Subacute sclerosing panencephalitis (SSPE) is a slowly progressive disease characterized by inflammatory lesions in many areas of the brain. It is a rare disease of **children** who were infected by **measles virus** several years earlier. SSPE begins with mild changes in personality and ends with dementia and death.

SSPE is a persistent infection by a variant of measles virus that cannot complete its replication. The evidence for this is as follows:

(1) Inclusion bodies containing helical nucleocapsids, which react with antibody to measles virus, are seen in the affected neurons.

(2) A virus very similar to measles virus can be induced from these cells by cocultivation with permissive cells in culture. The induced virus has a different matrix protein; this protein is important in viral assembly.

(3) Patients have high titers of measles antibody in the blood and spinal fluid.

(4) SSPE has virtually disappeared in the United States since the onset of widespread immunization with measles vaccine.

A progressive panencephalitis can also occur in patients with congenital rubella.

Acquired Immunodeficiency Syndrome (AIDS) AIDS is caused by human immunodeficiency virus (HIV), a member of the lentivirus group of retroviruses. AIDS is a disease with a long latent period and a progressive course and can involve the central nervous system. See Chapter 45 for more information.

DISEASES CAUSED BY UNCONVENTIONAL AGENTS

Kuru In contrast to the agents of PML and SSPE, no conventional virus is associated with kuru. This fatal disease is characterized by progressive tremors and ataxia but not dementia. It occurs **only** among the **Fore tribes in New Guinea.** It was transmitted during a ritual in which the skulls of the dead were opened and the brains eaten. It is suspected that transmission occurred through cuts in the skin during preparation rather than by eating the brain, because the women who prepared the brains were affected more frequently than the men who ate them. Since the practice was stopped, kuru has almost disappeared. The agents of kuru and Creutzfeldt-Jakob disease (see below) have been transmitted serially in primates.

Creutzfeldt-Jakob Disease Pathologic examination of the brains of patients with Creutzfeldt-Jakob disease (CJD) and kuru reveals a **spongiform** (sponge or swiss-cheese) appearance similar to that associated with scrapie in sheep (see below). **Prions** cause scrapie and have been found in the brains of CJD patients; they appear to cause CJD and kuru as well. A variant form of CJD and its relationship to "mad-cow" disease is described below in the section on bovine spongiform encephalopathy.

In contrast to kuru, CJD is **found sporadically worldwide** and affects both sexes. This rare disease is characterized by presenile dementia and ataxia, progressing to coma and death. It is not highly transmissible; an increased incidence within families is rare. It has been transmitted **iatrogenically,** eg, in a corneal transplant, via intracerebral electrodes, and in hormones extracted from human pituitaries. Proper sterilization of CJD agent-contaminated material consists of either auto-claving or treating with sodium hypochlorite.

Although most cases of CJD are sporadic, about 10% are hereditary. In these patients, a point mutation in codon 102 of the prion protein gene occurs. The same mutation is found in patients with Gerstmann-Straussler-Scheinker (GSS) syndrome, another slow central nervous system disease of humans. The hereditary forms of these diseases may be prevented by the detection of carriers and genetic counseling. The origin of these spongiform encephalopathies is three-fold: **infectious, hereditary, and sporadic.** The term sporadic refers to the appearance of the disease in the absence of either an infectious or a hereditary etiology.

SLOW VIRUS DISEASES OF ANIMALS

There are two slow virus diseases of animals, scrapie and visna, that are important models for human diseases.

Scrapie   Scrapie is a disease of sheep, characterized by tremors, ataxia, and itching, in which the sheep scrape off their wool against fence posts. It has an incubation period of many months. Spongiform degeneration without inflammation is seen in the brain tissue of affected animals. It has been transmitted to mice and other animals via a brain extract that contained no recognizable virus particles. Studies of mice revealed that the infectivity is associated with a 27,000-molecular-weight protein known as a prion (see pp 153–154).

Visna   Visna is a disease of sheep that is characterized by pneumonia and demyelinating lesions in the brain. It is caused by visna virus, a member of the lentivirus subgroup of retroviruses. As such, it has a single-stranded, diploid RNA genome and an RNA-dependent DNA polymerase in the virion. It is thought that integration of the DNA provirus into the host cell DNA may be important in the persistence of the virus within the host and, consequently, in its long incubation period and prolonged, progressive course.

Bovine Spongiform Encephalopathy   A third slow virus disease of animals is bovine spongiform encephalopathy (BSE), also known as "mad cow" disease. Cattle acquire BSE by eating feed supplemented with organs, eg, brains, obtained from sheep infected with scrapie prions. BSE is endemic in Great Britain and has not occurred in the United States. Supplementation of feed with sheep organs was banned in Great Britain in 1988. In 1996, several cases of Creutzfeldt-Jakob disease occurred in Great Britain which are attributed to the ingestion of beef. These cases are a new variant of CJD because they occurred in much younger people than usual and had certain clinical and pathologic findings different from those found in the typical form of the disease. The prions isolated from the "variant CJD" cases in humans chemically resemble the prions isolated from mad cow disease more than they resemble other prions, which is evidence to support the hypothesis that variant CJD originated by eating beef.

Review Questions

1. To what does the term "slow virus" refer?
2. Contrast the etiology and pathogenesis of PML and SSPE.
3. What are prions, and what is the evidence that they may be involved in human disease?
4. Contrast the transmission of kuru and Creutzfeldt-Jakob disease.
5. Contrast the causative agents of scrapie and visna.

Human Immunodeficiency Virus

45

Disease   Human immunodeficiency virus (HIV)* is the cause of acquired immunodeficiency syndrome (AIDS). Both HIV-1 and HIV-2 cause AIDS, but HIV-1 is found worldwide whereas HIV-2 is found primarily in West Africa. This chapter refers to HIV-1 unless otherwise noted.

Important Properties   HIV is one of the human T cell lymphotrophic retroviruses (human T cell leukemia virus types I and II are others). HIV preferentially infects and **kills helper (CD4) T lymphocytes,** resulting in the loss of cell-mediated immunity and a high probability that the host will develop **opportunistic infections.** Other cells, eg, macrophages and monocytes, that have CD4 proteins on their surfaces can be infected also.

HIV belongs to the lentivirus subgroup of retroviruses, which cause "slow" infections with long incubation periods (see Chapter 44). HIV has a bar-shaped (type D) core surrounded by an envelope containing virus-specific glycoproteins (gp120 and gp41) (Fig 45–1). The genome of HIV consists of two identical molecules of single-stranded, positive-polarity RNA and is said to be **diploid.** The HIV genome is the most complex of the known retroviruses (Fig 45–2). In addition to the three typical retroviral genes *gag, pol,* and *env,* which encode the structural proteins, the genome RNA has at least five other genes, several of which are regulatory genes.

The *gag* gene encodes the internal "core" proteins, the most important of which is p24, an antigen used in serologic tests. The *pol* gene encodes several proteins including the virion "reverse transcriptase," which synthesizes DNA by using the genome RNA as a template, an integrase that integrates the viral DNA into the cellular DNA, and a protease that cleaves the various viral precursor proteins. The *env* gene encodes gp160, a precursor glycoprotein that is cleaved to form the two envelope (surface) glycoproteins, gp120 and gp41.

On the basis of differences in the base sequence of the gene that encodes gp120, HIV has been subdivided into subtypes **(clades)** A through I. The B clade is the most common subtype in North America. Subtype B preferentially infects mononuclear cells and appears to be passed readily during anal sex, whereas subtype E preferentially infects female genital tract cells and appears to be passed readily during vaginal sex.

Three enzymes are located within the nucleocapsid of the virion: reverse transcriptase, integrase, and protease. Reverse transcriptase is the RNA-dependent DNA polymerase that is the source of the family name, retroviruses. This enzyme transcribes the RNA genome into the proviral DNA. Reverse transcriptase is a bifunctional enzyme; it also has ribonuclease H activity. Ribonuclease H degrades RNA when it is in the form of an RNA-DNA hybrid molecule. The degradation of the viral RNA genome is an essential step in the synthesis of the double-stranded proviral DNA. Integrase, another important enzyme within the virion, mediates the integration of the proviral DNA into the host cell DNA. The viral protease cleaves the precursor polyproteins into functional viral polypeptides.

One important regulatory gene is the *tat* (transactivation of transcription)† gene, which encodes a protein that enhances viral (and perhaps cellular) gene transcription. The Tat protein and another HIV-encoded regulatory protein called Nef repress the synthesis of class I MHC proteins, thereby reducing the ability of cytotoxic T cells to kill HIV-infected cells.

There are several important antigens of HIV.

(1) gp120 and gp41 are the **type-specific envelope glycoproteins.** gp120 protrudes from the surface and interacts with the CD4 receptor (and a second protein, a chemokine receptor) on the cell surface. gp41 is embedded in the envelope and mediates the fusion of the viral envelope with the cell membrane at the time of infection. The gene that encodes gp120 mutates rapidly, resulting in many **anti-**

---

*Formerly known as human T lymphotropic virus type 3 (HTLV-III), lymphadenopathy-associated virus (LAV), and AIDS-related virus (ARV).

†Transactivation refers to activation of transcription of genes distant from the gene, ie, other genes on the same proviral DNA or on cellular DNA. One site of action of the *tat* protein is the long terminal repeat at the 5′ end of the viral genome.

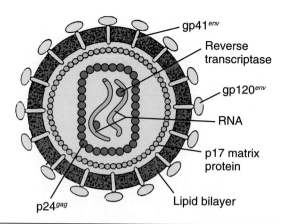

Figure 45–1. Cross-section of HIV. In the interior, two molecules of viral RNA are shown associated with reverse transcriptase. Surrounding those structures is a rectangular nucleocapsid composed of p24 proteins. On the exterior are the two envelope proteins, gp120 and gp41, which are embedded in the lipid bilayer derived from the cell membrane. (Modified and reproduced, with permission, from Greene WC: *N Engl J Med* 1993; **328:**330.)

genic variants. The most immunogenic region of gp120 is called the V3 loop; it is one of the sites that varies antigenically to a significant degree. Antibody against gp120 neutralizes the infectivity of HIV, but the rapid appearance of gp120 variants will make production of an effective vaccine difficult. The high mutation rate may be due to lack of an editing function in the reverse transcriptase.

(2) The group-specific antigen, p24, is located in the core and is not known to vary. Antibodies against p24 do not neutralize HIV infectivity but serve as important serologic markers of infection.

The natural host range of HIV is limited to humans, although certain primates can be infected in the laboratory. HIV is **not an endogenous virus** of humans; ie, no HIV sequences are found in normal human cell DNA. The origin of HIV and how it entered the human population remains uncertain. There has been speculation that monkeys or other primates were the source, but the issue is unresolved.

Viruses similar to HIV have been isolated. Examples are listed below.

(1) Human immunodeficiency virus type 2 (HIV-2) was isolated from AIDS patients in West Africa in 1986. The proteins of HIV-2 are only about 40% identical to those of the original HIV isolates. HIV-2 remains localized primarily to West Africa and is much less transmissible than HIV-1.

(2) Simian immunodeficiency virus (SIV) was isolated from monkeys with an AIDS-like illness. Antibodies in some African women cross-react with SIV. The proteins of SIV resemble those of HIV-2 more closely than they resemble those of the original HIV isolates.

(3) HTLV-IV infects T cells but does not kill them and is not associated with any disease.

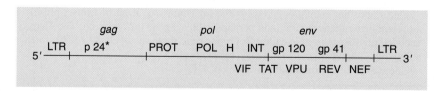

Figure 45–2. The genome of HIV. Above the line are the three genes for the main structural proteins: (1) *gag* encodes the internal group-specific antigens, eg, p24; (2) *pol* encodes the polymerase protein (reverse transcriptase), which has four enzymatic activities: protease (PROT), polymerase (POL), RNAse H (H), and integrase (INT); (3) *env* encodes the two envelope glycoproteins, gp120 and gp41. Below the line are five regulatory genes: viral infectivity factor (VIF), transactivating protein (TAT), viral protein U (VPU), regulator of expression of virion protein (REV), and negative regulatory factor (NEF). At both ends are long terminal repeats (LTR), which are transcription initiation sites. Within the 5′ LTR is the binding site for the TAT protein, called the trans-activation response element (TAR). TAT enhances the initiation and elongation of viral mRNA transcription.

* p24 and other smaller proteins such as p17, p9, and p7 are encoded by the *gag* gene.

Summary of Replicative Cycle   The details of the replicative cycle are incomplete, but it is thought to follow the typical retroviral cycle (see Fig 45–3). The initial step in the entry of HIV into the cell is the binding of the virion gp120 envelope protein to the CD4 protein on the cell surface. The virion gp120 protein then interacts with a second protein on the cell surface, one of the chemokine receptors. Next the virion gp41 protein mediates fusion of the viral envelope with the cell membrane, and the virion enters the cell.

Chemokine receptors, such as fusin and CCR5 proteins, are required for the entry of HIV into CD4-positive cells. The T-cell-tropic strains of HIV bind to fusin, whereas the macrophage-tropic strains bind to CCR5. Mutations in the gene encoding CCR5 endow the individual with protection from infection with HIV. Approximately 1% of people of Western European ancestry have homozygous mutations in this gene.

After uncoating, the virion RNA-dependent DNA polymerase transcribes the genome RNA into double-stranded DNA, which integrates into the host cell DNA. The viral DNA can integrate at different sites in the host cell DNA, and multiple copies of viral DNA can integrate. Integration is mediated by a virus-encoded endonuclease (integrase). Viral mRNA is transcribed from the proviral DNA by host cell RNA polymerase and translated into several large polyproteins, which are then cleaved by the virus-encoded protease to form the virion structural proteins, namely the reverse transcriptase, the core proteins, and the two envelope glycoproteins. The virions assemble in the cytoplasm and are released from the cell by budding. Much of the virus remains cell-associated and may be difficult to neutralize with antibody.

Transmission & Epidemiology   Transmission of HIV occurs primarily by sexual contact and by transfer of infected blood. Perinatal transmission from infected mother to neonate also occurs, either at birth or via breast milk. Infection occurs by the transfer of either HIV-infected cells or free HIV (ie, HIV that is not cell-associated). Although small amounts of virus have been found in other fluids, eg, saliva and tears, there is no evidence that they play a role in infection. In general, transmission of HIV follows the pattern of hepatitis B virus, except that HIV infection is much less efficiently transferred; ie, the dose of HIV required to cause infection is much higher than that of HBV.

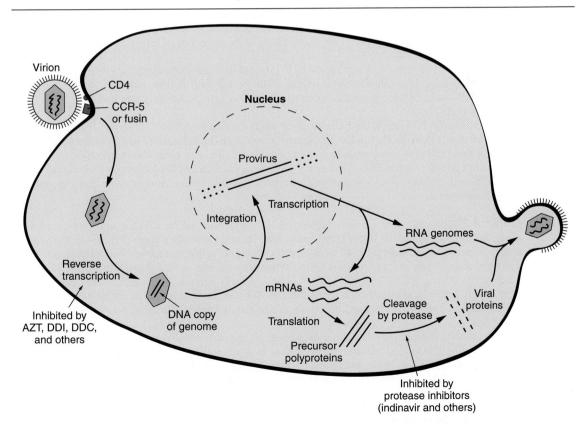

Figure 45–3. Replicative cycle of HIV. The sites of action of the important antiviral drugs are indicated. (Modified and reproduced, with permission, from Ryan K et al: *Sherris Medical Microbiology,* 3rd ed. Appleton & Lange, 1994.)

Since 1981, when AIDS was first reported, and the year 1995, between 1 and 2 million people in the United States have been infected with HIV. During this time, approximately 500,000 cases of AIDS have been reported in the United States and half of those people have died. Worldwide, it is estimated that more than 30 million people are infected, mostly in Sub-Saharan Africa. Three regions, Africa, Asia, and Latin America have the highest rates of new infections.

In the United States and Europe during the 1980s, HIV infection and AIDS occurred primarily in promiscuous homosexual men, intravenous drug abusers, and hemophiliacs. Heterosexual transmission was rare in these regions in the 1980s but is now rising significantly. Heterosexual transmission is the predominant mode of infection in African countries. Very few health care personnel have been infected despite prolonged exposure and needle-stick injuries, supporting the view that the infectious dose of HIV is high. In 1990, it was reported that a dentist may have infected five of his patients. It is thought that transmission of HIV from health care personnel to patients is exceedingly rare.

Pathogenesis & Immunity   HIV infects helper T cells and kills them, resulting in **suppression of cell-mediated immunity.** This predisposes the host to various opportunistic infections and certain cancers such as Kaposi's sarcoma and lymphoma. However, HIV genes are not found in these cancer cells, so HIV does not directly cause these tumors. (The DNA of human herpesvirus 8 has been detected in Kaposi's sarcoma cells, but whether this virus is the cause of this cancer has yet to be determined.) HIV also infects brain monocytes and macrophages, producing multinucleated giant cells and significant central nervous system symptoms. The fusion of HIV-infected cells in the brain and elsewhere mediated by gp41 is one of the main pathologic findings. The cells recruited into the syncytia ultimately die. The death of HIV-infected cells may also be the result of immunologic attack by cytotoxic CD8 lymphocytes or antibody. Effectiveness of the cytotoxic T cells may be limited by the ability of the viral *tat* gene to reduce class I MHC protein synthesis.

Another mechanism hypothesized to explain the death of helper T cells is that HIV acts as a "superantigen," which indiscriminately activates many helper T cells and leads to their demise. The finding that another retrovirus, mouse mammary tumor virus, can act as a superantigen lends support to this theory. Superantigens are described in Chapter 58.

Persistent noncytopathic infection of T lymphocytes also occurs. Persistently infected cells continue to produce HIV, which may help to sustain the infection in vivo. A person infected with HIV is considered to be infected for life. This seems likely to be the result of integration of viral DNA into the DNA of infected cells.

In 1995, it was reported that a group of HIV-infected individuals has lived for many years without opportunistic infections and without a reduction in the number of their helper T (CD4) cells. The strain of HIV isolated from them has mutations in the *nef* gene, indicating that this gene plays a role in pathogenesis.

Approximately 90% of AIDS patients have antibodies against HIV. However, these antibodies, which are detected by ELISA in the laboratory, **neutralize the infectivity of the virus poorly.** This indicates that immunity is incomplete and that infectious virus and antibodies can coexist.

In addition to the detrimental effects on T cells, abnormalities of B cells occur. Polyclonal activation of B cells is seen, with resultant high immunoglobulin levels. Autoimmune diseases, such as thrombocytopenia, occur.

Clinical Findings   The clinical picture of HIV infection can be divided into three stages: an early, acute stage; a middle, latent stage; and a late, immunodeficiency stage (Fig 45–4). In the acute stage, which usually begins 2–4 weeks after infection, a mononucleosislike picture of fever, lethargy, sore throat, and generalized lymphadenopathy occurs. A maculopapular rash is also seen. Leukopenia occurs, but the number of CD4 cells is usually normal. Antibodies to HIV typically appear within 2 months after infection. Note that this delay in the appearance of antibodies can result in "false-negative" serologic tests; ie, the person is infected, but antibodies are not detectable at the time of the test.

In the middle stage, a long latent period, measured in years, usually ensues. The patient is asymptomatic during this period. Although the patient is asymptomatic and viremia is low or absent, a large amount of HIV is being produced by lymph node cells but remains sequestered within the lymph nodes. This indicates that during this period of clinical latency, the virus itself does not enter a latent state.

It is estimated that an infected person produces 10 billion new virions each day. This viral load can be estimated by using an assay for viral RNA in the patient's plasma, and the amount of viral RNA serves to guide treatment decisions and the prognosis. For example, if a drug regimen fails to

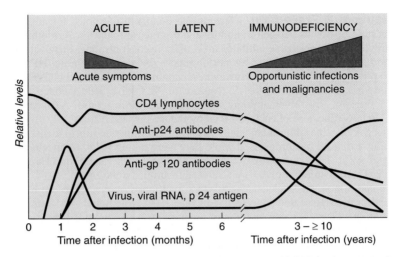

Figure 45–4. Time course of HIV infection. The three main stages of HIV infection, acute, latent, and immunodeficiency, are shown in conjunction with several important laboratory findings. Note that the levels of virus and viral RNA (viral load) are high early in the infection, become low for several years, and then rise during the immunodeficiency stage. The level of CD4 lymphocytes remains more or less normal for many years but then falls. This results in the immunodeficiency stage, which is characterized by opportunistic infections and malignancies. (Modified and reproduced, with permission, from Feinberg M: *Curr Opin Infect Dis* 1992; **5:**214.)

reduce the viral load, the drugs should be changed. As far as the prognosis is concerned, a patient with more than 100,000 copies of viral RNA/mL of plasma is significantly more likely to progress to AIDS than a patient with fewer than 100,000 copies.

A syndrome called AIDS-related complex (ARC) can occur during the latent period. The most frequent manifestations are persistent fevers, fatigue, weight loss, and lymphadenopathy. ARC often progresses to AIDS.

The late stage of HIV infection is AIDS, manifested by a decline in the number of CD4 cells to below 400/mm³ and an increase in the frequency and severity of opportunistic infections.

The two most characteristic manifestations of AIDS are *Pneumocystis* pneumonia and Kaposi's sarcoma. However, many other opportunistic infections occur with some frequency. These include viral infections such as disseminated herpes simplex, herpes zoster, and cytomegalovirus infections and progressive multifocal leukoencephalopathy; fungal infections such as thrush (caused by *Candida albicans*), cryptococcal meningitis, and disseminated histoplasmosis; protozoal infections such as toxoplasmosis and cryptosporidiosis; and bacterial infections such as disseminated *Mycobacterium avium-intracellulare* and *Mycobacterium tuberculosis* infections. Many AIDS patients have severe neurologic problems, eg, dementia and neuropathy, which can be due either to HIV infection of the brain or to many of these opportunistic organisms.

In 1992, patients with AIDS who had no evidence of infection by HIV-1 or HIV-2 were reported. At present, it is unknown whether another virus can cause AIDS.

Laboratory Diagnosis   The presumptive diagnosis of HIV infection is made by the detection of antibodies by **ELISA.** Because there are some false-positive results with this test, the definitive diagnosis is made by **"Western blot"** analysis, in which the viral proteins are displayed by acrylamide gel electrophoresis, transferred to nitrocellulose paper (the blot), and reacted with the patient's serum. If antibodies are present, they will bind to the viral proteins (predominantly to the gp41 or p24 protein). Enzymatically labeled antibody to human IgG is then added. A color reaction reveals the presence of the HIV antibody in the infected patient's serum.

HIV can be grown in culture from clinical specimens, but this procedure is available only at a few medical centers. The polymerase chain reaction (PCR) is a very sensitive and specific technique that can be used to detect HIV DNA within infected cells. Some individuals who do not have detectable antibodies have been shown by this test to be infected.

During the first month or two after infection, antibody tests are frequently negative. The presence of HIV can be detected during that period by either viral culture, p24 antigen test, or PCR assay.

Treatment & Prevention   The current treatment of choice for advanced disease is a regimen consisting of two nucleoside inhibitors and a protease inhibitor. Azidothymidine (AZT, zidovudine, Retrovir) is the nucleoside inhibitor most often used. It prolongs survival and reduces the number of opportunistic infections but does not eliminate the virus. It inhibits HIV replication by interfering with proviral DNA synthesis. However, it cannot cure an infected cell of an already integrated copy of proviral DNA. Strains of HIV resistant to AZT have been isolated from patients on long-term AZT therapy. Severe hematologic side effects can limit its use. AZT can be combined with ddI or ddC to lower the dose of each and thereby reduce the side effects.

Dideoxyinosine (ddI, didanosine, Videx) is recommended for patients who are intolerant of AZT or whose disease has progressed while they were taking AZT. Its mechanism of action is similar to that of AZT. Three other drugs, dideoxycytidine (ddC, zalcitabine, Hivid), d4T (stavudine, Zerit), and 3TC (lamivudine, Epivir) are also used in similar situations.

In addition to the nucleoside inhibitors mentioned above, there are non-nucleoside inhibitors of reverse transcriptase that are effective against HIV. Nevirapine (Viramune) is the currently approved drug in this class. The combination of nevirapine, AZT, and ddI lowers viral RNA levels and raises CD4 counts significantly more than the two-drug regimen of AZT and ddI.

Protease inhibitors, such as saquinavir (Invirase), ritonavir (Norvir), and indinavir (Crixivan), when combined with nucleoside analogues, such as AZT, are very effective in inhibiting viral replication and increasing CD4 cell counts. Mutants of HIV resistant to protease inhibitors have been isolated from patients only infrequently and are not a major clinical problem at present. Resistance to one of these drugs conveys resistance to all.

No vaccine for human use is available. A vaccine containing recombinant gp120 protects nonhuman primates against challenge by HIV and by HIV-infected cells. The success of a vaccine containing a live, attenuated mutant of SIV in protecting monkeys against challenge by a large dose of SIV may encourage a similar effort with a mutant of HIV in humans.

Prevention consists of taking measures to avoid exposure to the virus, eg, using condoms, not sharing needles, and discarding donated blood that is contaminated with HIV. Infection following a needle-stick injury may be prevented in some individuals by use of two drugs, AZT and 3TC, to which a third, indinavir, can be added. Two steps can be taken to reduce the number of HIV-infected children: AZT should be given perinatally to HIV-infected mothers and neonates, and HIV-infected mothers should not breast feed.

Several drugs are commonly taken by those in the advanced stages of AIDS to prevent certain opportunistic infections. Some examples are trimethoprim-sulfamethoxazole to prevent *Pneumocystis* pneumonia, fluconazole to prevent recurrences of cryptococcal meningitis, ganciclovir to prevent recurrences of retinitis caused by cytomegalovirus, and oral preparations of antifungal drugs, such as clotrimazole, to prevent thrush caused by *Candida albicans*.

Review Questions

1. Describe the genome of HIV, its genes, and their function.
2. What is the unusual characteristic of the envelope glycoprotein of HIV that may impede development of a vaccine?
3. What are the two important modes of transmission of HIV to adults? to newborns?
4. Which type of cell does HIV primarily infect? Why?
5. What is the effect of HIV on these cells?
6. Describe the three stages of clinical findings in HIV infection.
7. Which two tests for what components of the virus are used to determine whether HIV infection has occurred?
8. What is the mode of action of azidothymidine and dideoxyinosine?
9. How can HIV infection be prevented?

Minor Viral Pathogens

46

These viruses are presented in alphabetical order. They are listed in Table 46–1 in terms of their nucleic acid and presence of an envelope.

Astroviruses   Astroviruses are nonenveloped RNA viruses similar in size to polioviruses. They have a characteristic five- or six-pointed morphology. These viruses cause watery diarrhea, especially in children. Most adults have antibodies against astroviruses, suggesting that infection occurs commonly. No antiviral drugs or preventive measures are available.

Coronaviruses   Coronaviruses are enveloped, single-stranded, positive-polarity RNA viruses with club-shaped surface spikes that resemble a "corona." They cause **upper respiratory tract infection** (colds) in adults. Although the incidence varies from year to year, approximately 20% of colds are caused by these viruses. Laboratory diagnosis is rarely made. No antiviral drugs or preventive measures are available.

Ebola Virus   Ebola virus is named for the river in Zaire that was the site of an outbreak of **hemorrhagic fever** in 1976. The disease begins with fever, headache, vomiting, and diarrhea. Later, bleeding into the gastrointestinal tract occurs, followed by shock and disseminated intravascular coagulation. The hemorrhages are caused by severe thrombocytopenia. The mortality rate associated with this virus approaches 100%. Most cases arise by secondary transmission from contact with the patient's blood or secretions, eg, in hospital staff.

Ebola virus is a member of the filovirus family. The natural reservoir of this virus is unknown. Monkeys can be infected but, because they become sick, are unlikely to be the reservoir. Diagnosis is made by isolating the virus or by detecting a rise in antibody titer. (Extreme care must be taken when handling specimens in the laboratory.) No antiviral therapy is available. Prevention centers on limiting secondary spread by proper handling of patient's secretions and blood.

Hantaviruses   Hantaviruses are members of the bunyavirus family. The prototype virus is Hantaan virus, the cause of Korean hemorrhagic fever (KHF). KHF is characterized by headache, petechial hemorrhages, shock, and renal failure. It occurs in Asia and Europe but not North America and has a mortality rate of about 10%. Hantaviruses are part of a heterogeneous group of viruses called Roboviruses which stands for "*ro*dent-*bo*rne" viruses. Roboviruses are transmitted from rodents directly (without an arthropod vector) whereas Arboviruses are "*ar*thropod-*bo*rne."

In 1993, an outbreak of a new disease, characterized by influenza-like symptoms followed rapidly by acute respiratory failure, occurred in the western United States, centered in New Mexico and Arizona. This disease, now called Hantavirus pulmonary syndrome, is caused by a hantavirus (Sin Nombre virus) endemic in deer mice (*Peromyscus*) and is acquired by inhalation of aerosols of the rodent's urine and feces. It is not transmitted from person to person. Very few people have antibody to the virus, indicating that asymptomatic infections are not common. The diagnosis is made by detecting viral RNA in lung tissue with the polymerase chain reaction (PCR) assay, by performing im-

Table 46–1. Minor viral pathogens.

Characteristics	Representative Viruses
DNA enveloped viruses	Herpes B virus, human herpesvirus 6, human herpesvirus 8 (Kaposi's sarcoma-associated herpesvirus), molluscum contagiosum virus, cowpox virus, monkeypox virus
DNA nonenveloped viruses	
RNA enveloped viruses	Coronaviruses, Ebola virus, Hantaviruses, Japanese encephalitis virus, Lassa fever virus, lymphocytic choriomeningitis virus, Marburg virus, spumaviruses, Tacaribe complex of viruses (eg, Junin and Machupo viruses)
RNA nonenveloped viruses	Astroviruses, encephalomyocarditis virus, Norwalk virus

munohistochemistry on lung tissue, or by detecting IgM antibody in serum. The mortality rate is very high, approximately 60%.

There is no effective drug; ribavirin has been used but appears to be ineffective. There is no vaccine for any hantavirus.

Herpes B Virus   This virus (monkey B virus or herpesvirus simiae) causes a rare, often fatal **encephalitis** in persons in close contact with monkeys or their tissues, eg, zookeepers or cell culture technicians. The virus causes a latent infection in monkeys that is similar to HSV-1 infection in humans.

Herpes B virus and HSV-1 cross-react antigenically, but antibody to HSV-1 does not protect from herpes B encephalitis. The presence of HSV-1 antibody can, however, confuse serologic diagnosis by making the interpretation of a rise in antibody titer difficult. The diagnosis can therefore be made only by recovering the virus. Acyclovir may be beneficial. Prevention consists of using protective clothing and masks to prevent exposure to the virus. Immune globulin containing antibody to herpes B virus should be given after a monkey bite.

Human Herpesvirus 6   This herpesvirus is the cause of exanthem subitum (roseola infantum), a common disease in infants that is characterized by a high fever and a transient rash. The virus is found worldwide, and up to 80% of people are seropositive. The virus is lymphotropic and infects both T and B cells. It remains latent within these cells but can be reactivated in immunocompromised patients and cause pneumonia. Many virologic and clinical features of HHV-6 are similar to those of cytomegalovirus, another member of the herpesvirus family.

Human Herpesvirus 8 (Kaposi's Sarcoma-Associated Herpesvirus)   In 1994, it was reported that a new herpesvirus, now known as human herpesvirus 8 (HHV-8) or Kaposi's sarcoma-associated herpesvirus (KSHV), may be the cause of Kaposi's sarcoma (KS), the most common cancer in patients with AIDS. The initial evidence for this association was that most sarcoma cells taken from AIDS patients contain the DNA of this virus but tissues taken from AIDS patients without KS had very little viral DNA. The DNA of this virus was also found in KS cells that arose in non-HIV-infected patients. Based on DNA analysis, KSHV resembles the lymphotropic herpesviruses, eg, Epstein-Barr virus and herpesvirus saimiri, more than it does the neurotropic herpesviruses, such as herpes simplex virus and varicella-zoster virus.

Additional support was provided by serologic studies showing that most HIV-infected patients with KS had antibodies to KSHV whereas many fewer HIV-infected patients without KS had antibodies to the virus and very few patients with other sexually transmitted diseases, but who were not HIV-infected, had these antibodies. The current estimate of KSHV infection in the general population is about 2%.

Japanese Encephalitis Virus   This virus is the most common cause of **epidemic encephalitis.** The disease is characterized by fever, headache, nuchal rigidity, altered states of consciousness, tremors, incoordination, and convulsions. The mortality rate is high, and neurologic sequelae are severe and can be detected in the majority of survivors. The disease occurs throughout Asia but is most prevalent in Southeast Asia. The rare cases seen in the United States have occurred in travelers returning from that continent. American military personnel in Asia have been affected.

Japanese encephalitis virus is a member of the flavivirus family. It is transmitted to humans by certain species of *Culex* mosquitoes endemic to Asian rice fields. There are two main reservoir hosts, birds and pigs. The diagnosis can be made by isolating the virus, by detecting IgM antibody in serum or spinal fluid, or by staining brain tissue with fluorescent antibody. There is no antiviral therapy. Prevention consists of an inactivated vaccine and pesticides to control the mosquito vector. Immunization is recommended for individuals living in areas of endemic infection for several months or longer.

Lassa Fever Virus   Lassa fever virus was first seen in 1969 in the Nigerian town of that name. It causes a severe, often fatal **hemorrhagic fever** characterized by multiple-organ involvement. The disease begins slowly with fever, headache, vomiting, and diarrhea and progresses to involve the lungs, heart, kidneys, and brain. A petechial rash and gastrointestinal tract hemorrhage ensue, followed by death from vascular collapse.

Lassa fever virus is a member of the arenavirus family, which includes other infrequent human pathogens such as lymphocytic choriomeningitis virus and certain members of the Tacaribe group.

Arenaviruses ("arena" means sand) are united by their unusual appearance in the electron microscope. Their most striking feature is the "sandlike" particles on their surface, which are ribosomes. The function, if any, of these ribosomes is unknown. Arenaviruses are enveloped viruses with surface spikes, a helical nucleocapsid, and single-stranded RNA with negative polarity.

The natural host for Lassa fever virus is the small rodent *Mastomys,* which undergoes a chronic, lifelong infection. The virus is transmitted to humans by contamination of food or water with animal urine. Secondary transmission among hospital personnel occurs also. Asymptomatic infection is widespread in areas of endemic infection.

The diagnosis is made either by isolating the virus or by detecting a rise in antibody titer. Ribavirin reduces the mortality rate if given early, and hyperimmune serum, obtained from persons who have recovered from the disease, has been beneficial in some cases. No vaccine is available, and prevention centers around proper infection control practices and rodent control.

Lymphocytic Choriomeningitis Virus   Lymphocytic choriomeningitis virus is a member of the arenavirus family. It is a rare cause of aseptic meningitis and cannot be distinguished clinically from the more frequent viral causes, eg, echovirus, coxsackievirus, or mumps virus. The usual picture consists of fever, headache, vomiting, stiff neck, and changes in mental status. Spinal fluid shows an increased number of cells, mostly lymphocytes, with an elevated protein level and a normal or low sugar level.

The virus is endemic in the mouse population, in which chronic infection occurs. Animals infected transplacentally become healthy lifelong carriers. The virus is transmitted to humans via food or water contaminated by mouse urine or feces. There is no human-to-human spread: ie, humans are accidental dead-end hosts. Diagnosis is made by isolating the virus from the spinal fluid or by detecting an increase in antibody titer. No antiviral therapy or vaccine is available.

This disease is the prototype used to illustrate **immunopathogenesis** and immune-complex disease. If immunocompetent adult mice are inoculated, meningitis and death ensue. If, however, newborn mice or x-irradiated immunodeficient adults are inoculated, no meningitis occurs despite extensive viral replication. If sensitized T cells are transplanted to the immunodeficient adults, meningitis and death occur. The immunodeficient adult mice, who are apparently well, slowly develop immune-complex glomerulonephritis. It appears that the mice are partially tolerant to the virus in that their cell-mediated immunity is inactive but sufficient antibody is produced to cause immune complex disease.

Marburg Virus   Marburg virus and Ebola virus are similar in that they both cause **hemorrhagic fevers** and are members of the filovirus family; however, they are antigenically distinct. Marburg virus was first recognized as a cause of human disease in 1967 in Marburg, Germany. The common feature of the infected individuals was their exposure to African green monkeys that had recently arrived from Uganda.

The clinical picture of this hemorrhagic fever is as described for Ebola virus (see p 257). No cases of disease caused by either Ebola or Marburg virus have occurred in the United States. The diagnosis is made by isolating the virus or detecting a rise in antibody titer. No antiviral therapy or vaccine is available. As with Ebola virus, secondary cases among medical personnel have occurred; therefore, stringent infection control practices must be instituted to prevent nosocomial spread.

Molluscum Contagiosum Virus   This virus is one of the two causes of **warts** in the adult genital region, the other being the human papillomavirus (see p 203). The lesions are a few millimeters long and are soft, pink, and rounded. In children the warts are most often found on the face and body. The virus is transmitted by direct skin contact. Transmission during sexual intercourse accounts for the frequency of genital lesions.

Molluscum contagiosum virus is classified as a member of the poxvirus family on the basis of its morphology when visualized in the electron microscope. Typical cytoplasmic inclusion bodies are seen in the cells of the malpighian layer. The virus has not been grown in cell culture, and little is known about its life cycle.

Lesions are usually removed by surgery, electrocautery, or cryotherapy. Even if untreated, the lesions will resolve spontaneously in a few years.

Norwalk Virus   Norwalk virus is one cause of outbreaks of **gastroenteritis,** usually in settings such as schools, camps, cruise ships, and similar confined populations. It is named for an outbreak in a school in Norwalk, Ohio, in 1969. The virus was first identified in the stool by immunoelectron microscopy; antibody from a patient who had recovered from the disease was used to aggregate the virus into clumps that contained particles of small (27-nm) icosahedral viruses without envelopes. Subsequent study showed that the genome was a single-stranded, positive-polarity RNA and that the capsid contained only one protein. This description is sufficient to classify it as a member of the calicivirus family.

The clinical picture consists of nausea, vomiting, and diarrhea that resolve spontaneously in 12–24 hours. The virus is transmitted by the fecal-oral route and occurs worldwide. In contrast to most viruses transmitted by the fecal-oral route, it is uncommon in children, and antibody response peaks in young adulthood.

Immunity following infection is relatively brief, ie, less than 2 years. Laboratory diagnosis is not performed for this disease. If, for epidemiologic reasons, a specific viral diagnosis is required, either immunoelectron microscopy or radioimmunoassay can be used. No antiviral therapy is indicated, and no preventive measures other than hand-washing are available.

Poxviruses of Animal Origin   Four poxviruses cause disease in animals and also cause pox-like lesions in humans on rare occasions. They are transmitted by contact with the infected animals, usually in an occupational setting.

Cowpox virus causes vesicular lesions on the udders of cows and can cause similar lesions on the skin of persons who milk cows. Pseudocowpox virus causes a similar picture but is antigenically distinct. Orf virus is the cause of contagious pustular dermatitis in sheep and of vesicular lesions on the hands of sheepshearers.

Monkeypox virus is different from the other three; it causes a human disease that resembles smallpox. In 1997, an outbreak of monkeypox disease that resembled smallpox occurred in Central Africa. Any new case of smallpoxlike disease must be precisely diagnosed to ensure that it is not due to smallpox virus. There has not been a case of smallpox in the world since 1977,* and smallpox immunization has been allowed to lapse, so it is important to ensure that new cases are due to monkeypox virus. Monkeypox virus can be distinguished from smallpox virus in the laboratory both antigenically and by the distinctive lesions it causes on the chorioallantoic membrane of chicken eggs.

Spumaviruses   Spumaviruses are a subfamily of retroviruses, which cause a foamy appearance in cultured cells. They can present a problem in the production of viral vaccines if they contaminate the cell cultures used to make the vaccine. There are no known human pathogens.

Tacaribe Complex of Viruses   The Tacaribe† complex contains several human pathogens, all of which cause **hemorrhagic fever.** The best known are Sabia virus in Brazil, Junin virus in Argentina, and Machupo virus in Bolivia. Hemorrhagic fevers, as the name implies, are characterized by fever and bleeding into the gastrointestinal tract, skin, and other organs. The bleeding is due to thrombocytopenia. Death occurs in up to 20% of cases, and outbreaks can involve thousands of people. Agricultural workers are particularly at risk.

Similar to other arenaviruses such as Lassa fever virus and lymphocytic choriomeningitis virus, these viruses are endemic in the rodent population and are transmitted to humans by accidental contamination of food and water by rodent excreta. The diagnosis can be made either by isolating the virus or by detecting a rise in antibody titer. In a laboratory-acquired Sabia virus infection, ribavirin was an effective treatment. No vaccine is available.

---

*With the exception of two laboratory-acquired cases in 1978.
†Tacaribe virus was isolated from bats in Trinidad in 1956. It does not cause human disease.

Part V: Mycology

Basic Mycology   47

STRUCTURE & GROWTH

Because fungi (yeasts and molds) are **eukaryotic** organisms whereas bacteria are prokaryotic, they differ in several fundamental respects (Table 47–1). Two fungal cell structures are important medically:

(1) The fungal cell wall consists primarily of chitin* (not peptidoglycan as in bacteria); thus, fungi are insensitive to antibiotics, such as penicillin, that inhibit peptidoglycan synthesis.

(2) The fungal cell membrane contains ergosterol and zymosterol, in contrast to human cell membranes, which contain cholesterol. The selective action of amphotericin B and azole drugs, such as fluconazole and ketoconazole, on fungi is based on this difference in membrane sterols.

There are 2 types of fungi: yeasts and molds. **Yeasts** grow as **single cells** that reproduce by asexual budding. **Molds** grow as **long filaments (hyphae)** and form a mat **(mycelium).** Some hyphae form transverse walls **(septate hyphae),** whereas others do not **(nonseptate hyphae).** Nonseptate hyphae are multinucleated (coencytic).

Several medically important fungi are thermally **dimorphic;** ie, they form different structures at different temperatures. They exist as molds in the saprophytic, free-living state at ambient temperature and as yeasts in host tissues at body temperature.

Most fungi are obligate aerobes; some are facultative anaerobes; but none are obligate anaerobes. All fungi require a preformed organic source of carbon, hence their frequent association with decaying matter. The natural habitat of most fungi is, therefore, the **environment.** An important exception is *Candida albicans,* which is part of the human normal flora.

Some fungi reproduce sexually by mating and forming sexual spores, eg, **zygospores, ascospores,** and **basidiospores.** Zygospores are single large spores with thick walls; ascospores are formed in a sac called ascus; and basidiospores are formed externally on the tip of a pedestal called a basidium. The classification of these fungi is based on their sexual spores. Fungi that do not form sexual spores are termed "imperfect" and are classified as **Fungi Imperfecti.**

Most fungi of medical interest propagate asexually by forming **conidia** (asexual spores) from the sides or ends of specialized structures (Fig 47–1). The shape, color, and arrangement of conidia aid in the identification of fungi. Some important conidia are (1) **arthrospores,**† which arise by fragmentation of the ends of hyphae and are the mode of transmission of *Coccidioides immitis;* (2) **chlamydospores,** which are rounded, thick-walled, and quite resistant (the terminal chlamydospores of *C albicans* aid in its identification); (3) **blastospores,** which are formed by the budding process by which yeasts reproduce asexually (some yeasts, eg, *C albicans,* can form multiple buds that do not detach, thus producing sausagelike chains called **pseudohyphae,** which can be used for identification); and (4) **sporangiospores,** which are formed within a sac (sporangium) on a stalk by molds such as *Rhizopus* and *Mucor.*

Although this book focuses on the fungi that are human pathogens, it should be remembered that fungi are used in the production of important foods, eg, bread, cheese, wine, and beer. Fungi are

---

*Chitin is a homopolymer of *N*-acetylglucosamine.
†The term "spores" can be replaced by "conidia," eg, arthroconidia.

Table 47–1. Comparison of fungi and bacteria.

Feature	Fungi	Bacteria
Diameter	Approximately 4 μm (*Candida*)	Approximately 1 μm (*Staphylococcus*)
Nucleus	Eukaryotic	Prokaryotic
Cytoplasm	Mitochondria and endoplasmic reticulum present	Mitochondria and endoplasmic reticulum absent
Cell membrane	Sterols present	Sterols absent (except *Mycoplasma*)
Cell wall content	Chitin	Peptidoglycan
Spores	Sexual and asexual spores for reproduction	Endospores for survival, not for reproduction
Thermal dimorphism	Yes (some)	No
Metabolism	Require organic carbon; no obligate anaerobes	Many do not require organic carbon; many obligate anaerobes

also responsible for the spoilage of certain foods. Because molds can grow in a drier, more acidic, and higher-osmotic-pressure environment than bacteria, they tend to be involved in the spoilage of fruits, grains, vegetables, and jams.

PATHOGENESIS

The response to infection with many fungi is the formation of **granulomas.** Granulomas are produced in the major systemic fungal diseases, eg, coccidioidomycosis, histoplasmosis, and blastomycosis, as well as several others. The cell-mediated immune response is involved in granuloma formation. Acute suppuration, characterized by the presence of neutrophils in the exudate, also occurs in certain fungal diseases such as aspergillosis and sporotrichosis. Fungi do not have endotoxin in their cell walls and do not produce bacterial-type exotoxins.

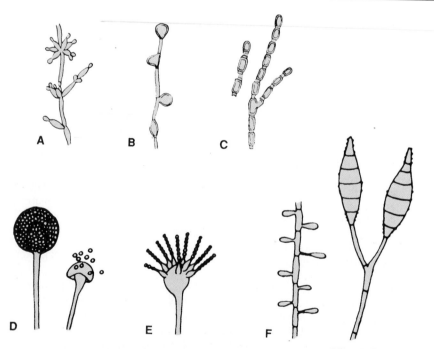

Figure 47–1. Asexual spores. **A:** Blastoconidia and pseudohyphae (*Candida*). **B:** Chlamydospores (*Candida*). **C:** Arthrospores (*Coccidioides*). **D:** Sporangia and sporangiospores (*Mucor*). **E:** Microconidia (*Aspergillus*). **F:** Microconidia and macroconidia (*Microsporum*). (Modified and reproduced, with permission, from Conant NF et al: *Manual of Clinical Mycology,* 3rd ed. Saunders, 1971.)

Activation of the cell-mediated immune system results in a **delayed hypersensitivity skin test** response to certain fungal antigens injected intradermally. A positive skin test indicates exposure to the fungal antigen. It does *not* imply current infection, because the exposure may have occurred in the past. A negative skin test makes the diagnosis unlikely unless the patient is immunocompromised. Because most people carry *Candida* as part of the normal flora, skin testing with *Candida* antigens can be used to determine whether cell-mediated immunity is normal.

The transmission and geographic locations of some important fungi are described in Table 47–2.

Intact skin is an effective host defense against certain fungi (eg, *Candida,* dermatophytes), but if the skin is damaged, organisms can become established. Fatty acids in the skin inhibit dermatophyte growth, and hormone-associated skin changes at puberty limit ringworm of the scalp caused by *Trichophyton.* The normal flora of the skin and mucous membranes suppress fungi. When the normal flora is inhibited, eg, by antibiotics, overgrowth of fungi such as *C albicans* can occur.

In the respiratory tract, the important host defenses are the mucous membranes of the nasopharynx, which trap inhaled fungal spores, and alveolar macrophages. Circulating IgG and IgM are produced in response to fungal infection, but their role in protection from disease is uncertain. The cell-mediated immune response is protective; its suppression can lead to reactivation and dissemination of asymptomatic fungal infections and to disease caused by opportunistic fungi.

FUNGAL TOXINS & ALLERGIES

In addition to mycotic infections, there are two other kinds of fungal disease: (1) **mycotoxicoses,** caused by ingested toxins, and (2) **allergies** to fungal spores. The best-known mycotoxicosis occurs after eating *Amanita* mushrooms. These fungi produce five toxins, two of which—amanitin and phalloidin—are among the most potent hepatotoxins. Another mycotoxicosis, ergotism, is caused by the mold *Claviceps purpura,* which infects grains and produces alkaloids (eg, ergotamine and lysergic acid diethylamide [LSD]) that cause pronounced vascular and neurologic effects. Other ingested toxins, **aflatoxins,** are coumarin derivatives produced by *Aspergillus flavus* that cause liver damage and tumors in animals and are suspected of causing hepatic carcinoma in humans. Aflatoxins are ingested with spoiled grains and peanuts and are metabolized by the liver to the epoxide, a potent carcinogen. Allergies to fungal spores, particularly those of *Aspergillus,* are manifested primarily by an asthmatic reaction (rapid bronchoconstriction mediated by IgE), eosinophilia, and a "wheal and flare" immediate skin test reaction.

LABORATORY DIAGNOSIS

There are four approaches to the laboratory diagnosis of fungal diseases: (1) direct microscopic examination, (2) culture of the organism, (3) DNA probe tests, and (4) serologic tests. Direct micro-

Table 47–2. Transmission and location of some important fungi.

Genus	Habitat	Form of Organism Transmitted	Portal of Entry	Endemic Geographic Location
Coccidioides	Soil	Arthrospores	Inhalation into lungs	Southwestern United States and Latin America
Histoplasma	Soil (associated with bird feces)	Microconidia	Inhalation into lungs	Mississippi and Ohio River valleys in United States; many other countries
Blastomyces	Soil	Microconidia	Inhalation into lungs	States east of Mississippi River in United States; Africa
Paracoccidioides	Soil	Uncertain	Inhalation into lungs	Latin America
Cryptococcus	Soil (associated with pigeon feces)	Yeast	Inhalation into lungs	Worldwide
Aspergillus	Soil and vegetation	Conidia	Inhalation into lungs	Worldwide
Candida	Human body	Yeast	Normal flora of skin, mouth, gastrointestinal tract, and vagina	Worldwide

scopic examination of clinical specimens such as sputum, lung biopsy material, and skin scrapings depends on finding characteristic asexual spores, hyphae, or yeasts in the light microscope. The specimen is either treated with 10% KOH to dissolve tissue material, leaving the alkali-resistant fungi intact, or stained with special fungal stains. Some examples of diagnostically important findings made by direct examination are (1) the spherules of *Coccidioides immitis* and (2) the wide capsule of *Cryptococcus neoformans* seen in India ink preparations of spinal fluid. Calciflor white is a fluorescent dye that binds to fungal cell walls and is useful in the identification of fungi in tissue specimens.

Tests involving DNA probes can identify colonies growing in culture at an earlier stage of growth than can tests based on visual detection of the colonies. As a result, the diagnosis can be made more rapidly. At present, DNA probe tests are available for *Coccidioides, Histoplasma, Blastomyces,* and *Cryptococcus.*

Fungi are frequently cultured on Sabouraud's agar, which facilitates the appearance of the slow-growing fungi by inhibiting the growth of bacteria in the specimen. Inhibition of bacterial growth is due to the low pH of the medium and to the chloramphenicol and cycloheximide that are frequently added. The appearance of the mycelium and the nature of the asexual spores are frequently sufficient to identify the organism.

Tests for the presence of antibodies in the patient's serum or spinal fluid are useful in diagnosing the systemic mycoses but less so in diagnosing other fungal infections. As is the case for bacterial and viral serologic testing, a significant rise in the antibody titer must be observed to confirm a diagnosis. The complement fixation test is most frequently used in suspected cases of coccidioidomycosis, histoplasmosis, and blastomycosis. In cryptococcal meningitis, the presence of the polysaccharide capsular antigens of *Cryptococcus neoformans* in the spinal fluid can be detected by the latex agglutination test.

ANTIFUNGAL THERAPY

The drugs used to treat bacterial diseases have no effect on fungal diseases. For example, penicillins and aminoglycosides inhibit the growth of many bacteria but do not affect the growth of fungi. This difference is explained by the presence of certain structures in bacteria, eg, peptidoglycan and 70S ribosomes, that are absent in fungi.

The most effective antifungal drugs exploit the presence of **ergosterol** in fungal cell membranes that is not found in bacterial or human cell membranes. These drugs, ie, amphotericin B and the various azoles, are discussed in Chapter 10. There is no clinically significant resistance to antifungal drugs.

Review Questions

1. How do fungal and bacterial cell walls differ?
2. How do fungal and human cell membranes differ?
3. Describe dimorphism.
4. In general, what is the natural habitat of fungi? How does *Candida albicans* differ?
5. Contrast sexual and asexual reproduction of fungi.
6. Describe budding in yeasts.
7. What type of lesions are formed in most of the systemic fungal diseases? What is the pathogenesis of these lesions?
8. In the laboratory diagnosis of fungi, why is Sabouraud's agar used?
9. Why is amphotericin B selectively toxic for fungi?

Cutaneous & Subcutaneous Mycoses 48

Medical mycoses can be divided into four categories: (1) **cutaneous,** (2) **subcutaneous,** (3) **systemic,** and (4) **opportunistic.** Some features of the important fungal diseases are described in Table 48–1. Cutaneous and subcutaneous mycoses are discussed below; systemic and opportunistic mycoses are discussed in later chapters.

CUTANEOUS MYCOSES

Dermatophytoses   Dermatophytoses are caused by fungi (**dermatophytes**) that infect only superficial keratinized structures (skin, hair, and nails), not deeper tissues. The most important dermatophytes are classified in three genera: *Epidermophyton, Trichophyton,* and *Microsporum.* They are spread from infected persons by direct contact. *Microsporum* is also spread from animals such as dogs and cats. This indicates that to prevent reinfection, the animal must be treated also.

Dermatophytoses (tinea, ringworm) are chronic infections favored by heat and humidity, eg, athlete's foot and jock itch.* They are characterized by pruritic papules and vesicles, broken hairs, and thickened, broken nails. *Trichophyton tonsurans* is the most common cause of outbreaks of tinea capitis in children and is the main cause of endothrix (inside the hair) infections. *T rubrum* is also a very common cause of tinea capitis. *T schoenleinii* is the cause of favus, a form of tinea capitis in which crusts are seen on the scalp.

In some infected persons, hypersensitivity causes **dermatophytid ("id")** reactions, eg, vesicles on the fingers. Id lesions are a response to circulating fungal antigens; the lesions do not contain hyphae. Patients with tinea infections show positive skin tests with fungal extracts, eg, trichophytin.

Scrapings of skin or nail placed in 10% KOH on a glass slide show hyphae under microscopy. Cultures on Sabouraud's agar at room temperature develop typical hyphae and conidia. Tinea capitis lesions caused by *Microsporum* species can be detected by seeing fluorescence when the lesions are exposed to ultraviolet light from a Wood's lamp. Treatment involves local antifungal creams (undecylenic acid, miconazole, tolnaftate, etc) or oral griseofulvin. Prevention centers on keeping skin dry and cool.

Tinea Versicolor   Tinea versicolor (pityriasis versicolor), a superficial skin infection of cosmetic importance only, is caused by *Malassezia furfur.* The lesions are usually noticed as hypopigmented areas, especially on tanned skin in the summer. There may be slight scaling or itching, but usually the infection is asymptomatic. It occurs more frequently in hot, humid weather. The lesions contain both budding yeast cells and hyphae. Diagnosis is usually made by observing this mixture in KOH preparations of skin scrapings. Culture is not usually done. The treatment of choice is topical miconazole, but the lesions have a tendency to recur and a permanent cure is difficult to achieve.

Tinea Nigra   Tinea nigra is an infection of the keratinized layers of the skin. It appears as a brownish spot due to the melaninlike pigment in the hyphae. The causative organism, *Cladosporium werneckii,* is found in the soil and transmitted during injury. In the United States, the disease is seen in the southern states. Diagnosis is made by microscopic examination and culture of skin scrapings. The infection is treated with a topical keratolytic agent, eg, salicylic acid.

SUBCUTANEOUS MYCOSES

These are caused by fungi that grow in soil and on vegetation and are introduced into subcutaneous tissue through **trauma.**

---

*These infections are also known as tinea pedis and tinea cruris, respectively.

Table 48–1. Features of important fungal diseases.

Type	Anatomic Location	Representative Disease	Genus of Causative Organism(s)	Seriousness of Illness
Cutaneous	Dead layer of skin	Tinea versicolor	*Malassezia*	1 +
	Epidermis, hair, nails	Dermatophytosis (ringworm)	*Microsporum, Trichophyton, Epidermophyton*	2 +
Subcutaneous	Subcutis	Sporotrichosis	*Sporothrix*	2 +
		Mycetoma	Several genera	2 +
Systemic	Internal organs	Coccidioidomycosis	*Coccidioides*	4 +
		Histoplasmosis	*Histoplasma*	4 +
		Blastomycosis	*Blastomyces*	4 +
		Paracoccidioidomycosis	*Paracoccidioides*	4 +
Opportunistic	Internal organs	Cryptococcosis	*Cryptococcus*	4 +
		Candidiasis	*Candida*	2 + to 4 +
		Aspergillosis	*Aspergillus*	4 +
		Mucormycosis	*Mucor, Rhizopus*	4 +

Sporotrichosis   *Sporothrix schenckii* is a **dimorphic** fungus that lives on vegetation. When introduced into the skin, typically by a thorn, it causes a local pustule or ulcer with nodules along the draining lymphatics. There is little systemic illness. Lesions may be chronic.

In the clinical laboratory, round or cigar-shaped budding yeasts are seen in tissue specimens. In culture, hyphae occur bearing oval conidia in clusters at the tip of slender conidiophores (resembling a daisy). The disease is treated with itraconazole or oral potassium iodide. It can be prevented by protecting skin when touching plants, moss, and wood.

Chromomycosis   This is a slowly progressive granulomatous infection that is caused by several soil fungi (*Fonsecaea, Phialophora, Cladosporium,* etc) when introduced into the skin through trauma. These fungi are collectively called **dematiaceous** fungi, so named because they produce melanin-like pigments. Wartlike lesions with crusting abscesses extend along the lymphatics. The disease occurs mainly in the tropics and is found on bare feet and legs. In the clinical laboratory, dark brown, round fungal cells are seen in leukocytes or giant cells. The disease is treated with oral flucytosine or thiabendazole, plus local surgery.

Mycetoma   Soil organisms (*Petriellidium, Madurella*) enter through wounds on the feet, hands, or back and cause abscesses, with pus discharged through sinuses. The pus contains compact colored granules. Actinomycetes such as *Nocardia* can cause similar lesions (actinomycotic mycetoma). Sulfonamides may help the actinomycotic form. There is no effective drug against the fungal form; surgical excision is recommended.

Review Questions

1. Which part of the skin do the dermatophytes infect?
2. How are dermatophytes spread?
3. Describe the typical tinea lesion.
4. How is the diagnosis of tinea infections usually made?
5. What is the "id" reaction?
6. How is sporotrichosis acquired?

Systemic Mycoses

49

These infections result from **inhalation** of the spores of **dimorphic** fungi that have their saprophytic **mold** forms in the **soil.** Within the **lungs,** the spores differentiate into **yeasts** or other specialized forms. Most lung infections are asymptomatic and self-limited. However, some persons develop disseminated disease in which the organisms grow in other organs, cause destructive lesions, and may result in death. Infected persons do *not* communicate these diseases to others.

COCCIDIOIDES

Disease   *Coccidioides immitis* causes coccidioidomycosis.

Properties   *C immitis* is a **dimorphic** fungus that exists as a **mold** in soil and as a **spherule** in tissue (Fig 49–1).

Transmission & Epidemiology   The fungus is **endemic** in arid regions of the **southwestern United States** and **Latin America.** In soil, it forms hyphae with alternating **arthrospores** and empty cells. Arthrospores are very light and are carried by the wind. They can be **inhaled** and infect the lungs.

Pathogenesis   In the lungs, arthrospores form spherules that are large (30 μm in diameter), have a thick, doubly refractive wall, and are filled with **endospores.** Upon rupture of the wall, endospores are released and differentiate to form new spherules. The organism can spread within a person by direct extension or via the bloodstream. Granulomatous lesions can occur in virtually any organ but are found primarily in bones and the central nervous system (meningitis). **Dissemination** indicates some defect in cell-mediated immunity. Most persons who develop a positive skin test to infection develop immunity to spread and to reinfection. However, if their cellular immunity is suppressed by drugs or disease, dissemination can occur at any time.

Clinical Findings   Infection of the lungs is often asymptomatic and is evident only by a positive skin test and the presence of antibodies. Some infected persons have an influenzalike illness with fever and cough. About 50% have changes in the lungs as seen in x-rays, and 10% develop erythema nodosum (see below) or arthralgias. This syndrome is called "valley fever" (in the San Joaquin Valley of California) or "desert rheumatism" (in Arizona); it tends to subside spontaneously.

Disseminated disease can occur in almost any organ; the meninges, bone, and skin are important sites. The overall incidence of dissemination in persons infected with *C immitis* is 1%, although the incidence in Filipinos and African Americans is 10 times higher. Pregnant women in the third trimester also have a markedly increased incidence of dissemination.

Erythema nodosum (EN) manifests as red, tender nodules on extensor surfaces such as the shins. It is a delayed (cell-mediated) hypersensitivity response to fungal antigens and thus is an indicator of a good prognosis. There are no organisms in these lesions; they are not a sign of disseminated disease. EN is not specific for coccidioidomycosis; it occurs in other granulomatous diseases, eg, histoplasmosis, tuberculosis, and leprosy.

Laboratory Diagnosis   In tissue specimens, spherules are seen microscopically. Cultures on Sabouraud's agar incubated at 25 °C show hyphae with arthrospores. (*Caution:* Cultures are highly infectious; precautions against inhaling arthrospores must be taken.) In infected persons, **skin tests** with fungal extracts (coccidioidin or spherulin) cause at least a 5-mm induration 48 hours after injection (delayed hypersensitivity reaction). Skin tests become positive within 2–4 weeks of infection and remain so for years but are often negative (anergy) in patients with disseminated disease. In serologic tests, IgM and IgG precipitins appear within 2–4 weeks of infection and then decline in

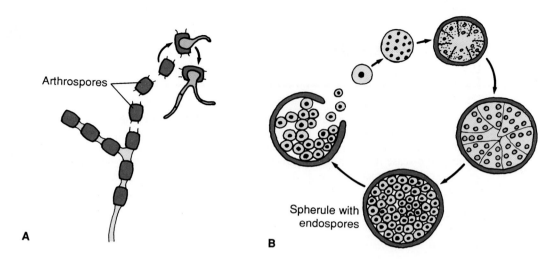

Arthrospores

Spherule with
endospores

A

B

Figure 49–1. Stages of *Coccidioides immitis*. **A:** Arthrospores form at the ends of hyphae in the soil. They germinate in the soil to form new hyphae. If inhaled, the arthrospores differentiate into spherules. **B:** Endospores form within spherules in tissue. When spherules rupture, endospores disseminate and form new spherules. (Modified and reproduced, with permission, from Brooks GF et al: *Medical Microbiology,* 20th ed. Appleton & Lange, 1995.)

subsequent months. Complement-fixing antibodies occur at low titer initially, but the titer rises greatly if dissemination occurs.

Treatment & Prevention   No treatment is needed in asymptomatic or mild primary infection. Amphotericin B (Fungizone) is used for persisting lung lesions or disseminated disease. Ketoconazole is also effective in lung disease. If meningitis occurs, fluconazole is the drug of choice. Intrathecal amphotericin B may be required and may induce remission, but long-term results are often poor. There are no means of prevention except avoiding travel to endemic areas.

HISTOPLASMA

Disease   *Histoplasma capsulatum* causes histoplasmosis.

Properties   *H capsulatum* is a **dimorphic** fungus that exists as a **mold** in soil and as a **yeast** in tissue. It forms two types of asexual spores (Fig 49–2): (1) **tuberculate macroconidia,** with typical

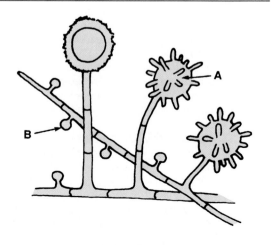

Figure 49–2. Asexual spores of *Histoplasma capsulatum*. **A:** Tuberculate macroconidia. **B:** Microconidia. (Reproduced, with permission, from Brooks GF et al: *Medical Microbiology,* 19th ed. Appleton & Lange, 1991.)

thick walls and fingerlike projections that are important in laboratory identification, and (2) **microconidia,** which are smaller, thin, smooth-walled spores that, if inhaled, transmit the infection.

Transmission & Epidemiology   This fungus occurs in many parts of the world. In the United States it is **endemic** in central and eastern states, especially in the **Ohio and Mississippi River valleys.** It grows in soil, particularly if the soil is heavily contaminated with **bird droppings,** especially from starlings. Although the birds are not infected, bats can be infected and can excrete the organism in their guano. In areas of endemic infection, excavation of the soil during construction or exploration of bat-infested caves has resulted in a significant number of infected individuals.

Pathogenesis & Clinical Findings   **Inhaled spores** are engulfed by **macrophages** and develop into yeast forms. In tissues, *H capsulatum* occurs as an **oval budding yeast inside macrophages** (Fig 49–3). The organisms spread widely throughout the body, especially to the liver and spleen, but most infections remain asymptomatic and the small granulomatous foci heal by calcification. With intense exposure (eg, in a chicken house or bat-infested cave), pneumonia may become clinically manifest. Severe disseminated histoplasmosis develops in a small minority of infected persons, especially infants and individuals with reduced cell-mediated immunity, such as AIDS patients. In AIDS patients, ulcerated lesions on the tongue are typical of disseminated histoplasmosis.

Laboratory Diagnosis   In tissue biopsy specimens or bone marrow aspirates, oval yeast cells **within macrophages** are seen microscopically. Cultures on Sabouraud's agar show hyphae with tuberculate macroconidia. Tests that detect *Histoplama* antigens by radioimmunoassay and *Histoplasma* RNA with DNA probes are also useful.

Two serologic tests are useful for diagnosis: complement fixation (CF) and immunodiffusion (ID). An antibody titer of 1:32 in the CF test with yeast phase antigens is considered to be diagnostic. However, cross-reactions with other fungi, especially *Blastomyces,* occur. CF titers fall when the disease becomes inactive and rise in disseminated disease. The ID test detects precipitating antibodies (precipitins) by forming two bands, M and H, in an agar-gel diffusion assay. The ID test is more specific but less sensitive than the CF test.

A skin test using histoplasmin (a mycelial extract) becomes positive, ie, shows at least 5 mm of induration, within 2–3 weeks after infection and remains positive for many years. However, because there are many false-positive reactions (due to cross-reactivity) and many false-negative reactions (in disseminated disease), the skin test is not useful for diagnosis. Furthermore, the skin test can stimulate an antibody response and confuse the serological tests. The skin test is useful for epidemiologic studies, and up to 90% of individuals are positive in areas of endemic infection.

Treatment & Prevention   No therapy is needed in asymptomatic or mild primary infections. With progressive lung lesions, oral itraconazole is beneficial. In disseminated disease, amphotericin B is the treatment of choice. In meningitis, fluconazole is often used because it penetrates the spinal fluid well. Oral itraconazole is used to treat pulmonary or disseminated disease, as well as for chronic suppression in patients with AIDS. There are no means of prevention except avoiding exposure in areas of endemic infection.

BLASTOMYCES

Disease   *Blastomyces dermatitidis* causes blastomycosis, also known as North American blastomycosis.

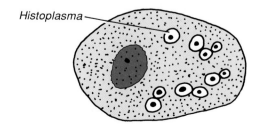

Figure 49–3. *Histoplasma capsulatum.* Yeasts are located within the macrophage. (Reproduced, with permission, from Brooks GF et al: *Medical Microbiology,* 19th ed. Appleton & Lange, 1991.)

Properties   *B dermatitidis* is a **dimorphic** fungus that exists as a mold in soil and as a yeast in tissue. The yeast is round with a doubly refractive wall and a single **broad-based bud** (Fig 49–4).

Transmission & Epidemiology   This fungus is **endemic** in **North and Central America** and in Africa. It grows in moist soil rich in organic material, forming hyphae with small pear-shaped conidia. Inhalation of the conidia causes human infection.

Pathogenesis & Clinical Findings   Infection occurs mainly via the respiratory tract. Asymptomatic or mild cases are rarely recognized. Dissemination may result in ulcerated granulomas of skin, bone, or other sites.

Laboratory Diagnosis   In tissue biopsy specimens, thick-walled yeast cells with single broad-based buds are seen microscopically. Hyphae with small pear-shaped conidia are visible on culture. The skin test lacks specificity and has little value. Serologic tests have little value.

Treatment & Prevention   Itraconazole is the drug of choice for most patients, but amphotericin B should be used to treat severe disease. Surgical excision may be helpful. There are no means of prevention.

PARACOCCIDIOIDES

Disease   *Paracoccidioides brasiliensis* causes paracoccidioidomycosis, also known as South American blastomycosis.

Properties   *P brasiliensis* is a **dimorphic** fungus that exists as a mold in soil and as a yeast in tissue. The yeast is thick-walled with **multiple buds,** in contrast to *B dermatitidis,* which has a single bud (Fig 49–5).

Transmission & Epidemiology   This fungus grows in the soil and is endemic in rural Latin America. Disease occurs only in that region.

Pathogenesis & Clinical Findings   The spores are **inhaled,** and early lesions occur in the lungs. Asymptomatic infection is common. Alternatively, oral mucous membrane lesions, lymph node enlargement, and sometimes dissemination to many organs develops.

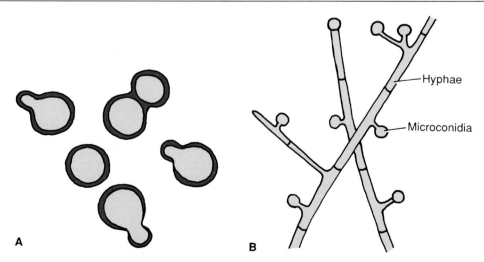

Figure 49–4. *Blastomyces dermatidis.* **A:** Yeast with a broad-based bud at 37 °C. **B:** Mold with microconidia at 20 °C. (Reproduced, with permission, from Brooks GF et al: *Medical Microbiology,* 19th ed. Appleton & Lange, 1991.)

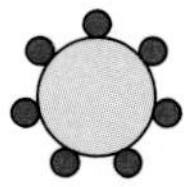

Figure 49–5. *Paracoccidioides brasiliensis.* Note the multiple buds of the yeast form of *Paracoccidioides,* in contrast to the single bud of *Blastomyces.*

Laboratory Diagnosis   In pus or tissues, yeast cells with multiple buds are seen microscopically. A specimen cultured for 2–4 weeks may grow typical organisms. Skin tests are rarely helpful. Serologic testing shows that when significant antibody titers (by immunodiffusion or complement fixation) are found, active disease is present.

Treatment & Prevention   The drug of choice is itraconazole taken orally for several months. There are no means of prevention.

Review Questions

In regard to coccidioidomycosis, histoplasmosis, and blastomycosis:
1. Which of the causative organisms are dimorphic?
2. What is the geographic distribution of the disease?
3. How is the infection acquired? What is the site of the initial lesions?
4. What is the morphology of the organism in the body?
5. What is the role of skin tests?
6. What is the role of complement-fixing antibodies?
7. What is the treatment for mild primary disease? for disseminated disease?

Opportunistic Mycoses

50

Opportunistic fungi fail to induce disease in most normal persons but may do so in those with **impaired** host defenses.

CANDIDA

Diseases   *Candida albicans,* the most important species of *Candida,* causes thrush, vaginitis, and chronic mucocutaneous candidiasis, as well as other diseases.

Properties   *C albicans* is an **oval yeast with a single bud.** It is part of the **normal flora** of mucous membranes of the upper respiratory, gastrointestinal, and female genital tracts. In tissues it may appear as yeasts or as **"pseudohyphae"** (Fig 50–1). Pseudohyphae are elongated yeasts that visually resemble hyphae but are not true hyphae. Carbohydrate fermentation reactions differentiate it from other species, eg, *Candida tropicalis, Candida parapsilosis, Candida krusei,* and *Torulopsis glabrata.*

Transmission   As a member of the normal flora, it is not transmitted.

Pathogenesis & Clinical Findings   When local or systemic host defenses are impaired, disease may result. Overgrowth of *C albicans* in the mouth produces white patches (thrush). Vulvovaginitis with itching and discharge is favored by high pH, diabetes, or use of antibiotics. Skin invasion occurs in warm, moist areas, which be-come red and weeping. Fingers and nails become involved when repeatedly immersed in water; persons employed as dishwashers in restaurants and institutions are commonly affected. Thickening or loss of the nail can occur. In immunosuppressed individuals, *Candida* may disseminate to many organs or cause chronic mucocutaneous candidiasis. Intravenous drug abuse and hyperalimentation also predispose to disseminated candidiasis, especially right-sided endocarditis. *C albicans* is the most common species to cause disseminated disease in these patients, but *C tropicalis* and *C parapsilosis* are important pathogens also.

Laboratory Diagnosis   In exudates or tissues, budding yeasts and pseudohyphae are seen microscopically. Such specimens grow typical yeasts when cultured. **Germ tubes** form in serum at 37 °C, which serves to distinguish *C albicans* from most other *Candida* species (Fig 50–1). **Chlamydospores** are typically formed by *C albicans* but not by other species of *Candida*. Serologic testing is rarely helpful.

Skin tests with *Candida* antigens are uniformly positive in normal adults and are used as an indicator of competent cellular immunity. A person who does not respond to *Candida* antigens in the skin test is presumed to have deficient cell-mediated immunity. Such a person is **anergic,** and other skin tests cannot be interpreted. Thus, if a person has a negative *Candida* skin test, a negative PPD skin test for tuberculosis could be a false-negative result.

Treatment & Prevention   The drug of choice for oropharyngeal or esophageal thrush is fluconazole. Treatment of skin infections consists of topical antifungal drugs, eg, clotrimazole or nystatin. Mucocutaneous candidiasis can be controlled by ketoconazole. Treatment of disseminated candidiasis consists of either amphotericin B or fluconazole. These two drugs can be used with or without flucytosine. Treatment of candidal infections with antifungal drugs should be supplemented by reduction of predisposing factors. Certain candidal infections, eg, thrush, can be prevented by oral clotrimazole troches or nystatin "swish and swallow." There is no vaccine.

CRYPTOCOCCUS

Disease   *Cryptococcus neoformans* causes cryptococcosis, especially cryptococcal meningitis.

Properties   *C neoformans* is an **oval, budding yeast** surrounded by a **wide polysaccharide capsule** (Fig 50–2). It is not dimorphic.

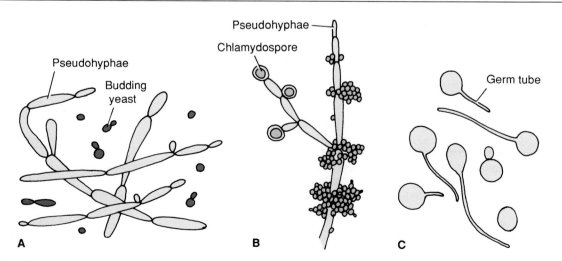

Figure 50–1. *Candida albicans.* **A:** Budding yeasts and pseudohyphae in tissues or exudate. **B:** Pseudohyphae and chlamydospores in culture at 20 °C. **C:** Germ tubes at 37 °C. (Reproduced, with permission, from Brooks GF et al: *Medical Microbiology,* 20th ed. Appleton & Lange, 1995.)

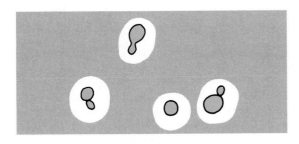

Figure 50–2. *Cryptococcus neoformans.* India ink preparation shows budding yeasts with a wide capsule. India ink forms a dark background; it does not stain the yeast itself. (Reproduced, with permission, from Brooks GF et al: *Medical Microbiology,* 19th ed. Appleton & Lange, 1991.)

Transmission   This yeast occurs widely in nature and grows abundantly in **soil containing bird (especially pigeon) droppings.** The birds are not infected. Human infection results from **inhalation** of the organism. There is no human-to-human transmission.

Pathogenesis & Clinical Findings   Lung infection is often asymptomatic or may produce pneumonia. Disease occurs mainly in patients with reduced cell-mediated immunity, especially AIDS patients, in whom the organism disseminates to the central nervous system (meningitis) and other organs. However, roughly half the patients with cryptococcal meningitis fail to show evidence of immunosuppression.

Laboratory Diagnosis   In spinal fluid mixed with **India ink,** the yeast cell is seen microscopically surrounded by a wide, unstained capsule. The organism can be cultured from spinal fluid and other specimens. Serologic tests can be done for both antibody and antigen. In infected spinal fluid, **capsular antigen** occurs in high titer and can be detected by the **latex particle agglutination** test.

Treatment & Prevention   Combined treatment with amphotericin B and flucytosine is used in meningitis or other disseminated disease. There are no specific means of prevention. Fluconazole is used in AIDS patients for long-term suppression of cryptococcal meningitis.

ASPERGILLUS

Disease   *Aspergillus* species, especially *Aspergillus fumigatus,* cause infections of the skin, eyes, ears, and other organs; "fungus ball" in the lungs; and allergic bronchopulmonary aspergillosis.

Properties   *Aspergillus* species exist **only as molds;** they are not dimorphic. They have **septate hyphae** that form V-shaped (dichotomous) branches (Fig 50–3). The walls are more or less parallel, in contrast to *Mucor* and *Rhizopus* walls, which are irregular (Fig 50–3; also see below). The conidia of *Aspergillus* form radiating chains, in contrast to those of *Mucor* and *Rhizopus,* which are enclosed within a sporangium (Fig 50–4; also see below).

Transmission   These molds are widely distributed in nature. They grow on decaying vegetation, producing chains of conidia. Transmission is by **airborne conidia.**

Pathogenesis & Clinical Findings   *Aspergillus fumigatus* can colonize and later invade abraded skin, wounds, burns, the cornea, the external ear, or paranasal sinuses. In immunocompromised persons, especially those with neutropenia, it can invade the lungs and other organs, producing hemoptysis and granulomas. Aspergilli can grow in pulmonary cavities (eg, those due to tuberculosis) and produce an aspergilloma (**"fungus ball"**), which can be seen on x-ray. Allergic bronchopulmonary aspergillosis (ABPA) is an infection of the bronchi by *Aspergillus* species. Patients with ABPA have asthmatic symptoms and a high IgE titer against *Aspergillus* antigens, and they expectorate bronchial plugs containing hyphae. Asthma caused by the inhalation of airborne conidia, especially in certain occupational settings, also occurs. *Aspergillus flavus* growing on cereals or nuts produces aflatoxins that may be carcinogenic or acutely toxic.

Laboratory Diagnosis   Biopsy specimens show **septate, branching hyphae** invading tissue (Fig 50–3). Cultures show colonies with characteristic radiating chains of conidia (Fig 50–4). How-

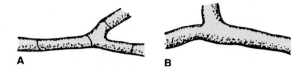

Figure 50–3. *Aspergillus* and *Mucor* in tissue. **A:** *Aspergillus* has septate hyphae with V-shaped branching. **B:** *Mucor* has nonseptate hyphae with right-angle branching.

ever, positive cultures do not prove disease because colonization is common. In persons with invasive aspergillosis, there may be high titers of galactomannan antigen in serum. Patients with ABPA have high levels of IgE specific for *Aspergillus* antigens. IgG precipitins are also present.

Treatment & Prevention   Invasive aspergillosis is treated with amphotericin B, but results may be poor. A fungus ball growing in a sinus or in a pulmonary cavity can be surgically removed. Patients with ABPA can be treated with steroids and antifungal agents. There are no specific means of prevention.

MUCOR & RHIZOPUS

Mucormycosis (zygomycosis, phycomycosis) is a disease caused by saprophytic **molds** (eg, *Mucor, Rhizopus,* and *Absidia*) found widely in the environment. They are not dimorphic. These organisms are transmitted by airborne asexual spores and invade tissues of patients with reduced host defenses. They proliferate in the walls of blood vessels, particularly of the paranasal sinuses, lungs, or gut, and cause infarction and necrosis of tissue distal to the blocked vessel. Patients with **diabetic ketoacidosis,** burns, or leukemias are particularly susceptible. In biopsy specimens, organisms are seen microscopically as **nonseptate hyphae** with broad, irregular walls and branches that form more or less at right angles. Cultures show colonies with spores contained within a sporangium. If diagnosis is made early, treatment of the underlying disorder, plus administration of amphotercin B and surgical removal of necrotic infected tissue, has resulted in some remissions and cures.

PSEUDALLESCHERIA BOYDII

Pseudallescheria boydii is a mold that causes disease primarily in immunocompromised patients. The clinical findings and the microscopic appearance of the septate hyphae in tissue closely resemble those of *Aspergillus.* In culture, the appearance of the conidia (pear-shaped) and the color of the mycelium (brownish-gray) of *P boydii* are different from those of *Aspergillus.* The drug of choice is either ketoconazole or itraconazole because the response to amphotercin B is poor. Debridement of necrotic tissue is important as well.

PNEUMOCYSTIS

Pneumocystis carinii is classified as a yeast on the basis of molecular analysis, but medically it is still considered a member of the protozoa. It is therefore discussed in Chapter 52 with the blood and tissue protozoa.

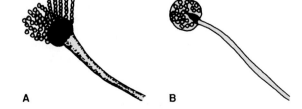

Figure 50–4. *Aspergillus* and *Mucor* in culture. **A:** *Aspergillus* spores form in radiating columns. **B:** *Mucor* spores are contained within a sporangium.

Review Questions

1. Where is *Candida albicans* usually found as part of the normal flora?
2. What factors predispose to candidal invasion or infection?
3. Contrast the appearance of *C albicans* when it is part of the normal flora and when it is the cause of invasive disease.
4. What is the role of serologic and skin tests in the diagnosis of candidiasis?
5. What is the most striking structural feature of *Cryptococcus neoformans?*
6. What are the natural habitat and mode of transmission of *C neoformans?*
7. What is the main predisposing factor to cryptococcal meningitis?
8. Which two tests are used in the diagnosis of cryptococcal meningitis?
9. Contrast the appearance of (a) hyphae and (b) spores of *Aspergillus* and *Mucor.*
10. What are the predisposing factors to aspergillosis? To mucormycosis?

Part VI: Parasitology

Parasites occur in two distinct forms: single-celled **protozoa** and multicellular metazoa called **helminths** or worms. For medical purposes, protozoa can be subdivided into four groups: Sarcodina (amebas), Sporozoa (sporozoans), Mastigophora (flagellates), and Ciliata (ciliates). Metazoa are subdivided into two phyla: the Platyhelminthes (flatworms) and the Nemathelminthes (roundworms or nematodes). The phylum Platyhelminthes contains two medically important classes: Cestoda (tapeworms) and Trematoda (flukes). This classification is diagrammed in Fig 1.

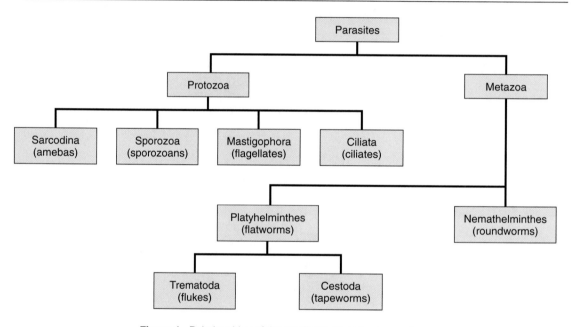

Figure 1. Relationships of the medically important parasites.

51   Intestinal & Urogenital Protozoa

In this book, the major protozoan pathogens are grouped according to the location in the body where they most frequently cause disease. The intestinal and urogenital protozoa are described in this chapter, and the blood and tissue protozoa are described in Chapter 52.

(1) Within the intestinal tract, three organisms—the ameba *Entamoeba histolytica,* the flagellate *Giardia lamblia,* and the sporozoan *Cryptosporidium* species—are the most important.

(2) In the urogenital tract, the flagellate *Trichomonas vaginalis* is the important pathogen.

(3) The blood and tissue protozoa are a varied group consisting of the flagellates *Trypanosoma* and *Leishmania* and the sporozoans *Plasmodium* and *Toxoplasma*. The important opportunistic lung pathogen *Pneumocystis* will be discussed in this group, although there is recent molecular evidence that it should be classified as a fungus.

The major and minor pathogenic protozoa are listed in Table 51–1.

Although immigrants and Americans returning from abroad can present to physicians in the United States with any parasitic disease, certain parasites are much more likely to occur outside the United States. The features of the medically important protozoa, including their occurrence in the United States, are described in Table 51–2.

Intestinal Protozoa

ENTAMOEBA

Diseases   *Entamoeba histolytica* causes amebic dysentery and liver abscess.

Important Properties   The life cycle of *E histolytica* has two stages: the motile **ameba (trophozoite)** and the nonmotile **cyst** (Fig 51–1A and B). The trophozoite is found within the intestinal and extraintestinal lesions and in diarrheal stools. The cyst predominates in nondiarrheal stools. These cysts are not highly resistant and are readily killed by boiling but not by chlorination of water supplies. They are removed by filtration of water.

The cyst has **four nuclei,** an important diagnostic criterion. Upon excystation in the intestinal tract, an ameba with four nuclei emerges and then divides to form eight trophozoites. The mature

Table 51–1. Major and minor pathogenic protozoa.

Type and Location	Species	Disease
Major protozoa Intestinal tract	*Entamoeba histolytica* *Giardia lamblia* *Cryptosporidium parvum*	Ambiasis Giardiasis Cryptosporidiosis
Urogenital tract	*Trichomonas vaginalis*	Trichomoniasis

Blood and tissue	*Plasmodium* species
	Toxoplasma gondii
	Pneumocystis carinii
	Trypanosoma species
	    T cruzi
	    T gambiense[1]
	    T rhodesiense[1]
	Leishmania species
	    L donovani
	    L tropica
	    L mexicana
	    L braziliensis
		Malaria
		Toxoplasmosis
		Pneumonia
		Trypanosomiasis
		    Chagas' disease
		    Sleeping sickness
		    Sleeping sickness
		Leishmaniasis
		    Kala-azar
		    Cutaneous leishmaniasis[2]
		    Cutaneous leishmaniasis[2]
		    Mucocutaneous leishmaniasis

Minor protozoa Intestinal tract	*Balantidium coli* *Isospora belli* *Enterocytozoon bienusi* *Septata intestinalis* *Cyclospora cayetanensis*	Dysentery Isosporosis Microsporidiosis Microsporidiosis Cyclosporiasis
Blood and tissue	*Naegleria* species *Acanthamoeba* species *Babesia microti*	Meningitis Meningitis Babesiosis

[1]Also known as *T brucei gambiense* and *T brucei rhodesiense,* respectively.
[2]*L tropica* and *L mexicana* cause Old World and New World cutaneous leishmaniasis, respectively.

Table 51–2. Features of medically important protozoa.

Organism	Mode of Transmission	Occurrence in United States	Diagnosis	Treatment
Entamoeba	Ingestion of cysts in food.	Yes	Trophozoites or cysts in stool; serology.	Metronidazole plus iodoquinol.
Giardia	Ingestion of cysts in food.	Yes	Trophozoites or cysts in stools.	Metronidazole.
Cryptosporidium	Ingestion of cysts in food.	Yes	Cysts on acid-fast stain.	None.
Trichomonas	Sexual.	Yes	Trophozoites in wet mount.	Metronidazole.
Trypanosoma T cruzi	Reduviid bug.	Rare	Blood smear, bone marrow, xenodiagnosis.	Nifurtimox.
T gambiense, T rhodesiense	Tsetse fly.	No	Blood smear.	Suramin.[1]
Leishmania L donovani	Sand fly.	No	Bone marrow, spleen, or lymph node.	Stibogluconate.
L tropica, L mexicana, L braziliensis	Sand fly.	No	Fluid from lesion.	Stibogluconate.
Plasmodium P vivax, P ovale, P malariae	Anopheles mosquito.	Rare	Blood smear.	Chloroquine; also primaquine for P vivax and P ovale.
P falciparum	Anopheles mosquito.	No	Blood smear.	Chloroquine; mefloquine or quinine, sulfadoxine, and pyrimethamine if resistant.
Toxoplasma	Ingestion of cysts in raw meat; contact with soil contaminated by cat feces.	Yes	Serology; microscopic examination of tissue; mouse inoculation.	Sulfonamide and pyrimethamine for congenital disease and immunocompromised patients.
Pneumocystis	Inhalation.	Yes	Lung biopsy or lavage.	Trimethoprim-sulfamethoxazole. Also pentamidine or atovaquone.

[1]Melarsoprol is used if the central nervous system is involved.

trophozoite has a single nucleus with an even lining of peripheral chromatin and a prominent central nucleolus (karyosome).

Antibodies are formed against trophozoite antigens in invasive amebiasis, but they are not protective; prior infection does not prevent reinfection. The antibodies are useful, however, for serologic diagnosis.

Pathogenesis & Epidemiology   The organism is acquired by ingestion of cysts that are transmitted primarily by the **fecal-oral** route in contaminated food and water. Anal-oral transmission, eg, among male homosexuals, also occurs. There is **no animal reservoir.** The ingested cysts differentiate into trophozoites in the ileum but tend to colonize the cecum and colon.

The trophozoites invade the colonic epithelium and secrete enzymes that cause localized necrosis. Little inflammation occurs at the site. As the lesion reaches the muscularis layer, a typical **"teardrop" ulcer** forms that can undermine and destroy large areas of the intestinal epithelium. Progression into the submucosa leads to invasion of the portal circulation by the trophozoites. By far the most frequent site of systemic disease is the **liver,** where abscesses form.

Infection by *E histolytica* is found worldwide but occurs most frequently in tropical countries, especially in areas with poor sanitation. About 1–2% of people in the United States are affected. The disease is widely prevalent among male homosexuals.

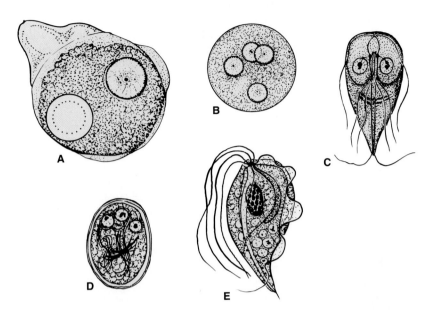

Figure 51–1. **A:** *E histolytica* trophozoite with one ingested red blood cell and one nucleus (circle with inner dotted line represents a red blood cell). **B:** *E histolytica* cyst with four nuclei. **C:** *G lamblia* trophozoite. **D:** *G lamblia* cyst. **E:** *T vaginalis* trophozoite. 1200 ×.

Clinical Findings   Acute intestinal amebiasis presents as **dysentery** (ie, bloody, mucus-containing diarrhea) accompanied by lower abdominal discomfort, flatulence, and tenesmus. Chronic amebiasis with low-grade symptoms such as occasional diarrhea, weight loss, and fatigue also occurs. Roughly 90% of those infected are asymptomatic carriers, whose feces contain cysts that can be transmitted to others.

   Amebic abscess of the liver is characterized by right-upper-quadrant pain, weight loss, fever, and a tender, enlarged liver. Right-lobe abscesses can penetrate the diaphragm and cause lung disease. Most cases of amebic liver abscess occur in patients who have not had overt intestinal amebiasis.

Laboratory Diagnosis   Diagnosis of intestinal amebiasis rests on finding either trophozoites in diarrheal stools or cysts in formed stools. Diarrheal stools should be examined within 1 hour of collection to see the ameboid motility of the trophozoite. Trophozoites characteristically contain ingested red blood cells. The most common error is to mistake fecal leukocytes for trophozoites. Because cysts are passed intermittently, at least three specimens should be examined. About half of the patients with extraintestinal amebiasis have negative stool examinations.

   E histolytica can be distinguished from other amebas by two major criteria. (1) The first is the nature of the **nucleus** of the trophozoite. The *E histolytica* nucleus has a small central nucleolus and fine chromatin granules along the border of the nuclear membrane. The nuclei of other amebas are quite different. (2) The second is **cyst size and number of its nuclei.** Mature cysts of *E histolytica* are smaller than those of *Entamoeba coli* and contain four nuclei, whereas *Entamoeba coli* cysts have eight nuclei.

   A complete examination for cysts includes a wet mount in saline, an iodine-stained wet mount, and a fixed, trichrome-stained preparation, each of which brings out different aspects of cyst morphology. These preparations are also helpful in distinguishing amebic from bacillary dysentery. In the latter, many inflammatory cells such as polymorphonuclear leukocytes are seen, whereas in amebic dysentery they are not.

   Serologic testing is useful for the diagnosis of invasive amebiasis. The indirect hemagglutination test is usually positive in patients with invasive disease but is frequently negative in asymptomatic individuals who are passing cysts.

Treatment   The treatment of choice for symptomatic intestinal amebiasis or hepatic abscesses is metronidazole (Flagyl) plus iodoquinol. Hepatic abscesses need not be drained. Asymptomatic cyst carriers should be treated with iodoquinol.

Prevention   Prevention involves avoiding fecal contamination of food and water and observing good personal hygiene such as hand-washing. Purification of municipal water supplies is usually effective, but outbreaks of amebiasis in city dwellers still occur when contamination is heavy. The use of "night soil" (human feces) for fertilization of crops should be prohibited. In areas of endemic infection, vegetables should be cooked.

GIARDIA

Disease   *Giardia lamblia* causes giardiasis.

Important Properties   The life cycle consists of two stages, the **trophozoite** and the **cyst** (Fig 51–1C and D). The trophozoite is pear-shaped with two nuclei, four pairs of flagella, and a suction disk with which it attaches to the intestinal wall. The oval cyst is thick-walled with four nuclei and several internal fibers. Each cyst gives rise to two trophozoites during excystation in the intestinal tract.

Pathogenesis & Epidemiology   Transmission occurs by ingestion of the cyst in **fecally contaminated** food and water. Excystation takes place in the duodenum, where the trophozoite attaches to the gut wall but does *not* invade. The trophozoite causes inflammation of the duodenal mucosa, leading to **malabsorption** of protein and fat.

The organism is found worldwide; about 5% of stool specimens in the United States contain *Giardia* cysts. Approximately half of those infected are asymptomatic carriers, who continue to excrete the cysts for years. IgA deficiency greatly predisposes to symptomatic infection.

In addition to being endemic, giardiasis occurs in outbreaks related to contaminated water supplies. Chlorination does not kill the cysts, but filtration removes them. Hikers who drink untreated stream water are frequently infected. Many species of mammals as well as humans act as the reservoirs. They pass cysts in the stool and contaminate water sources. Giardiasis is common in male homosexuals as a result of oral-anal contact. The incidence is high among children in day-care centers and among patients in mental hospitals.

Clinical Findings   **Nonbloody, foul-smelling diarrhea** is accompanied by nausea, anorexia, flatulence, and abdominal cramps persisting for weeks or months. There is no fever.

Laboratory Diagnosis   Diagnosis is made by finding trophozoites or cysts or both in diarrheal stools. In formed stools, eg, in asymptomatic carriers, only cysts are seen.

If microscopic examination of the stool is negative, the **string test,** which consists of swallowing a weighted piece of string until it reaches the duodenum, should be performed. The trophozoites adhere to the string and can be visualized after withdrawal of the string. No serologic test is available.

Treatment   The treatment of choice is metronidazole (Flagyl) or quinacrine hydrochloride.

Prevention   Prevention involves drinking boiled, filtered, or iodine-treated water in endemic areas and while hiking. No prophylactic drug or vaccine is available.

CRYPTOSPORIDIUM

Disease   *Cryptosporidium parvum* causes cryptosporidiosis, the main symptom of which is diarrhea. The diarrhea is most severe in **immunocompromised** patients, eg, those with AIDS.

Important Properties   Some aspects of the life cycle remain uncertain, but the following stages have been identified. Oocysts release sporozoites, which form trophozoites. Several stages ensue, involving the formation of schizonts and merozoites. Eventually microgametes and macrogametes form; these unite to produce a zygote, which differentiates into an oocyst. This cycle has several features in common with other sporozoa, eg, *Isospora*. Taxonomically, *Cryptosporidium* is in the subclass Coccidia.

Pathogenesis & Epidemiology   The organism is acquired by **fecal-oral** transmission of oocysts from either human or animal sources. The oocysts excyst in the small intestine, where the trophozoites (and other forms) attach to the gut wall. Invasion does not occur. The jejunum is the site most heavily infested. The pathogenesis of the diarrhea is unknown; no toxin has been identified.

Cryptosporidia cause diarrhea worldwide. Large outbreaks of diarrhea caused by cryptosporidia in several cities in the United States are attributed to inadequate purification of drinking water.

Clinical Findings   The disease in immunocompromised patients presents primarily as a watery, nonbloody **diarrhea** causing large fluid loss. Symptoms persist for long periods in immunocompromised patients, whereas they are self-limited in immunocompetent patients. Although immunocompromised patients usually do not die of cryptosporidiosis, the fluid loss and malnutrition are severely debilitating.

Laboratory Diagnosis   Diagnosis is made by finding oocysts in fecal smears when using a modified Kinyoun **acid-fast** stain. Serologic tests are not available.

Treatment & Prevention   There is no effective drug therapy. There is no vaccine or other specific means of prevention. Purification of the water supply, including filtration to remove the cysts, which are resistant to the chlorine used for disinfection, can prevent cryptosporidiosis.

Urogenital Protozoa

TRICHOMONAS

Disease   *Trichomonas vaginalis* causes trichomoniasis.

Important Properties   *T vaginalis* is a pear-shaped organism with a central nucleus and four anterior flagella (Fig 51–1E). It has an undulating membrane that extends about two-thirds of its length. It exists **only as a trophozoite;** there is no cyst form.

Pathogenesis & Epidemiology   The organism is transmitted by sexual contact, and hence there is no need for a durable cyst form. The primary locations of the organism are the vagina and the prostate.

Trichomoniasis is one of the most common infections worldwide. Roughly 25–50% of women in the United States harbor the organism. The frequency of symptomatic disease is highest among sexually active women in their 30s and lowest in postmenopausal women.

Clinical Findings   In women, a watery, foul-smelling, greenish discharge accompanied by itching and burning occurs. Infection in men is usually asymptomatic, but about 10% of infected men have urethritis.

Laboratory Diagnosis   In a wet mount of vaginal (or prostatic) secretions, the pear-shaped trophozoites have a typical jerky motion. There is no serologic test.

Treatment & Prevention   The drug of choice is metronidazole (Flagyl) for both partners to prevent reinfection. Maintenance of the low pH of the vagina is helpful. Condoms limit transmission. No prophylactic drug or vaccine is available.

Review Questions

1. What are the three important protozoa that cause intestinal tract disease?
2. What are the two stages in the life cycle of *Entamoeba histolytica?* of *Giardia lamblia?*

3. How is *E histolytica* transmitted? *G lamblia?* Is there an animal reservoir for either?
4. How is the laboratory diagnosis made for *E histolytica?* for *G lamblia?* How is *E histolytica* distinguished from *Entamoeba coli?*
5. How is *Cryptosporidium* transmitted? Is there an animal reservoir?
6. How is the laboratory diagnosis of cryptosporidiosis made?
7. What is the life cycle of *Trichomonas vaginalis?*
8. How is *T vaginalis* transmitted?
9. How is the laboratory diagnosis of trichomoniasis made?

52

Blood & Tissue Protozoa

The medically important organisms in this category of protozoa consist of the sporozoans *Plasmodium* and *Toxoplasma* and the flagellates *Trypanosoma* and *Leishmania*. *Pneumocystis* is discussed in this book as a protozoan because it is considered as such from a medical point of view. However, molecular data indicate that it is related to yeasts such as *Saccharomyces cerevisiae*.

PLASMODIUM

Disease   Malaria is caused by four plasmodia: *Plasmodium vivax, Plasmodium ovale, Plasmodium malariae,* and *Plasmodium falciparum. P vivax* and *P falciparum* are more common causes of malaria than are *P ovale* and *P malariae*.

Important Properties   The vector and definitive host for plasmodia is the **female *Anopheles* mosquito** (only the female takes a blood meal). There are two phases in the life cycle: the sexual cycle, which occurs primarily in mosquitoes, and the asexual cycle, which occurs in humans, the intermediate hosts.* The sexual cycle is called **sporogony** because sporozoites are produced, and the asexual cycle is called **schizogony** because schizonts are made.

The life cycle in humans begins with the introduction of sporozoites into the blood from the saliva of the biting mosquito. The sporozoites are taken up by hepatocytes within 30 minutes. This "exoerythrocytic" phase consists of cell multiplication and differentiation into **merozoites.** *P vivax* and *P ovale* produce a latent form **(hypnozoite)** in the liver; this form is the cause of relapses seen with vivax and ovale malaria.

Merozoites are released from the liver cells and infect red blood cells. During the erythrocytic phase, the organism differentiates into a ring-shaped trophozoite (Fig 52–1A–F). The ring form grows into an ameboid form and then differentiates into a schizont filled with merozoites. After release, the merozoites infect other erythrocytes. This cycle in the red blood cell repeats at regular intervals typical for each species. The periodic release of merozoites causes the typical recurrent symptoms of chills, fever, and sweats seen in malaria patients.

The sexual cycle begins in the human red blood cells when some merozoites develop into male and others into female gametocytes. The gametocyte-containing red blood cells are ingested by the female *Anopheles* mosquito and, within her gut, produce a female macrogamete and eight spermlike male microgametes. After fertilization, the diploid zygote differentiates into a motile ookinete that burrows into the gut wall, where it grows into an oocyst within which many haploid sporozoites are produced. The sporozoites are released and migrate to the salivary glands, ready to complete the cycle when the mosquito takes her next blood meal.

---

*The sexual cycle is initiated in humans with the formation of gametocytes within red blood cells (gametogony) and completed in mosquitoes with the fusion of the male and female gametes, oocyst formation, and production of many sporozoites (sporogony).

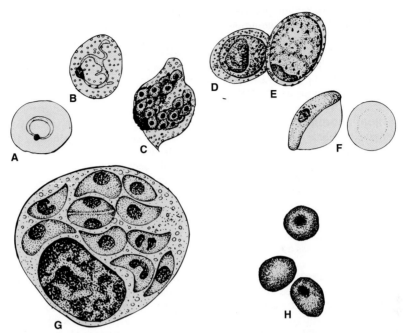

Figure 52–1. **A:** *P vivax* signet-ring trophozoite within a red blood cell. **B:** *P vivax* ameboid trophozoite within a red blood cell, showing Schüffner's dots. **C:** *P vivax* mature schizont with merozoites inside. **D:** *P vivax* microgametocyte. **E:** *P vivax* macrogametocyte. **F:** *P falciparum* "banana-shaped" gametocyte with attached red cell ghost. **G:** *T gondii* trophozoites within macrophage. **H:** *P carinii* cysts stained with methenamine-silver. **A–G,** 1200 ×; **H,** 800 ×.

Pathogenesis & Epidemiology Most of the pathologic findings of malaria are due to the **destruction of red blood cells.** Not only does the parasite rupture erythrocytes upon release of the merozoites, but the spleen sequesters and destroys many red cells also. The enlarged spleen characteristic of malaria is due to congestion of sinusoids with erythrocytes, coupled with hyperplasia of lymphocytes and macrophages.

Malaria caused by *P falciparum* is **more severe** than that caused by other plasmodia. It is characterized by infection of far more red cells than the other malarial species and by occlusion of the capillaries with aggregates of parasitized red cells. This leads to life-threatening hemorrhage and necrosis, particularly in the brain (cerebral malaria). Furthermore, extensive hemolysis and kidney damage occur, with resulting hemoglobinuria. The dark color of the patient's urine has given rise to the term "blackwater fever."

The timing of the fever cycle is 72 hours for *P malariae* and 48 hours for the other plasmodia. Disease caused by *P malariae* is called quartan malaria because it recurs every fourth day, whereas malaria caused by the others is called tertian malaria because it recurs every third day. Tertian malaria is subdivided into malignant malaria, caused by *P falciparum,* and benign malaria, caused by *P vivax* and *P ovale.*

P falciparum causes a high level of parasitemia, because it can infect red cells of all ages. In contrast, *P vivax* infects only reticulocytes and *P malariae* infects only mature red cells; therefore they produce much lower levels of parasites in the blood. Individuals with sickle cell trait (heterozygotes) are protected against malaria because their red cells have too little ATPase activity and cannot produce sufficient energy to support the growth of the parasite. People with homozygous sickle cell anemia are also protected but rarely live long enough to obtain much benefit.

Malaria is transmitted primarily by mosquito bites, but transmission across the placenta, in blood transfusions, and by intravenous drug abuse also occurs.

Partial immunity based on humoral antibodies that block merozoites from invading the red cells occurs in infected individuals. A low level of parasitemia and low-grade symptoms result; this condition is known as premunition.

More than 200 million people worldwide have malaria, and more than 1 million die from it each year, making it the most common lethal infectious disease. It occurs primarily in tropical and subtropical areas, especially in Asia, Africa, and Central and South America. Malaria in the United States is seen in Americans who travel to areas of endemic infection without adequate chemoprophylaxis and in immigrants from areas of endemic infection. It is not endemic in the United States. Certain regions in Southeast Asia, South America, and east Africa are particularly affected by chloroquine-resistant strains of *P falciparum*.

Clinical Findings   Malaria presents with abrupt onset of fever and chills, accompanied by headache, myalgias, and arthralgias, about 2 weeks after the mosquito bite. Fever may be continuous early in the disease; the typical periodic cycle does not develop for several days after onset. The fever spike, which can reach 41 °C, is frequently accompanied by nausea, vomiting, and abdominal pain. The fever is followed by drenching sweats. Splenomegaly is seen in most patients, and hepatomegaly occurs in roughly one-third. Anemia is prominent.

Untreated malaria caused by *P falciparum* is potentially life-threatening as a result of extensive brain and kidney damage. Malaria caused by the other three plasmodia is usually self-limited, with a low mortality rate. However, relapses of *P vivax* and *P ovale* malaria can occur up to several years after the initial illness as a result of hypnozoites latent in the liver.

Laboratory Diagnosis   Diagnosis rests on microscopic examination of blood, using both **thick** and **thin** Giemsa-stained smears. The thick smear is used to screen for the presence of organisms, and the thin smear is used for species identification. It is important to identify the species, because the treatment of different species can differ. Ring-shaped trophozoites can be seen within infected red blood cells. The gametocytes of *P falciparum* are crescent-shaped ("banana-shaped"), whereas those of the other plasmodia are spherical (Fig 52–1F).

Treatment   Chloroquine is the drug of choice for acute malaria caused by sensitive strains. Chloroquine kills the merozoites, thereby reducing the parasitemia, but does not affect the hypnozoites of *P vivax* and *P ovale* in the liver. These are killed by primaquine, which must be used to prevent relapses. For chloroquine-resistant strains of *P falciparum,* either mefloquine or a combination of quinine and Fansidar (sulfadoxine and pyrimethamine) is used.

Prevention   **Chemoprophylaxis** of malaria for travelers to areas where *P falciparum* is endemic consists of either mefloquine or a combination of chloroquine plus Fansidar, although the possibility of serious side effects resulting from the prolonged use of Fansidar limits its use as a prophylactic drug. Travelers to areas where the other plasmodia are found should take chloroquine starting 2 weeks before arrival and continuing for 6 weeks after departure. This should be followed by a 2-week course of primaquine if exposure was high.

Other preventive measures include the use of mosquito netting, window screens, protective clothing, and insect repellents. The mosquitoes feed from dusk to dawn, so protection is particularly important during the night. Communal preventive measures are directed against reducing the mosquito population. Many insecticide sprays, such as DDT, are no longer effective because the mosquitoes have developed resistance. Drainage of stagnant water in swamps and ditches reduces the breeding areas. There is no vaccine.

TOXOPLASMA

Disease   *Toxoplasma gondii* causes toxoplasmosis.

Important Properties   The definitive host is the **domestic cat** and other felines; humans and other mammals are intermediate hosts. Infection of humans begins with the **ingestion of cysts** in undercooked meat or from contact with cat feces. In the small intestine, the cysts rupture and release forms that invade the gut wall, where they are ingested by macrophages and differentiate into rapidly multiplying trophozoites **(tachyzoites),** which kill the cells and infect other cells (Fig 52–1G). Cell-mediated immunity usually limits the spread of tachyzoites, and the parasites enter host cells in the brain, muscle, and other tissues, where they develop into cysts in which the parasites multiply slowly. These forms are called **bradyzoites.** These tissue cysts are both an important diagnostic feature and a source of organisms when the tissue cyst breaks in an immunocompromised patient.

The cycle within the cat begins with the ingestion of cysts in raw meat, eg, mice. Bradyzoites are released from the cysts in the small intestine, infect the mucosal cells, and differentiate into male and female gametocytes, whose gametes fuse to form oocysts that are excreted in cat feces. The cycle is completed when soil contaminated with cat feces is accidentally ingested. Human infection usually occurs from eating undercooked meat, eg, lamb and pork, from animals that grazed in soil contaminated with infected cat feces.

Pathogenesis & Epidemiology   *T gondii* is usually acquired by **ingestion; transplacental transmission** from an infected mother to the fetus occurs also. Human-to-human transmission, other than transplacental transmission, does not occur. Following infection of the intestinal epithelium, the organisms spread to other organs, especially the brain, lungs, liver, and eyes. Progression of the infection is usually limited by a competent immune system. **Cell-mediated immunity** plays the major role, but circulating antibody enhances killing of the organism. Most initial infections are asymptomatic. When contained, the organisms persist as cysts within tissues. There is no inflammation, and the individual remains well unless immunosuppression allows activation of organisms in the cysts.

Congenital infection of the fetus occurs **only** when the mother is infected during pregnancy. If she is infected before the pregnancy, the organism will be in the cyst form and there will be no trophozoites to pass the placenta. The mother who is reinfected during pregnancy but who has immunity from a previous infection will not transmit the organism to her child. Roughly one-third of mothers infected during pregnancy give birth to infected infants, but only 10% of these infants are symptomatic.

Infection by *T gondii* occurs worldwide. Serologic surveys reveal that in the United States antibodies are found in 5–50% of people in various regions. Infection is usually sporadic, but outbreaks due to ingestion of raw meat or contaminated water occur. Approximately 1% of domestic cats in the United States shed *Toxoplasma* cysts.

Clinical Findings   Most primary infections in immunocompetent adults are asymptomatic, but some resemble infectious mononucleosis, except that the heterophil antibody test is negative. Congenital infection can result in abortion, stillbirth, or neonatal disease with encephalitis, **chorioretinitis,** and hepatosplenomegaly. Fever, jaundice, and **intracranial calcifications** are also seen. Most infected newborns are asymptomatic, but some will develop chorioretinitis or mental retardation months or years later. In immunosuppressed patients, life-threatening disseminated disease, primarily encephalitis, occurs.

Laboratory Diagnosis   For the diagnosis of acute and congenital infections, an immunofluorescence assay for **IgM antibody** is used. IgM is used to diagnose congenital infection, because IgG can be maternal in origin. Tests of IgG antibody can be used to diagnose acute infections if a significant rise in antibody titer in paired sera is observed.

Microscopic examination of Giemsa-stained preparations shows crescent-shaped trophozoites during acute infections. Cysts may be seen in the tissue. The organism can be grown in cell culture. Inoculation into mice can confirm the diagnosis.

Treatment   Congenital toxoplasmosis, whether symptomatic or asymptomatic, should be treated with a combination of sulfadiazine and pyrimethamine. These drugs also constitute the treatment of choice for disseminated disease in immunocompromised patients. Acute toxoplasmosis in an immunocompetent individual is usually self-limited, but any patient with chorioretinitis should be treated.

Prevention   The most effective means of preventing toxoplasmosis is to cook meat thoroughly to kill the cysts. Pregnant women should be especially careful to avoid undercooked meat and contact with cats. They should refrain from emptying cat litter boxes. Cats should not be fed raw meat.

PNEUMOCYSTIS

Disease   *Pneumocystis carinii* is an important cause of pneumonia in immunocompromised individuals.

Important Properties   The classification and life cycle of *Pneumocystis* are unclear. An analysis of rRNA sequences published in 1988 indicates that *Pneumocystis* should be classified as a **fungus** related to yeasts such as *Saccharomyces cerevisiae.* Subsequent analysis of mitochondrial DNA and of various enzymes supports the idea that it is a fungus. However, medically, it is still thought of as a protozoan. The findings that it does not grow on fungal media and that antifungal drugs are ineffective have delayed acceptance of its classification as a fungus. The organism has been found in domestic animals such as horses and sheep and in a variety of rodents, but it is not known whether these animals form a reservoir for human infection.

Pathogenesis & Epidemiology   Transmission occurs by **inhalation,** and infection is prominent in the lungs. The organism is *not* transmitted from person to person. The presence of cysts in the alveoli induces an inflammatory response, resulting in a frothy exudate that blocks oxygen exchange. The organism does not invade the lung tissue. Pneumonia occurs when host defenses, eg, the number of helper T cells, are reduced. This accounts for the prominence of *Pneumocystis* pneumonia in patients with AIDS and in premature or debilitated infants.

P carinii is distributed worldwide; perhaps 70% of people have been infected. Most 5-year-old children in the United States have antibodies to this organism. Asymptomatic infection is therefore quite common. Prior to the advent of immunosuppressive therapy, *Pneumocystis* pneumonia was rarely seen in the United States. Its incidence has paralleled the increase in immunosuppression and the rise in the number of AIDS cases.

Clinical Findings   The sudden onset of fever, cough, dyspnea, and tachypnea is typical of *Pneumocystis* pneumonia. Bilateral rales and rhonchi are heard, and the chest x-ray shows a diffuse interstitial pneumonia. In infants, the disease usually has a more gradual onset. Extrapulmonary *Pneumocystis* infections occur in the late stages of AIDS and affect primarily the liver, spleen, lymph nodes, and bone marrow. The mortality rate of untreated *Pneumocystis* pneumonia approaches 100%, but with treatment about half survive the first episode.

Laboratory Diagnosis   Diagnosis is made by microscopic examination of lung tissue obtained by bronchoscopy, bronchial lavage, or open lung biopsy. Sputum is usually less suitable. The cysts can be visualized with methenamine-silver, Giemsa, or other tissue stains (Fig 52–1H). Fluorescent-antibody staining is also commonly used for diagnosis. The organism stains poorly with Gram's stain. There is no serologic test, and the organism has not been grown in culture.

Treatment   The treatment of choice is a combination of trimethoprim and sulfamethoxazole. Pentamidine and atovaquone are alternative drugs.

Prevention   Trimethoprim-sulfamethoxazole or aerosolized pentamidine can be used as **chemoprophylaxis** in immunosuppressed patients.

TRYPANOSOMA

The genus *Trypanosoma* includes three major pathogens: *Trypanosoma cruzi, Trypanosoma gambiense,* and *Trypanosoma rhodesiense.**

1.   Trypanosoma cruzi

Disease   T cruzi is the cause of Chagas' disease (American trypanosomiasis).

Important Properties   The life cycle involves the **reduviid bug** (*Triatoma,* cone-nose or kissing bug) as the vector and both humans and animals as reservoir hosts. The animal reservoirs include domestic cats and dogs and wild species such as the armadillo, raccoon, and rat. The cycle in the reduviid bug begins with ingestion of trypomastigotes in the blood of the reservoir host. In the insect gut, they multiply and differentiate first into epimastigotes and then into trypomastigotes. When the bug bites again, the site is contaminated with feces containing trypomastigotes, which enter the blood of the per-

---

*Taxonomically, the last two organisms are morphologically identical species called *T brucei gambiense* and *T brucei rhodesiense,* but the shortened names are used here.

son (or other reservoir) and form nonflagellated amastigotes within host cells. Many cells can be affected, but myocardial, glial, and reticuloendothelial cells are the most frequent sites. To complete the cycle, amastigotes differentiate into trypomastigotes, which enter the blood and are taken up by the reduviid bug (Fig 52–2A–C).

Pathogenesis & Epidemiology   Chagas' disease occurs primarily in rural Central and South America and rarely in the southern United States. The reduviid bug lives in the walls of rural huts and feeds at night. It bites preferentially around the mouth or eyes, hence the name "kissing bug."

The amastigotes can kill cells and cause inflammation, consisting mainly of mononuclear cells. **Cardiac muscle** is the most frequently and severely affected tissue. In addition, neuronal damage leads to cardiac arrhythmias and loss of tone in the colon (**megacolon**) and esophagus (**megaesophagus**). During the acute phase, there are both trypomastigotes in the blood and amastigotes intracellularly in the tissues. In the chronic phase, the organism persists in the amastigote form.

Clinical Findings   The acute phase of Chagas' disease consists of facial edema and a nodule (chagoma) near the bite, coupled with fever, lymphadenopathy, and hepatosplenomegaly. The acute phase resolves in about 2 months. Most individuals then remain asymptomatic, but some progress to the chronic form with myocarditis and megacolon. Death from chronic Chagas' disease is usually due to cardiac arrhythmias and failure.

Laboratory Diagnosis   Acute disease is diagnosed by demonstrating the presence of trypomastigotes in thick or thin films of the patient's blood. Both stained and wet preparations should be examined, the latter for motile organisms. Because the trypomastigotes are not numerous in the blood, other diagnostic methods may be required, namely, (1) a stained preparation of a bone marrow aspirate or muscle biopsy specimen (which may reveal amastigotes); (2) culture of the organism on special medium; and (3) **"xenodiagnosis,"** which consists of allowing an uninfected, laboratory-raised reduviid bug to feed on the patient and, after several weeks, examining the intestinal contents of the bug for the organism.

Serologic tests can be helpful also. The indirect fluorescent-antibody test is the earliest to become positive. Indirect hemagglutination and complement fixation tests are also available. Diagnosis of chronic disease is difficult, because there are few trypomastigotes in the blood. Xenodiagnosis and serologic tests are used.

Treatment   The drug of choice for the acute phase is nifurtimox, which kills trypomastigotes in the blood but is much less effective against amastigotes in tissue. There is no effective drug against the chronic form.

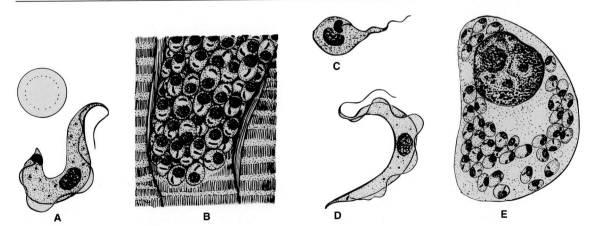

Figure 52–2. **A:** *T cruzi* trypomastigote found in human blood. 1200 ×. **B:** *T cruzi* amastigotes found in cardiac muscle. 850 ×. **C:** *T cruzi* epimastigote found in reduviid bug. 1200 ×. **D:** *T brucei gambiense* or *rhodesiense* trypomastigote found in human blood. 1200 ×. **E:** *L donovani* amastigotes within splenic macrophages. 1000 ×. (Circle with inner dotted line represents a red blood cell.)

Prevention   Prevention involves protection from the reduviid bite, improved housing, and insect control. No prophylactic drug or vaccine is available.

2. *Trypanosoma gambiense* & *Trypanosoma rhodesiense*

Disease   These pathogens cause sleeping sickness (African trypanosomiasis).

Important Properties   The morphology and life cycle of the two species are similar. The vector for both is the **tsetse fly,** *Glossina,* but different species of fly are involved for each. Humans are the reservoir for *T gambiense,* whereas *T rhodesiense* has reservoirs in both domestic animals, especially cattle, and wild animals, eg, antelopes.

The 3-week life cycle in the tsetse fly begins with ingestion of trypomastigotes in a blood meal from the reservoir host. They multiply in the insect gut and then migrate to the salivary glands, where they transform into epimastigotes, multiply further, and then form metacyclic trypomastigotes, which are transmitted by the tsetse fly bite. The organisms in the saliva are injected into the skin, where they enter the bloodstream, differentiate into blood-form trypomastigotes, and multiply, thereby completing the cycle (Fig 52–2D).

These trypanosomes exhibit remarkable **antigenic variation** of their surface glycoproteins, with hundreds of antigenic types found. One antigenic type will coat the surface of the parasites for approximately 10 days, followed by other types in sequence in the new progeny. This variation is due to sequential movement of the glycoprotein genes to a preferential location on the chromosome, where only that specific gene is transcribed into mRNA. These antigenic variations allow the organism to continually evade the host immune response.

Pathogenesis & Epidemiology   The trypomastigotes spread from the skin through the blood to the lymph nodes and the brain. The typical somnolence **(sleeping sickness)** progresses to coma as a result of a demyelinating encephalitis.

In the acute form, a cyclical fever spike (approximately every 2 weeks) occurs that is related to antigenic variation. As antibody-mediated agglutination and lysis of the trypomastigotes occur, the fever subsides. However, a few antigenic variants survive, multiply, and cause a new fever spike. This cycle repeats itself over a long period. The lytic antibody is directed against the surface glycoprotein.

The disease is endemic in sub-Saharan Africa, the natural habitat of the tsetse fly. Both sexes of fly take blood meals and can transmit the disease. The fly is infectious throughout its 2- to 3-month lifetime. *T gambiense* is the species that causes the disease along water courses in west Africa, whereas *T rhodesiense* is found in the arid regions of east Africa. Both species are found in central Africa.

Clinical Findings   Although both species cause sleeping sickness, the progress of the disease differs. *T gambiense*-induced disease runs a low-grade chronic course over a few years, whereas *T rhodesiense* causes a more acute, rapidly progressive disease that is usually fatal within several months.

The initial lesion is an indurated skin ulcer ("trypanosomal chancre") at the site of the fly bite. After the organisms enter the blood, intermittent weekly fever and lymphadenopathy develop. The encephalitis is characterized initially by headache, insomnia, and mood changes, followed by muscle tremors, slurred speech, and apathy that progress to somnolence and coma. Untreated disease is usually fatal as a result of pneumonia.

Laboratory Diagnosis   During the early stages, microscopic examination of the blood (either wet films or thick or thin smears) reveals trypomastigotes. An aspirate of the chancre or enlarged lymph node can also demonstrate the parasites. The presence of trypanosomes in the spinal fluid, coupled with an elevated protein level and pleocytosis, indicates that the patient has entered the late, encephalitic stage. Serologic tests, especially the ELISA for IgM antibody, can be helpful.

Treatment   Treatment must be initiated before the development of encephalitis, because suramin, the most effective drug, does not pass the blood-brain barrier well. Suramin will effect a cure if given early. Pentamidine is an alternative drug. If central nervous system symptoms are present, suramin (to clear the parasitemia) followed by melarsoprol should be given.

Prevention   The most important preventive measure is protection against the fly bite, using netting and protective clothing. Clearing the forest around villages and using insecticides are helpful. No vaccine is available.

LEISHMANIA

The genus *Leishmania* includes four major pathogens: *Leishmania donovani, Leishmania tropica, Leishmania mexicana,* and *Leishmania braziliensis.*

1. *Leishmania donovani*

Disease   *L donovani* is the cause of kala-azar (visceral leishmaniasis).

Important Properties   The life cycle involves the **sandfly*** as the vector and a variety of mammals such as dogs, foxes, and rodents as reservoirs. Only female flies are vectors because only they take blood meals (a requirement for egg maturation). When the sandfly sucks blood from an infected host, it ingests **macrophages containing amastigotes.**† After dissolution of the macrophages, the freed amastigotes differentiate into promastigotes in the gut. They multiply and then migrate to the pharynx, where they can be transmitted during the next bite. The cycle in the sandfly takes approximately 10 days.

Shortly after an infected sandfly bites a human, the promastigotes are engulfed by macrophages, where they transform into amastigotes (Fig 52–2E). The infected cells die and release progeny amastigotes that infect other macrophages and reticuloendothelial cells. The cycle is completed when the fly ingests macrophages containing the amastigotes.

Pathogenesis & Epidemiology   In visceral leishmaniasis, the organs of the **reticuloendothelial** system (liver, spleen, and bone marrow) are the most severely affected. Reduced bone marrow activity, coupled with cellular destruction in the spleen, results in anemia, leukopenia, and thrombocytopenia. This leads to secondary infections and a tendency to bleed. The striking **enlargement of the spleen** is due to a combination of proliferating macrophages and sequestered blood cells. The marked increase in IgG is neither specific nor protective.

Kala-azar occurs in three distinct epidemiologic patterns. In one area, which includes the Mediterranean basin, the Middle East, southern Russia, and parts of China, the reservoir hosts are primarily dogs and foxes. In sub-Saharan Africa, rats and small carnivores, eg, civets, are the main reservoirs. A third pattern is seen in India and neighboring countries (and Kenya), in which humans appear to be the only reservoir.

Clinical Findings   Symptoms begin with intermittent fever, weakness, and weight loss. Massive enlargement of the spleen is characteristic. Hyperpigmentation of the skin is seen in light-skinned patients (kala-azar means **"black sickness"**). The course of the disease runs for months to years. Initially, patients feel reasonably well despite persistent fever. As anemia, leukopenia, and thrombocytopenia become more profound, weakness, infection, and gastrointestinal bleeding occur. Untreated severe disease is nearly always fatal as a result of secondary infection.

Laboratory Diagnosis   Diagnosis is usually made by detecting amastigotes in a bone marrow, spleen, or lymph node biopsy or "touch" preparation. The organisms can also be cultured. Serologic (indirect immunofluorescence) tests are positive in most patients. Although not diagnostic, a very high concentration of IgG is indicative of infection. A skin test using a crude homogenate of promastigotes (leishmanin) as the antigen is available. The skin test is negative during active disease but positive in patients who have recovered.

Treatment   The treatment is sodium stibogluconate, a pentavalent antimony compound. With proper therapy, the mortality rate is reduced to near 5%. Recovery results in permanent immunity.

Prevention   Prevention involves protection from sandfly bites (use of netting, protective clothing, and insect repellents) and insecticide spraying.

---

*Phlebotomus species in the Old World; *Lutzomyia* species in South America.
†Amastigotes are nonflagellated, in contrast to promastigotes, which have a flagellum with a characteristic anterior kinetoplast.

2. *Leishmania tropica, Leishmania mexicana, & Leishmania braziliensis*

Disease *L tropica* and *L mexicana* both cause cutaneous leishmaniasis; the former organism is found in the Old World, whereas the latter is found only in the Americas. *L braziliensis* causes mucocutaneous leishmaniasis, which occurs only in Central and South America.

Important Properties Sandflies are the vectors for these three organisms, as they are for *L donovani,* and forest rodents are their main reservoirs. The life cycle of these parasites is essentially the same as that of *L donovani.*

Pathogenesis & Epidemiology The lesions are confined to the skin in cutaneous leishmaniasis and to the mucous membranes, cartilage, and skin in mucocutaneous leishmaniasis. A granulomatous response occurs, and a necrotic ulcer forms at the bite site. The lesions tend to become superinfected with bacteria.

Old World cutaneous leishmaniasis (Oriental sore, Delhi boil), caused by *L tropica,* is endemic in the Middle East, Africa, and India. New World cutaneous leishmaniasis (chicle ulcer, bay sore), caused by *L mexicana,* is found in Central and South America. Mucocutaneous leishmaniasis (espundia), caused by *L braziliensis,* occurs mostly in Brazil and Central America, primarily in forestry and construction workers.

Clinical Findings The initial lesion of cutaneous leishmaniasis is a red papule at the bite site, usually on an exposed extremity. This enlarges slowly to form multiple satellite nodules that coalesce and ulcerate. There is usually a single lesion that heals spontaneously in patients with a competent immune system. However, in certain individuals, if cell-mediated immunity does not develop, the lesions can spread to involve large areas of skin and contain enormous numbers of organisms. (Compare tuberculoid and lepromatous leprosy, Chapter 21.)

Mucocutaneous leishmaniasis begins with a papule at the bite site, but then metastatic lesions form, usually at the mucocutaneous junction of the nose and mouth. Disfiguring granulomatous, ulcerating lesions destroy nasal cartilage but not adjacent bone. These lesions heal slowly, if at all. Death can occur from secondary infection.

Laboratory Diagnosis Diagnosis is usually made microscopically by demonstrating the presence of **amastigotes** in a smear taken from the skin lesion. The leishmanin skin test becomes positive when the skin ulcer appears and can be used to diagnose cases outside the area of endemic infection.

Treatment The drug of choice is sodium stibogluconate, but the results are frequently unsatisfactory.

Prevention Prevention involves protection from sandfly bites by using netting, window screens, protective clothing, and insect repellents.

Review Questions

1. Distinguish between sporogony and schizogony in the life cycle of plasmodia.
2. What happens to the plasmodia during the (a) exoerythrocytic and (b) erythrocytic stages?
3. Where does the sexual cycle of plasmodia occur?
4. What is the main mode of transmission of plasmodia? their typical pathogenetic feature?
5. What is "blackwater fever"? Which *Plasmodium* species causes it? Why? How?
6. What causes the recurrent fever pattern seen in malaria?
7. How is the laboratory diagnosis of malaria made?
8. Describe the chemoprophylaxis of malaria and the problem of resistant strains.
9. Which animal is the reservoir for *Toxoplasma gondii?* How is it transmitted from animals to humans? What is the other important mode of transmission?
10. What are the differences between *Toxoplasma* infection in an immunocompetent adult and a newborn?

11. How is the laboratory diagnosis of toxoplasmosis made?
12. How can toxoplasmosis be prevented?
13. What is the mode of transmission of *Pneumocystis carinii?*
14. What is the predisposing factor to *Pneumocystis* pneumonia?
15. How is the laboratory diagnosis of *Pneumocystis* pneumonia made?
16. Which diseases are caused by *Trypanosoma cruzi? Trypanosoma gambiense?*
17. What is the vector for *T cruzi? T gambiense?*
18. In which geographic area does Chagas' disease primarily occur?
19. What is the pathogenesis of Chagas' disease? of sleeping sickness?
20. How is the laboratory diagnosis of these diseases made?
21. How do trypanosomes evade the host immune system?
22. Which diseases are caused by *Leishmania donovani? Leishmania tropica?*
23. What is the vector for *Leishmania* species?
24. In which geographic areas does kala-azar occur?
25. What types of cells are primarily affected in kala-azar? What is its pathogenesis?
26. How is the laboratory diagnosis of kala-azar made?

Minor Protozoan Pathogens 53

ACANTHAMOEBA & NAEGLERIA

Acanthamoeba and *Naegleria* are free-living **amebas** that cause **meningoencephalitis.** The organisms are found in warm freshwater lakes and in soil. Their life cycle involves trophozoite and cyst stages. Cysts are quite resistant and are not killed by chlorination.

Naegleria trophozoites usually enter the body through mucous membranes while an individual is **swimming.** They can penetrate the nasal mucosa and cribriform plate to produce a purulent meningitis and encephalitis that are usually rapidly fatal. *Acanthamoeba* is carried into the skin or eyes during trauma. *Acanthamoeba* infections occur primarily in immunocompromised individuals, whereas *Naegleria* infections occur in otherwise healthy persons, usually children. In the United States, these rare infections occur mainly in the southern states and California.

Diagnosis is made by finding amebas in the spinal fluid. The prognosis is poor even in treated cases. There is no effective therapy; occasionally, amphotericin B has resulted in recovery.

Acanthamoeba also causes keratitis, an inflammation of the cornea that occurs primarily in those who wear contact lenses.

BABESIA

Babesia microti causes babesiosis, a zoonosis acquired chiefly in the coastal areas and islands off the northeastern coast of the United States, eg, Nantucket Island. The sporozoan organism is endemic in rodents and is transmitted by the bite of the **tick** *Ixodes dammini* (renamed *I scapularis*), the same species of tick that transmits *Borrelia burgdorferi,* the agent of Lyme disease. *Babesia* infects red blood cells, causing them to lyse, but unlike plasmodia, it has no exoerythrocytic phase. Asplenic patients are affected more severely.

The influenzalike symptoms begin gradually and may last for several weeks. Hepatosplenomegaly and anemia occur. Diagnosis is made by seeing intraerythrocytic ring-shaped parasites on Giemsa-stained blood smears. Unlike the case with plasmodia, there is no pigment in the erythrocytes. Combined therapy with quinine and clindamycin may be effective. Prevention involves protection from tick bites and, if a person is bitten, prompt removal of the tick.

BALANTIDIUM

Balantidium coli is the **only ciliated protozoan** that causes human disease, ie, **diarrhea.** It is found worldwide but only infrequently in the United States. Domestic animals, especially pigs, are the main reservoir for the organism, and humans are infected after ingesting the cysts in food or water contaminated with animal or human feces. The trophozoites excyst in the small intestine, travel to the colon, and, by burrowing into the wall, cause an ulcer similar to that of *Entamoeba histolytica*. However, unlike the case with *E histolytica,* extraintestinal lesions do not occur.

Most infected individuals are asymptomatic; diarrhea rarely occurs. Diagnosis is made by finding large ciliated trophozoites or large cysts with a characteristic V-shaped nucleus in the stool. There are no serologic tests. The treatment of choice is tetracycline. Prevention consists of avoiding contamination of food and water by domestic-animal feces.

CYCLOSPORA

Cyclospora cayetanensis is an intestinal protozoan that causes watery diarrhea in both immunocompetent and immunocompromised individuals. It is classified as a member of the Coccidia.* The organism is acquired by fecal-oral transmission, especially via contaminated water supplies. One outbreak in the United States was attributed to the ingestion of contaminated raspberries. There is no evidence for an animal reservoir.

The diarrhea can be prolonged and relapsing, especially in immunocompromised patients. Infection occurs worldwide. The diagnosis is made microscopically by observing the spherical oocysts in a modified acid-fast stain of a stool sample. There are no serologic tests. The treatment of choice is trimethoprim-sulfamethoxazole.

ISOSPORA

Isospora belli is an intestinal protozoan that causes **diarrhea,** especially in **immunocompromised patients,** eg, those with AIDS. Its life cycle parallels that of other members of the Coccidia. The organism is acquired by fecal-oral transmission of oocysts from either human or animal sources. The oocysts excyst in the upper small intestine and invade the mucosa, causing destruction of the brush border.

The disease in immunocompromised patients presents as a chronic, profuse, watery diarrhea. The pathogenesis of the diarrhea is unknown. Diagnosis is made by finding the typical oocysts in fecal specimens. Serologic tests are not available. The treatment of choice is trimethoprim-sulfamethoxazole.

MICROSPORIDIA

Microsporidia are a group of protozoa characterized by obligate intracellular replication and spore formation. *Enterocytozoon bienusi* and *Septata intestinalis* are two important microsporidial species that cause severe, persistent, watery diarrhea in AIDS patients. The organisms are transmitted from human to human by the fecal-oral route. It is uncertain whether an animal reservoir exists. They are diagnosed by visualization of spores in stool samples or intestinal biopsy samples. The treatment of choice is albendazole.

---

*Coccidia is a subclass of Sporozoa.

Cestodes

54

Platyhelminthes (platy means flat; helminth means worm) are divided into two classes: Cestoda (tapeworms) and Trematoda (flukes). Tapeworms consist of a rounded head called a **scolex** and a flat body of multiple segments called **proglottids.** The scolex has specialized means of attaching to the intestinal wall, namely suckers, hooks, or sucking grooves. The worm grows by adding new proglottids from its germinal center next to the scolex. The oldest proglottids at the distal end are gravid and produce many eggs, which are excreted in the feces and transmitted to various intermediate hosts such as cattle, pigs, and fish. Humans usually acquire the infection when undercooked flesh containing the larvae is ingested. In certain instances, eg, cysticercosis and hydatid disease, the eggs are ingested and the resulting larvae cause the disease.

There are four medically important cestodes: *Taenia solium, Taenia saginata, Diphyllobothrium latum,* and *Echinococcus granulosus.* Their features are summarized in Table 54–1. Two cestodes of lesser importance, *Echinococcus multilocularis* and *Hymenolepis nana,* are described on p 297.

TAENIA

There are two important human pathogens in the genus *Taenia: T solium* (the pork tapeworm) and *T saginata* (the beef tapeworm).

1. Taenia solium

Diseases   The adult form of *T solium* causes taeniasis. *T solium* larvae cause cysticercosis.

Important Properties   *T solium* can be identified by its scolex with **four suckers and circle of hooks** and by its gravid proglottids, which have 5–10 primary uterine branches (Fig 54–1A and B). The eggs appear the same microscopically as those of *T saginata* and *Echinococcus* species (Fig 54–2A).

Humans are infected by eating raw or undercooked **pork** containing the larvae, called **cysticerci.** (A cysticercus consists of a pea-sized fluid-filled bladder with an invaginated scolex.) In the small intestine, the larvae attach to the gut wall and take about 3 months to grow into adult worms measuring up to 5 m. The gravid terminal proglottids detach daily, are passed in the feces, and are accidentally eaten by pigs. A six-hooked embryo (oncosphere) emerges from each egg in the pig's intestine. The embryos burrow into a blood vessel and are carried to skeletal muscle. They develop into cysticerci in the muscle, where they remain until eaten by a human. Humans are the definitive hosts, and pigs are the intermediate hosts.

A different and far more dangerous sequence occurs when a person **ingests the eggs** in food or water that has been fecally contaminated. The eggs hatch in the small intestine, and the oncospheres burrow through the wall into a blood vessel. They can disseminate to many organs, especially the eyes and brain, where they encyst to form cysticerci.

Pathogenesis & Epidemiology   The adult tapeworm attached to the intestinal wall causes little damage. The **cysticerci,** on the other hand, can become very large, especially in the **brain,** where they manifest as a **space-occupying lesion.** Living cysticerci do not cause inflammation, but when they die they can release substances that provoke an inflammatory response. Eventually, the cysticerci calcify and can be seen on x-ray.

The epidemiology of taeniasis and cysticercosis is related to the access of pigs to human feces and to consumption of raw or undercooked pork. The disease occurs worldwide but is endemic in areas of Asia, South America, and eastern Europe. Most cases in the United States are imported.

Clinical Findings   Most patients with adult tapeworms are asymptomatic, but anorexia and diarrhea can occur. Some may notice proglottids in the stools. Cysticercosis in the brain causes

Table 54–1. Features of medically important cestodes (tapeworms).

Cestode	Mode of Transmission	Intermediate Host(s)	Main Sites Affected in Human Body	Diagnosis	Treatment
Taenia solium	(A) Ingest larvae in undercooked pork	Pigs	Intestine	Proglottids in stool	Praziquantel
	(B) Ingest eggs in food or water contaminated with human feces		Brain and eyes (cysticerci)	Biopsy, CT scan	Praziquantel or surgical removal of cysticerci
Taenia saginata	Ingest larvae in undercooked beef	Cattle	Intestine	Proglottids in stool	Praziquantel
Diphyllobothrium latum	Ingest larvae in undercooked fish	Copepods and fish	Intestine	Operculated eggs in stool	Praziquantel
Echinococcus granulosus	Ingest eggs in food contaminated with dog feces	Sheep	Liver, lungs, and brain (hydatid cysts)	Biopsy, CT scan, serology	Albendazole or surgical removal of cyst

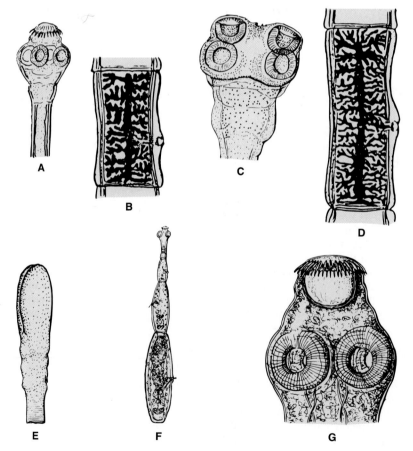

Figure 54–1. **A:** *T solium* scolex with suckers and hooks. 10 ×. **B:** *T solium* gravid proglottid. This has fewer uterine branches than does the proglottid of *T saginata* (see panel **D**). 2 ×. **C:** *T saginata* scolex with suckers. 10 ×. **D:** *T saginata* gravid proglottid. 2 ×. **E:** *D latum* scolex with sucking grooves. 7 ×. **F:** Entire adult worm of *E granulosus*. 7 ×. **G:** *E granulosis* adult scolex. 70 ×.

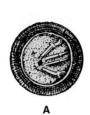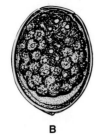

A   **B**

Figure 54–2. A: *T solium* egg containing oncosphere embryo. Four hooklets are visible. *T saginata* and *E granulosus* eggs are very similar to the *T solium* egg but do not have hooklets. **B:** *D latum* operculated egg. 300 ×.

headache, vomiting, and seizures. Cysticercosis in the eyes can appear as uveitis or retinitis, or the larvae can be visualized floating in the vitreous.

Laboratory Diagnosis   Identification of *T solium* consists of finding gravid proglottids with 5–10 primary uterine branches in the stools. In contrast, *T saginata* proglottids have 15–20 primary uterine branches. Eggs are found in the stools less often than are proglottids. Diagnosis of cysticercosis depends on demonstrating the presence of the cyst in tissue by x-ray or computed tomography (CT) scan.

Treatment   The treatment of choice for the intestinal worms is praziquantel. Although asymptomatic, patients should be treated to prevent autoinfection with the eggs, leading to cysticercosis. The treatment for cysticercosis is praziquantel, but surgical excision may be necessary. Albendazole is an alternative to praziquantel.

Prevention   Prevention of taeniasis involves cooking pork adequately and preventing pigs from ingesting human feces by disposing of waste properly. Prevention of cysticercosis consists of treatment of patients to prevent autoinfection plus observation of proper hygiene, including handwashing, to prevent contamination of food with the eggs.

2. *Taenia saginata*

Disease   *T saginata* causes taeniasis. *T saginata* larvae do not cause cysticercosis.

Important Properties   *T saginata* has a scolex with four suckers but, in contrast to *T solium*, **no hooklets.** Its gravid proglottids have 15–25 primary uterine branches, in contrast to *T solium* proglottids, which have 5–10 (Fig 54–1C and D). The eggs are morphologically indistinguishable from those of *T solium*.

Humans are infected by eating raw or undercooked **beef** containing larvae (cysticerci). In the small intestine, the larvae attach to the gut wall and take about 3 months to grow into adult worms measuring up to 10 m. The gravid proglottids detach, are passed in the feces, and are eaten by cattle. The embryos **(oncospheres)** emerge from the eggs in the cow's intestine and burrow into a blood vessel, where they are carried to skeletal muscle. In the muscle, they develop into cysticerci. The cycle is completed when the cysticerci are ingested. Humans are the definitive hosts and cattle the intermediate hosts. Unlike *T solium*, *T saginata* **does not cause cysticercosis** in humans.

Pathogenesis & Epidemiology   Little damage results from the presence of the adult worm in the small intestine. The epidemiology of taeniasis caused by *T saginata* is related to the access of cattle to human feces and to the consumption of raw or undercooked beef. The disease occurs worldwide but is endemic in Africa, South America, and eastern Europe. In the United States, most cases are imported.

Clinical Findings   Most patients with adult tapeworms are asymptomatic, but malaise and mild cramps can occur. In some, proglottids appear in the stools and may even protrude from the anus.

Laboratory Diagnosis   Identification of *T saginata* consists of finding gravid proglottids with 15–20 uterine branches in the stools. Eggs are found in the stools less often than are the proglottids.

Treatment   The treatment of choice is praziquantel.

Prevention   Prevention involves cooking beef adequately and preventing cattle from consuming human feces by disposing of waste properly.

DIPHYLLOBOTHRIUM

Disease   *Diphyllobothrium latum,* the fish tapeworm, causes diphyllobothriasis.

Important Properties   In contrast to the other cestodes, which have suckers, the scolex of *D latum* has two elongated **sucking grooves** by which the worm attaches to the intestinal wall (Fig 54–1E). The scolex has no hooks, unlike *T solium* and *Echinococcus.* The proglottids are wider than they are long, and the gravid uterus is in the form of a rosette. Unlike other tapeworm eggs, which are round, *D latum* eggs are oval and have a lidlike opening (**operculum**) at one end (Fig 54–2B). *D latum* is the longest of the tapeworms, measuring up to 13 m.

   Humans are infected by ingesting raw or undercooked **fish** containing larvae (called plerocercoid or sparganum larvae). In the small intestine, the larvae attach to the gut wall and develop into adult worms. Gravid proglottids release fertilized eggs through a genital pore, and the eggs are then passed in the stools. The immature eggs must be deposited in fresh water for the life cycle to continue. The embryos emerge from the eggs and are eaten by tiny copepod crustacea (first intermediate hosts). There, the embryos differentiate and form procercoid larvae in the body cavity. When the copepod is eaten by freshwater fish, eg, pike, trout, and perch, the larvae differentiate into plerocercoids in the muscle of the fish (second intermediate host). The cycle is completed when raw or undercooked fish is eaten by humans (definitive hosts).

Pathogenesis & Epidemiology   Infection by *D latum* causes little damage in the small intestine. In some individuals, megaloblastic anemia occurs as a result of vitamin B_{12} deficiency caused by preferential uptake of the vitamin by the worm.

   The epidemiology of *D latum* infection is related to the ingestion of raw or inadequately cooked fish and to contamination of bodies of fresh water with human feces. The disease is found worldwide but is endemic in areas where eating raw fish is the custom, such as Scandinavia, northern Russia, Japan, Canada, and certain north-central states of the United States.

Clinical Findings   Most patients are asymptomatic, but abdominal discomfort and diarrhea can occur.

Laboratory Diagnosis   Diagnosis depends on finding the typical eggs, ie, oval, yellow-brown eggs with an operculum at one end, in the stools. There is no serologic test.

Treatment   The treatment of choice is praziquantel.

Prevention   Prevention involves adequate cooking of fish and proper disposal of human feces.

ECHINOCOCCUS

Disease   The larva of *Echinococcus granulosus* (dog tapeworm) causes unilocular hydatid cyst disease. Multilocular hydatid disease is caused by *E multilocularis,* which is a minor pathogen and is discussed below.

Important Properties   *E granulosus* is composed of a scolex and only three proglottids, making it **one of the smallest tapeworms** (Fig 54–1F and G). **Dogs** are the most important definitive hosts. The intermediate hosts are usually **sheep.** Humans are almost always dead-end intermediate hosts.

   In the typical life cycle, worms in the dog's intestine liberate thousands of eggs, which are ingested by sheep (or humans). The oncosphere embryos emerge in the small intestine and migrate primarily to the liver but also to the lungs, bones, and brain. The embryos develop into large fluid-filled **hydatid cysts,** the inner germinal layer of which generates many protoscoleces within "brood capsules." The life cycle is completed when the entrails (eg, liver containing hydatid cysts) of slaughtered sheep are eaten by dogs.

Pathogenesis & Epidemiology   *E granulosus* usually forms one large fluid-filled cyst (unilocular) that contains thousands of individual scoleces as well as many daughter cysts within the large cyst. Individual scoleces lying at the bottom of the large cyst are called "hydatid sand." The cyst acts as a space-occupying lesion, putting pressure on adjacent tissue. The outer layer of the cyst is thick, fibrous tissue produced by the host. The cyst fluid contains parasite antigens, which can sensitize the host. Later, if the cyst ruptures spontaneously or during trauma or surgical removal, life-threatening **anaphylaxis** can occur. Rupture of a cyst can also spread protoscoleces widely.

The disease is found primarily in shepherds living in the Mediterranean region, the Middle East, and Australia. In the United States, the western states report the largest number of cases.

Clinical Findings   Many individuals with hydatid cysts are asymptomatic, but **liver cysts** may cause hepatic dysfunction. Cysts in the lungs can erode into a bronchus, causing bloody sputum, and cerebral cysts can cause headache and focal neurologic signs. Rupture of the cyst can cause fatal anaphylactic shock.

Laboratory Diagnosis   Diagnosis is based either on microscopic examination demonstrating the presence of brood capsules containing multiple protoscoleces or on serologic tests, eg, the indirect hemagglutination test.

Treatment   Treatment involves albendazole with or without surgical removal of the cyst. Extreme care must be exercised to prevent release of the protoscoleces during surgery. A protoscolicidal agent, eg, hypertonic saline, should be injected into the cyst to kill the organisms and prevent accidental dissemination. For medical therapy, albendazole is used.

Prevention   Prevention of human disease involves not feeding the entrails of slaughtered sheep to dogs.

CESTODES OF MINOR IMPORTANCE

Echinococcus multilocularis   Many of the features of this organism are the same as those of *E granulosus,* but the definitive hosts are mainly foxes and the intermediate hosts are various rodents. Humans are infected by accidental ingestion of food contaminated with fox feces. The disease occurs primarily in hunters and trappers and is endemic in northern Europe, Siberia, and the western provinces of Canada. In the United States, it occurs in North and South Dakota, Minnesota, and Alaska.

Within the human liver, the larvae form multiloculated cysts with few protoscoleces. No outer fibrous capsule forms, so the cysts continue to proliferate, producing a honeycomb effect of hundreds of small vesicles. The clinical picture usually involves jaundice and weight loss. The prognosis is poor. Albendazole treatment may be successful in some cases. Surgical removal may be feasible.

Hymenolepis nana   *H nana* (dwarf tapeworm) is the **most frequently** found tapeworm in the United States. It is only 3–5 cm long and is different from other tapeworms because its eggs are **directly infectious** for humans; ie, ingested eggs can develop into adult worms without an intermediate host. Within the duodenum, the eggs hatch and differentiate into cysticercoid larvae and then into adult worms. Gravid proglottids detach, disintegrate, and release fertilized eggs. The eggs either pass in the stool or can reinfect the small intestine (autoinfection). In contrast to infection by other tapeworms, where only one adult worm is present, many *H nana* worms (sometimes hundreds) are found.

Infection causes little damage, and most patients are asymptomatic. The organism is found worldwide, commonly in the tropics. In the United States, it is most prevalent in the southeastern states, usually in children. Diagnosis is based on finding eggs in stools. The characteristic feature of *H nana* eggs is the 8–10 polar filaments lying between the membrane of the six-hooked larva and the outer shell. The treatment is praziquantel. Prevention consists of good personal hygiene and avoidance of fecal contamination of food and water.

Review Questions

1. Which cestode causes cysticercosis?
2. What is the pathogenesis of cysticercosis?
3. How is *Taenia solium* transmitted? *Taenia saginata? Diphyllobothrium latum?*
4. What is the difference in appearance of the scoleces of *T solium, T saginata,* and *D latum?*
5. How is the laboratory diagnosis of these three cestodes made?
6. How can (a) taeniasis, (b) cysticercosis, and (c) diphyllobothriasis be prevented?
7. What is the treatment for these three diseases?
8. Which cestode causes unilocular hydatid cyst disease?
9. How is the agent of unilocular hydatid cyst disease acquired by humans? In which population is the disease endemic? Why? Which animal is the definitive host?
10. What is inside the hydatid cyst? Why is this important during surgical removal of the cyst? What is done to minimize risk during removal?

55

Trematodes

Trematoda (flukes) and Cestoda (tapeworms) are the two large classes of parasites in the phylum Platyhelminthes. The most important trematodes are *Schistosoma* species (blood flukes), *Clonorchis sinensis* (liver fluke), and *Paragonimus westermani* (lung fluke). Schistosomes have by far the greatest impact in terms of the number of people infected, morbidity, and mortality. Features of the medically important trematodes are summarized in Table 55–1. Three trematodes of lesser importance, *Fasciola hepatica, Fasciolopsis buski,* and *Heterophyes heterophyes,* are described later in the chapter.

The life cycle of the medically important trematodes involves a sexual cycle in humans and asexual reproduction in **freshwater snails** (intermediate hosts). Transmission to humans takes place either via penetration of the skin by the **free-swimming cercariae** of the schistosomes or via **ingestion of cysts** in undercooked (raw) fish or crabs in *Clonorchis* and *Paragonimus* infection, respectively.

Trematodes that cause human disease are not endemic in the United States. However, immigrants from tropical areas, especially Southeast Asia, are frequently infected.

SCHISTOSOMA

Disease   *Schistosoma* causes schistosomiasis. *Schistosoma mansoni* and *Schistosoma japonicum* affect the gastrointestinal tract,* whereas *Schistosoma haematobium* affects the urinary tract.

Important Properties   In contrast to the other trematodes, which are hermaphrodites, adult schistosomes exist as **separate sexes** but live attached to each other. The female resides in a groove in the male, the gynecophoric canal ("schist"), where he continuously fertilizes her eggs (Fig 55–1A). The three species can be distinguished by the appearance of their eggs in the microscope: *S mansoni* eggs have a **prominent lateral spine,** whereas *S japonicum* eggs have a very small lateral spine and *S haematobium* eggs have a **terminal spine** (Fig 55–2A and B). *S mansoni* and *S japonicum* adults live in the **mesenteric veins,** whereas *S haematobium* lives in the veins draining the **urinary bladder.** Schistosomes are therefore known as **"blood flukes."**

*As does *Schistosoma mekongi.*

Table 55–1. Features of medically important trematodes (flukes).

Trematode	Mode of Transmission	Main Sites Affected	Intermediate Host(s)	Diagnostic Features of Eggs	Endemic Area(s)	Treatment
Schistosoma mansoni	Penetrate skin	Veins of colon	Snail	Large lateral spine	Africa, Latin America (Caribbean)	Praziquantel
Schistosoma japonicum	Penetrate skin	Veins of small intestine, liver	Snail	Small lateral spine	Orient	Praziquantel
Schistisoma haematobium	Penetrate skin	Veins of urinary bladder	Snail	Large terminal spine	Africa, Middle East	Praziquantel
Clonorchis sinensis	Ingested with raw fish	Liver	Snail and fish	Operculated	Orient	Praziquantel
Paragonimus westermani	Ingested with raw crab	Lung	Snail and crab	Operculated	Orient, India	Praziquantel

Humans are infected when the free-swimming, fork-tailed **cercariae** penetrate the skin (Fig 55–1D). They differentiate to larvae (schistosomula), enter the blood, and are carried via the veins into the arterial circulation. Those that enter the superior mesenteric artery pass into the portal circulation and reach the liver, where they mature into adult flukes. *S mansoni* and *S japonicum* adults migrate against the portal flow to reside in the mesenteric venules. *S haematobium* adults reach the bladder veins through the venous plexus between the rectum and the bladder.

In their definitive venous site, the female lays fertilized eggs, which penetrate the vascular endothelium and enter the gut or bladder lumen, respectively. The eggs are excreted in the stools or urine and must enter fresh water to hatch. Once hatched, the ciliated larvae (miracidia) penetrate **snails** and undergo further development and multiplication to produce many cercariae. (The three schistosomes use different species of snails as intermediate hosts.) Cercariae leave the snails, enter fresh water, and complete the cycle by penetrating human skin.

Pathogenesis & Epidemiology Most of the pathologic findings are due to the presence of eggs in the liver, spleen, or wall of the gut or bladder. Eggs in the liver induce granulomas, which lead to fibrosis, hepatomegaly, and portal hypertension. The granulomas are formed in response to antigens secreted by the eggs. Hepatocytes are usually undamaged, and liver function tests remain normal. Portal hypertension leads to **splenomegaly.**

S mansoni eggs damage the wall of the distal colon (inferior mesenteric venules), whereas *S japonicum* eggs damage the walls of both the small and large intestines (superior and inferior mesen-

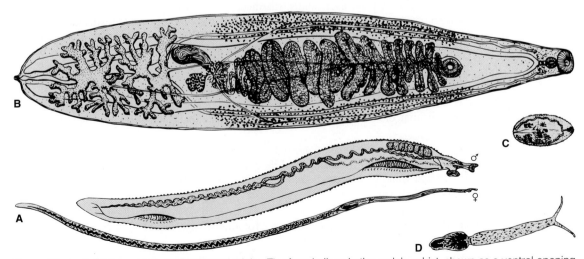

Figure 55–1. **A:** Male and female *S mansoni* adults. The female lives in the male's schist, shown as a ventral opening. 6 ×. **B:** *C sinensis* adult. 6 ×. **C:** *P westermani* adult. 0.6 ×. **D:** *S mansoni* cercaria. 300 ×.

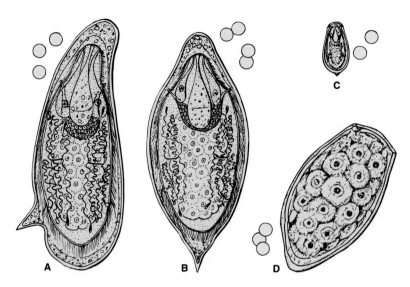

Figure 55–2. *A: S mansoni* ovum with lateral spine. *B: S haematobium* ovum with terminal spine. *C: C sinensis* ovum with operculum. *D: P westermani* ovum with operculum. 300 ×. (Circles represent red blood cells.)

teric venules). The damage is due both to digestion of tissue by proteolytic enzymes produced by the egg and to the host inflammatory response. The eggs of *S haematobium* in the wall of the bladder induce granulomas and fibrosis, which can lead to **carcinoma of the bladder.**

Schistosomes have evolved a remarkable process for **evading the host defenses.** There is evidence that their surface becomes coated with host antigens, thereby limiting the ability of the immune system to recognize them as foreign.

The epidemiology of schistosomiasis depends on the presence of the specific freshwater snails that serve as intermediate hosts. *S mansoni* is found in Africa and Latin America (including Puerto Rico), whereas *S haematobium* is found in Africa and the Middle East. *S japonicum* is found only in the Orient and is the only one for which domestic animals, eg, water buffalo and pigs, act as important reservoirs. More than 150 million people in the tropical areas of Africa, Asia, and Latin America are affected.

Clinical Findings   Most patients are asymptomatic, but chronic infections may become symptomatic. The acute stage, which begins shortly after cercarial penetration, consists of itching and dermatitis followed 2–3 weeks later by fever, chills, diarrhea, lymphadenopathy, and hepatosplenomegaly. Eosinophilia is seen in response to the migrating larvae. This stage usually resolves spontaneously.

The chronic stage can cause significant morbidity and mortality. In patients with *S mansoni* or *S japonicum* infection, gastrointestinal hemorrhage, hepatomegaly, and massive splenomegaly can develop. The most common cause of death is exsanguination from ruptured esophageal varices. Patients infected with *S haematobium* have hematuria as their chief early complaint. Superimposed bacterial urinary tract infections occur frequently.

"Swimmer's itch," a frequent problem in many lakes in the United States, is due to penetration of the skin by the cercariae of nonhuman schistosomes, which are incapable of replicating in humans.

Laboratory Diagnosis   Diagnosis depends on finding the characteristic ova in the feces or urine. The large lateral spine of *S mansoni* and the rudimentary spine of *S japonicum* are typical, as is the large terminal spine of *S haematobium* (Fig 55–2A and B). Serologic tests are not useful. Moderate eosinophilia occurs.

Treatment   Praziquantel is the treatment choice for all three species.

Prevention   Prevention involves proper disposal of human waste and eradication of the snail host when possible. Swimming in areas of endemic infection should be avoided.

CLONORCHIS

Disease   *Clonorchis sinensis* causes clonorchiasis (Oriental liver fluke infection).

Important Properties   Humans are infected by eating raw or undercooked **fish** containing the encysted larvae (metacercariae). Following excystation in the duodenum, immature flukes enter the **biliary ducts** and differentiate into adults (Fig 55–1B). The hermaphroditic adults produce eggs, which are excreted in the feces (Fig 55–2C). Upon reaching fresh water, the eggs are ingested by snails, which are the first intermediate hosts. The eggs hatch within the gut and differentiate first into larvae (rediae) and then into many free-swimming cercariae. Cercariae encyst under the scales of certain freshwater fish (second intermediate hosts), which are then eaten by humans.

Pathogenesis & Epidemiology   In some infections, the inflammatory response can cause hyperplasia and fibrosis of the biliary tract, but often there are no lesions. Clonorchiasis is endemic in China, Japan, Korea, and Indochina, where it affects about 20 million people. It is seen in the United States among immigrants from these areas.

Clinical Findings   Most infections are asymptomatic. In patients with a heavy worm burden, upper abdominal pain, anorexia, hepatomegaly, and eosinophilia can occur.

Laboratory Diagnosis   Diagnosis is made by finding the typical small, brownish, operculated eggs in the stool (Fig 55–2C). Serologic tests are not useful.

Treatment   Praziquantel is an effective drug.

Prevention   Prevention centers on adequate cooking of fish and proper disposal of human waste.

PARAGONIMUS

Disease   *Paragonimus westermani,* the lung fluke, causes paragonimiasis.

Important Properties   Humans are infected by eating raw or undercooked **crab meat** containing the encysted larvae (metacercariae). Following excystation in the small intestine, immature flukes penetrate the intestinal wall and migrate through the diaphragm into the **lung** parenchyma. They differentiate into hermaphroditic adults (Fig 55–1C) and produce eggs that enter the bronchioles and are coughed up or swallowed (Fig 55–2D). Eggs in either sputum or feces that reach fresh water hatch into miracidia, which enter snails (first intermediate hosts). There, they differentiate first into larvae (rediae) and then into many free-swimming cercariae. The cercariae infect and encyst in freshwater crabs (second intermediate hosts). The cycle is completed when undercooked infected crabs are eaten by humans.

Pathogenesis & Epidemiology   Within the lung, the worms exist in a fibrous capsule that communicates with a bronchiole. Secondary bacterial infection frequently occurs, resulting in bloody sputum. Paragonimiasis is endemic in the Orient and India. In the United States, it occurs in immigrants from these areas.

Clinical Findings   The main symptom is a chronic cough with bloody sputum. Dyspnea, pleuritic chest pain, and recurrent attacks of bacterial pneumonia occur. The disease can resemble tuberculosis.

Laboratory Diagnosis   Diagnosis is made by finding the typical operculated eggs in sputum or feces (Fig 55–2D). Serologic tests are not useful.

Treatment   Praziquantel is the treatment of choice.

Prevention   Cooking crabs properly is the best method of prevention.

TREMATODES OF MINOR IMPORTANCE

Fasciola   *Fasciola hepatica,* the sheep liver fluke, causes disease primarily in sheep and other domestic animals in Latin America, Africa, Europe, and China. Humans are infected by **eating watercress** (or other aquatic plants) contaminated by larvae (metacercariae) that excyst in the duodenum, penetrate the gut wall, and reach the liver, where they mature into adults. Hermaphroditic adults in the bile ducts produce eggs, which are excreted in the feces. The eggs hatch in fresh water, and miracidia enter the snails. Miracidia develop into cercariae, which then encyst on aquatic vegetation. Sheep and humans eat the plants, thus completing the life cycle.

Symptoms are due primarily to the presence of the adult worm in the biliary tract. In early infection, right-upper-quadrant pain, fever, and hepatomegaly can occur, but most infections are asymptomatic. Months or years later, obstructive jaundice can occur. Halzoun is a painful pharyngitis caused by the presence of adult flukes on the posterior pharyngeal wall. The adult flukes are acquired by eating raw sheep liver.

Diagnosis is made by identification of eggs in the feces. There is no serologic test. Praziquantel and bithional are effective drugs. Adult flukes in the pharynx and larynx can be removed surgically. Prevention involves not eating wild aquatic vegetables or raw sheep liver.

Fasciolopsis   *Fasciolopsis buski* is an intestinal parasite of humans and pigs that is endemic to Asia and India. Humans are infected by **eating aquatic vegetation** that carries the cysts. After excysting in the small intestine, the parasites attach to the mucosa and differentiate into adults. Eggs are passed in the feces; on reaching fresh water, they differentiate into miracidia. The ciliated miracidia penetrate snails and, after several stages, develop into cercariae that encyst on aquatic vegetation. The cycle is completed when plants carrying the cysts are eaten.

Pathology is due to damage of the intestinal mucosa by the adult fluke. Most infections are asymptomatic, but ulceration, abscess formation, and hemorrhage can occur. Diagnosis is based on finding typical eggs in the feces. Praziquantel is the treatment of choice. Prevention consists of proper disposal of human sewage.

Heterophyes   *Heterophyes heterophyes* is an intestinal parasite of people living in Africa, the Middle East, and Asia who are infected by **eating raw fish** containing cysts. Larvae excyst in the small intestine, attach to the mucosa, and develop into adults. Eggs are passed in the feces and, on reaching brackish water, are ingested by snails. After several developmental stages, cercariae are produced that encyst under the scales of certain fish. The cycle is completed when fish carrying the infectious cysts are eaten.

Pathology is due to inflammation of the intestinal epithelium as a result of the presence of the adult flukes. Most infections are asymptomatic, but abdominal pain and nonbloody diarrhea can occur. Diagnosis is based on finding the typical eggs in the feces. Praziquantel is the treatment of choice. Prevention consists of proper disposal of human sewage.

Review Questions

1. The life cycle of *Schistosoma, Clonorchis,* and *Paragonimus* involves asexual reproduction in which animal?
2. What is the difference in the mode of transmission between *Schistosoma, Clonorchis,* and *Paragonimus?*
3. How do the three species of *Schistosoma* differ in (a) location of adults in the human body and (b) appearance of eggs?
4. What is the cause of swimmer's itch?
5. How is the laboratory diagnosis of (a) the three *Schistosoma* species, (b) *Clonorchis,* and (c) *Paragonimus* made?
6. What is the treatment of choice for (a) *Schistosoma,* (b) *Clonorchis,* and (c) *Paragonimus?* How can infection by these trematodes be prevented?
7. In general, which of the trematodes are found in (a) Latin America, (b) Africa, and (c) the Orient?

Nematodes

56

Nematodes (also known as Nemathelminthes) are roundworms with a cylindrical body and a complete digestive tract including a mouth and an anus. The body is covered with a noncellular, highly resistant coating called a cuticle. Nematodes have separate sexes; the female is usually larger than the male. The male typically has a coiled tail.

The medically important nematodes can be divided into two categories according to their primary location in the body, namely, **intestinal** and **tissue** nematodes.

(1) The intestinal nematodes include *Enterobius* (pinworm), *Trichuris* (whipworm), *Ascaris* (giant roundworm), *Necator* and *Ancylostoma* (the two hookworms), *Strongyloides* (small roundworm), and *Trichinella. Enterobius, Trichuris,* and *Ascaris* are transmitted by ingestion of eggs; the others are transmitted as larvae. There are two larval forms: the first- and second-stage **(rhabditiform)** larvae are noninfectious, feeding forms; the third-stage **(filariform)** larvae are the infectious, nonfeeding forms. As adults, these nematodes live within the human body, except for *Strongyloides,* which can also exist in the soil.

(2) The important tissue nematodes *Wuchereria, Onchocerca,* and *Loa* are called the "filarial worms," because they produce motile embryos called **microfilariae** in blood and tissue fluids. These organisms are transmitted from person to person by bloodsucking mosquitoes or flies. A fourth species is the guinea worm, *Dracunculus,* whose larvae inhabit tiny crustaceans (copepods) and are ingested in drinking water.

The nematodes described above cause disease as a result of the presence of adult worms within the body. In addition, several species cannot mature to adults in human tissue but their larvae can cause disease. The most serious of these diseases is visceral larva migrans, caused primarily by the larvae of the dog ascarid, *Toxocara canis.* Cutaneous larva migrans, caused mainly by the larvae of the dog and cat hookworm, *Ancylostoma caninum,* is less serious. A third disease, anisakiasis, is caused by the ingestion of *Anisakis* larvae in raw seafood.

In infections caused by certain nematodes that migrate through tissue, eg, *Strongyloides, Trichinella, Ascaris,* and the two hookworms *Ancylostoma* and *Necator,* marked **eosinophilia** occurs. Eosinophils do not ingest the organisms; rather, they attach to the surface of the parasite via IgE and secrete cytotoxic enzymes contained within their eosinophilic granules. Host defenses against helminths are stimulated by interleukins synthesized by the Th-2 subset of helper T cells; eg, the production of IgE is increased by interleukin-4, and the number of eosinophils is increased by interleukin-5 (see Chapter 58). Cysteine proteases produced by the worms to facilitate their migration through tissue are the stimuli for IL-5 production.

Features of the medically important nematodes are summarized in Table 56–1.

Intestinal Nematodes

ENTEROBIUS

Disease   *Enterobius vermicularis* causes pinworm infection.

Important Properties   The life cycle is **confined to humans.** The infection is acquired by ingesting the worm eggs. The eggs hatch in the small intestine, where the larvae differentiate into adults and migrate to the colon. The adult male and female worms live in the colon, where mating occurs (Fig 56–1A). At night, the female migrates from the anus and releases thousands of fertilized eggs on the perianal skin and into the environment. Within 6 hours, the eggs develop into larvae and

Table 56–1. Features of medically important nematodes.

Primary Location	Species	Common Name or Disease	Mode of Transmission	Endemic Areas	Diagnosis	Treatment
Intestines	Enterobius	Pinworm	Ingestion of eggs	Worldwide.	Eggs on skin.	Mebendazole or pyrantel pamoate
	Trichuris	Whipworm	Ingestion of eggs	Worldwide, especially tropics.	Eggs in stools.	Mebendazole
	Ascaris	Ascariasis	Ingestion of eggs	Worldwide, especially tropics.	Eggs in stools.	Mebendazole or pyrantel pamoate
	Ancylostoma and Necator	Hookworm	Larval penetration of skin	Worldwide, especially tropics (Ancylostoma), United States (Necator).	Eggs in stools.	Mebendazole or pyrantel pamoate
	Strongyloides	Strongyloidiasis	Larval penetration of skin, also autoinfection	Tropics primarily.	Larvae in stools.	Thiabendazole
	Trichinella	Trichinosis	Larvae in undercooked meat	Worldwide.	Larvae encysted in muscle; serology.	Thiabendazole against adult worm
	Anisakis	Anisakiasis	Larvae in undercooked seafood	Japan, United States, Netherlands.	Clinical.	No drug available
Tissue	Wuchereria	Filariasis	Mosquito bite	Tropics primarily.	Blood smear.	Diethylcarbamazine
	Onchocerca	Onchocerciasis (river blindness)	Blackfly bite	Africa, Central America.	Skin biopsy.	Ivermectin
	Loa	Loiasis	Deer fly bite	Tropical Africa.	Blood smear.	Diethylcarbamazine
	Dracunculus	Guinea worm	Ingestion of copepods in water	Tropical Africa and Asia.	Clinical.	Niridazole prior to extracting worm
	Toxocara larvae	Visceral larva migrans	Ingestion of eggs	Worldwide.	Clinical and serologic.	Diethylcarbamazine
	Ancylostoma larvae	Cutaneous larva migrans	Penetration of skin	Worldwide.	Clinical.	Thiabendazole

become infectious. Reinfection can occur if they are carried to the mouth by fingers after scratching the itching skin.

Pathogenesis & Clinical Findings **Perianal pruritus** is the most prominent symptom. Scratching predisposes to secondary bacterial infection.

Epidemiology *Enterobius* is found worldwide and is the **most common** helminth in the United States. Children under 12 years of age are the most commonly affected group.

Laboratory Diagnosis The eggs are recovered from perianal skin by using the **"Scotch tape"** technique and can be observed microscopically (Fig 56–2A). Unlike those of other intestinal nematodes, these **eggs are not found in the stools.** The small, whitish adult worms can be found in the stools or near the anus of diapered children. No serologic tests are available.

Treatment Either mebendazole or pyrantel pamoate is effective. They kill the adult worms in the colon but not the eggs, so that retreatment in 2 weeks is suggested. Reinfection is very common.

Prevention There are no means of prevention.

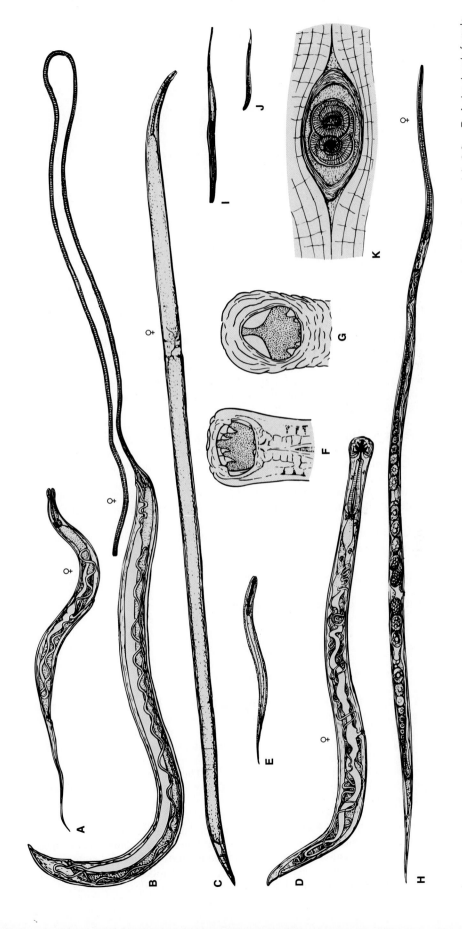

Figure 56–1. A: *E vermicularis* female adult. 6 ×. **B:** *T trichura* female adult. Note the thin anterior (whiplike) end. 6 ×. **C:** *A lumbricoides* female adult. 0.6 ×. **D:** *A duodenale* female adult. 6 ×. **E:** *A duodenale* filariform larva. 60 ×. **F:** *A duodenale* head with teeth. 60 ×. **G:** *N americanus* head with cutting plates. 25 ×. **H:** *S stercoralis* female adult. 60 ×. **I:** *S stercoralis* filariform larva. 60 ×. **J:** *S stercoralis* rhabditiform larva. 60 ×. **K:** *T spiralis* cyst containing two larvae in muscle. 60 ×.

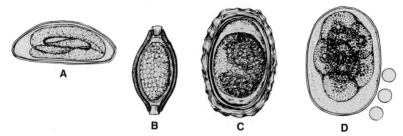

Figure 56–2. *A:* E vermicularis ovum. *B:* T trichura ovum. *C:* A lumbricoides ovum. *D:* A duodenale or N americanus ovum. 300 ×. (Circles represent red blood cells.)

TRICHURIS

Disease *Trichuris trichiura* causes whipworm infection.

Important Properties Humans are **infected by eating eggs in soil** contaminated with human feces. The eggs hatch in the small intestine, where the larvae differentiate into immature adults. These forms migrate to the colon, where they mature, mate, and produce thousands of fertilized eggs daily, which are passed in the feces. Eggs deposited in warm, moist soil form embryos. When the embryonated eggs are ingested, the cycle is completed. Figure 56–1B illustrates the characteristic "whiplike" appearance of the adult worm.

Pathogenesis & Clinical Findings Although adult *Trichuris* worms burrow their hairlike anterior ends into the intestinal mucosa, they do not cause a significant anemia, unlike the hookworms. *Trichuris* may cause diarrhea, but most infections are asymptomatic.

Epidemiology Whipworm infection occurs worldwide, especially in the tropics; more than 500 million people are affected. In the United States, it occurs mainly in the southern states.

Laboratory Diagnosis Diagnosis is based on finding the typical eggs, ie, barrel-shaped with a plug at each end, in the stool (Fig 56–2B).

Treatment Mebendazole is the drug of choice.

Prevention Proper disposal of feces prevents transmission.

ASCARIS

Disease *Ascaris lumbricoides* causes ascariasis.

Important Properties Humans are **infected by eating eggs in soil** contaminated with human feces. The eggs hatch in the small intestine, and the larvae migrate through the gut wall into the bloodstream and then to the lungs. They enter the alveoli, pass up the bronchi and trachea, and are swallowed. Within the small intestine, they become adults (Fig 56–1C). They live in the lumen, do not attach to the wall, and derive their sustenance from ingested food. The adults are the **largest intestinal nematodes,** often growing to 25 cm or more. Thousands of eggs are laid daily, are passed in the feces, and form embryos in warm, moist soil (Fig 56–2C). Ingestion of the embryonated eggs completes the cycle.

Pathogenesis & Clinical Findings The major damage occurs during larval migration rather than from the presence of the adult worm in the intestine. The principal sites of tissue reaction are the **lungs,** where inflammation with an **eosinophilic exudate** occurs in response to larval antigens. Because the adults derive their nourishment from ingested food, a heavy worm burden may contribute to malnutrition, especially in children in developing countries.

Most infections are asymptomatic. *Ascaris* **pneumonia** with fever, cough, and eosinophilia can occur with a heavy larval burden. Abdominal pain and even obstruction can result from the presence of adult worms in the intestine.

Epidemiology   *Ascaris* infection is very common, especially in the tropics; hundreds of millions of people are infected. In the United States, most cases occur in the southern states.

Laboratory Diagnosis   Diagnosis is usually made microscopically by detecting eggs in the stools. The egg is oval with an irregular surface (Fig 56–2C). Occasionally, the patient sees adult worms in the stools.

Treatment   Both mebendazole and pyrantel pamoate are effective.

Prevention   Proper disposal of feces can prevent ascariasis.

ANCYLOSTOMA & NECATOR

Disease   *Ancylostoma duodenale* (Old World hookworm) and *Necator americanus* (New World hookworm) cause hookworm infection.

Important Properties   Humans are infected when **filariform larvae in moist soil penetrate the skin,** usually of the feet or legs (Fig 56–1E). They are carried by the blood to the lungs, migrate into the alveoli and up the bronchi and trachea, and then are swallowed. They develop into adults in the small intestine, attaching to the wall with either cutting plates (*Necator*) or teeth (*Ancylostoma*) (Fig 56–1D, F, and G). They feed on blood from the capillaries of the intestinal villi. Thousands of eggs per day are passed in the feces (Fig 56–2D). Eggs develop first into noninfectious, feeding (rhabditiform) larvae and then into third-stage, infectious, nonfeeding (filariform) larvae (Fig 56–1E), which penetrate the skin to complete the cycle.

Pathogenesis & Clinical Findings   The major damage is due to the **loss of blood** at the site of attachment in the small intestine. Up to 0.1–0.3 mL per worm can be lost per day. Blood is consumed by the worm and oozes from the site in response to an anticoagulant made by the worm. Weakness and pallor accompany the microcytic anemia caused by blood loss. These symptoms occur in patients whose nutrition cannot compensate for the blood loss. "Ground itch," a pruritic papule or vesicle, can occur at the site of entry of the larvae into the skin. Pneumonia with eosinophilia can be seen during larval migration through the lungs.

Epidemiology   Hookworm is found worldwide, especially in tropical areas. In the United States, *Necator* is endemic in the rural southern states.

Laboratory Diagnosis   Diagnosis is made microscopically by observing the eggs in the stools (Fig 56–2D). Occult blood in the stools is frequent. Eosinophilia is typical.

Treatment   Both mebendazole and pyrantel pamoate are effective.

Prevention   Disposing of sewage properly and wearing shoes are effective means of prevention.

STRONGYLOIDES

Disease   *Strongyloides stercoralis* causes strongyloidiasis.

Important Properties   *S stercoralis* has **two distinct life cycles,** one within the human body and the other free-living in the soil. The life cycle in the human body begins with the **penetration of the skin,** usually of the feet, by **infectious (filariform) larvae** (Fig 56–1I) and their migration to the lungs. They enter the alveoli, pass up the bronchi and trachea, and then are swallowed. In the small intestine, the larvae molt into adults (Fig 56–1H) that enter the mucosa and produce eggs.

The eggs usually hatch within the mucosa, forming rhabditiform larvae (Fig 56–1J) that are passed in the feces. Some larvae molt to form filarial larvae, which penetrate the intestinal wall directly without leaving the host and migrate to the lungs (**autoinfection**). In immunocompetent patients, this is an infrequent, clinically unimportant event, but in T cell-deficient, eg, AIDS, or malnourished patients, it can lead to **massive reinfection,** with larvae passing to many organs and with severe, sometimes fatal consequences.

If larvae are passed in the feces and enter warm, moist soil, they molt through successive stages to form adult male and female worms. After mating, the entire life cycle of egg, larva, and adult can occur in the soil. After several free-living cycles, filarial larvae are formed. When they contact skin, they penetrate and again initiate the parasitic cycle within humans.

Pathogenesis & Clinical Findings Most patients are asymptomatic, especially those with a low worm burden. Adult female worms in the wall of the small intestine can cause inflammation, resulting in watery diarrhea. In autoinfection, the penetrating larvae may cause sufficient damage to the intestinal mucosa that sepsis due to enteric bacteria can occur. Larvae in the lungs can produce a pneumonitis similar to that caused by *Ascaris.* Pruritus (ground itch) can occur at the site of larval penetration of the skin, as with hookworm.

Epidemiology Strongyloidiasis occurs primarily in the tropics, especially in Southeast Asia. Its geographic pattern is similar to that of hookworm because the same type of soil is required. In the United States, *Strongyloides* is endemic in the southeastern states.

Laboratory Diagnosis Diagnosis depends on finding larvae in the stool. As with all migratory nematode infections, **eosinophilia can be striking.** Serologic tests are not useful.

Treatment Thiabendazole is the drug of choice.

Prevention Prevention involves disposing of sewage properly and wearing shoes.

TRICHINELLA

Disease *Trichinella spiralis* causes trichinosis.

Important Properties Any mammal can be infected, but **pigs** are the most important reservoirs of human disease in the United States (except in Alaska, where bears constitute the reservoir). Humans are infected by **eating raw** or **undercooked meat** containing larvae encysted in the muscle (Fig 56–1K). The larvae excyst and mature into adults within the mucosa of the small intestine. Eggs hatch within the adult females, and larvae are released and distributed via the bloodstream to many organs; however, they develop only in **striated muscle cells.** Within these "nurse cells," they encyst within a fibrous capsule and can remain viable for several years but eventually calcify.

The parasite is maintained in nature by cycles within reservoir hosts, primarily swine and rats. Humans are **end-stage hosts,** because the infected flesh is not consumed by other animals.

Pathogenesis & Clinical Findings A few days after eating undercooked meat, usually pork, the patient experiences gastroenteritis followed 1–2 weeks later by **fever, muscle pain, periorbital edema,** and **eosinophilia.** Signs of cardiac and central nervous system disease are frequent, because the larvae migrate to these tissues as well. Death, which is rare, is usually due to congestive heart failure or respiratory paralysis.

Epidemiology Trichinosis occurs worldwide, especially in eastern Europe and west Africa. In the United States, it is related to eating home-prepared sausage, usually on farms where the pigs are fed uncooked garbage. Bear and seal meat also are sources.

Laboratory Diagnosis Muscle biopsy reveals **larvae within striated muscle** (Fig 56–1K). Serologic tests, especially the bentonite flocculation test, become positive 3 weeks after infection.

Treatment There is no treatment for trichinosis, but for patients with severe symptoms, steroids plus mebendazole can be tried. Thiabendazole is effective against the adult intestinal worms early in infection.

Prevention The disease can be prevented by properly cooking pork and by feeding pigs only cooked garbage.

Tissue Nematodes

WUCHERERIA

Disease   *Wuchereria bancrofti* causes filariasis.*

Important Properties   Humans are infected when the **female mosquito** (especially *Anopheles* and *Culex* species) deposits infective larvae on the skin while biting. The larvae penetrate the skin, enter a lymph node, and, after a year, mature to adults that produce **microfilariae** (Fig 56–3A). These circulate in the blood, chiefly at night, and are ingested by biting mosquitoes. Within the mosquito, the microfilariae produce infective larvae that are transferred with the next bite. Humans are the only definitive hosts.

Pathogenesis & Clinical Findings   Adult worms in the lymph nodes cause inflammation that eventually obstructs the lymphatic vessels, causing edema. Microfilariae do not cause symptoms. Early infections are asymptomatic. Later, fever, lymphangitis, and cellulitis develop. Gradually, the obstruction leads to edema of the legs and genitalia. **Elephantiasis** occurs mainly in patients who have been repeatedly infected over a long period.

Epidemiology   This disease occurs in the tropics. The species of mosquito that acts as the vector varies from area to area. Altogether, 200–300 million people are infected.

Laboratory Diagnosis   Thick blood smears taken from the patient at night reveal the microfilariae. Serologic tests are not useful.

Treatment   Diethylcarbamazine is effective only against microfilariae; no drug therapy for adult worms is available.

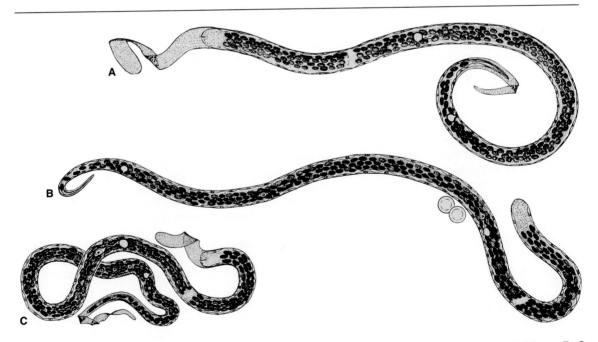

Figure 56–3. **A:** *W bancrofti* microfilaria in blood. Note that the pointed tail is free of nuclei. 225–300 × 8–10 μm. **B:** *O volvulus* microfilaria in skin (rare in blood). 300–350 × 5–9 μm. **C:** *L loa* microfilaria in blood. Note that the pointed tail contains nuclei. 250–300 × 6–9 μm. (Circles represent red blood cells.)

Brugia malayi causes filariasis in Malaysia.

Prevention   Prevention involves mosquito control with insecticides and the use of protective clothing, mosquito netting, and repellents.

ONCHOCERCA

Disease   *Onchocerca volvulus* causes onchocerciasis.

Important Properties   Humans are infected when the **female blackfly,** *Simulium,* deposits infective larvae while biting. The larvae enter the wound and migrate into the subcutaneous tissue, where they differentiate into adults, usually within **dermal nodules.** The female produces microfilariae (Fig 56–3B) that are ingested when another blackfly bites. The microfilariae develop into infective larvae in the fly to complete the cycle. Humans are the only definitive hosts.

Pathogenesis & Clinical Findings   Inflammation occurs in subcutaneous tissue, and pruritic papules and nodules form in response to the adult worm proteins. Microfilariae migrate through subcutaneous tissue, ultimately concentrating in the eyes. There they cause lesions that can lead to blindness.

Epidemiology   Millions of people are affected in Africa and Central America. The disease is a major cause of blindness. It is called **"river blindness,"** because the blackflies develop in rivers and people who live along those rivers are affected. Infection rates are often over 80% in areas of endemic infection.

Laboratory Diagnosis   Biopsy of the affected skin reveals microfilariae (Fig 56–3B). Examination of the blood is not useful, because microfilariae do not circulate in the blood. Serologic tests are also not helpful.

Treatment   Ivermectin is effective against microfilariae but not adults. Suramin kills adults but is quite toxic and is used particularly in those with eye disease. Skin nodules can be removed surgically, but new nodules can develop; therefore, a surgical cure is unlikely in areas of endemic infection.

Prevention   Prevention involves control of the blackfly with insecticides. Ivermectin prevents the disease.

LOA

Disease   *Loa loa* causes loiasis.

Important Properties   Humans are infected by the bite of the **deer fly** (mango fly), *Chrysops,* which deposits infective larvae on the skin. The larvae enter the bite wound, wander in the body, and develop into adults. The females release microfilariae (Fig 56–3C) that enter the blood, particularly during the day. The microfilariae are taken up by the fly during a blood meal and differentiate into infective larvae, which continue the cycle when the fly bites the next person.

Pathogenesis & Clinical Findings   There is no inflammatory response to the microfilariae or adults, but a hypersensitivity reaction causes transient, localized, nonerythematous, subcutaneous edema (Calabar swellings). The most dramatic finding is an adult worm **crawling across the conjunctiva** of the eye, a harmless but disconcerting event.

Epidemiology   The disease is found only in tropical central and west Africa, the habitat of the vector *Chrysops.*

Laboratory Diagnosis   Diagnosis is made by visualization of the microfilariae in a blood smear (Fig 56–3C). There are no useful serologic tests.

Treatment   Diethylcarbamazine eliminates the microfilariae and may kill the adults. Worms in the eyes may require surgical excision.

Prevention   Control of the fly by insecticides can prevent the disease.

DRACUNCULUS

Disease   *Dracunculus medinensis* (guinea fire worm) causes dracunculiasis.

Important Properties   Humans are infected when tiny **crustaceans** (copepods) containing infective larvae are **swallowed in drinking water.** The larvae are released in the small intestine and migrate into the body, where they develop into adults. Meter-long adult females cause the skin to ulcerate and then release motile larvae into fresh water. Copepods eat the larvae, which molt to form infective larvae. The cycle is completed when these are ingested in the water.

Pathogenesis & Clinical Findings   The adult female produces a substance that causes inflammation, blistering, and ulceration of the skin, usually of the lower extremities. The inflamed papule **burns and itches,** and the ulcer can become secondarily infected. Diagnosis is usually made clinically by finding the **head of the worm in the skin ulcer.**

Epidemiology   The disease occurs over large areas of tropical Africa, the Middle East, and India. Tens of millions of people are infected.

Laboratory Diagnosis   The laboratory usually does not play a role in diagnosis.

Treatment   The time-honored treatment consists of gradually extracting the worm by winding it up on a stick over a period of days. Niridazole or metronidazole makes the worm easier to extract.

Prevention   Prevention consists of filtering or boiling drinking water.

Nematodes Whose Larvae Cause Disease

TOXOCARA

Disease   *Toxocara canis* is the major cause of visceral larva migrans. *T cati* and several other related nematodes also cause this disease.

Important Properties   The definitive host for *T canis* is the dog. The adult *T canis* female in the dog intestine produces eggs that are passed in the feces into the soil. Humans ingest soil containing the eggs, which hatch into larvae in the small intestine. The larvae migrate to many organs, especially the liver, brain, and eyes. The larvae eventually are encapsulated and die. The life cycle is not completed in humans; humans are therefore accidental, dead-end hosts.

Pathogenesis & Clinical Findings   Pathology is related to the granulomas that form around the dead larvae as a result of a delayed hypersensitivity response to larval proteins. The most serious clinical finding is blindness due to retinal involvement. Fever, hepatomegaly, and eosinophilia are common.

Epidemiology   Young children are primarily affected, because they are likely to ingest soil containing the eggs. *T canis* is a common parasite of dogs in the United States.

Laboratory Diagnosis   Serologic tests are commonly used, but the definitive diagnosis depends on visualizing the larvae in tissue. The presence of hypergammaglobulinemia and eosinophilia supports the diagnosis.

Treatment   The treatment of choice is diethylcarbamazine.

Prevention   Dogs should be dewormed, and children should be prevented from eating soil.

ANCYLOSTOMA

Cutaneous larva migrans is caused by the filariform larvae of *Ancylostoma caninum* (dog hookworm) and *Ancylostoma braziliense* (cat hookworm), as well as other nematodes. The organism cannot complete its life cycle in humans. The larvae penetrate the skin and **migrate through subcutaneous tissue,** causing an inflammatory response. The lesions ("creeping eruption") are extremely pruritic. The disease occurs primarily in the southern United States, in children and construction workers who are exposed to infected soil. The diagnosis is made clinically; the laboratory is of little value. Oral or topical thiabendazole is usually effective.

ANISAKIS

A third human disease caused by the larvae of a nematode is anisakiasis. *Anisakis simplex* larvae are **ingested in raw seafood** and can penetrate the submucosa of the stomach or intestine. Gastroenteritis, eosinophilia, and occult blood in the stool typically occur. Acute infection can resemble appendicitis, and chronic infection can resemble gastrointestinal cancer.

Most cases in the United States have been traced to eating sushi and sashimi (especially salmon and red snapper) in Japanese restaurants. The diagnosis is typically made endoscopically or on laparotomy. Microbiologic and serologic tests are not helpful in the diagnosis. There are no effective drugs. Surgical removal may be necessary. Prevention consists of cooking seafood adequately or freezing it for 24 hours before eating.

Another member of the Anisakid family of nematodes is *Pseudoterranova decepiens,* whose larvae cause a noninvasive form of anisakiasis. The larvae are acquired by eating undercooked fish and cause vomiting and abdominal pain. The diagnosis is made by finding the larvae in the intestinal tract or in the vomitus. There is no drug treatment. The larvae can be removed during endoscopy.

Review Questions

1. Which of the intestinal nematodes are transmitted by ingestion of eggs?
2. Which of the intestinal nematodes are acquired by penetration of the skin?
3. Which of the tissue nematodes are transmitted by mosquitoes or flies?
4. In pinworm infection, how do the *Enterobius* eggs reach the environment?
5. How is the laboratory diagnosis of pinworms made?
6. In (a) whipworm infection and (b) *Ascaris* infection, how is the disease transmitted and how is the laboratory diagnosis made?
7. What is the pathogenesis of *Ascaris* pneumonia?
8. In hookworm infection, what is the mode of transmission and how is the laboratory diagnosis made?
9. What is the pathogenesis of anemia caused by hookworms?
10. Contrast the free-living and the non-free-living life cycles of *Strongyloides.*
11. In strongyloidiasis, what is the mode of transmission and how is the laboratory diagnosis made?
12. What is the pathogenesis of the severe clinical consequences of strongyloidiasis in a T cell-deficient, eg, AIDS, patient?
13. In trichinosis, what is the mode of transmission, how is the laboratory diagnosis usually made, and how can the disease be prevented?
14. Why are humans end-stage hosts for *Trichinella?*
15. Contrast visceral with cutaneous larva migrans regarding (a) the organism, (b) transmission, (c) location of lesions, and (d) laboratory diagnosis.
16. In filariasis, what is the mode of transmission and how is the laboratory diagnosis made?
17. What is the pathogenesis of elephantiasis?
18. In onchocerciasis, what is the mode of transmission and how is the laboratory diagnosis made?
19. What is the pathogenesis of river blindness? Why is the term "river" used?
20. Contrast *Loa* and *Dracunculus* regarding (a) mode of transmission, (b) laboratory diagnosis, and (c) location of the adult worms.

21. Which nematodes are found worldwide? For those that are not found worldwide, where do they primarily occur?
22. For which nematodes is (a) mebendazole, (b) thiabendazole, (c) diethylcarbamazine, or (d) ivermectin the appropriate treatment?

Part VII: Immunology

57   Immunity

INTRODUCTION

The main function of the immune system is to **prevent or limit infections** by microorganisms such as bacteria, viruses, fungi, and parasites. Protection is provided primarily by the **cell-mediated** and **antibody-mediated (humoral)** arms of the immune system. Two other major components of the immune system are complement and phagocytes. Complement is described in Chapter 63 and phagocytes in Chapter 8. An overview of the interactions and functions of these components is provided in Figure 57–1.

The cell-mediated arm consists primarily of **T lymphocytes** (eg, helper T cells and cytotoxic T cells) whereas the antibody-mediated arm consists of **B lymphocytes** (and plasma cells). Some of the major functions of T cells and B cells are shown in Table 57–1. The main functions of antibodies are (1) to **neutralize toxins and viruses** and (2) to **opsonize bacteria,** making them easier to phagocytize. Cell-mediated immunity, on the other hand, inhibits organisms such as fungi, parasites, and certain intracellular bacteria; it also kills **virus-infected cells** and **tumor cells.**

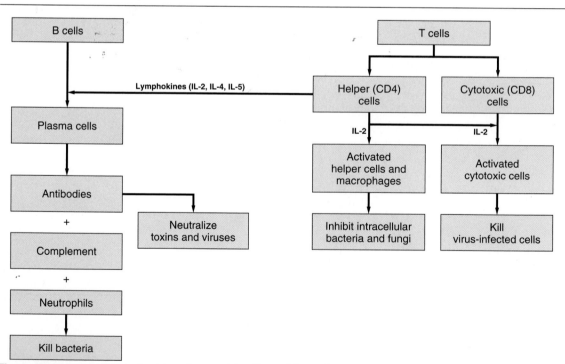

Figure 57–1. Introduction to the interactions and functions of the major components of the immune system. **Left:** Antibody-mediated (humoral) immunity. This is our main defense against extracellular, encapsulated, pyogenic bacteria such as staphylococci and streptococci. Antibodies also neutralize toxins, such as tetanus toxin, as well as viruses, such as hepatitis B virus. **Right:** Cell-mediated immunity. There are two distinct components. (1) Helper T cells and macrophages are our main defense against intracellular bacteria, such as *Mycobacterium tuberculosis,* and fungi, such as *Histoplasma capsulatum.* (2) Cytotoxic T cells are an important defense against viruses and act by destroying virus-infected cells.

Table 57–1. Major functions of T cells and B cells.

Antibody-Mediated Immunity (B Cells)	Cell-Mediated Immunity (T Cells)
1. Host defense against infection (opsonize bacteria, neutralize toxins and viruses) 2. Allergy, eg, hay fever 3. Autoimmunity	1. Host defense against infection (especially *M tuberculosis,* viruses, and fungi) 2. Allergy, eg, poison oak 3. Graft and tumor rejection 4. Regulation of antibody response (help and suppression)

Both the cell-mediated and antibody-mediated responses are characterized by three important features: (1) they exhibit remarkable **diversity** (ie, they can respond to millions of different antigens); (2) they have a long **memory** (ie, they can respond many years after the initial exposure because memory T cells and memory B cells are produced); and (3) they exhibit exquisite **specificity** (ie, their actions are specifically directed against the antigen that initiated the response).

The combined effects of certain cells (eg, T cells, B cells, macrophages, and neutrophils) and certain proteins (eg, antibodies and complement) produce an **inflammatory response,** one of the body's main defense mechanisms. The process by which these components interact to cause inflammation is described in Chapter 8.

SPECIFICITY OF THE IMMUNE RESPONSE

(handwritten: ① recognition of non-self ② activation ③ response.)

Cell-mediated immunity and antibody are both highly specific for the invading organism. How do these specific protective mechanisms originate? The process by which these host defenses originate can be summarized by three actions: the **recognition** of the foreign organism by specific immune cells, the **activation** of these immune cells to produce a specific response (eg, antibodies), and the **response** that specifically targets the organism for destruction. The following examples briefly describe how specific immunity to microorganisms occurs. An overview of these processes with a viral infection as the model is shown in Figure 57–2. A detailed description is presented in Chapter 58.

1. Cell-mediated Immunity

(handwritten: snippet of bacterial protein = epitope = antigen)

In the following example, a bacterium, eg, *Mycobacterium tuberculosis,* enters the body and is ingested by a macrophage. The bacterium is broken down, and fragments of it called **antigens** or **epitopes** appear on the surface of the macrophage in association with **class II major histocompatibility complex (MHC)** proteins. The antigen–class II MHC protein complex interacts with an antigen-specific receptor on the surface of a **helper T lymphocyte.** Activation and clonal proliferation of this antigen-specific helper T cell occur as a result of the production of **interleukins,** the most important of which are interleukin-1 (produced by macrophages) and interleukin-2 (produced by lymphocytes). These activated helper T cells, aided by activated macrophages, mediate one important component of cellular immunity, ie, a **delayed hypersensitivity reaction** specifically against *M tuberculosis.*

(handwritten left margin: macrophage presents w/ MHC)

(handwritten left margin: Class II – helper T/CD4)

(handwritten left margin: Class I – cytotoxic T/ CD8)

Cytotoxic T lymphocytes are also specific effectors of the cellular immune response, particularly against virus-infected cells. In this example, a virus, eg, influenza virus, is inhaled and infects a cell of the respiratory tract. Viral envelope glycoproteins appear on the surface of the infected cell in association with **class I MHC** proteins. A cytotoxic T cell binds via its antigen-specific receptor to the viral antigen–class I MHC protein complex and is stimulated to grow into a clone of cells by interleukin-2 produced by helper T cells. These cytotoxic T cells specifically kill influenza virus-infected cells (and not cells infected by other viruses) by recognizing viral antigen–class-I MHC protein complexes on the cell surface and releasing perforins that destroy the membrane of the infected cell.

2. Antibody-mediated Immunity

(handwritten: IL-2 → t cell growth factor! IL-4 → B " " ")

Antibody synthesis typically involves the cooperation of three cells: **macrophages, helper T cells, and B cells.** After processing by a macrophage, fragments of antigen appear on the surface of the macrophage in association with **class II MHC** proteins. The antigen–class II MHC protein complex binds to specific receptors on the surface of a helper T cell, which then produces interleukins such as interleukin-2 (T cell growth factor), interleukin-4 (B cell growth factor), and interleukin-5 (B cell

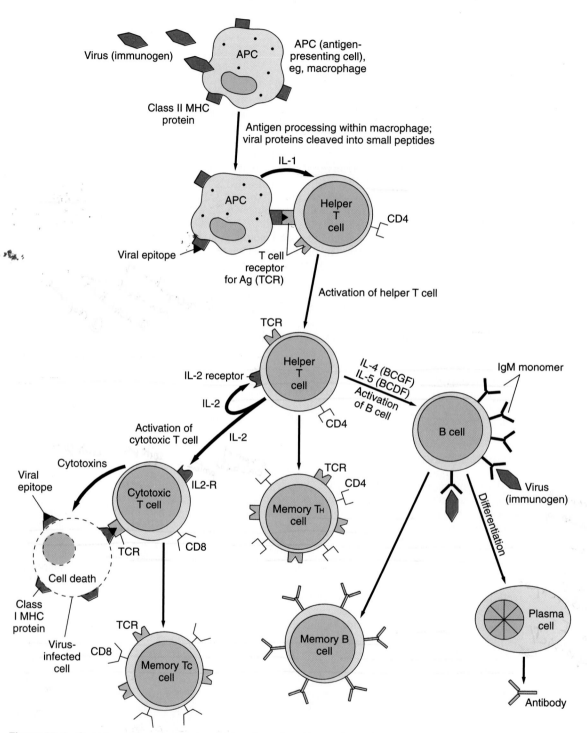

Figure 57–2. Overview of the process by which cell-mediated immunity and antibody-mediated immunity are induced by exposure to a virus. (Modified and reproduced, with permission, from Stites D, Terr A, Parslow T [editors]: *Basic & Clinical Immunology*, 9th ed. Appleton & Lange, 1997).

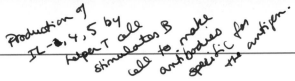

[handwritten: Production of IL-2,4,5 by helper T cell stimulates B cell to make antibodies specific for the antigen.]

[handwritten margin note: Immunoglobulin = Antibody.]

differentiation factor). These factors activate the B cell capable of producing antibodies specific for that antigen. (Note that the interleukins are nonspecific; the specificity lies in the T cells and B cells and is mediated by the antigen receptors on the surface of these cells.) The activated B cell proliferates and differentiates to form many plasma cells that secrete large amounts of **immunoglobulins** (antibodies). Although antibody formation usually involves helper T cells, certain antigens, eg, bacterial polysaccharides, can activate B cells directly, without the help of T cells, and are called T cell-independent antigens.

Figure 57–3 summarizes the human host defenses against virus-infected cells and illustrates the close interaction of various cells in mounting a coordinated attack against the pathogen. The specificity of the response is provided by the antigen receptor (T cell receptor [TCR]) on the surface of both the CD4-positive T cell and the CD8-positive T cell and by the antigen receptor (IgM) on the surface of the B cell. The interleukins, on the other hand, are **not specific.**

NATURAL & ACQUIRED IMMUNITY

[handwritten: natural — non specific — constant — no memory — present all the time]

[handwritten: acquired — specific — increases w/ exposure — memory. — present upon exposure]

Immunity may be **natural (innate)** or **acquired (adaptive).**

(1) Natural immunity is resistance not acquired through contact with an antigen. It is **nonspecific** and includes host defenses such as barriers to infectious agents (eg, skin and mucous membranes), certain cells (eg, natural killer cells), certain proteins (eg, the complement cascade and interferons), and other processes such as phagocytosis and inflammation (Table 57–2). Natural immunity **does not improve after exposure** to the organism, in contrast to acquired immunity, which does. In addition, **natural immune processes have no memory,** whereas acquired immunity is characterized by long-term memory.

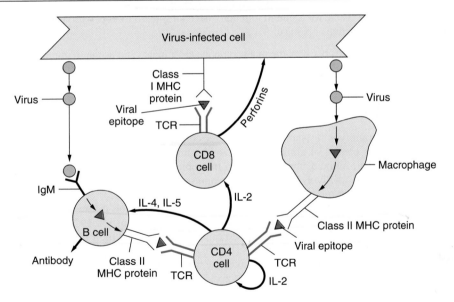

Figure 57–3. Induction of cell-mediated immunity and antibody against a viral infection. ***Right:*** Virus released by an infected cell is ingested and processed by an antigen-presenting cell (APC), eg, a macrophage. The viral epitope is presented in association with a class II MHC protein to the virus-specific T cell receptor (TCR) on the CD4 cell. The macrophage makes IL-1, which helps to activate the CD4 cell. The activated CD4 cell makes interleukins (eg, IL-2, which activates the CD8 cell to attack the virus-infected cell, and IL-4 and IL-5, which activate the B cell to produce antibody). The specificity of the cytotoxic response mounted by the CD8 cell is provided by its TCR, which recognizes the viral epitope presented by the virus-infected cell in association with a class I MHC protein. ***Left:*** Virus released by an infected cell interacts with the antigen receptor (IgM monomer) specific for that virus located on the surface of a B cell. The virus is internalized, and the viral proteins are broken down into small peptides. B cells (as well as macrophages) can present viral epitopes in association with class II MHC proteins and activate CD4 cells. The CD4-positive helper cell produces IL-4 and IL-5, which induce the B cell to differentiate into a plasma cell that produces antibody specifically against this virus.

Table 57–2. Natural immunity.

Mechanism	Factor
Entry of microorganism limited	Keratin layer of intact skin (mechanical barrier) Lysozyme in tears and other secretions (degrades peptidoglycan in bacterial cell wall) Fatty acids of the skin (inhibit growth of microorganisms) Respiratory cilia (elevate mucus containing trapped organisms) Normal flora of throat, colon, and vagina (inhibits colonization by pathogens) Low pH of vagina and stomach (inhibits or kills certain pathogens) Surface phagocytes, eg, alveolar macrophages
Growth of microorganism in body limited	Natural killer cells (kill virus-infected cells) Phagocytes, eg, neutrophils (ingest and kill bacteria) Interferons (inhibit virus replication) Transferrin and lactoferrin (sequester iron required for bacterial growth) Complement (C3b is an opsonin; membrane attack complex kills bacteria) Elevated body temperature (may retard growth of organisms) Inflammatory response (limits spread of organisms)

The **acute-phase response,** which consists of an increase in the levels of various plasma proteins, eg, C-reactive protein and mannose-binding protein, is also part of natural immunity. These proteins are synthesized by the liver and are nonspecific responses to microorganisms and other forms of tissue injury. The liver synthesizes these proteins in response to certain cytokines, namely, interleukin-1, interleukin-6, and tumor necrosis factor, produced by the macrophage after exposure to microorganisms. Some acute-phase proteins bind to the surface of bacteria and activate complement which can kill the bacteria.

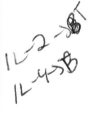

(2) Acquired immunity occurs **after exposure** to an agent, **improves upon repeated exposure,** and is **specific.** It is mediated by antibody and by T lymphocytes, namely, helper T cells and cytotoxic T cells. The cells responsible for acquired immunity have **long-term memory** for a specific antigen. Acquired immunity can be active or passive.

The relationships between the main components of innate and acquired immunity and the humoral (antibody-mediated) and cell-mediated arms of the immune system are depicted in Table 57–3.

ACTIVE & PASSIVE IMMUNITY

Active immunity is resistance induced **after contact** with foreign antigens, eg, microorganisms. This contact may consist of clinical or subclinical infection, immunization with live or killed infectious agents or their antigens, or exposure to microbial products (eg, toxins and toxoids). In all these instances, the host actively produces an immune response consisting of antibodies and activated helper and cytotoxic T lymphocytes.

The main advantage of active immunity is that resistance is **long-term** (Table 57–4). Its major disadvantage is its **slow onset,** especially the primary response (see Chapter 60).

Passive immunity is resistance based on antibodies **preformed** in another host. Administration of antibody against diphtheria, tetanus, botulism, etc, makes large amounts of antitoxin immediately available to neutralize the toxins. Likewise, preformed antibodies to certain viruses (eg, rabies and hepatitis A and B viruses) can be injected during the incubation period to limit viral multiplication.

Table 57–3. Main components of innate and acquired immunity that contribute to humoral (antibody-mediated) immunity and cell-mediated immunity.

	Humoral Immunity	Cell-mediated Immunity
Innate	Complement Neutrophils	Macrophages
Acquired	B cells Plasma cells	Helper T cells Cytotoxic T cells

Table 57–4. Characteristics of active and passive immunity.

	Mediators	Advantages	Disadvantages
Active immunity	Antibody and T cells	Long duration (years)	Slow onset
Passive immunity	Antibody only	Immediate availability	Short duration (months)

Other forms of passive immunity are IgG passed from mother to fetus during pregnancy and IgA passed from mother to newborn during breast-feeding.

The main advantage of passive immunization is the **prompt availability** of large amounts of antibody; disadvantages are the **short life-span** of these antibodies and possible hypersensitivity reactions if globulins from another species are used.

Passive-active immunity involves giving both preformed antibodies (immune globulins) to provide immediate protection and a vaccine to provide long-term protection. These preparations should be given at different sites in the body to prevent the antibodies from neutralizing the immunogens in the vaccine. This approach is used in the prevention of tetanus (see Chapters 12 and 17), rabies (see Chapters 36 and 39) and hepatitis B (see Chapters 36 and 41).

ANTIGENS

Antigens are molecules that react with antibodies, whereas immunogens are molecules that induce an immune response. In most cases, antigens are immunogens and the terms are used interchangeably. However, there are certain important exceptions, eg, haptens. A **hapten** is a molecule that is not immunogenic by itself but can react with specific antibody. Haptens are usually small molecules, but some high-molecular-weight nucleic acids are haptens as well. Many drugs, eg, penicillins, are haptens and the catechol in the plant oil that causes poison oak and poison ivy is a hapten.

Haptens are not immunogenic, because they cannot activate helper T cells. The failure of haptens to activate is due to their inability to bind to MHC proteins; they cannot bind because they are not polypeptides and only polypeptides can be presented by MHC proteins. Furthermore, haptens are univalent and therefore cannot activate B cells by themselves. (Compare to the T-independent response of multivalent antigens in Chapter 58.) Although haptens cannot stimulate a primary or secondary response by themselves, they can do so when covalently bound to a "carrier" protein (Fig. 57–4). In this process, the hapten interacts with an IgM receptor on the B cell and the hapten-carrier protein complex is internalized. A peptide of the carrier protein is presented in association with class II MHC protein to the helper T cells. The activated helper T cell then produces interleukins, which stimulate the B cells to produce antibody to the hapten (see Chapter 58, p 327, for additional information).

The interaction of antigen and antibody is highly specific, and this characteristic is frequently used in the diagnostic laboratory to identify microorganisms. Antigen and antibody bind by **weak forces** such as hydrogen bonds and van der Waals' forces rather than by covalent bonds. The strength of the binding (the affinity) is proportionate to the fit of the antigen with its antibody-combining site, ie, its ability to form more of these bonds. The affinity of antibodies increases with successive exposures to the specific antigen (see Chapter 60). Another term, avidity, is also used to express certain aspects of binding. It need not concern us here.

The features of molecules that determine **immunogenicity** are as follows.

A. Foreignness: In general, molecules recognized as "self" are not immunogenic; ie, we are tolerant to those self-molecules (see Chapter 66). To be immunogenic, molecules must be recognized as "nonself," ie, foreign.

B. Molecular Size: The most potent immunogens are proteins with high molecular weights, ie, above 100,000. Generally, molecules with molecular weight below 10,000 are weakly immunogenic, and very small ones, eg, an amino acid, are nonimmunogenic. Certain small molecules, eg, haptens, become immunogenic only when linked to a carrier protein.

C. Chemical-Structural Complexity: A certain amount of chemical complexity is required; eg, amino acid homopolymers are less immunogenic than heteropolymers containing two or three different amino acids.

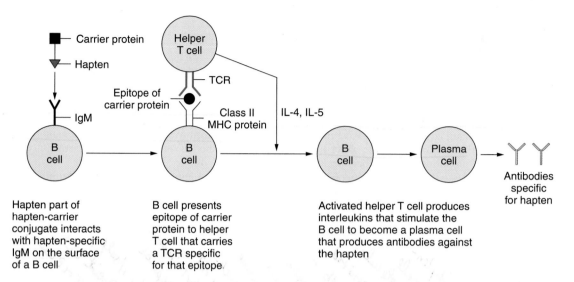

Figure 57–4. Hapten-carrier conjugate induces antibody against the hapten. A hapten covalently bound to a carrier protein can induce antibody to a hapten by the mechanism depicted in the figure. A hapten alone cannot induce antibody, because the helper T cells are not activated by the hapten. Although the hapten alone (without the carrier protein) can bind to the IgM receptor on the B cell surface, the interleukins essential for the B cell to become a plasma cell are not made. Note that a secondary response is induced by the carrier protein, not by the hapten.

D. Antigenic Determinants (Epitopes): Epitopes are small chemical groups on the antigen molecule that can elicit and react with antibody. An antigen can have one or more determinants. Most antigens have many determinants; ie, they are multivalent. In general, a determinant is roughly 5 amino acids or sugars in size. The overall three-dimensional structure is the main criterion of antigenic specificity.

E. Dosage, Route, and Timing of Antigen Administration: These also affect immunogenicity. In addition, the genetic constitution of the host (HLA genes) determines whether a molecule is immunogenic. Different strains of the same species of animal may respond differently to the same antigen.

Adjuvants enhance the immune response to an immunogen. They are chemically unrelated to the immunogen and may act by nonspecifically stimulating the immunoreactive cells or by releasing the immunogen slowly. Some human vaccines contain adjuvants such as aluminum hydroxide or lipids.

AGE & THE IMMUNE RESPONSE

Immunity is **less than optimal** at both ends of life, ie, in the **newborn** and the **elderly.** The reason for the relatively poor immune response in newborns is unclear, but they appear to have less effective T cell function than do adults. In newborns, antibodies are provided primarily by the transfer of maternal IgG across the placenta. Maternal antibody decays so that little remains by 3–6 months of age, and the risk of infection in the child is high. Colostrum also contains antibodies, especially secretory IgA, which can protect the newborn against various respiratory and intestinal infections.

The fetus can mount an IgM response to certain (probably T cell-independent) antigens, eg, to *Treponema pallidum,* the cause of syphilis, which can be acquired congenitally. IgG and IgA begin to be made shortly after birth. The response to certain protein antigens is good; hence, poliovirus immunization can begin at 2 months of age. However, young children respond poorly to certain polysaccharide antigens; therefore, vaccines for protection from certain pathogens, eg, *Streptococcus pneumoniae,* should not be given until 18–24 months of age.

In the elderly, immunity generally declines. There is a reduced IgG response to certain antigens, fewer T cells, and a reduced delayed hypersensitivity response. As in the very young, the frequency and severity of infections are high. The frequency of autoimmune diseases is also high in the elderly, possibly because of a decline in the number of regulatory T cells, which allows autoreactive T cells to proliferate and cause disease.

Review Questions

1. What are the major protective functions of (a) antibodies? (b) cell-mediated immunity?
2. Describe how (a) antibodies and (b) cellular immunity specific for a certain antigen arise.
3. What are the mediators of natural and acquired immunity?
4. Distinguish between active and passive immunity. What are the advantages and disadvantages of each?
5. What are the main attributes that make a substance a good antigen?
6. What is (a) a hapten? (b) an epitope? (c) an adjuvant?
7. What is the nature of the interaction between antigen and antibody?
8. How does humoral immunity in the newborn differ from that in the adult?

Cellular Basis of the Immune Response

58

ORIGIN OF IMMUNE CELLS

during development, precursors in fetal liver + yolk sac
postnatal —reside in bone marrow. differentiate in thymus

The capability of responding to immunologic stimuli rests mainly with lymphoid cells. During embryonic development, blood cell precursors originate mainly in the fetal liver and yolk sac; in postnatal life, the stem cells reside in the bone marrow. Stem cells differentiate into cells of the erythroid, myeloid, or lymphoid series. The latter evolve into two main lymphocyte populations: **T cells** and **B cells** (Fig 58–1 and Table 58–1). The ratio of T cells to B cells is approximately 3:1.

T cell precursors differentiate into immunocompetent T cells within the thymus. Stem cells lack antigen receptors and CD3, CD4, and CD8 molecules on their surface, but during passage through the thymus they differentiate into T cells that can express these glycoproteins. The stem cells, which initially express neither CD4 nor CD8 (double-negatives), first differentiate to express **both** CD4 and CD8 (double-positives) and then proceed to express **either** CD4 or CD8. A double-positive cell will differentiate into a CD4-positive cell if it contacts a cell bearing class II MHC proteins but will differentiate into a CD8-positive cell if it contacts a cell bearing class I MHC proteins. (Mutant mice that do not make class II MHC proteins will not make CD4-positive cells, indicating that this interaction is required for differentiation into single-positive cells to occur.) The double-negative cells and the double-positive cells are located in the cortex of the thymus, whereas the single-positive cells are located in the medulla, from which they migrate outside of the thymus.

Within the thymus, two very important processes called **thymic education** occur.

self-reactive cells are removed via negative selection clonal deletion → tolerance

1. CD4-positive, CD8-positive cells, bearing antigen receptors, antigen receptors for "self" proteins, are killed (**clonal deletion**) by a process of "programmed cell death" called **apoptosis** (Fig. 58–2). The removal of these self-reactive cells, a process called **negative selection,** results in **tolerance** to our own proteins, ie, self-tolerance, and prevents autoimmune reactions (see Chapter 66).

2. CD4-positive, CD8-positive cells, bearing antigen receptors, that do not react with self MHC proteins (see the section on activation, below) are also killed. This results in a **positive selection** for T cells that react well with self MHC proteins. *kill cells that don't react properly.*

These two processes produce cells that are selected for their ability to react both with foreign antigens via their antigen receptors and with self MHC proteins. Both of these features are required for an effective immune response by T cells.

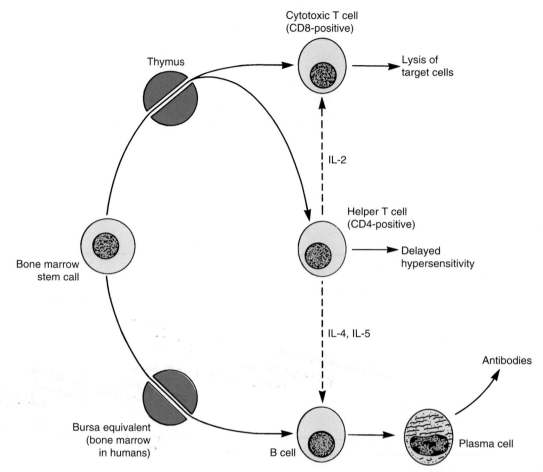

Figure 58–1. Origin of T and B cells. Stem cells in the bone marrow (or fetal liver) are the precursors of both T and B lymphocytes. Stem cells differentiate into T cells in the thymus, whereas they differentiate into B cells in the bone marrow. Within the thymus, T cells become either CD4-positive (helper) cells or CD8-positive (cytotoxic) cells. B cells can differentiate into plasma cells that produce large amounts of antibodies (immunoglobulins). Dotted lines indicate interactions mediated by interleukins. (Modified and reproduced, with permission, from Brooks GF et al: *Medical Microbiology,* 20th ed. Appleton & Lange, 1995.)

Table 58–1. Comparison of T cells and B cells.

Feature	T Cells	B Cells
Antigen receptors on surface	Yes	Yes
IgM on surface	No	Yes
CD3 proteins on surface	Yes	No
Clonal expansion after contact with specific antigen	Yes	Yes
Immunoglobulin synthesis	No	Yes
Regulator of antibody synthesis	Yes	No
IL-2, IL-4, IL-5, and gamma interferon synthesis	Yes	No
Effector of cell-mediated immunity	Yes	No
Maturation in thymus	Yes	No
Maturation in bursa or its equivalent	No	Yes

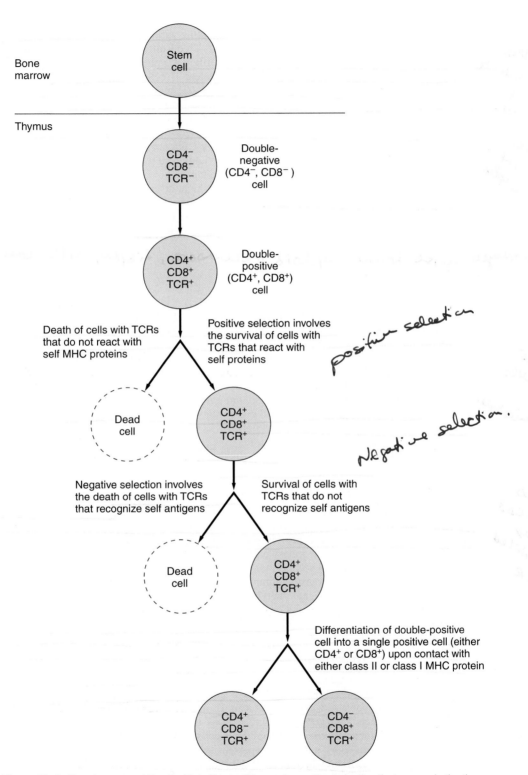

Figure 58–2. Development of T cells. Note the positive and negative selection that occurs in the thymus.

During their passage through the thymus, each double-positive T cell synthesizes a different, highly specific antigen receptor. The rearrangement of the variable, diversity, and joining genes (see Chapter 59) that encode the receptor occurs early in T cell differentiation and accounts for the remarkable ability of T cells to recognize millions of different antigens.

B cell precursors differentiate into immunocompetent B cells in the bone marrow; they do not pass through the thymus. B cells also undergo clonal deletion of those cells bearing antigen receptors for self proteins, a process that induces tolerance and reduces the occurrence of autoimmune diseases (see Chapter 66). The site of clonal deletion of B cells is uncertain, but it is not the thymus.

Natural killer (NK) cells are large granular lymphocytes that do not pass through the thymus, do not have an antigen receptor, and do not bear CD4 or CD8 proteins. They recognize and kill target cells, such as virus-infected cells and tumor cells, without the requirement that the antigens be presented in association with class I or class II MHC proteins.

In contrast to T cells, B cells, and NK cells, which differentiate from lymphoid stem cells, macrophages arise from myeloid precursors. Macrophages have two important functions, namely, phagocytosis and antigen presentation. They do not pass through the thymus and do not have an antigen receptor. On their surface, they display class II MHC proteins, which play an essential role in antigen presentation to helper T cells.

T CELLS

T cells perform several important functions, which can be divided into two main categories, namely, **regulatory** and **effector.** The regulatory functions are mediated primarily by **helper** (CD4-positive) T cells, which produce **interleukins.** For example, helper T cells make (1) interleukin-4 (IL-4) and IL-5, which help B cells produce antibodies; (2) IL-2, which activates CD4 and CD8 cells; and (3) gamma interferon, which activates macrophages, the main mediators of delayed hypersensitivity against intracellular organisms such as *Mycobacterium tuberculosis.* (Suppressor T cells are postulated to down-regulate the immune response, but evidence to support the existence of these cells is lacking.) The effector functions are carried out primarily by cytotoxic (CD8-positive) T cells, which kill virus-infected cells, tumor cells, and allografts.

CD4 & CD8 Types of T Cells   Within the thymus, perhaps within the outer cortical epithelial cells (nurse cells), T cell progenitors differentiate under the influence of thymic hormones (thymosins and thymopoietins) into T cell subpopulations. These cells are characterized by certain surface glycoproteins, eg, CD3, CD4, and CD8. **All T cells have CD3** proteins on their surface in association with antigen receptors (T cell receptor [see below]). The CD3 complex of five transmembrane proteins is involved with transmitting, from the outside of the cell to the inside, the information that the **antigen receptor is occupied.** One of the CD3 transmembrane proteins, the zeta chain, is linked to a tyrosine kinase called *fyn,* which is involved with signal transduction. The signal is transmitted via several second messengers, which are described in the section on activation (see below). CD4 is a single transmembrane polypeptide whereas CD8 consists of two transmembrane polypeptides. They may signal via tyrosine kinase (the *lck* kinase) also.

T cells are subdivided into two major categories on the basis of whether they have CD4 or CD8 proteins on their surface. Mature T cells have either CD4 or CD8 proteins but not both.

CD4 lymphocytes perform the following **helper functions:** (1) they help B cells develop into antibody-producing plasma cells; (2) they help CD8 T cells to become activated cytotoxic T cells; and (3) they help macrophages effect delayed hypersensitivity (eg, limit infection by *M tuberculosis*). These functions are performed by 2 subpopulations of CD4 cells: **Th-1 cells** help the delayed hypersensitivity response by producing primarily IL-2 and gamma interferon, whereas **Th-2 cells** perform the B cell helper function by producing primarily IL-4 and IL-5 (Fig 58–3). One important regulator of the balance between Th-1 cells and Th-2 cells is interleukin-12 (IL-12), which is produced by macrophages. IL-12 increases the number of Th-1 cells, thereby enhancing host defenses against organisms that are controlled by a delayed hypersensitivity response (Table 58–2). Another important regulator is gamma interferon which inhibits the production of Th-2 cells. CD4 cells make up about 65% of peripheral T cells and predominate in the thymic medulla, tonsils, and blood.

CD8 lymphocytes perform cytotoxic functions; that is, they kill virus-infected, tumor, and allograft cells. They kill by either of two mechanisms, namely, the release of perforins, which destroy cell membranes, or the induction of programmed cell death (apoptosis). CD8 cells predominate in human bone marrow and gut lymphoid tissue and constitute about 35% of peripheral T cells.

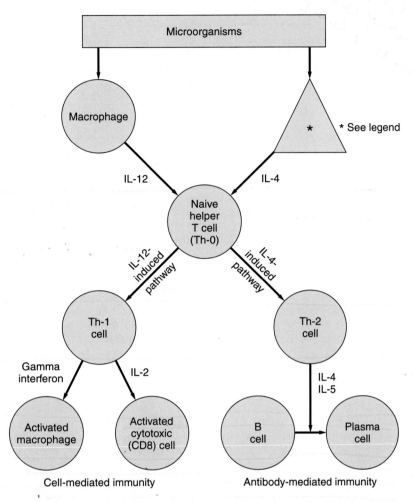

Figure 58–3. The origin of Th-1 and Th-2 cells. On the **left** side, the origin of Th-1 cells is depicted. Microorganisms are ingested by macrophages and IL-12 is produced. IL-12 induces naive Th-0 cells to become Th-1 cells that produce gamma interferon and IL-2. These interleukins activate macrophages and cytotoxic T cells, respectively, and cell-mediated immunity occurs. On the **right** side, the origin of Th-2 cells is depicted. Microorganisms are ingested by an unknown type of cell (see footnote below) and IL-4 is produced. IL-4 induces naive Th-0 cells to become Th-2 cells that produce IL-4 and IL-5. These interleukins activate B cells to become plasma cells and antibodies are produced.

Not shown in the figure is an important regulatory step, namely, that IL-10 produced by Th-2 cells inhibits IL-12 production by macrophages and drives the system toward an antibody response and away from a cell-mediated response.

* The human cell that produces the IL-4 which induces naive helper T cells to become Th-2 cells has not been identified.

Activation of T Cells   The activation of **helper T cells** requires that they recognize a complex on the surface of antigen-presenting cells (APCs), eg, macrophages* consisting of **both the antigen and a class II MHC protein.** Within the cytoplasm of the macrophage, the foreign protein is cleaved into small peptides that associate with the class II MHC proteins. The complex is transported to the surface of the macrophage, where the antigen, in association with a class II MHC protein, is presented to the receptor on the CD4-positive helper cell. Similar events occur within a virus-infected cell, ex-

Class II MHC activates receptor on CD4 + helper Tcell.

*Macrophages are the most important antigen-presenting cells, but B cells, dendritic cells in the spleen, and Langerhans cells on the skin also present antigen, ie, have class II proteins on their surface.

[Handwritten margin note, top: "Rule of Eight: CD4 interact w/ class II (4×2=8). CD8 interacts w/ class I (8×1=8)"]

Table 58–2. Comparison of Th-1 cells and Th-2 cells.

Property	Th-1 Cells	Th-2 Cells
Produces IL-2 and gamma interferon	Yes	No
Produces IL-4, IL-5, IL-6, and IL-10	No	Yes
Enhances cell-mediated immunity and delayed hypersensitivity primarily	Yes	No
Enhances antibody production primarily	No	Yes
Stimulated by IL-12	Yes	No
Stimulated by IL-4	No	Yes

cept that the cleaved viral peptide associates with a **class I** rather than a class II MHC protein. The complex is transported to the surface, where the viral antigen is presented to the receptor on a **CD8-positive cytotoxic cell.** Remember the rule of eight: CD4 cells interact with class II (4 x 2 = 8), and CD8 cells interact with class I (8 x 1 = 8).

There are many different alleles within the class I and class II MHC genes; hence, there are many different MHC proteins. These various MHC proteins bind to different peptide fragments. The polymorphism of the MHC genes and the proteins they encode are a means of presenting many different antigens to the T cell receptor. Note that class I and class II MHC proteins can *only* present peptides; other types of molecules do not bind and therefore cannot be presented. MHC proteins can present peptides derived from self proteins as well as from foreign proteins; therefore whether an immune response occurs is determined by whether a T cell bearing a receptor specific for that peptide has survived the positive and negative selection processes in the thymus.

[Handwritten margin note: "1st step in activation is Ag: Ab interaction"]

The first step in the activation process is the interaction of the antigen with the T cell receptor specific for that antigen (Fig 58–4). **IL-1** produced by the macrophage is also necessary for efficient helper T cell activation. Note that when the T cell receptor interacts with the antigen-MHC protein complex, the CD4 protein on the surface of the helper T cell also interacts with the class II MHC protein. In addition to the binding of the CD4 protein with the MHC class II protein, other proteins interact to help stabilize the contact between the T cell and the APC; eg, LFA-1 protein* on T cells (both CD4-positive and CD8-positive) binds to ICAM-1 protein* on APCs.

[Handwritten margin note: "CD28/B7 interaction is essential for proper"]

For full activation of helper T cells, an additional **"costimulatory" signal** is required; that is, **B7 protein on the APC must interact with CD28 protein** on the helper T cell (Fig 58–4). If the costimulatory signal occurs, IL-2 is made by the helper T cell, and it is this step that is crucial to producing a helper T cell capable of performing its regulatory, effector, and memory functions. If, on the other hand, the T cell receptor interacts with its antigen (epitope) and the costimulatory signal does not occur, a state of unresponsiveness called **anergy** ensues (see Chapter 66). The anergic state is specific for that epitope, since other helper T cells specific for other epitopes are not affected. (A second costimulatory protein called CTLA-4 serves a similar function to CD28 but is expressed only on activated T cells.)

T cells recognize *only* polypeptide antigens. Furthermore, they recognize those polypeptides only when they are presented in association with MHC proteins. Helper T cells recognize antigen in association with class II MHC proteins, whereas cytotoxic T cells recognize antigen in association with class I MHC proteins. This is called **MHC restriction;** ie, the two types of T cells (CD4 helper and CD8 cytotoxic) are "restricted" because they are able to recognize antigen *only* when the antigen is presented with the proper class of MHC protein. This restriction is mediated by specific binding sites primarily on the T cell receptor, but also on the CD4 and CD8 proteins that bind to specific regions on the class II and class I MHC proteins, respectively.

[Handwritten margin note: "Class I MHC present endogenous proteins. Class II MHC present antigens of extracellular organisms that have been taken up by macrophg."]

Generally speaking, class I MHC proteins present **endogenously synthesized** antigens, eg, viral proteins, whereas class II MHC proteins present the antigens of **extracellular** microorganisms that have been phagocytized, eg, bacterial proteins. One important consequence of these observations is that killed viral vaccines do not activate the cytotoxic (CD8-positive) T cells, because the virus does not replicate within cells and therefore viral epitopes are not presented in association with class I MHC proteins. Class I and class II proteins are described in more detail in Chapter 62.

*LFA proteins belong to a family of cell surface proteins called **integrins,** which mediate adhesion to other cells. Integrin proteins are embedded in the surface membrane and have both extracellular and intracellular domains. Hence they interact with other cells externally and with the cytoplasm internally. Abbreviations: LFA, lymphocyte function-associated antigen; ICAM, intercellular adhesion molecule.

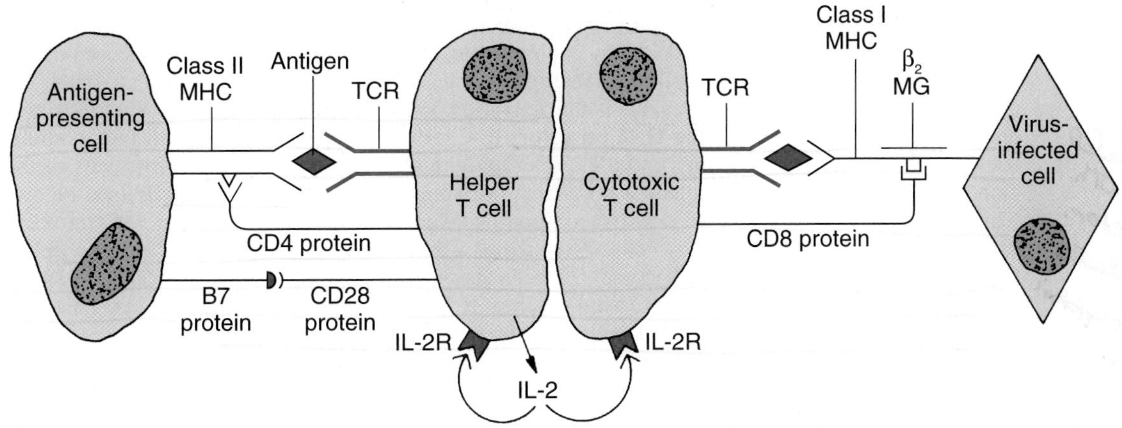

Figure 58–4. Activation of T cells. **Left:** An antigen-presenting cell (APC) presents processed antigen in association with a class II MHC protein. The antigen is recognized by the T cell receptor (TCR) specific for that antigen, and the helper T cell is activated to produce interleukin-2 (IL-2). IL-2 binds to its receptor on the helper T cell and further activates it. Note that CD4 protein on the helper T cell binds to the MHC class II protein on the APC, which stabilizes the interaction between the two cells, and that B7 on the APC must interact with CD28 on the helper T cell for full activation of helper T cells to occur. **Right:** A virus-infected cell presents viral antigen in association with class I MHC protein. The viral antigen is recognized by the TCR specific for that antigen and, in conjunction with IL-2 produced by the helper T cell, the cytotoxic T cell is activated to kill the virus-infected cell. The CD8 protein on the cytotoxic T cell binds to the class I protein on the virus-infected cell, which stabilizes the interaction between the two cells. Note that the class II MHC protein consists of two polypeptides, both of which are encoded by genes in the HLA locus. The class I protein, in contrast, consists of one polypeptide encoded by the HLA locus and β_2-microglobulin (β_2 MG), which is encoded elsewhere.

This distinction between endogenously synthesized and extracellularly acquired proteins is achieved by **processing the proteins in different compartments** within the cytoplasm. The endogenously synthesized proteins, eg, viral proteins, are cleaved by a proteasome, and the peptide fragments associate with a **"TAP transporter"** that transports the fragment into the **rough endoplasmic reticulum,** where it associates with the class I MHC protein. The complex of peptide fragment and class I MHC protein then migrates via the Golgi apparatus to the cell surface. In contrast, the extracellularly acquired proteins are cleaved to peptide fragments within an **endosome,** where the fragment associates with class II MHC proteins. This complex then migrates to the cell surface.

An additional protection that prevents endogenously synthesized proteins from associating with class II MHC proteins is the presence of an **"invariant chain"** that is attached to the class II MHC proteins when these proteins are outside of the endosome. The invariant chain is degraded by proteases within the endosome, allowing the peptide fragment to attach to the class II MHC proteins only within that compartment.

B cells, on the other hand, can interact directly with antigens via their surface immunoglobulins (IgM and IgD). Antigens do *not* have to be presented to B cells in association with class II MHC proteins, unlike T cells. Note that B cells can then present the antigen, after internalization and processing, to helper T cells in association with class II MHC proteins located on the surface of the B cells (see the section on B cells, below). Unlike the antigen receptor on T cells, which recognizes only peptides, the antigen receptors on B cells (IgM and IgD) recognize many different types of molecules, such as peptides, polysaccharides, nucleic acids, and small chemicals, eg, penicillin.

These differences between T cells and B cells explain the hapten-carrier relationship described in Chapter 57. To stimulate hapten-specific antibody, the hapten must be covalently bound to the carrier protein. A B cell specific for the hapten internalizes the hapten-carrier conjugate, processes the carrier protein, and presents a peptide to a helper T cell bearing a receptor for that peptide. The helper T cell then secretes lymphokines that activate the B cell to produce antibodies to the hapten.

When the antigen-MHC protein complex on the APC interacts with the T cell receptor, a signal is transmitted by the CD3 protein complex through several pathways that eventually lead to a large influx of calcium into the cell. (The details of the signal transduction pathway are beyond the scope of this book, but it is known that stimulation of the T cell receptor activates a series of phosphokinases which then activate phospholipase C, which cleaves phosphoinositide to produce inositol triphosphate, which opens the calcium channels.) Calcium activates calcineurin, a serine phosphatase. Calcineurin moves to the nucleus and is involved in the activation of the genes for IL-2 and the IL-2 receptor. (Calcineurin function is blocked by cyclosporine, one of the most effective drugs used to prevent rejection of organ transplants [see Chapter 62].)

The end result of this series of events is the activation of the helper T cell to produce various lymphokines, eg, **IL-2,** as well as the **IL-2 receptor,** IL-2, also known as T cell growth factor, stimulates the helper T cell to multiply into a clone of antigen-specific helper T cells. Most cells of this clone perform effector and regulatory functions, but some become **"memory"** cells (see below), which are capable of being rapidly activated upon exposure to antigen at a later time. (Cytotoxic T cells and B cells also form memory cells.) Note that IL-2 stimulates CD8 cytotoxic T cells as well as CD4 helper T cells. Activated CD4-positive T cells also produce another lymphokine called **gamma interferon,** which increases the expression of class II MHC proteins on APCs. This enhances the ability of APCs to present antigen to T cells and upregulates the immune response.

The process of activating T cells does not function as a simply "on-off" switch. The binding of an epitope to the T cell receptor can result in full activation, partial activation in which only certain lymphokines are made, or no activation, depending on which of the signal transduction pathways is stimulated by that particular epitope. This important observation may have profound implications for our understanding of how helper T cells shape our response to infectious agents.

There are three genes at the class I locus (A, B, and C) and three genes at the class II locus (DP, DQ, and DR). We inherit one set of class I and one set of class II genes from each parent. Therefore, our cells can express as many as six different class I and six different class II proteins (see Chapter 62). Furthermore, there are multiple alleles at each gene locus. Each of these MHC proteins can present peptides with a different amino acid sequence. This explains, in part, our ability to respond to many different antigens.

Memory T Cells

Memory T (and B) cells, as the name implies, endow our host defenses with the ability to respond rapidly and vigorously for many years after the initial exposure to a microbe or other foreign material. This memory response to a specific antigen is due to several features: (1) many memory cells are produced, so that the secondary response is greater than the primary response, in which very few cells respond; (2) memory cells live for many years or have the capacity to reproduce themselves; (3) memory cells are activated by smaller amounts of antigen and require less costimulation than do naive, unactivated T cells; and (4) activated memory cells produce greater amounts of interleukins than do naive T cells when they are first activated.

T Cell Receptor

The T cell receptor (TCR) for antigen consists of two polypeptides, alpha and beta,* which are associated with CD3 proteins. TCR proteins are **similar** to immunoglobulin heavy chains in that (1) the genes that code for them are formed by rearrangement of multiple regions of DNA (see Chapter 59); (2) there are V (variable), D (diversity), J (joining), and C (constant) segments that rearrange to provide diversity, giving rise to an estimated number of more than 10^7 different receptor proteins; (3) each T cell has a unique T cell receptor on its surface; and (4) activated T cells, like activated B cells, clonally expand to yield large numbers of cells specific for that antigen.

Although TCRs and immunoglobulins are analogous in that they both interact with antigen in a highly specific manner, the T cell receptor is different in two important ways: (1) it has two chains rather than four; and (2) it recognizes antigen only in conjunction with MHC proteins, whereas immunoglobulins recognize free antigen.

Effect of Superantigens on T Cells

Certain proteins, particularly staphylococcal enterotoxins and toxic shock syndrome toxin, act as "superantigens" (Fig 58–5). In contrast to the usual antigen, which activates one (or a few) helper T cell, superantigens activate a large number of helper T cells. For example, toxic shock syndrome toxin binds directly to class II MHC proteins without internal processing of the toxin. This complex interacts with the variable portion of the beta chain (Vβ) of the T cell receptor of many T cells.† This activates the T cells, causing the release of IL-2 from the T cells and IL-1 from macrophages. These interleukins account for many of the findings

---

*Some TCRs have a different set of polypeptides called gamma and delta. Some of the T cells bearing these TCRs are involved in cell-mediated immunity against *M tuberculosis*.

†Each superantigen, eg, the different staphylococcal enterotoxins, interacts with different Vβ chains. This explains why many but not all helper T cells are activated by the various superantigens.

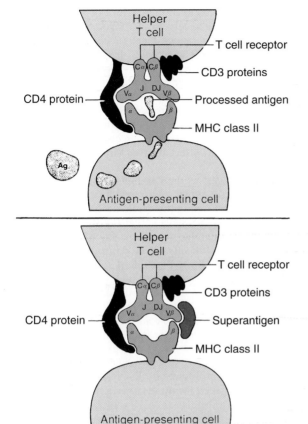

Figure 58–5. Activation of helper T cells by superantigen. **Top:** The helper T cell is activated by the presentation of processed antigen in association with class II MHC protein to the antigen-specific portion of the T cell receptor. Note that superantigen is not involved and that only one or a small number of helper T cells specific for the antigen are activated. **Bottom:** The helper T cell is activated by the binding of superantigen to the Vβ portion of the T cell receptor outside of its antigen-specific site without being processed by the antigen-presenting cell. Because it bypasses the antigen-specific site, super-antigen can activate many helper T cells. (Modified and reproduced, with permission, from Pantaleo G et al: *N Engl J Med* 1993; **328:**327.)

seen in toxin-mediated staphylococcal diseases. Certain viral proteins, eg, those of mouse mammary tumor virus (a retrovirus), also possess superantigen activity.

Features of T Cells   T cells constitute 65–80% of the recirculating pool of small lymphocytes. Within lymph nodes, they are located in the inner, subcortical region, not in the germinal centers. (B cells make up most of the remainder of the pool of small lymphocytes and are found primarily in the germinal centers of lymph nodes.) The life span of T cells is long: months or years. They can be stimulated to divide when exposed to certain mitogens, eg, phytohemagglutinin or concanavalin A (endotoxin, a lipopolysaccharide found on the surface of gram-negative bacteria, is a mitogen for B cells but not T cells). Most human T cells have receptors for sheep erythrocytes on their surface and can form "rosettes" with them; this finding serves as a means of identifying T cells in a mixed population of cells.

Effector Functions of T Cells   There are two important components of host defenses mediated by T cells: delayed hypersensitivity and cytotoxicity.

A. Delayed Hypersensitivity: Delayed hypersensitivity reactions are produced particularly against antigens of **intracellular microorganisms** including certain fungi, eg, *Histoplasma* and *Coccidioides,* and certain intracellular bacteria, eg, mycobacteria. Delayed hypersensitivity is mediated by **macrophages and CD4 cells,** in particular by the Th-1 subset of CD4 cells. Important lymphokines for these reactions include gamma interferon, macrophage activation factor, and macrophage migration inhibition factor. CD4 cells produce the interleukins, and macrophages are the ultimate effectors of delayed hypersensitivity. A deficiency of cell-mediated immunity manifests itself as a marked susceptibility to infection by such microorganisms.

B. Cytotoxicity: The **cytotoxic response** is concerned primarily with **graft rejection** and with destroying **virus-infected cells and tumor cells.** In response to virus-infected cells, the CD8 lymphocytes must recognize both viral antigens and class I molecules on the surface of infected cells. To kill the virus-infected cell, the cytotoxic T cell must also receive a cytokine stimulus from a helper T cell. To become activated to produce these cytokines, helper T cells recognize viral antigens bound to class II molecules on an APC, eg, a macrophage. The activated helper T cells secrete cytokines such as IL-2, which stimulates the virus-specific cytotoxic T cell to form a clone of activated cytotoxic T cells. These cytotoxic T cells kill the virus-infected cells by inserting "**perforins**" and degradative enzymes called **granzymes** into the infected cell. Perforins form a channel through the membrane, the cell contents are lost, and the cell dies. Granzymes are proteases that degrade proteins in the cell membrane, which also leads to the loss of cell contents and hence to cell death. After killing the virus-infected cell, the cytotoxic T cell itself is not damaged and can continue to kill other cells infected with the same virus. Cytotoxic T cells have no effect on free virus, only on virus-infected cells.

A third mechanism by which cytotoxic T cells kill target cells is the **Fas-Fas ligand (FasL)** interaction. Fas is a protein displayed on the surface of many cells. When a cytotoxic T cell receptor recognizes an epitope on the surface of a target cell, FasL is induced in the cytotoxic T cell. When Fas and FasL interact, apoptosis (death) of the target cell occurs. NK cells can also kill target cells by Fas-FasL-induced apoptosis.

In addition to direct killing by cytotoxic T cells, virus-infected cells can be destroyed by a combination of IgG and phagocytic cells. In this process, called **antibody-dependent cellular cytotoxicity (ADCC)**, antibody bound to the surface of the infected cell is recognized by IgG receptors on the surface of phagocytic cells, eg, macrophages or NK cells, and the infected cell is killed. The ADCC process can also kill helminths (worms). In this case, IgE is the antibody involved and eosinophils are the effector cells. IgE binds to surface proteins on the worm, and the surface of eosinophils displays receptors for the epsilon heavy chain. The major basic protein located in the granules of the eosinophils is released and damages the surface of the worm.

Many tumor cells develop new antigens on their surface. These antigens bound to class I proteins are recognized by cytotoxic T cells, which are stimulated to proliferate by IL-2. The resultant clone of cytotoxic T cells can kill the tumor cells, a phenomenon called **immune surveillance.**

In response to allografts, cytotoxic (CD8) cells recognize the class I MHC molecules on the surface of the foreign cells. Helper (CD4) cells recognize the foreign class II molecules on certain cells in the graft, eg, macrophages and lymphocytes. The activated helper cells secrete IL-2, which stimulates the cytotoxic cell to form a clone of cells. These cytotoxic cells kill the cells in the allograft.

Regulatory Functions of T Cells

T cells play a central role in regulating both the humoral (antibody) and cell-mediated arms of the immune system.

A. Antibody Production: Antibody production by B cells usually requires the participation of helper T cells (**T cell-dependent response**), but antibodies to some antigens, eg, polymerized (multivalent) macromolecules such as bacterial capsular polysaccharide, are **T cell-independent.** These polysaccharides are long chains consisting of repeated subunits of several sugars. The **repeated subunits act as a multivalent antigen** that cross-links the IgM antigen receptors on the B cell and activates it in the absence of help from CD4 cells.

In the following example illustrating the T cell-dependent response, B cells are used as the APC, although macrophages commonly perform this function. In this instance, antigen binds to surface IgM or IgD, is internalized within the B cell, and is fragmented. Some of the fragments return to the surface in association with class II MHC molecules (Fig 58–6A).* These interact with the receptor on the helper T cell, and, if the costimulatory signal is given by the B7 protein on the B cell interacting with CD28 protein on the helper T cell, the helper T cell is then stimulated to produce lymphokines, eg, IL-2, B cell growth factor (IL-4), and B cell differentiation factor (IL-5). IL-4 and IL-5 induce "class switching" from IgM, which is the first class of immunoglobulins produced, to other classes, namely, IgG, IgA, and IgE (see the end of Chapter 59). These factors stimulate the B cell to divide and differentiate into many antibody-producing plasma cells.

Note that interleukins alone are *not* sufficient to activate B cells. A membrane protein on activated helper T cells, called CD40 ligand (CD40L), must interact with a protein called CD40 on the

---

*Note that one important difference between B cells and T cells is that B cells recognize antigen itself, whereas T cells recognize antigen only in association with MHC proteins.

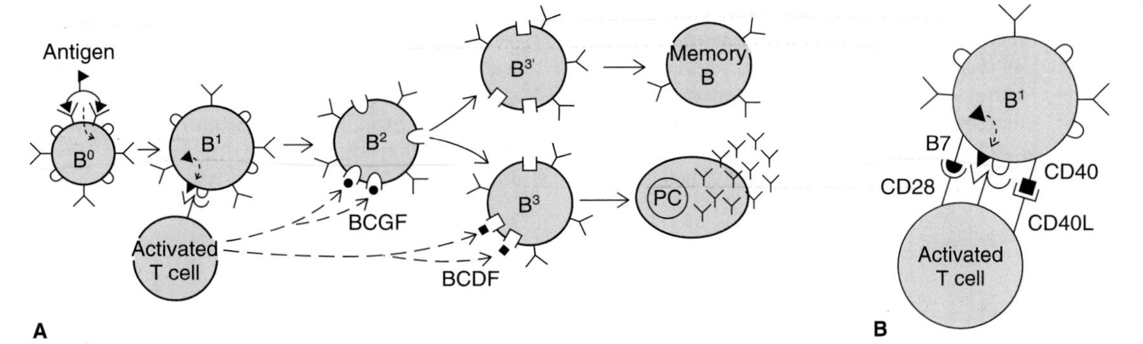

Figure 58–6. **A.** B cell activation by helper T cells. B^0 is a resting B cell to which a multivalent antigen ( ) is attaching to monomer IgM receptors (Y). The antigen is internalized, and a fragment (▲) is returned to the surface in conjunction with a class II molecule (△). A receptor on an activated T cell recognizes the complex on the B cell surface and the T cell produces B cell growth factor (BCGF, IL-4; ●) and B cell differentiation factor (BCDF, IL-5; ■). These factors cause the progression of the B^1 cell to form B^2 and B^3 cells, which differentiate into antibody-producing (eg, pentamer IgM) plasma cells (PC). Memory B cells are also produced. (Modified and reproduced, with permission, from Stites DP, Terr A [editors]: *Basic & Clinical Immunology,* 7th ed. Appleton & Lange, 1991.) **B.** Inducible protein B7 on the B cell must interact with CD28 protein on the helper T cell in order for the helper T cell to be fully activated, and CD40L (CD40 ligand) on the helper T cell must interact with CD40 on the B cell for the B cell to be activated and synthesize the full range of antibodies.

surface of the resting B cells to stimulate the differentiation of B cells into antibody-producing plasma cells (Fig 58–6B). Furthermore, other proteins on the surface of these cells serve to strengthen the interaction between the helper T cell and the antigen-presenting B cell; eg, CD28 on the T cell interacts with B7 on the B cell and LFA-1 on the T cell interacts with ICAM-1 on the B cell. (There are also ICAM proteins on the T cell that interact with LFA proteins on the B cell.)

In the T cell-dependent response, all classes of antibody are made (IgG, IgM, IgA, etc), whereas in the **T cell-independent response, primarily IgM is made.** This indicates that lymphokines produced by the helper T cell are needed for class switching. The T cell-dependent response generates memory B cells whereas the T cell-independent response does not, so a secondary antibody response (see Chapter 60) does not occur in the latter. The T cell-independent response is the main response to bacterial capsular polysaccharides, because these molecules are not effectively processed and presented by APCs and hence do not activate helper T cells. The most likely reason for this is that polysaccharides do not bind to class II MHC proteins whereas peptide antigens do.

B. Cell-Mediated Immunity: In the cell-mediated response, the initial events are similar to those described above for antibody production. The antigen is processed by macrophages, is fragmented, and is presented in conjunction with class II MHC molecules on the surface. These interact with the receptor on the helper T cell, which is then stimulated to produce lymphokines such as IL-2 (T cell growth factor), which stimulates the specific helper and cytotoxic T cells to grow.

C. Suppression of Certain Immune Responses: Certain T cells can suppress antibody production. Failure of such regulation may result in unrestrained antibody production to self antigens, which can cause autoimmune diseases. There may not be a specific population of T cells that mediates suppression. There is evidence that in some situations CD8 cells can suppress, but inhibitory lymphokines produced by CD4 cells also can play this role.

When there is an imbalance in numbers or activity between CD4 and CD8 cells, cellular immune mechanisms are greatly impaired. For example, in lepromatous leprosy there is unrestrained multiplication of *Mycobacterium leprae,* a lack of delayed hypersensitivity to *M leprae* antigens, a lack of cellular immunity to that organism, and an excess of CD8 cells in lesions. Removal of some CD8 cells can restore cellular immunity in such patients and limit *M leprae* multiplication. In acquired immunodeficiency syndrome (AIDS), the normal ratio of CD4:CD8 cells (> 1.5) is greatly reduced. Many CD4 cells are destroyed by the human immunodeficiency virus (HIV), and the number of CD8 cells increases. This imbalance, ie, a loss of helper activity and an increase in suppressor activity, results in a susceptibility to opportunistic infections and certain tumors.

↓ interferon ⟶ ↑ Class I + II MHC proteins.

One important part of the host response to infection is the increased expression of class I and class II MHC proteins induced by various cytokines, especially interferons such as gamma interferon. The increased amount of MHC proteins leads to increased antigen presentation and a more vigorous immune response. However, certain viruses can suppress the increase in MHC protein expression, thereby enhancing their survival. For example, hepatitis B virus, adenovirus, and cytomegalovirus can prevent an increase in class I MHC protein expression, thereby reducing the cytotoxic T cell response against cells infected by these viruses.

B CELLS

B cells perform two important functions: (1) They differentiate into plasma cells and produce antibodies, and (2) they are antigen-presenting cells (APCs).

Origin   During embryogenesis, B cell precursors are recognized first in the fetal liver. From there they migrate to the **bone marrow,** which is their main location during adult life. Unlike T cells, they **do not require the thymus for maturation.** Pre-B cells lack surface immunoglobulins and light chains but do have μ heavy chains in the cytoplasm. The maturation of B cells has two phases: the antigen-independent phase consists of stem cells, pre-B cells, and B cells, whereas the antigen-dependent phase consists of the cells that arise subsequent to the interaction of antigen with the B cells, eg, activated B cells and plasma cells (Fig 58–7). B cells display surface IgM, which serves as a receptor for antigens. This surface IgM is a monomer, in contrast to circulating IgM, which is a pentamer. Surface IgD on some B cells may also be an antigen receptor.

fetal liver ↓ bone marrow.

B cells constitute about 30% of the recirculating pool of small lymphocytes, and their life span is short, ie, days or weeks. Approximately 10^9 B cells are produced each day. Within lymph nodes, they are located in germinal centers; within the spleen, they are found in the white pulp. They are also found in the gut-associated lymphoid tissue, eg, Peyer's patches.

Clonal Selection   How do antibodies arise? Does the antigen "instruct" the B cell to make an antibody, or does the antigen "select" a B cell endowed with the preexisting capacity to make the antibody?

It appears that the latter alternative, ie, **clonal selection,** accounts for antibody formation. Each individual has a large pool of B lymphocytes (about 10^7). Each immunologically responsive B cell bears a surface receptor (either IgM or IgD) that can react with one antigen (or closely related group of antigens); ie, there are about 10^7 different specificities. An antigen interacts with the B lymphocyte that shows the best "fit" with its immunoglobulin surface receptor. After the antigen binds, the B cell is stimulated to proliferate and form a clone of cells. These selected B cells soon become plasma cells and secrete antibody specific for the antigen. Plasma cells synthesize the immunoglobulins with the same antigenic specificity (ie, they have the same heavy chain and the same light chain)

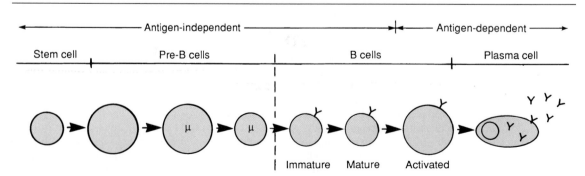

Figure 58–7. Maturation of B cells. B cells arise from stem cells and differentiate into pre-B cells expressing μ heavy chains in the cytoplasm and then into B cells expressing monomer IgM on the surface. This occurs independent of antigen. Activation of B cells and differentiation into plasma cells is dependent on antigen. μ, mu heavy chains in cytoplasm; Y, IgM. (Modified and reproduced, with permission, from Stites DP, Terr A [editors]: *Basic and Clinical Immunology,* 7th ed. Appleton & Lange, 1991.)

as those carried by the selected B cell. Antigenic specificity does *not* change when heavy-chain class switching occurs (see Chapter 59).

Note that **clonal selection also occurs with T cells.** The antigen interacts with a specific receptor located on the surface of either a CD4-positive or a CD8-positive T cell. This "selects" this cell and activates it to expand into a clone of cells with the same specificity.

Activation of B Cells   In the following example, the B cell is the APC. Multivalent antigen binds to surface IgM (or IgD) and cross-links adjacent immunoglobulin molecules. The immunoglobulins aggregate to form "patches" and eventually migrate to one pole of the cell to form a cap. Endocytosis of the capped material follows, the antigen is processed, and epitopes appear on the surface in conjunction with class II MHC proteins. This complex is recognized by a helper T cell with a receptor for the antigen on its surface.* The T cell now produces various lymphokines (IL-2, IL-4, and IL-5) that stimulate the growth and differentiation of the B cell.

The activation of B cells to produce the full range of antibodies requires two other interactions in addition to recognition of the epitope by the T cell antigen receptor and the production of IL-4 and IL-5 by the helper T cell. These **costimulatory** interactions which occur between surface proteins on the T and B cells, are as follows: (1) CD28 on the T cell must interact with B7 on the B cell, and (2) CD40L on the T cell must interact with CD40 on the B cell. The CD28-B7 interaction is required for activation of the T cell to produce IL-2, and the CD40L-CD40 interaction is required for class switching from IgM to IgG and other immunoglobulin classes to occur.

Many **plasma cells** that produce large amounts of immunoglobulins specific for the epitope are the end result. Plasma cells secrete thousands of antibody molecules per second for a few days and then die. Some activated B cells form **memory cells,** which can remain quiescent for long periods but are capable of being activated rapidly upon reexposure to antigen. Most memory B cells have surface IgG that serves as the antigen receptor, but some have IgM. Memory T cells secrete interleukins that enhance antibody production by the memory B cells. The presence of these cells explains the rapid appearance of antibody in the secondary response (see Chapter 60).

MACROPHAGES

Macrophages have three main functions: phagocytosis, antigen presentation, and cytokine production.

(1) Phagocytosis. Macrophages ingest bacteria, viruses, and other foreign particles. They have surface Fc receptors that interact with the Fc portion of immunoglobulins, thereby enhancing the uptake of opsonized organisms.†

(2) Antigen presentation. Foreign material is ingested and degraded, and fragments of antigen are presented on the macrophage cell surface (in conjunction with class II MHC molecules) for interaction with the TCR. Degradation of the foreign protein stops when the fragment associates with the class II MHC protein in the cytoplasm. The complex is then transported to the cell surface by specialized "transporter" proteins.

(3) Cytokine production. Macrophages produce several cytokines (macrokines, monokines), the most important of which are IL-1 and tumor necrosis factor (TNF). IL-1 plays an essential role in the activation of helper T cells, and TNF is an important inflammatory mediator (see below).

Macrophages are derived from bone marrow histiocytes and exist both free, eg, monocytes, and fixed in tissues, eg, Kupffer cells of the liver. Macrophages migrate to the site of inflammation, attracted by certain mediators, especially C5a, an anaphylatoxin released in the complement cascade.

---

*Macrophages bearing antigen bound to class II MHC proteins can also present antigen to the T cell, resulting in antibody formation. In general, B cells are poor activators of "virgin" T cells in the primary response because B cells do not make IL-1. B cells are, however, very good activators of memory T cells because little, if any, IL-1 is needed.
†Macrophages have receptors for complement also.

NATURAL KILLER CELLS — active w/o prior viral exposure.

Natural killer (NK) cells play an important role in the innate host defenses. They specialize in killing virus-infected cells and tumor cells by secreting cytotoxins (perforins and granzymes) similar to those of cytotoxic T lymphocytes and by participating in Fas-Fas ligand-mediated apoptosis. They are called "natural" killer cells because they are active without prior exposure to the virus, are not enhanced by exposure, and are not specific for any virus. They can kill without antibody, but antibody enhances their effectiveness, a process called antibody-dependent cellular cytotoxicity (ADCC) (see the section on effector functions of T cells [above]). IL-12 and gamma interferon are potent activators of NK cells. From 5 to 10% of peripheral lymphocytes are NK cells.

IL-12 +
γ-Interferon
potent activators
of NK cells

NK cells are lymphocytes with some T cell markers, but they do not have to pass through the thymus in order to mature. They have no immunologic memory and, unlike cytotoxic T cells, have no T cell receptor; also, killing does not require recognition of MHC proteins. IL-2-activated NK cells (LAK cells) are being used for the treatment of certain cancers.

POLYMORPHONUCLEAR NEUTROPHILS

These cells and the process of phagocytosis are described in Chapter 8.

IMPORTANT CYTOKINES

The important functions of the main cytokines are described in Table 58–3.

Mediators Affecting Lymphocytes

(1) IL-1 is a protein produced mainly by macrophages. It activates a wide variety of target cells, eg, T and B lymphocytes, neutrophils, epithelial cells, and fibroblasts, to grow, differentiate, or synthesize specific products. For example, it stimulates helper T cells to differentiate and produce IL-2 (see below). In addition, it is **"endogenous pyrogen,"** which acts on the hypothalamus to cause the fever associated with infections and other inflammatory reactions. (Exogenous pyrogen is endotoxin, a lipopolysaccharide found in the cell wall of gram-negative bacteria [see Chapter 7].)

(2) IL-2 is a protein produced mainly by helper T cells that **stimulates both helper and cytotoxic T cells to grow.** Resting T cells are stimulated by antigen (or other stimulators) both to produce IL-2 and to form IL-2 receptors on their surface, thereby acquiring the capacity to respond to IL-2. Interaction of IL-2 with its receptor stimulates DNA synthesis. IL-2 acts synergistically with IL-4 (see below) to stimulate the growth of B cells.

Table 58–3. Important functions of the main cytokines.

Cytokine	Major Source	Important Functions
Interleukin-1	Macrophages	Activates helper T cells. Causes fever.
Interleukin-2	Th-1 subset of helper T cells	Activates helper and cytotoxic T cells. Also activates B cells.
Interleukin-4	Th-2 subset of helper T cells	Stimulates B cell growth. Increases isotype switching and IgE. Increases Th-2 subset of helper T cells.
Interleukin-5	Th-2 subset of helper T cells	Stimulates B cell differentiation. Increases eosinophils and IgA.
Gamma interferon	Th-1 subset of helper T cells	Stimulates phagocytosis and killing by macrophages and NK cells. Increases class I and II MHC protein expression.
Tumor necrosis factor	Macrophages	Low concentration: activates neutrophils and increases their adhesion to endothelial cells. High concentration: mediates septic shock, acts as cachectin, causes necrosis of tumors.

made by TH₂

(3) __IL-4 and IL-5__ are proteins produced by helper T cells; they promote the growth and differentiation of B cells, respectively. IL-4 enhances humoral immunity by increasing the number of Th-2 cells, the subset of helper T cells that produces IL-4 and IL-5 (Fig 58–3). IL-4 is required for class (isotype) switching, ie, the switching from one class of antibody to another, within the antibody-producing cell (see Chapter 59). It also enhances the synthesis of IgE and hence may predispose to type I (anaphylactic) hypersensitivity. IL-5 enhances the synthesis of IgA and stimulates the production and activation of eosinophils. Eosinophils are an important host defense against many helminths (worms), eg, *Strongyloides* (see Chapter 56) and are increased in immediate hypersensitivity (allergic) reactions (see Chapter 65).

(4) Other interleukins (IL-6 through IL-12) have been described. IL-6 is produced by helper T cells and macrophages. It stimulates B cells to differentiate, induces fever by affecting the hypothalamus, and induces the production of acute-phase proteins by the liver.

th -1 delayed hypersensitivity

IL-10 and IL-12 regulate the production of Th-1 cells, the cells that mediate delayed hypersensitivity (Fig 58–3). IL-12 is produced by macrophages and promotes the development of Th-1 cells, whereas IL-10 is produced by Th-2 cells and inhibits the development of Th-1 cells by limiting gamma interferon production. (Gamma interferon is described below.) The relative amounts of IL-4, IL-10, and IL-12 drive the differentiation of Th-1 and Th-2 cells and therefore enhance either cell-mediated or humoral immunity, respectively. This is likely to have important medical consequences because the main host defense against certain infections is either cell-mediated or humoral immunity. For example, *Leishmania* infections in mice are lethal if a humoral response predominates but are controlled if a vigorous cell-mediated response occurs. The other lymphokines are of lesser medical importance than those discussed above.

(5) The main function of transforming growth factor-β (TGF-β) is to **inhibit** the growth and activities of T cells. It is viewed as an "anti-cytokine" because, in addition to its action on T cells, it can inhibit many functions of macrophages, B cells, neutrophils, and natural killer cells by counteracting the action of other activating factors. Although it is a "negative regulator" of the immune response, it stimulates wound healing by enhancing the synthesis of collagen. It is produced by many types of cells, including T cells, B cells, and macrophages. In summary, the role of TGF-β is to dampen or suppress the immune response when it is no longer needed after an infection and to promote the healing process.

Mediators Affecting Macrophages & Monocytes   Chemokines are a group of cytokines that can attract either macrophages or neutrophils to the site of infection. The term "chemokine" is a contraction of **chemo**tactic and cyto**kine.** Approximately 50 chemokines have been identified; they are small polypeptides ranging in size from 68 to 120 amino acids. The alpha-chemokines have two adjacent cysteines (Cys-Cys) whereas the beta-chemokines have two cysteines separated by another amino acid (Cys-X-Cys) (Table 58–4).

The alpha-chemokines attract neutrophils and are produced by activated mononuclear cells. IL-8 is a very important member of this group. The beta-chemokines attract macrophages and monocytes and are produced by activated T cells. RANTES and MCAF are important beta-chemokines.

There are specific receptors for chemokines on the surface of cells, such as neutrophils and monocytes. Interaction of the chemokine with its receptor results in changes in cell surface proteins that allow the cell to adhere to and migrate through the endothelium to the site of infection.

Mediators Affecting Polymorphonuclear Leukocytes

(1) Tumor necrosis factor activates the phagocytic and killing activities of neutrophils and increases the synthesis of adhesion molecules by endothelial cells. The adhesion molecules mediate the attachment of neutrophils at the site of infection.

(2) Leukocyte-inhibitory factor inhibits migration of neutrophils, analogous to migration-inhibitory factor (above).

(3) Chemotactic factors for neutrophils, basophils, and eosinophils selectively attract each cell type. (See the discussion of chemokines [above] and Table 58–4).

Table 58–4. Chemokines of medical importance.

Class	Chemistry	Attracts	Produced by	Examples
Alpha	C-X-C	Neutrophils	Activated mononuclear cells	Interleukin-8
Beta	C-C	Monocytes	Activated T cells	RANTES,[1] MCAF[2]

[1]RANTES is an abbreviation for *r*egulated upon *a*ctivation, *n*ormal *T* expressed and *s*ecreted.
[2]MCAF is an abbreviation for *m*acrophage *c*hemoattractant and *a*ctivating factor.

Mediators Affecting Stem Cells   IL-3 is made by activated helper T cells and supports the growth and differentiation of bone marrow stem cells. Granulocyte-macrophage colony-stimulating factor (GM-CSF, sargramostim) is made by T lymphocytes and macrophages. It stimulates the growth of granulocytes and macrophages and enhances the antimicrobial activity of macrophages. It is used clinically to improve regeneration of these cells after bone marrow transplantation. Granulocyte colony-stimulating factor (G-CSF, filgrastim) is made by various cells, eg, macrophages, fibroblasts, and endothelial cells. It enhances the development of neutrophils from stem cells and is used clinically to prevent infections in patients who have received cancer chemotherapy. The stimulation of neutrophil production by G-CSF and GM-CSF results in the increased number of these cells in the peripheral blood after infection.

Mediators With Other Effects

(1) Interferons are glycoproteins that block virus replication and exert many immunomodulating functions. Alpha interferon (from leukocytes) and beta interferon (from fibroblasts) are induced by viruses (or double-stranded RNA) and have antiviral activity (see Chapter 33). **Gamma interferon** is a lymphokine produced primarily by the Th-1 subset of helper T cells. It is one of the most potent activators of the phagocytic activity of macrophages, NK cells, and neutrophils, thereby enhancing their ability to kill microorganisms and tumor cells. For example, it greatly increases the killing of intracellular bacteria, such as *M tuberculosis*, by macrophages. It also increases the synthesis of class I and II MHC proteins in a variety of cell types. This enhances antigen presentation by these cells.

(2) Tumor necrosis factor (TNF-α) is an **inflammatory mediator** released primarily by macrophages. It has many important effects that differ depending on the concentration. At low concentrations, it increases the synthesis of adhesion molecules by endothelial cells, which allows neutrophils to adhere to blood vessel walls at the site of infection. It also activates the respiratory burst within neutrophils, thereby enhancing the killing power of these phagocytes. It increases lymphokine synthesis by helper T cells and stimulates the growth of B cells. At high concentrations, it is an important mediator of **endotoxin-induced septic shock;** antibody to TNF-α prevents the action of endotoxin. TNF-α is also known as **cachectin** because it inhibits lipoprotein lipase in adipose tissue, thereby reducing the utilization of fatty acids. This results in cachexia. TNF-α, as its name implies, causes the **death and necrosis of certain tumors** in experimental animals. It may do this by promoting intravascular coagulation that causes infarction of the tumor tissue. The role of TNF-α in the death of human tumor cells is unclear.

(3) Lymphotoxin (also known as TNF-β) is made by activated T lymphocytes and causes effects similar to those of TNF-α. It binds to the same receptor as TNF-α and hence has the same effects as TNF-α.

(4) Nitric oxide (NO) is an important mediator made by macrophages in response to the presence of endotoxin, a lipopolysaccharide found in the cell wall of gram-negative bacteria. NO causes vasodilation and therefore may be an important mediator of the hypotension seen in septic shock. Inhibitors of NO synthase, the enzyme that catalyzes the synthesis of NO from arginine, can prevent the hypotension associated with septic shock.

Review Questions

1. Describe the process by which stem cells differentiate into CD4-positive T cells and CD8-positive T cells.
2. What is the goal of thymic education?
3. What are the functions of CD4-positive T cells? of CD8-positive T cells?
4. To activate T cells, two molecules must be recognized on the antigen-presenting cell. One is antigen. What is the other?
5. Which cells contribute to cell-mediated immunity?
6. Which cells have a cytotoxic effect on foreign grafts?
7. How do helper T cells regulate antibody production?
8. How do helper T cells regulate the cell-mediated immune response?
9. Contrast the antigen receptor on the surface of B cells with that on T cells.
10. In regard to antibody synthesis, what does the term "clonal selection" mean?
11. What are the main functions of (a) macrophages? (b) NK cells?
12. Contrast the functions of IL-1 and IL-2. Which cells make these interleukins?
13. What are the main differences between the functions of alpha interferon and those of gamma interferon?
14. What are the four important biologic effects of tumor necrosis factor?

Antibodies

59

Antibodies are globulin proteins (immunoglobulins) that react specifically with the antigen that stimulated their production. They make up about 20% of the protein in blood plasma. Blood contains three types of globulins, alpha, beta, and gamma, based on their electrophoretic migration rate. Antibodies are gamma globulins. There are five classes of antibodies: IgG, IgM, IgA, IgD, and IgE.

Antibodies that arise in an animal in response to typical antigens are heterogeneous, because they are formed by several different clones of plasma cells; ie, they are **polyclonal.** Antibodies that arise from a single clone of cells, eg, in a plasma cell tumor (myeloma),* are homogeneous; ie, they are **monoclonal.** Monoclonal antibodies also can be made in the laboratory by fusing a myeloma cell with an antibody-producing cell (Fig 59–1; also see box [below]). Such **hybridomas** produce virtually unlimited quantities of monoclonal antibodies that are useful in diagnostic tests and in research (see box on p 328).

IMMUNOGLOBULIN STRUCTURE

Immunoglobulins are glycoproteins made up of **light (L) and heavy (H)** polypeptide chains. The terms "light" and "heavy" refer to molecular weight; light chains have a molecular weight of about 25,000, whereas heavy chains have a molecular weight of 50,000–70,000. The simplest antibody

---

*Multiple myeloma is a malignant disease characterized by an overproduction of plasma cells (B cells). All the myeloma cells in a patient produce the same type of immunoglobulin molecule (M protein), which indicates that all the cells arose from a single progenitor. Excess κ or λ L chains are synthesized and appear as dimers in the urine. These are known as Bence Jones proteins and have the unusual attribute of precipitating at 50–60 °C but dissolving when the temperature is raised to the boiling point.

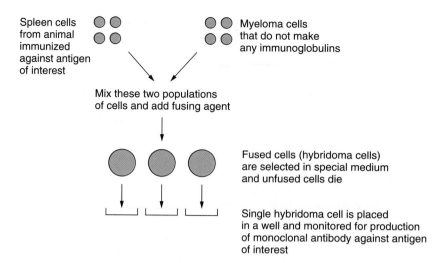

Spleen cells
from animal
immunized
against antigen
of interest

Myeloma cells
that do not make
any immunoglobulins

Mix these two populations
of cells and add fusing agent

Fused cells (hybridoma cells)
are selected in special medium
and unfused cells die

Single hybridoma cell is placed
in a well and monitored for production
of monoclonal antibody against antigen
of interest

Figure 59–1. Production of monoclonal antibodies.

molecule has a Y shape (Fig 59–2) and consists of four polypeptide chains: two H chains and two L chains. The four chains are linked by disulfide bonds. An individual antibody molecule always consists of **identical** H chains and **identical** L chains. This is primarily the result of two phenomena: allelic exclusion (see p 345) and regulation within the B cell, which ensure the synthesis of either kappa (κ) or lambda (λ) L chains but not both.

L and H chains are subdivided into **variable** and **constant** regions. The regions are composed of three-dimensionally folded, repeating segments called domains. An L chain consists of one variable (VL) and one constant (CL) domain. Most H chains consist of one variable (VH) and three constant (CH) domains. (IgG and IgA have three CH domains, whereas IgM and IgE have four.) Each do-

---

Hybridomas & Monoclonal Antibodies

One of the most important scientific advances of this century is the hybridoma cell, which has the remarkable ability to produce large quantities of a single molecular species of immunoglobulin. These immunoglobulins, which are known as monoclonal antibodies, are called "monoclonal" because they are made by a clone of cells that arose from a single cell. Note, however, that this single cell is, in fact, formed by the fusion of two different cells; ie, it is a hybrid, hence the term "hybridoma."

Hybridoma cells are made in the following manner: (1) An animal, eg, a mouse, is immunized with the antigen of interest. (2) Spleen cells from this animal are grown in a culture dish in the presence of mouse myeloma cells. The strain of myeloma cells chosen has two important attributes: it grows indefinitely in culture, and it does not produce immunoglobulins. (3) Fusion of the cells is encouraged by adding certain chemicals, eg, polyethylene glycol. (4) The cells are grown in a special culture medium (HAT medium) that supports the growth of the fused, hybrid cells but not of the "parental" cells. (5) The resulting clones of cells are screened for the production of antibody to the antigen of interest.

Chimeric monoclonal antibodies consisting of mouse variable regions and human constant regions are being made for use in treating human diseases such as leukemia. The advantages of the human constant chain are that human complement is activated (whereas it is not if the constant region is mouse-derived) and that antibodies against the monoclonal antibody are not formed (whereas antibodies are formed if the constant region is mouse-derived). The advantage of the mouse variable region is that it is much easier to obtain monoclonal antibodies against, for example, a human tumor antigen by inoculating a mouse with the tumor cells. Chimeric antibodies can kill tumor cells either by complement-mediated cytotoxicity or by delivering toxins, eg, diphtheria toxin, specifically to the tumor cell.

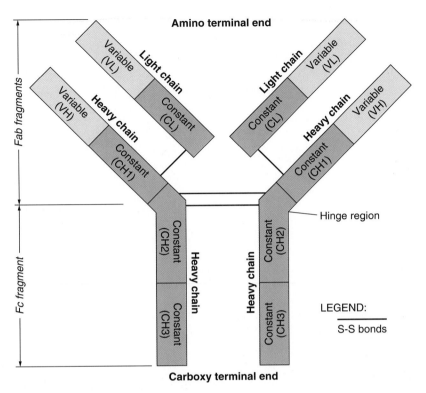

Amino terminal end

Carboxy terminal end

Figure 59–2. Structure of IgG. The Y-shaped IgG molecule consists of two light chains and two heavy chains. Each light chain consists of a variable region and a constant region. Each heavy chain consists of a variable region and a constant region that is divided into three domains: CH1, CH2, and CH3. The CH2 domain contains the complement-binding site, and the CH3 domain is the site of attachment of IgG to receptors on neutrophils and macrophages. The antigen-binding site is formed by the variable regions of both the light and heavy chains. The specificity of the antigen-binding site is a function of the amino acid sequence of the hypervariable regions (see Fig 59–3). (Modified and reproduced, with permission, from Brooks GF et al: *Medical Microbiology,* 20th ed. Appleton & Lange, 1995.)

main is approximately 110 amino acids long. The **variable** regions are responsible for **antigen-binding,** whereas the **constant** regions are responsible for **various biologic functions,** eg, complement activation and binding to cell surface receptors.

The variable regions of both L and H chains have three extremely variable ("**hypervariable**") amino acid sequences at the amino-terminal end that form the antigen-binding site (Fig 59–3). Only 5–10 amino acids in each hypervariable region form the antigen-binding site. Antigen-antibody binding involves electrostatic and van der Waals' forces and hydrogen and hydrophobic bonds rather than covalent bonds. The remarkable specificity of antibodies is due to these hypervariable regions (see the discussion of idiotypes on p 343).

L chains belong to one of two types, κ **(kappa)** or λ **(lambda),** on the basis of amino acid differences in their constant regions. Both types occur in all classes of immunoglobulins (IgG, IgM, etc), but any one immunoglobulin molecule contains only one type of L chain.* The amino-terminal portion of each L chain participates in the antigen-binding site. H chains are distinct for each of the five immunoglobulin classes and are designated γ, α, μ, ε, and δ (Table 59–1). The amino-terminal portion of each H chain participates in the antigen-binding site; the carboxy terminal forms the Fc fragment, which has the biologic activities described above and in Table 59–1.

If an antibody molecule is treated with a proteolytic enzyme such as papain, peptide bonds in the "hinge" region are broken, producing two identical **Fab fragments,** which carry the antigen-binding sites, and one **Fc fragment,** which is involved in placental transfer, complement fixation, attachment site for various cells, and other biologic activities (Fig 59–2).

*In humans, the ratio of immunoglobulins containing κ chains to those containing λ chains is approximately 2:1.

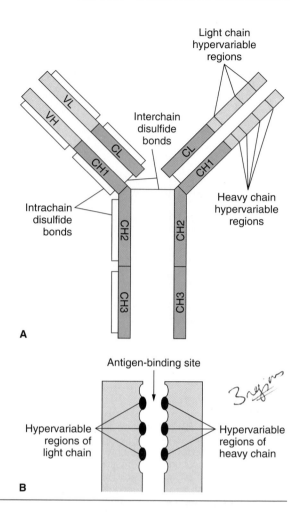

Figure 59–3. The antigen-binding site is formed by the hypervariable regions. **A:** Hypervariable regions on IgG. **B:** Magnified view of antigen-binding site. (Modified and reproduced, with permission, from Stites DP, Terr A, Parslow T [editors]: *Basic & Clinical Immunology*, 8th ed. Appleton & Lange, 1994.)

Table 59–1. Properties of human immunoglobulins.

Property	IgG	IgA	IgM	IgD	IgE
Percentage of total immunoglobulin in serum (approx)	75	15	9	0.2	0.004
Serum concentration (mg/dL) (approx)	1000	200	120	3	0.05
Sedimentation coefficient	7S	7S or 11S[1]	19S	7S	8S
Molecular weight (× 1000)	150	170 or 400[1]	900	180	190
Structure	Monomer	Monomer or dimer	Monomer or pentamer	Monomer	Monomer
H-chain symbol	γ	α	μ	δ	ε
Complement fixation	+	−	+	−	−
Transplacental passage	+	−	−	?	−
Mediation of allergic responses	−	−	−	−	+
Found in secretions	−	+	−	−	−
Opsonization	+	−	−[2]	−	−
Antigen receptor on B cell	−	−	+	?	−
Polymeric form contains J chain	−	+	+	−	−

[1]The 11S form is found in secretions (eg, saliva, milk, and tears) and fluids of the respiratory, intestinal, and genital tracts.
[2] IgM opsonizes indirectly by activating complement. This produces C3b, which is an opsonin.

IMMUNOGLOBULIN CLASSES

IgG   Each IgG molecule consists of two L chains and two H chains linked by disulfide bonds (molecular formula H2L2). Because it has two identical antigen-binding sites, it is said to be **divalent.** There are four subclasses, IgG1–IgG4, based on antigenic differences in the H chains and on the number and location of disulfide bonds. IgG1 makes up most (65%) of the total IgG. IgG2 antibody is directed against polysaccharide antigens and is an important host defense against encapsulated bacteria.

IgG is the predominant antibody in the **secondary response** and constitutes an important defense against bacteria and viruses (Table 59–2). IgG is the only antibody to **cross the placenta;** only its Fc portion binds to receptors on the surface of placental cells. It is therefore the **most abundant immunoglobulin in newborns.** IgG is one of the two immunoglobluins that can activate complement; IgM is the other (see Chapter 63).

IgG is the immunoglobulin that **opsonizes.** It can opsonize, ie, enhance phagocytosis, because there are receptors for the γ H chain on the surface of phagocytes. IgM does not opsonize directly, because there are no receptors on the phagocyte surface for the μ H chain. However, IgM activates complement, and the resulting C3b can opsonize because there are binding sites for C3b on the surface of phagocytes.

IgA   IgA is the main immunoglobulin in **secretions** such as colostrum, saliva, tears, and respiratory, intestinal, and genital tract secretions. It prevents attachment of microorganisms, eg, bacteria and viruses, to mucous membranes. Each secretory IgA molecule consists of two H2L2 units plus one molecule each of J (joining) chain* and secretory component (Fig 59–4). The secretory component is a polypeptide synthesized by epithelial cells that provides for IgA passage to the mucosal surface. It also protects IgA from being degraded in the intestinal tract. In serum, some IgA exists as monomeric H2L2.

IgM   IgM is the main immunoglobulin produced early in the **primary response.** It is present as a monomer on the surface of virtually all B cells, where it functions as an antigen-binding receptor.† In serum, it is a **pentamer** composed of 5 H2L2 units plus one molecule of J (joining) chain (Fig 59–4). Because the pentamer has 10 antigen-binding sites, it is the **most efficient** immunoglobulin in agglutination, complement fixation (activation), and other antibody reactions and is important in defense against bacteria and viruses. It can be produced by the fetus in certain infections. It has the **highest avidity** of the immunoglobulins; its interaction with antigen can involve all 10 of its binding sites.

Table 59–2. Important functions of immunoglobulins.

Immunoglobulin	Major Functions
IgG	Main antibody in the secondary response. Opsonizes bacteria, making them easier to phagocytize. Fixes complement, which enhances bacterial killing. Neutralizes bacterial toxins and viruses. Crosses the placenta.
IgA	Secretory IgA prevents attachment of bacteria and viruses to mucous membranes. Does not fix complement.
IgM	Produced in the primary response to an antigen. Fixes complement. Does not cross the placenta. Antigen receptor on the surface of B cells.
IgD	Uncertain. Found on the surface of many B cells as well as in serum.
IgE	Mediates immediate hypersensitivity by causing release of mediators from mast cells and basophils upon exposure to antigen (allergen). Defends against worm infections by causing release of enzymes from eosinophils. Does not fix complement. Main host defense against helminth infections.

*Only IgA and IgM have J chains. Only these immunoglobulins exist as multimers (dimers and pentamers, respectively). The J chain initiates the polymerization process, and the multimers are held together by disulfide bonds between their Fc regions.

†The surface monomer IgM has a different heavy chain from that of the serum IgM. The heavy chain of the surface IgM has a hydrophobic sequence that mediates binding within the cell membrane.

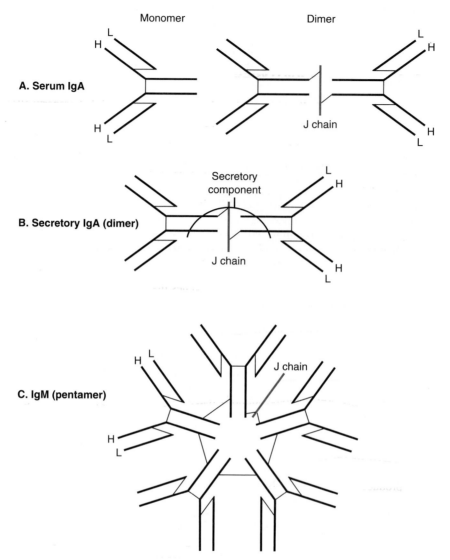

Figure 59–4. Structure of serum IgA, secretory IgA, and IgM. Note that both IgA and IgM have a J chain but that only secretory IgA has a secretory component. (Reproduced, with permission, from Stites D, Terr A, Parslow T [editors]: *Basic & Clinical Immunology,* 8th ed. Appleton & Lange, 1994.)

IgD This immunoglobulin has no known antibody function but may function as an antigen receptor; it is present on the surface of many B lymphocytes. It is present in small amounts in serum.

IgE IgE is medically important for two reasons: (1) it mediates immediate (anaphylactic) hypersensitivity (see Chapter 65), and (2) it participates in host defenses against certain parasites, eg, helminths (worms) (see Chapter 56). The Fc region of IgE binds to the surface of mast cells and basophils. Bound IgE serves as a receptor for antigen (allergen), and this antigen-antibody complex triggers **allergic** responses of the **immediate (anaphylactic)** type through the release of mediators (see Chapter 65). Although IgE is present in **trace** amounts in normal serum (approximately 0.004%), persons with allergic reactivity have greatly increased amounts, and IgE may appear in external secretions. IgE does not fix complement and does not cross the placenta.

IgE is the main host defense against certain important helminth (worm) infections, such as *Strongyloides, Trichinella, Ascaris,* and the hookworms. The serum IgE level is usually increased in these infections. Because worms are too large to be ingested by phagocytes, they are killed by eosinophils that release worm-destroying enzymes. IgE specific for worm proteins binds to receptors on eosinophils, triggering the antibody-dependent cellular cytotoxicity (ADCC) response.

ISOTYPES, ALLOTYPES, & IDIOTYPES

Because immunoglobulins are proteins, they are antigenic, and that property allows them to be subdivided into isotypes, allotypes, and idiotypes. *all isotypes in all humans.*

(1) Isotypes are defined by antigenic (amino acid) differences in their constant regions. Although different antigenically, all isotypes are found in all normal humans. For example, IgG and IgM are different isotypes; the constant region of their H chains (γ and μ) is different antigenically (the five immunoglobulin classes—IgG, IgM, IgA, IgD, and IgE—are different isotypes; their H chains are antigenically different). The IgG isotype is subdivided into four subtypes, IgG1, IgG2, IgG3, and IgG4, based on antigenic differences of their heavy chains. Similarly, IgA1 and IgA2 are different isotypes (the antigenicity of the constant region of their H chains is different), and κ and λ chains are different isotypes (their constant regions also differ antigenically).

(2) Allotypes, on the other hand, are additional antigenic features of immunoglobulins that vary among individuals. They vary because the genes that code for the L and H chains are polymorphic, and individuals can have different alleles. For example, the γ H chain contains an allotype called Gm, which is due to a one- or two-amino-acid difference that provides a different antigenicity to the molecule. Each individual inherits different allelic genes that code for one or another amino acid at the Gm site.*

(3) Idiotypes are the antigenic determinants formed by the specific amino acids in the hypervariable region.† Each idiotype is unique for the immunoglobulin produced by a specific clone of antibody-producing cells. Anti-idiotype antibody reacts only with the hypervariable region of the specific immunoglobulin molecule that induced it. *each idiotype, per specific IG.*

IMMUNOGLOBULIN GENES

To produce the very large number of different immunoglobulin molecules (10^6–10^9) without requiring excessive numbers of genes, special genetic mechanisms, eg, **DNA rearrangement** and **RNA splicing,** are used.

Each immunoglobulin chain consists of a distinct variable (V) and constant (C) region. For each type of immunoglobulin chain, ie, kappa light chain (κL), lambda light chain (λL), and the five heavy chains (γ H, α H, μ H, ε H, and δ H), there is a separate pool of gene segments located on different chromosomes.‡ Each pool contains a set of different V gene segments widely separated from the D (diversity, seen only in H chains), J (joining), and C gene segments (Fig 59–5). In the synthesis of an H chain, for example, a particular V region is translocated to lie close to a D segment, several J segments, and a C region. These genes are transcribed into mRNA, and all but one of the J segments are removed by splicing the RNA. During B cell differentiation the first translocation brings a VH gene near a Cμ gene, leading to the formation of IgM as the first antibody produced in a primary response. Note that the J (joining) gene does *not* encode the J chain found in IgM and IgA.

The V region of each L chain is encoded by two gene segments (V + J). The V region of each H chain is encoded by three gene segments (V + D + J). These various segments are united into one functional V gene by DNA rearrangement. Each of these assembled V genes is then transcribed with the appropriate C genes and spliced to produce an mRNA that codes for the complete peptide chain. L and H chains are synthesized separately on polysomes and then assembled in the cytoplasm by means of disulfide bonds to form H2L2 units. Finally, an oligosaccharide is added to the constant region of the heavy chain and the immunoglobulin molecule is released from the cell.

*Allotypes related to γ H chains are called Gm (an abbreviation of gamma); allotypes related to κ L chains are called Inv (an abbreviation of a patient's name).
†Any one of these antigen determinants is called an idiotope.
‡The genes for κL, λL, and the five heavy chains are on chromosomes 2, 22, and 14, respectively.

Embryonic/germ line
Heavy chain gene

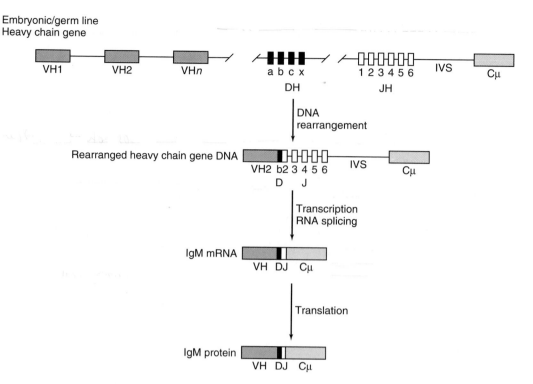

Figure 59–5. Gene rearrangement to produce a μ H chain. V, variable regions; D, diversity segments; J, joining segments; C, constant region; IVS, intervening sequence. (Modified and reproduced, with permission, from Stites DP, Terr A, Parslow T [editors]: *Basic & Clinical Immunology,* 8th ed. Appleton & Lange, 1994.)

The gene organization mechanism outlined above permits the assembly of a very large number of different molecules. Antibody **diversity** depends on (1) multiple gene segments, (2) their rearrangement into different sequences, (3) the combining of different L and H chains in the assembly of immunoglobulin molecules, and (4) mutations. A fifth mechanism called junctional diversity applies primarily to the antibody heavy chain. Junctional diversity occurs by the addition of new nucleotides at the splice junctions between the V-D and D-J gene segments.

The diversity of the T cell antigen receptor is also dependent on the joining of V, D, and J gene segments and the combining of different alpha and beta polypeptide chains. However, unlike antibodies, mutations do *not* play a significant role in the diversity of the T cell receptor.

IMMUNOGLOBULIN CLASS SWITCHING (ISOTYPE SWITCHING)

Initially, all B cells carry IgM specific for an antigen and produce IgM antibody in response to exposure to that antigen. Later, gene rearrangement permits the elaboration of antibodies of the same antigenic specificity but of different immunoglobulin classes (Fig 59–6). Note that the antigenic specificity **remains the same** for the lifetime of the B cell and plasma cell because the specificity is determined by the variable region genes (V, D, and J genes on the heavy chain and V and J genes on the light chain) no matter which heavy chain constant region is being utilized.

In **class switching,** the same assembled VH gene can sequentially associate with different CH genes so that the immunoglobulins produced later (IgG, IgA, or IgE) are specific for the same antigen as the original IgM but have different biologic characteristics. This is illustrated in the "class switch" section of Fig 59–6. A different molecular mechanism is involved in the switching from IgM to IgD. In this case, a single mRNA consisting of VDJ CμCδ is initially transcribed and is then spliced into separate VDJ Cμ and VDJ Cδ mRNAs. Mature B cells can, in this manner, express both IgM and IgD (see Fig 59–6, alternative RNA splicing). Note that once a B cell has "class" switched past a certain H-chain gene, it can no longer make that class of H chain because the intervening

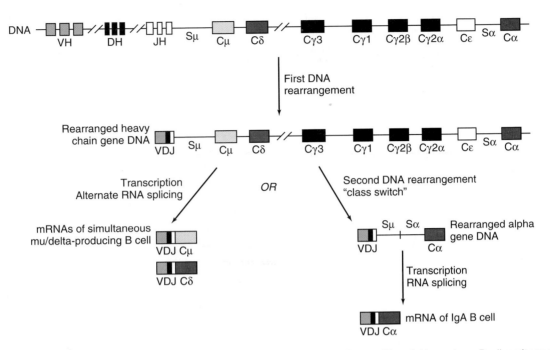

Figure 59–6. Gene rearrangement to produce different immunoglobulin classes. V, variable regions; D, diversity segments; J, joining segments; C, constant regions; S, switch sites. (Modified and reproduced, with permission, from Stites DP, Terr A, Parslow T [editors]: *Basic & Clinical Immunology,* 8th ed. Appleton & Lange, 1994.)

DNA is excised and discarded. Class switching occurs only with heavy chains; light chains do not undergo class switching.

The control of class switching is dependent on at least two factors. One is the concentration of various interleukins. For example, IL-4 enhances the production of IgE whereas IL-5 increases IgA (Table 58–2). The other is the interaction of the CD40 protein on the B cell with CD40 ligand protein on the helper T cell. In hyper-IgM syndrome, the failure to interact properly results in an inability of the B cell to switch to the production of either IgG, IgA, or IgE. Therefore, only IgM is made (see Chapter 68).

A single B cell expresses only one L-chain (either κ or λ) and one H-chain allele; ie, either the paternal or maternal set is expressed but not both. This is called **allelic exclusion.** Each individual contains a mixture of B cells, some expressing the paternal genes and others the maternal ones. The mechanism of this exclusion is unknown.

Review Questions

1. What are monoclonal antibodies, and which cells make them? Describe how these cells are produced.
2. Contrast the structure of an IgG, IgM, and IgA molecule.
3. What forms the antigen-binding site?
4. To which portion of the immunoglobulin molecule does complement bind?
5. What do the terms constant, variable, and hypervariable refer to?
6. What are domains, and where are they located?
7. Distinguish between the terms isotype, allotype, and idiotype.
8. Which immunoglobulin class (a) makes up more than half the immunoglobulin in adult serum? (b) is present in the highest concentration in newborn serum? (c) has the highest avidity? (d) is secreted on mucosal surfaces? (e) triggers anaphylaxis? (f) is on the mast cell surface? (g) can cross the placenta? (h) opsonizes bacteria?

9. Describe the structure of the immunoglobulin genes and how a large number of antibody specificities are produced from a relatively small number of genes.
10. Which class of immunoglobulin is produced first in response to antigen? Describe the process by which other classes are made.

60

Humoral Immunity

Humoral (antibody-mediated) immunity is directed primarily against (1) toxin-induced diseases, (2) infections in which virulence is related to polysaccharide capsules (eg, pneumococci, meningococci, *Haemophilus influenzae*), and (3) certain viral infections. In this chapter the kinetics of antibody synthesis, ie, the primary and secondary responses, are described. The functions of the various immunoglobulins are summarized in this chapter and described in detail in Chapter 59.

THE PRIMARY RESPONSE

When an antigen is first encountered, antibodies are detectable in the serum after a **longer lag period** than occurs in the secondary response. The lag period is typically **7–10 days** but can be longer depending on the nature and dose of the antigen and the route of administration (eg, parenteral or oral). A small clone of B cells and plasma cells specific for the antigen is formed. The serum antibody concentration continues to rise for several weeks, then declines and may drop to very low levels (Fig 60–1). The **first** antibodies to appear are **IgM** followed by IgG or IgA. IgM levels decline earlier than IgG levels.

THE SECONDARY RESPONSE

When there is a second encounter with the same antigen or a closely related (or cross-reacting) one, months or years after the primary response, there is a **rapid** antibody response (the lag period is typically only **3–5 days**) to **higher** levels than the primary response. This is attributed to the persistence of antigen-specific "memory cells" after the first contact. These memory cells proliferate to form a large clone of specific B cells and plasma cells, which mediate the secondary antibody response.

During the secondary response, the amount of IgM produced is similar to that after the first contact with antigen. However, a much **larger** amount of **IgG** antibody is produced and the levels tend to persist much **longer** than in the primary response.

With each succeeding exposure to the antigen, the antibodies tend to bind antigen more firmly. Antibody binding improves because mutations occur in the DNA that encodes the antigen-binding site. Some mutations result in the insertion of different amino acids in the hypervariable region that result in a better fit and cause the antigen to be bound more strongly. The subset of plasma cells with these improved hypervariable regions are more strongly (and frequently) selected by antigen and therefore constitute an increasingly larger part of the population of antibody-producing cells. This process is called **affinity maturation.**

RESPONSE TO MULTIPLE ANTIGENS ADMINISTERED SIMULTANEOUSLY

When two or more antigens are administered at the same time, the host reacts by producing antibodies to all of them. Competition of antigens for antibody-producing mechanisms occurs experimentally but appears to be of little significance in medicine. Combined immunization is widely used, eg, the diphtheria, pertussis, tetanus (DPT) vaccine or the measles, mumps, rubella (MMR) vaccine.

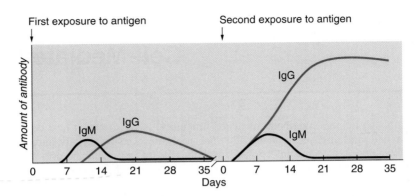

Figure 60–1. Antibody synthesis in the primary and secondary responses. In the primary response, IgM is the first type of antibody to appear. In the secondary response, IgG appears earlier and shows a more rapid rise and a higher final concentration than in the primary response. If at the time of the second exposure to the antigen (Ag1), a second, non-cross-reacting antigen (Ag2) was injected, a primary response to Ag2 would occur while a secondary response to Ag1 was occurring.

FUNCTION OF ANTIBODIES

The primary function of antibodies is to protect against infectious agents or their products (see Table 59–2). Antibodies provide resistance because they can (1) **neutralize** toxins and viruses and (2) **opsonize** microorganisms. Opsonization is the process by which antibodies make microorganisms more easily ingested by phagocytic cells. This occurs by either of two reactions: (1) The Fc portion of IgG interacts with its receptors on the phagocyte surface to facilitate ingestion; or (2) IgG or IgM activates complement to yield C3b, which interacts with its receptors on the surface of the phagocyte.

Antibodies can be induced **actively** in the host or acquired **passively** and are thus immediately available for defense. In medicine, passive immunity is used in the neutralization of the toxins of diphtheria, tetanus, and botulism by antitoxins and in the inhibition of such viruses as rabies and hepatitis A and B viruses early in the incubation period.

ANTIBODIES IN THE FETUS

IgM is the antibody made in greatest amounts by the fetus. Small amounts of fetal IgG and IgA are made also. Note, however, that the fetus has more total IgG than IgM because maternal IgG passes the placenta in large amounts.

TESTS FOR EVALUATION OF HUMORAL IMMUNITY

Evaluation of humoral immunity consists primarily of measuring the amount of each of the three important immunoglobulins, ie, IgG, IgM, and IgA, in the patient's serum. This is usually done by radial immunodiffusion. Immunoelectrophoresis can also provide valuable information. These techniques are described in Chapter 64.

Review Questions

1. Compare the primary and secondary responses from the following points of view: (a) time for antibody to appear, (b) quantity of antibody produced, (c) class of antibody produced, and (d) duration of antibody production.
2. Two important functions of antibodies are neutralization and opsonization. Describe these processes.

61 Cell-Mediated Immunity

Although humoral (antibody-mediated immunity) is an important host defense against many bacterial and viral diseases, in many other bacterial infections (especially intracellular infections such as tuberculosis) and viral infections, it is primarily the cell-mediated arm that imparts resistance and aids in recovery. Furthermore, cell-mediated immunity is important in defense against fungi, parasites, and tumors and in the rejection of organ transplants. The strongest evidence for the importance of cell-mediated immunity comes from clinical situations in which its suppression (by immunosuppressive drugs or disease, eg, AIDS) results in overwhelming infections or tumors.

The constituents of the cell-mediated immune system include several cell types: (1) **macrophages,** which present the antigen to T cells; (2) **helper T cells,** which participate in antigen recognition and in regulation (helper and suppressor) functions (see Chapter 58); (3) **natural killer (NK) cells,** which can inactivate pathogens; and (4) **cytotoxic T cells,** which can kill virus-infected cells with or without antibody. Macrophages and helper T cells produce cytokines that activate helper and cytotoxic T cells, leading to the killing of the pathogen or tumor cell.

Infection with some viruses, namely, measles virus and cytomegalovirus, can suppress cell-mediated immunity against other microorganisms. In particular, measles virus infection in people infected with *M tuberculosis* can result in a loss of PPD skin test reactivity, reactivation of dormant organisms, and clinical disease. A proposed explanation for these findings is that when measles virus binds to its receptor on the surface of human macrophages, the production of IL-12 by the macrophages, which is necessary for cell-mediated immunity to occur, is supressed.

The terms primary and secondary response are associated primarily with antibody formation as described in Chapter 60, but the timing of the T cell response also follows the same pattern. After the initial exposure to the antigen, the specific T cell proliferates to form a small clone of cells; ie, a primary response occurs. Then, on subsequent exposure to the antigen, the small clone expands and many more specific T cells are formed. These cells constitute the secondary response.

Although the interactions between various cells and various cytokines are complex, the result is relatively simple: In the person with competent cellular immunity, opportunistic pathogens rarely or never cause disease, and the spread of other agents—for example, certain viruses (eg, herpesviruses) or tumors (eg, Kaposi's sarcoma)—is limited. The assessment of the competence of cell-mediated immunity is therefore important.

TESTS FOR EVALUATION OF CELL-MEDIATED IMMUNITY

Evaluation of the immunocompetence of persons depends either on the demonstration of delayed-type hypersensitivity to universally present antigens (equating the ability to respond with the competence of cell-mediated immunity) or on laboratory assessments of T cells.

In Vivo Tests for Lymphoid Cell Competence (Skin Tests)

A. Skin Tests for the Presence of Delayed-Type Hypersensitivity: Most normal persons respond with delayed-type reactions to skin test antigens of *Candida,* streptokinase-streptodornase, or mumps because of past exposure to these antigens. Absence of reactions to several of these skin tests suggests impairment of cell-mediated immunity.

B. Skin Tests for the Ability to Develop Delayed-Type Hypersensitivity: Most normal persons readily develop reactivity to simple chemicals (eg, dinitrochlorobenzene [DNCB]) applied to their skin in lipid solvents. When the same chemical is applied to the same area 7–14 days later, they respond with a delayed-type skin reaction. Immunocompromised persons with incompetent cell-mediated immunity fail to develop such delayed-type hypersensitivity.

In Vitro Tests for Lymphoid Cell Competence

A. Lymphocyte Blast Transformation: When sensitized T lymphocytes are exposed to the specific antigen, they transform into large blast cells with greatly increased DNA synthesis, as measured by incorporation of tritiated thymidine. This *specific* effect involves relatively few cells. A larger number of T cells undergo *nonspecific* blast transformation when exposed to certain mitogens. The mitogens phytohemagglutinin and concanavalin A are plant extracts that stimulate T cells specifically. (Bacterial endotoxin, a lipopolysaccharide, stimulates B cells specifically.)

B. Macrophage Migration Inhibitory Factor: Macrophage migration inhibitory factor is elaborated by cultured T cells when exposed to the antigen to which they are sensitized. Its effect can be measured by observing the reduced migration of macrophages in the presence of the factor compared with the level in controls.

C. Enumeration of T Cells, B Cells, and Subpopulations: The number of each type of cell can be counted by use of a machine called a fluorescence-activated cell sorter (FACS) (see Chapter 64). In this approach, cells are labeled with monoclonal antibody tagged with a fluorescent dye, such as fluorescein or rhodamine. Single cells are passed through a laser light beam, and the number of cells that fluoresce is registered.

 Flow cytometry

B cells (and plasma cells) making different classes of antibodies can be detected by using monoclonal antibodies against the various heavy chains. The total number of B cells can be counted by using fluorescein-labeled antibody against all immunoglobulin classes. Specific monoclonal antibodies directed against T cell markers permit the enumeration of T cells, CD4 helper cells, CD8 suppressor cells, and others. The normal ratio of CD4 to CD8 cells is 1.5 or greater, whereas in some immunodeficiencies (eg, AIDS) it is less than 1.

ROLE OF ADJUVANTS & LIPIDS IN ESTABLISHING CELL-MEDIATED REACTIVITY

Weak antigens or simple chemicals tend not to elicit cell-mediated hypersensitivity when administered alone, but they do so when given as a mixture with an adjuvant. The role of the **adjuvant** is presumably to enhance the uptake of the antigen by antigen-presenting cells, eg, macrophages. A common experimental adjuvant is a mixture of mineral oil, lanolin, and killed mycobacteria (Freund's adjuvant), which stimulates the formation of local granulomas. It is prohibited for human use. Cell wall lipids (wax D) of mycobacteria serve as adjuvants for tuberculoprotein to establish cell-mediated reactivity.

Review Questions

1. Contrast the role of cell-mediated immunity in defense against infection with the role of humoral (antibody) immunity.
2. Describe the cells involved in cell-mediated immunity and their functions.
3. How can you evaluate the competency of a patient's cell-mediated immune system?
4. What role do adjuvants play in cell-mediated immunity?

62

Major Histocompatibility Complex & Transplantation

The success of tissue and organ transplants depends on the donor's and recipient's **human leukocyte antigens** (HLA) encoded by the HLA genes. These proteins are alloantigens; ie, they differ among members of the same species. If the HLA proteins on the donor's cells differ from those on the recipient's cells, an immune response occurs in the recipient. The genes for the HLA proteins are clustered in the major histocompatibility complex (MHC), located on the short arm of chromosome 6.* Three of these genes (HLA-A, HLA-B, and HLA-C) code for the class I MHC proteins. Several HLA-D loci determine the class II MHC proteins, ie, DP, DQ, and DR (Fig 62–1).

Each person has two **haplotypes,** ie, two sets of these genes, one on the paternal and the other on the maternal chromosome 6. These genes are very diverse **(polymorphic)** (ie, there are many alleles of the class I and class II genes). For example, there are at least 47 HLA-A genes, 88 HLA-B genes, 29 HLA-C genes, and more than 300 HLA-D genes, but any individual inherits only a single allele at each locus from each parent and thus can make no more than two class I and II proteins at each gene locus. Expression of these genes is **codominant;** ie, the proteins encoded by *both* the paternal and maternal genes are produced. Each person can make as many as 12 HLA proteins: 3 at class I loci and 3 at class II loci, from both chromosomes.

In addition to the major antigens encoded by the HLA genes, there are an unknown number of **minor** antigens encoded by genes at sites other than the HLA locus. These minor antigens can induce a weak immune response that can result in slow rejection of a graft. The cumulative effect of several minor antigens can lead to a more rapid rejection response. There are no laboratory tests for minor antigens.

Between the class I and class II gene loci is a third locus (Fig 62–1), sometimes called class III. This locus contains several immunologically important genes, encoding two cytokines (tumor necrosis factor and lymphotoxin) and two complement components (C2 and C4), but it does not have any genes that encode histocompatibility antigens.

MHC PROTEINS

Class I MHC Proteins
These are glycoproteins found on the **surface of virtually all nucleated cells.** There are approximately 20 different proteins encoded by the allelic genes at the A locus, 40 at the B locus, and 8 at the C locus. The complete class I protein is composed of a 45,000-molecular-weight heavy chain noncovalently bound to a β_2-microglobulin. The heavy chain is highly polymorphic and is similar to an immunoglobulin molecule; it has hypervariable regions in its N-terminal region. The **polymorphism** of these molecules is important in the **recognition of self and nonself.** Stated another way, if these molecules were more similar, our ability to accept foreign grafts would be correspondingly improved. The heavy chain also has a constant region where the CD8 protein of the cytotoxic T cell binds.

Class I proteins are detected in the laboratory by reacting lymphocytes (as antigen) with a battery of specific antibodies plus complement.† If lymphocyte and antibody match, the cell is lysed. This test, along with the test for class II proteins (see below), is used to identify the haplotypes of donors being considered for transplant surgery. Some laboratories use nucleotide sequencing of the class I and II MHC genes to determine the haplotype.

Class II MHC Proteins
These are glycoproteins found on the **surface of certain cells,** including macrophages, B cells, dendritic cells of the spleen, and Langerhans cells of the skin. They are

---

*In addition to these major antigens, there are "weak" minor antigens coded for by genes located at sites other than the MHC.

†The antibodies are obtained primarily from multiparous women who have been exposed to the father's antigens on fetal lymphocytes that cross the placenta during pregnancy. Some monoclonal antibodies are available also.

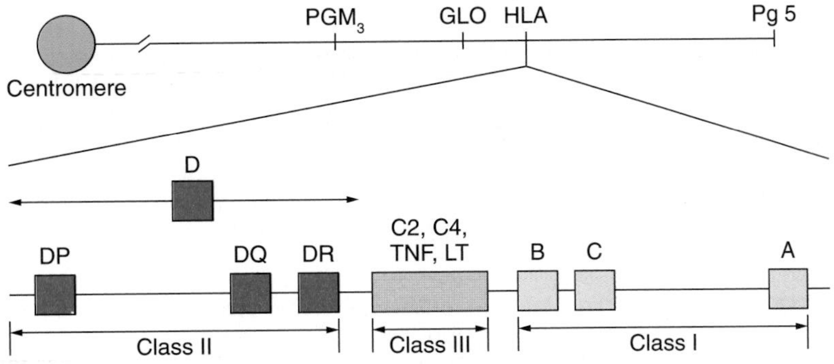

Figure 62–1. The human leukocyte antigen (HLA) gene complex. A, B, and C are class I loci. DP, DQ, and DR are class II loci. C2 and C4 are complement loci. TNF is tumor necrosis factor, LT is lymphotoxin. PGM₃, GLO, and Pg 5 are adjacent, unrelated genes. (Reproduced, with permission, from Stites DP, Terr A, Parslow T [editors]: *Basic & Clinical Immunology,* 9th ed. Appleton & Lange, 1997.)

highly polymorphic glycoproteins composed of two polypeptides (MW 33,000 and 28,000) that are noncovalently bound. Like class I proteins, they have hypervariable regions that provide much of the polymorphism. Unlike class I proteins, which have only one chain encoded by the MHC locus (β_2-microglobulin is encoded on chromosome 15), both chains of the class II proteins are encoded by the MHC locus. The two peptides also have a constant region where the CD4 proteins of the helper T cells bind.

Class II proteins were first demonstrated by the **mixed-leukocyte reaction** (mixed-lymphocyte reaction, MLR). In this test, "stimulator" lymphocytes from a potential donor are first killed by irradiation and then mixed with live "responder" lymphocytes from the recipient; the mixture is incubated in cell culture to permit DNA synthesis, which is measured by incorporation of tritiated thymidine. The greater the amount of DNA synthesis in the responder cells, the more foreign are the class II MHC proteins of the donor cells. A large amount of DNA synthesis indicates an unsatisfactory "match"; ie, donor and recipient class II (HLA-D) MHC proteins are *not* similar, and the graft is likely to be rejected. The best donor is, therefore, the person whose cells stimulated the incorporation of the **least** amount of tritiated thymidine in the recipient cells. Currently, clinical laboratories can determine the important class II proteins (DR loci) by using serologic tests analogous to those used for the class I proteins.

BIOLOGIC IMPORTANCE OF MHC

The ability of T cells to recognize antigen is dependent on association of the antigen with either class I or class II proteins. For example, cytotoxic T cells respond to antigen in association with class I MHC proteins. Thus, a cytotoxic T cell that kills a virus-infected cell will not kill a cell infected with the same virus if the cell does not also express the appropriate class I proteins. This finding was determined, using inbred animals, by mixing virus-infected cells and cytotoxic T cells bearing different class I proteins and observing that no killing of the virus-infected cells occurred. Helper T cells recognize class II proteins. Helper-cell activity depends in general on *both* the recognition of the antigen on antigen-presenting cells *and* the presence on these cells of "self" class II MHC proteins. This requirement to recognize antigen in association with a "self" MHC protein is called **MHC restriction.** Note that T cells recognize antigens only when the antigens are presented on the surface of cells (in association with either class I or II MHC proteins), whereas B cells do not have that requirement and can recognize soluble antigens in plasma with their surface monomer IgM acting as the antigen receptor.

MHC genes and proteins are also important in two other medical contexts. One is that many autoimmune diseases occur in people who carry certain MHC genes (see Chapter 66), and the other is that the success of organ transplants is, in large part, determined by the compatibility of the MHC genes of the donor and recipient (see below).

TRANSPLANTATION

An **autograft** (transfer of an individual's own tissue) is always accepted. A **syngeneic graft*** is a transfer of tissue between genetically identical individuals, ie, identical twins, and almost always "takes" permanently. A **xenograft,*** a transfer of tissue between different species, is always rejected by an immunocompetent recipient. An **allograft*** is a graft between genetically different members of the same species, eg, from one human to another. Allografts are usually rejected unless the recipient is given immunosuppressive drugs. The severity and rapidity of the rejection will vary depending on the degree of the differences between the donor and the recipient at the MHC loci.

Allograft Rejection   Unless immunosuppressive measures are taken, allografts are rejected by a process called the **allograft reaction.** In an acute allograft reaction, vascularization of the graft is normal initially but in 11–14 days, marked reduction in circulation and mononuclear cell infiltration occurs, with eventual necrosis.† This is called a **primary ("first-set")** reaction. A **T cell-mediated reaction is the main cause of rejection** of many types of grafts, eg, skin, but antibodies contribute to the rejection of certain transplants, especially bone marrow. In experimental animals, rejection of most types of grafts can be transferred by cells, not serum. Also, T cell-deficient animals do not reject grafts but B cell-deficient animals do. The role of cytotoxic T cells in allograft rejection is described on page 330.

If a second allograft from the same donor is applied to a sensitized recipient, it is rejected in 5–6 days. This **accelerated ("second-set")** reaction is caused primarily by presensitized cytotoxic T cells.

The acceptance or rejection of a transplant is determined, in large part, by the class I and class II MHC proteins on the donor cells, with **class II** playing the **major** role. The proteins encoded by the DR locus are especially important. These alloantigens activate T cells, both helper and cytotoxic, which bear T cell receptors specific for the alloantigens. The activated T cells proliferate and then react against the alloantigens on the donor cells. CD8-positive cytotoxic T cells do most of the killing of the allograft cells. Foreign MHC proteins typically activate many more T cells (ie, they elicit a much stronger reaction) than do foreign proteins that are not MHC proteins. The reason for the different strengths of the responses is unclear.

The allograft rejection process can be activated by two mechanisms: (1) antigen-presenting cells (eg, macrophages and dendritic cells) in the graft can present self (the donors) proteins in association with their class I and class II MHC proteins and activate the recipient's immune response, or (2) the donor's self proteins and class I and class II MHC proteins can be shed and subsequently processed by the recipient's antigen-presenting cells, which activates the recipient's immune response. There is evidence for both of these mechanisms contributing to rejection of the allograft.

Prior to transplantation surgery, laboratory tests, commonly called **"tissue typing,"** are performed to determine the closest match of MHC proteins in the donor and recipient. Class I proteins and certain class II proteins, especially DR, are detected by using a panel of known antibodies plus complement to lyse donor lymphocytes or by nucleotide sequencing. Additional information regarding the compatibility of the class II proteins can be determined by the mixed leukocyte reaction with cultured cells. In addition to the tests used for matching, preformed cytotoxic antibodies in the recipient's serum reactive against the graft are detected by observing the lysis of donor lymphocytes by the recipient's serum plus complement. This is called **crossmatching** and is done to prevent hyperacute rejections from occurring. (The donor and recipient are also matched for the compatibility of their ABO blood groups.)

Among siblings in a single family, there is a 25% chance for both haplotypes to be shared, a 50% chance for one haplotype to be shared, and a 25% chance for no haplotypes to be shared. For example, if the father is haplotype AB, the mother is CD, and the recipient child is AC, there is a 25% chance for a sibling to be AC, ie, a two-haplotype match, a 50% chance for a sibling to be either BC or AD, ie, a one-haplotype match, and a 25% chance for a sibling to be BD, ie, a zero-haplotype match.

---

*Previously used synonyms for these terms include isograft (syngeneic graft), heterograft (xenograft), and homograft (allograft).

†Two other types of graft rejection also can occur: (1) hyperacute (white graft) rejection, in which the graft is rejected very rapidly as a result of the presence of large amounts of preformed antibodies, eg, anti-ABO antibodies; and (2) chronic rejection, which can take months or years and is probably due to incompatibility of the weak (minor) histocompatibility antigens.

Results of Organ Transplants   If the donor and recipient are well matched by mixed-lymphocyte culture and histocompatibility antigen typing, the long-term survival of a transplanted organ or tissue is greatly enhanced. In 1986, the 5-year survival rate of two-haplotype-matched kidney transplants from related donors was near 95%, that of one-haplotype-matched kidney transplants was near 80%, and that of transplant of kidneys from cadaver donors was near 60%. The survival rate of the last category was higher if the graft recipient had had several previous blood transfusions. The reason for this is unknown (but may be associated with tolerance). The heart transplant survival rate for 5 years is near 50–60%; the liver transplant rate is lower. Corneas are easily grafted because they are avascular and the lymphatic supply of the eye prevents many antigens from triggering an immune response; consequently, the proportion of "takes" is very high. Because corneal transplants elicit a weak rejection response, immunosuppression is usually necessary for only a year. In contrast, most other transplants require lifelong immunosuppression, although the dose of immunosuppressive drugs typically decreases with time and in some recipients a state of tolerance ensues and the drugs can be stopped.

Graft-Versus-Host Reaction   Well-matched transplants of bone marrow may establish themselves initially in 85% of recipients, but subsequently a **graft-versus-host (GVH)** reaction develops in about two-thirds of them.* This reaction occurs because grafted immunocompetent T cells proliferate in the irradiated, immunocompromised host and reject cells with "foreign" proteins, resulting in severe organ dysfunction. The donor's cytotoxic T cells play a major role in destroying the recipient's cells. Among the main symptoms are maculopapular rash, jaundice, hepatosplenomegaly, and diarrhea. Many GVH reactions end in overwhelming infections and death.

   There are three requirements for a GVH reaction to occur: (1) the graft must contain immunocompetent T cells; (2) the host must be immunocompromised; and (3) the recipient must express antigens (eg, MHC proteins) foreign to the donor; ie, the donor T cells recognize the recipient cells as foreign. Note that even when donor and recipient have identical class I and class II MHC proteins, ie, identical haplotypes, a GVH reaction can occur because it can be elicited by differences in minor antigens. The GVH reaction can be reduced by treating the donor tissue with antithymocyte globulin or monoclonal antibodies before grafting; this eliminates mature T cells from the graft. Cyclosporine (see below) is also used to reduce the GVH reaction.

EFFECT OF IMMUNOSUPPRESSION ON GRAFT REJECTION

   To reduce the chance of rejection of transplanted tissue, immunosuppressive measures, eg, cyclosporine, tacrolimus (FK506), rapamycin, corticosteroids, azathioprine, OKT3 antibody and radiation, are used. Cyclosporine prevents the activation of T lymphocytes by inhibiting signal transduction within T cells. It interrupts signal transduction by inhibiting calcineurin, a protein (a serine phosphatase) involved in the activation of the genes for IL-2 and the IL-2 receptor. Cyclosporine is well-tolerated and is remarkably successful in preventing the rejection of transplants. Cyclosporine and tacrolimus have the same mode of action; tacrolimus is more immunosuppressive but causes more side effects. Rapamycin also inhibits signal transduction but at a site different from that of cyclosporine and tacrolimus. Unfortunately, immunosuppression greatly enhances the recipient's susceptibility to opportunistic infections and neoplasms. The incidence of cancer is as much as 100-fold increased in transplant recipients. Immunosuppressive drugs, eg, cyclosporine, also reduce GVH reactions.

   Corticosteroids act primarily by inhibiting cytokine (eg, IL-1 and TNF) production by macrophages and by lysing certain types of T cells. Azathioprine is an inhibitor of DNA synthesis and blocks the growth of T cells. OKT3 is a monoclonal antibody against the CD3 protein that can block T cell function as well as lyse T cells.

---

*GVH reactions can also occur in immunodeficient patients given a blood transfusion, because there are immunocompetent T cells in the donor's blood that react against the recipient's cells.

Review Questions

1. Describe the genes that constitute the major histocompatibility complex.
2. Each person has two haplotypes with codominant genes. Explain this sentence.
3. Compare class I and class II MHC proteins from the following points of view: (a) type of cells on which they are located, (b) laboratory test used to detect them, and (c) role in antigen recognition by CD4 and CD8 T cells.
4. Distinguish between an autograft, a syngeneic graft, an allograft, and a xenograft.
5. What is an allograft reaction?
6. What are the differences between a "first-set" and a "second-set" allograft reaction?
7. Describe how a prospective kidney donor is tested for compatibility with the recipient prior to transplant surgery.
8. Under which circumstances does a graft-versus-host reaction occur? Describe the reaction.

63

Complement

The complement system consists of approximately 20 proteins that are present in normal human (and other animal) serum. The term "complement" refers to the ability of these proteins to complement, ie, augment, the effects of other components of the immune system, eg, antibody. Complement is an important component of our innate host defenses.

There are three main effects of complement: (1) **lysis** of cells such as bacteria, allografts, and tumor cells; (2) **generation of mediators** that participate in inflammation and attract neutrophils; and (3) **opsonization,** ie, enhancement of phagocytosis. Complement proteins are synthesized mainly by the liver. Complement is heat-labile; ie, it is inactivated by heating serum at 56 °C for 30 minutes. Immunoglobulins are not inactivated at this temperature.

ACTIVATION

Several complement components are proenzymes, which must be cleaved to form active enzymes. Activation of the complement system can be initiated either by antigen-antibody complexes or by a variety of nonimmunologic molecules, eg, endotoxin.

Sequential activation of complement components (Fig 63–1) occurs via one of two pathways: the classic pathway and the alternative pathway (see below). Of the two pathways, the **alternative one is more important the first time** we are infected by a microorganism, since the antibody required to trigger the classic pathway is not present. Both pathways lead to the production of **C3b, the central molecule** of the complement cascade. C3b has two important functions: (1) It combines with other complement components to generate C5 convertase, the enzyme that leads to the production of the membrane attack complex, and (2) it opsonizes bacteria because phagocytes have receptors for C3b on their surface.

(1) In the **classic** pathway, antigen-antibody complexes* activate C1† to form a protease, which cleaves C2 and C4 to form a C4b2b complex. The latter is C3 convertase, which cleaves C3 mole-

---

*Only IgM and IgG fix complement. One molecule of IgM can activate complement; however, activation by IgG requires two cross-linked IgG molecules. C1 is bound to a site located in the Fc region of the heavy chain. Of the IgGs, only IgG1, IgG2, and IgG3 subclasses fix complement; IgG4 does not.

†C1 is composed of three proteins, C1q, C1r, and C1s. C1q is an aggregate of 18 polypeptides that binds to the Fc portion of IgG and IgM. It is multivalent and can cross-link several immunoglobulin molecules. C1s is a proenzyme that is cleaved to form an active protease. Calcium is required for the activation of C1.

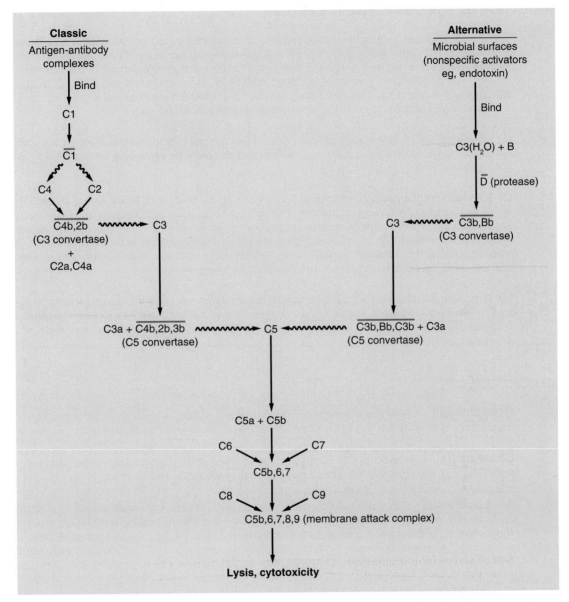

Figure 63–1. The classic and alternative pathways of the complement system. ∿➤ indicates that proteolytic cleavage of the molecule at the tip of the arrow has occurred; a line over a complex indicates that it is enzymatically active.

cules into two fragments, C3a and C3b. C3a, an **anaphylatoxin,** is discussed below. C3b forms a complex with C4b2b, producing a new enzyme, C5 convertase (C4b2b3b), which cleaves C5 to form C5a and C5b. C5a is an anaphylatoxin and a chemotactic factor (see below). C5b binds to C6 and C7 to form a complex that interacts with C8 and C9 to produce the **"membrane attack"** complex (C5b6789), which causes cytolysis. Note that the "b" fragment continues in the main pathway whereas the "a" fragment is split off and has other activities.

(2) In the **alternative** pathway, many unrelated cell surface substances, eg, bacterial lipopolysaccharides (endotoxin), fungal cell walls, and viral envelopes, can initiate the process by binding C3(H₂O) and factor B. This complex is cleaved by a protease, factor D, to produce C3bBb. This acts as a C3 convertase to generate more C3b. $\quad$ C3 tick over.

REGULATION OF THE COMPLEMENT SYSTEM

The first regulatory step in the classic pathway is at the level of the antibody itself. The complement-binding site on the heavy chain of IgM and IgG is unavailable to the C1 component of complement if antigen is not bound to these antibodies. This means that complement is not activated by IgM and IgG despite being present in the blood at all times. However, when antigen binds to its specific antibody, a conformational shift occurs and the C1 component can bind and initiate the cascade.

Several serum proteins regulate the complement system at different stages.

(1) C1 inhibitor is an important regulator of the classic pathway. It inactivates the protease activity of C1. Activation of the classic pathway proceeds past this point by generating sufficient C1 to overwhelm the inhibitor.

(2) Regulation of the alternative pathway is mediated by the binding of factor H to C3b and cleavage of this complex by factor I, a protease. This reduces the amount of C5 convertase available. The alternative pathway can proceed past this regulatory point if sufficient C3b attaches to cell membranes. Attachment of C3b to cell membranes protects it from degradation by factors H and I. Another component that enhances activation of the alternative pathway is properdin, which protects C3b and stabilizes the C3 convertase.

(3) Protection of human cells from lysis by the membrane attack complex of complement is mediated by **decay-accelerating factor (DAF)**, a glycoprotein located on the surface of human cells. DAF acts by destabilizing C3 convertase and C5 convertase. This prevents the formation of the membrane attack complex.

BIOLOGIC EFFECTS

Opsonization   Cells, antigen-antibody complexes, and viruses are phagocytized much better in the presence of C3b. This is due to the presence of C3b receptors on the surface of many phagocytes.

Chemotaxis   C5a and the C567 complex attract neutrophils. They migrate especially well toward C5a. C5a also enhances the adhesiveness of neutrophils to the endothelium.

Anaphylatoxin   C3a, C4a, and C5a cause degranulation of mast cells with release of mediators, eg, histamine, leading to increased vascular permeability and smooth muscle contraction, especially contraction of the bronchioles leading to bronchospasm. C5a is, by far, the most potent of these anaphylatoxins. Anaphylaxis caused by these complement components is less common than anaphylaxis caused by type I (IgE-mediated) hypersensitivity (see Chapter 65).

Cytolysis   Insertion of the C5b6789 complex into the cell membrane leads to killing or lysis of many types of cells including erythrocytes, bacteria, and tumor cells. Cytolysis is not an enzymatic process; rather, it appears that insertion of the complex results in disruption of the membrane and the entry of water and electrolytes into the cell.

Enhancement of Antibody Production   The binding of C3b to its receptors on the surface of activated B cells greatly enhances antibody production compared with that by B cells that are activated by antigen alone. The clinical importance of this is that patients who are deficient in C3b produce significantly less antibody than do those with normal amounts of C3b. The low concentration of both antibody and C3b significantly impairs host defenses, resulting in multiple, severe pyogenic infections.

CLINICAL ASPECTS

(1) Inherited (or acquired) deficiency of some complement components, especially C5–C8, greatly enhances susceptibility to *Neisseria* **bacteremia** and other infections. A deficiency of C3 leads to severe, recurrent pyogenic sinus and respiratory tract infections.

(2) Inherited deficiency of C1 esterase inhibitor results in **angioedema.** When the amount of inhibitor is reduced, an overproduction of esterase occurs. This leads to an increase in anaphylatoxins, which cause capillary permeability and edema.

(3) Acquired deficiency of decay-accelerating factor on the surface of cells results in an increase in complement-mediated hemolysis. Clinically, this appears as the disorder paroxysmal nocturnal hemoglobinuria (see Chapter 68).

(4) In transfusion mismatches, eg, when type A blood is given by mistake to a person who is type B, antibody to the A antigen in the recipient binds to A antigen on the donor red cells, complement is activated, and large amounts of anaphylatoxins and membrane attack complexes are generated. The anaphylatoxins cause shock, and the membrane attack complexes cause red cell hemolysis.

(5) Immune complexes bind complement, and thus complement levels are low in immune complex diseases, eg, acute glomerulonephritis and systemic lupus erythematosus. Binding (activating) complement attracts polymorphonuclear leukocytes, which release enzymes that damage tissue.

Review Questions

1. What are the three major biologic effects of complement?
2. Compare the classic and alternative pathways of complement activation. What is the nature of the substances that activate? What is the molecule that serves as the common entry point for both pathways to the rest of the sequence?
3. What is a convertase, and what role does it play?
4. Which components of complement facilitate (a) opsonization? (b) chemotaxis? (c) anaphylaxis? (d) cytolysis?
5. What is the membrane attack complex, and what is its biologic effect?

Antigen-Antibody Reactions in the Laboratory

64

Reactions of antigens and antibodies are highly specific. An antigen will react only with antibodies elicited by itself or by a closely related antigen. Because of the great specificity, reactions between antigens and antibodies are suitable for identifying one by using the other. This is the basis of serologic reactions. However, cross-reactions between related antigens can occur, and these can limit the usefulness of the test. The results of many immunologic tests are expressed as a **titer,** which is defined as the highest dilution of the specimen, eg, serum, that gives a positive reaction in the test. Note that a patient's serum with an antibody titer of, for example, 1/64 contains **more** antibodies, i.e., is a higher titer, than a serum with a titer of, for example, 1/4.

Microorganisms and other cells possess a variety of antigens and thus induce antisera containing many different antibodies; ie, the antisera are polyclonal. Monoclonal antibodies excel in the identification of antigens because cross-reacting antibodies are absent; ie, monoclonal antibodies are highly specific.

TYPES OF DIAGNOSTIC TESTS

Many types of diagnostic tests are performed in the immunology laboratory. Most of these tests can be designed to determine the presence of either antigen or antibody. To do this, one of the components, either antigen or antibody, is known and the other is unknown. For example, with a known antigen such as influenza virus, a test can determine whether antibody to the virus is present in the patient's serum. Alternatively, with a known antibody, such as antibody to herpes simplex virus, a test can determine whether viral antigens are present in cells taken from the patient's lesions.

Agglutination   In this test, the antigen is **particulate** (eg, bacteria and red blood cells)* or is an inert particle (latex beads) coated with an antigen. Antibody, because it is divalent or multivalent, cross-links the antigenically multivalent particles and forms a latticework, and clumping (agglutination) can be seen. This reaction can be done in a small cup or tube or with a drop on a slide. One very commonly used agglutination test is the test that determines a person's ABO blood group (Fig 64–1; see the section on blood groups at the end of this chapter).

Precipitation (Precipitin)   In this test, the antigen is **in solution.** The antibody cross-links antigen molecules in variable proportions, and aggregates (precipitates) form. In the **zone of equivalence,** optimal proportions of antigen and antibody combine; the maximal amount of precipitates forms, and the supernatant contains neither an excess of antibody nor an excess of antigen (Fig 64–2). In the **zone of antibody excess,** there is too much antibody for efficient lattice formation, and precipitation is less than maximal.† In the **zone of antigen excess,** all antibody has combined but precipitation is reduced because many antigen-antibody complexes are too small to precipitate; ie, they are "soluble."

Precipitin tests can be done in solution or in semisolid medium (agar).

A.   Precipitation in Solution: This reaction can be made quantitative; ie, antigen or antibody can be measured in terms of micrograms of nitrogen present. It is used primarily in research.

B.   Precipitation in Agar: This is done as either single or double diffusion. It can also be done in the presence of an electric field.

1.   Single diffusion: In single diffusion, antibody is incorporated into agar and antigen is measured into a well. As the antigen diffuses with time, precipitation rings form depending on the antigen concentration. The greater the amount of antigen in the well, the farther the ring will be from the well. By calibrating the method, such **radial immunodiffusion** is used to measure IgG, IgM, complement components, and other substances in serum. (IgE cannot be measured because its concentration is too low.)

2.   Double diffusion: In double diffusion, antigen and antibody are placed in different wells in agar and allowed to diffuse and form concentration gradients. Where optimal proportions (see

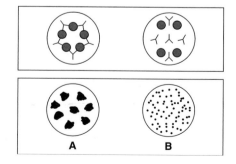

Figure 64–1. Agglutination test to determine ABO blood type. On the slide at the bottom of the figure, a drop of the patient's blood was mixed with antiserum against either type A **(left)** or type B **(right)** blood cells. Agglutination (clumping) has occurred in the drop on the left containing the type A antiserum but not in the drop containing the type B antiserum, indicating that the patient is type A, ie, has A antigen on the red cells. The slide at the top shows that the red cells (circles) are cross-linked by the antibodies (Y-shapes) in the drop on the left but not in the drop on the right. If agglutination had occurred in the right side as well, it would indicate that the patient was producing B antigen as well as A and was type AB.

---

*When red cells are used, the reaction is called hemagglutination.

†The term "prozone" refers to the failure of a precipitate or flocculate to form because too much antibody is present. For example, a false-negative serologic test for syphilis (VDRL) is occasionally reported because the antibody titer is too high. Dilution of the serum yields a positive result.

whether antigen or antibody alone fixes complement are needed to make the test results valid. If antigen or antibody alone fixes complement, it is said to be anticomplementary.

Neutralization Tests   These use the ability of antibodies to block the effect of toxins or the infectivity of viruses. They can be used in cell culture (eg, inhibition of cytopathic effect and plaque-reduction assays) or in host animals (eg, mouse protection tests).

Immune Complexes   Immune complexes in tissue can be stained with fluorescent complement. Immune complexes in serum can be detected by binding to C1q or by attachment to certain (eg, Raji lymphoblastoid) cells in culture.

Hemagglutination Tests   Many viruses clump red blood cells from one species or another (active hemagglutination). This can be inhibited by antibody specifically directed against the virus (hemagglutination inhibition) and can be used to measure the titer of such antibody. Red blood cells also can absorb many antigens and, when mixed with matching antibodies, will clump (this is known as **passive hemagglutination,** because the red cells are passive carriers of the antigen).

Antiglobulin (Coombs) Test   Some patients with certain diseases, eg, hemolytic disease of the newborn (Rh incompatibility) and drug-related hemolytic anemias, become sensitized but do not exhibit symptoms of disease. In these patients, antibodies against the red cells are formed and bind to the red cell surface but do not cause hemolysis. These cell-bound antibodies can be detected by the direct antiglobulin (Coombs) test, in which antiserum against human immunoglobulin is used to agglutinate the patient's red cells. In some cases, antibody against the red cells is not bound to the red cells but is in the serum and the indirect antiglobulin test for antibodies in the patient's serum should be performed. In the indirect Coombs test, the patient's serum is mixed with normal red cells and antiserum to human immunoglobulins is added. If antibodies are present in the patient's serum, agglutination occurs.

Western Blot   This test is typically used to determine whether a positive result in a screening immunologic test is a true-positive or a false-positive. For example, patients who are positive in the screening ELISA for HIV infection or for Lyme disease should have a Western blot test performed. Figure 64–9 illustrates a Western blot test for the presence of HIV antibodies in the patient's serum. In this test, HIV proteins are separated electrophoretically in a gel, resulting in discrete bands of viral protein. These proteins are then transferred from the gel, ie, blotted, onto filter paper, and the person's serum is added. If antibodies are present, they bind to the viral proteins (primarily gp41 and p24) and can be detected by

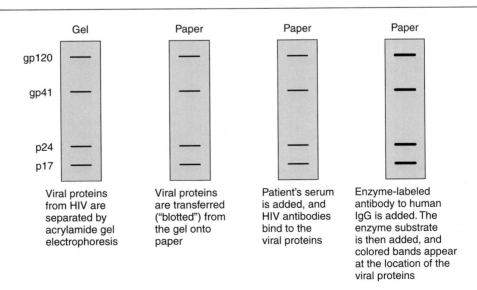

Figure 64–9. Western blot.

adding antibody to human IgG labelled with either radioactivity or an enzyme such as horseradish peroxidase, which produces a visible color change.

Fluorescence-Activated Cell Sorting (Flow Cytometry)
This test is commonly used to measure the number of the various types of immunologically active blood cells (Fig 64–10). For example, it is used in HIV-infected patients to determine the number of CD4-positive T cells. In this test, the patient's cells are labeled with monoclonal antibody to the protein specific to the cell of interest, eg, CD4 protein if the number of helper T cells is to be determined. The monoclonal antibody is tagged with a fluorescent dye, such as fluorescein or rhodamine. Single cells are passed through a laser light beam, and the number of cells that fluoresce is counted by use of a machine called a fluorescence-activated cell sorter (FACS).

ANTIGEN-ANTIBODY REACTIONS INVOLVING RED BLOOD CELL ANTIGENS

Many different blood group systems exist in humans. Each system consists of a gene locus specifying antigens on the erythrocyte surface. The two most important blood groupings, ABO and Rh, are described below.

The ABO Blood Groups & Transfusion Reactions
All human erythrocytes contain alloantigens (ie, antigens that vary among individual members of a species) of the ABO group. This is an important system, which is the basis for blood typing and transfusions. The A and B genes encode enzymes that add specific sugars to the end of a polysaccharide chain on the surface of many cells, including red cells (Fig 64–11). People who inherit neither gene are type O. The genes are codominant, so people who inherit both genes are type AB. People who are either homozygous AA or heterozygous AO are type A, and, similarly, people who are either homozygous BB or heterozygous BO are type B.

The A and B antigens are carbohydrates that differ by a single sugar. Despite this small difference, A and B antigens do not cross-react. Erythrocytes have three terminal sugars in common on their surface: N-acetylglucosamine, galactose, and fucose. These three sugars form the H antigen (Fig 64–11). Type A cells have an additional N-acetylgalactosamine, whereas type B cells have an additional galactose. The A and B genes code for transferases that add the respective sugars. Type O cells have only the H antigen.

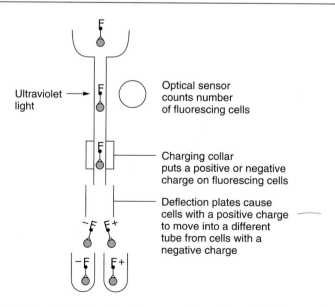

Figure 64–10. Flow cytometry. At the top of the figure, a cell has interacted with monoclonal antibody labeled with a fluorescent dye. As the cell passes down the tube, ultraviolet light causes the dye to fluoresce and a sensor counts the cell. Farther down the tube, an electrical charge can be put on the cell, which allows it to be deflected into a test tube and subjected to additional analysis.

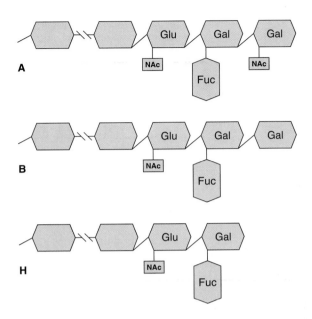

Figure 64–11. ABO blood groups. Structures of the terminal sugars that determine ABO blood groups are shown. (Reproduced, with permission, from Stites DP, Stobo JD, Wells JV [editors]: *Basic & Clinical Immunology,* 6th ed. Appleton & Lange, 1987.)

There are four combinations of the A and B antigens called A, B, AB, and O (Table 64–1). A person's blood group is determined by mixing the person's blood with antiserum against A antigen on one area on a slide and with antiserum against B antigen on another area (Fig 64–1). If agglutination occurs only with A antiserum, the blood group is A; if it occurs only with B antiserum, the blood group is B; if it occurs with both A and B antisera, the blood group is AB; and if it occurs with neither A nor B antisera, the blood group is O.

The plasma contains antibody against the absent antigens ie, people with blood group A have antibodies to B in their plasma. These antibodies are formed agsinst cross-reacting bacterial or food antigens, are first detectable at 3 to 6 months of age, and are of the IgM class. Individuals are tolerant to their own blood group antigens, so that a person with blood group A does not form antibodies to A antigen. The end result is that antigen and corresponding antibody do *not* coexist in the same person's blood. Transfusion reactions occur when incompatible donor red blood cells are transfused, eg, if group A blood were transfused into a group B person (because anti-A antibody is present). The red cell-antibody complex activates complement and a reaction consisting of shock caused by large amounts of C3a and C5a (anaphylatoxins) and hemolysis caused by C5, C6, C7, C8, and C9 (membrane attack complex) occurs.

To avoid antigen-antibody reactions that would result in transfusion reactions, all blood for transfusions must be carefully **"matched"**; ie, erythrocytes are typed for their surface antigens by specific sera. As shown in Table 64–1, persons with group O blood have no A or B antigens on their red cells and so are **"universal donors"**; ie, they can give blood to people in all four groups (Table 64–2). Note that type O blood has A and B antibodies. Therefore when type O blood is given to a person with type A, B, or AB blood, you might expect a reaction to occur. A clinically detectable reaction does not occur because the donor antibody is rapidly diluted below a significant level. Persons with group AB blood have neither A nor B antibody and thus are **"universal recipients."**

Table 64–1. ABO blood groups.

Group	Antigen on Red Cell	Antibody in Plasma
A	A	Anti-B
B	B	Anti-A
AB	A and B	No anti-A or anti-B
O	No A or B	Anti-A and anti-B

Table 64–2. Compatibility of blood transfusions between ABO blood groups.

Donor	Recipient			
	O	**A**	**B**	**AB**
O	Yes	Yes	Yes	Yes
A (AA or AO)	No	Yes	No	Yes
B (BB or BO)	No	No	Yes	Yes
AB	No	No	No	Yes

[1]Yes indicates that a blood transfusion from a donor with that blood group to a recipient with that blood group is compatible, ie, that no hemolysis will occur. No indicates that the transfusion is incompatible and that hemolysis of the donor's cells will occur.

In addition to red blood cells, the A and B antigens appear on the cells of many tissues. Furthermore, these antigens can be secreted in saliva and other body fluids. Secretion is controlled by a secretor gene. Approximately 85% of people carry the dominant form of the gene, which allows secretion to occur.

ABO blood group differences can lead to neonatal jaundice and anemia, but the effects on the fetus are usually less severe than those seen in Rh incompatibility (see below). For example, mothers with blood group O have antibodies against both A and B antigens. These IgG antibodies can pass the placenta and, if the fetus is blood group A or B, cause lysis of fetal red cells. Mothers with either blood group A or B have a lower risk of having a neonate with jaundice because these mothers produce antibodies to either B or A antigens, respectively, that are primarily IgM, and IgM does not pass the placenta.

Rh Blood Type & Hemolytic Disease of the Newborn

About 85% of humans have erythrocytes that express the Rh(D) antigen, ie, are Rh(D)$^+$. When an Rh(D)$^-$ person is transfused with Rh(D)$^+$ blood or when an Rh(D)$^-$ woman has an Rh(D)$^+$ fetus (the D gene being inherited from the father), the Rh(D) antigen will stimulate the development of antibodies (Table 64–3). This occurs most often when the Rh(D)$^+$ erythrocytes of the fetus leak into the maternal circulation during delivery of the first Rh(D)$^+$ child. Subsequent Rh(D)$^+$ pregnancies are likely to be affected by the mother's anti-D antibody, and hemolytic disease of the newborn (**erythroblastosis fetalis**) often results. This disease results from the passage of maternal IgG anti-Rh(D) antibodies through the placenta to the fetus, with subsequent lysis of the fetal erythrocytes. The direct antiglobulin (Coombs) test is typically positive (see above for a description of the Coombs test). The problem can be prevented by administration of **high-titer Rh(D) immune globulins (Rho-Gam)** to an Rh(D)$^-$ mother at 28 weeks of gestation and immediately upon the delivery of an Rh(D)$^+$ child. These antibodies promptly attach to Rh(D)$^+$ erythrocytes and prevent their acting as sensitizing antigen. This prophylaxis is widely practiced and effective.

Table 64–3. Rh status and hemolytic disease of the newborn.

Rh Status			Hemolysis[1]
Father	**Mother**	**Child**	
+	+	+ or −	No
+	−	+	No (1st child) Yes (2nd child and subsequent children)
+	−	−	No
−	+	+ or −	No
−	−	−	No

[1]No indicates that hemolysis of the newborn's red cells will not occur and that hemolytic disease will therefore not occur. Yes indicates that hemolysis of the newborn's red cells is likely to occur and that symptoms of hemolytic disease will therefore probably occur.

Review Questions

1. Contrast agglutination and precipitation reactions.
2. In the precipitin reaction, what happens in (a) the zone of antibody excess? (b) the zone of antigen excess? (c) the zone of equivalence?
3. What is the principle of (a) the RIA? (b) the ELISA?
4. What is the difference between the direct and indirect fluorescent-antibody assays?
5. Describe the procedure used in the complement fixation test. If the red cells lyse, is that a positive or a negative test? Why?
6. Contrast the direct and indirect Coombs tests. What are these tests used for?
7. What determines the ABO blood groups?
8. If group A blood is transfused into a group B person, what will happen and why?
9. If group O blood is transfused into a group B person, what will happen and why?
10. If group A blood is transfused into a group AB person, what will happen and why?
11. Which blood group is present in universal donors? Why? In universal recipients? Why?
12. Why is there a high risk of problems in children whose father is $Rh(D)^+$ and whose mother is $Rh(D)^-$?
13. How can the induction of Rh antibodies in the mother in question 12 be prevented?

Hypersensitivity (Allergy)   65

harmful.

When an immune response results in exaggerated or inappropriate reactions harmful to the host, the term **hypersensitivity** or **allergy** is used. The clinical manifestations of these reactions are typical in a given individual and occur on contact with the specific antigen to which the individual is hypersensitive. The first contact of the individual with the antigen sensitizes, ie, induces the antibody, and then the subsequent contacts elicit the allergic response.

Hypersensitivity reactions can be subdivided into four main types. Types I, II, and III are **antibody-mediated,** whereas type IV is **cell-mediated** (Table 65–1). Type I reactions are mediated by IgE, whereas types II and III are mediated by IgG.

TYPE I: IMMEDIATE (ANAPHYLACTIC) HYPERSENSITIVITY

An immediate hypersensitivity reaction occurs when antigen binds to IgE on the surface of mast cells with the consequent release of several mediators (see list of mediators below) (Fig 65–1). The process begins when an antigen induces the formation of **IgE antibody,** which binds firmly by its Fc portion to basophils and mast cells. Reexposure to the same antigen results in cross-linking of the cell-bound IgE and release of pharmacologically active mediators within minutes ("immediate reaction"). Cyclic nucleotides and calcium play essential roles in release of the mediators.*

The clinical manifestations of type I hypersensitivity can appear in various forms, eg, urticaria (also known as hives), eczema, rhinitis and conjunctivitis (also known as hay fever), and asthma. The most severe form is systemic **anaphylaxis,** in which severe bronchoconstriction and hypotension (shock) can be life-threatening. No single mediator accounts for all the manifestations of type I hypersensitivity reactions. Some important mediators and their effects are as follows:

---

*An increase in cyclic GMP within these cells increases mediator release, whereas an increase in cyclic AMP decreases the release. Therefore, drugs that increase intracellular cyclic AMP, such as epinephrine, are used to treat type I reactions. Epinephrine also has sympathomimetic activity, which is useful in treating type I reactions.

Table 65–1. Hypersensitivity reactions.

Mediator	Type	Reaction
Antibody (IgE)	I (immediate, anaphylactic)	IgE antibody is induced by allergen and binds to mast cells and basophils. When exposed to the allergen again, the allergen cross-links the bound IgE, which induces degranulation and release of mediators, eg, histamine.
Antibody (IgG)	II (cytotoxic)	Antigens on a cell surface combine with antibody; this leads to complement-mediated lysis, eg, tranfusion or Rh reactions, or autoimmune hemolytic anemia.
Antibody (IgG)	III (immune complex)	Antigen-antibody immune complexes are deposited in tissues, complement is activated, and polymorphonuclear cells are attracted to the site. They release lysosomal enzymes, causing tissue damage.
Cell	IV (delayed)	Helper T lymphocytes sensitized by an antigen release lymphokines upon second contact with the same antigen. The lymphokines induce inflammation and activate macrophages, which, in turn, release various mediators.

Arthus reaction

mast cells & basophils

(1) Histamine occurs in granules of tissue mast cells and basophils in a preformed state. Its release causes vasodilation, increased capillary permeability, and smooth-muscle contraction. Clinically, disorders such as allergic rhinitis (hay fever), urticaria, and angioedema can occur. The bronchospasm so prominent in acute anaphylaxis is due, in part, to histamine release. Antihistamine drugs block histamine receptor sites and can be relatively effective in allergic rhinitis but not in asthma (see below).

not preformed.

(2) Slow-reacting substance of anaphylaxis (SRS-A) consists of several **leukotrienes,** which do not exist in a preformed state but are produced during anaphylactic reactions. This accounts for the slow onset of the effect of SRS-A. Leukotrienes are formed from arachidonic acid by the lipoxygenase pathway and cause increased vascular permeability and smooth-muscle contraction. They are the principal mediators in the bronchoconstriction of asthma and are not influenced by antihistamines.

mast cells

(3) Eosinophil chemotactic factor of anaphylaxis (ECF-A) is a tetrapeptide that exists preformed in mast cell granules. When released during anaphylaxis, it attracts eosinophils that are prominent in immediate allergic reactions. The role of eosinophils in type I hypersensitivity reactions is uncertain, but they do release histaminase and arylsulfatase, which degrade two important mediators, histamine and SRS-A, respectively. Eosinophils may therefore reduce the severity of the type I response.

serotonin

(4) Serotonin (hydroxytryptamine) is preformed in mast cells and blood platelets. When released during anaphylaxis, it causes capillary dilation, increased vascular permeability, and smooth-muscle contraction but is of minor importance in human anaphylaxis.

cross link allergen release mediators from granules

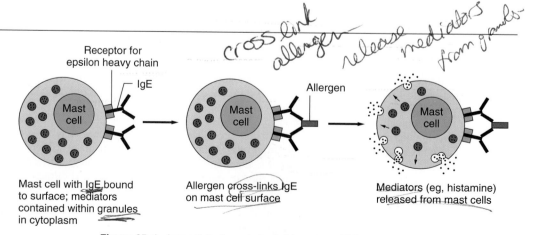

Receptor for epsilon heavy chain

IgE

Mast cell

Allergen

Mast cell

Mast cell

Mediators (eg, histamine) released from mast cells

Mast cell with IgE bound to surface; mediators contained within granules in cytoplasm

Allergen cross-links IgE on mast cell surface

Figure 65–1. Immediate (anaphylactic) hypersensitivity.

(5) Prostaglandins and thromboxanes are related to leukotrienes. They are derived from arachidonic acid via the cyclooxygenase pathway. Prostaglandins cause dilation and increased permeability of capillaries and bronchoconstriction. Thromboxanes aggregate platelets.

The above-mentioned mediators are active only for a few minutes after release; they are enzymatically inactivated and resynthesized slowly. Manifestations of anaphylaxis vary among species, because mediators are released at different rates in different amounts and tissues vary in their sensitivity to them. For example, the respiratory tract (bronchospasm, laryngeal edema) is a principal shock organ in humans but the liver (hepatic veins) plays that role in dogs.

In contrast to anaphylactic reactions, which are IgE-mediated, **anaphylactoid** reactions, which appear clinically similar to anaphylactic ones, are not IgE-mediated. In anaphylactoid reactions, the inciting agents, usually drugs or iodinated contrast media, directly induce the mast cells and basophils to release their mediators without the involvement of IgE.

Atopy Atopic disorders are immediate-hypersensitivity reactions that exhibit a strong **familial predisposition** and are associated with **elevated IgE levels.** Several processes seem likely to play a role in atopy, for example, failure of regulation at the T cell level (eg, increased production of interleukin-4 leads to increased IgE synthesis), enhanced uptake and presentation of environmental antigens, and hyperreactivity of target tissues.

The predisposition to atopy is genetic, and symptoms are induced by exposure to the specific allergens. These antigens are typically found in the environment (eg, pollens and house dust) or in foods (eg, shellfish and nuts). Exposure of nonatopic individuals to these substances does not elicit an allergic reaction. Common clinical manifestations include hay fever, asthma, eczema, and urticaria. Many sufferers give immediate-type reactions to skin tests (injection, patch, or scratch) containing the offending antigen.

Atopic hypersensitivity is transferable by serum (ie, it is antibody-mediated), not by lymphoid cells. In the past, this observation was used for diagnosis in the passive cutaneous anaphylaxis (Prausnitz-Küstner) reaction, which consists of taking serum from the patient and injecting it into the skin of a normal person. Some hours later the test antigen, injected into the "sensitized" site, will yield an immediate wheal-and-flare reaction. This test is now impractical because of the danger of transmitting certain viral infections. Radioallergosorbent tests (RAST) permit the identification of specific IgE against potentially offending allergens if suitable specific antigens for in vitro tests are available.

The cause of atopy is uncertain. Reduced numbers of suppressor T cells and a predisposition to an abnormally high IgE response have been proposed.

Drug Hypersensitivity Drugs, particularly antimicrobial agents such as penicillin, are now among the most common causes of hypersensitivity reactions. Usually it is not the intact drug that induces antibody formation. Rather, a metabolic product of the drug, which acts as a hapten and binds to a body protein, does so. The resulting antibody can react with the hapten or the intact drug to give rise to type I hypersensitivity.* When reexposed to the drug, the person may exhibit rashes, fevers, or local or systemic anaphylaxis of variable severity. Reactions to very small amounts of the drug can occur, eg, in a skin test with the hapten. A clinically useful example is the skin test using penicilloyl-polylysine to reveal an allergy to penicillin.

Desensitization Major manifestations of anaphylaxis occur when large amounts of mediators are suddenly released as a result of a massive dose of antigen abruptly combining with IgE on many mast cells. This is systemic anaphylaxis, which is potentially fatal. Desensitization can prevent systemic anaphylaxis.

Acute desensitization involves the administration of very small amounts of antigen at 15-minute intervals. Antigen-IgE complexes form on a small scale, and not enough mediator is released to produce a major reaction. This permits the administration of a drug or foreign protein to a hypersensitive person, but hypersensitivity is restored days or weeks later.

Chronic desensitization involves the long-term administration at weekly intervals of the antigen to which the person is hypersensitive. This stimulates the production of IgG-blocking antibodies in the serum, which can prevent subsequent antigen from reaching IgE on mast cells, thus preventing a reaction.

*Some drugs are involved in cytotoxic hypersensitivity reactions (type II) and in serum sickness (type III).

Treatment & Prevention of Anaphylactic Reactions   Treatment includes drugs to counteract the action of mediators, maintenance of an airway, and support of respiratory and cardiac function. Epinephrine, antihistamines, corticosteroids, or cromolyn sodium, either singly or in combination, should be given. Cromolyn sodium prevents release of mediators, eg, histamine, from mast cell granules. Prevention relies on identification of the allergen by a skin test and avoidance of that allergen.

TYPE II: CYTOTOXIC HYPERSENSITIVITY   Blood transfusion.

Cytotoxic hypersensitivity occurs when antibody directed at antigens of the **cell membrane** activates complement (Fig 65–2). This generates a membrane attack complex (see Chapter 63), which damages the cell membrane. The antibody (IgG or IgM) attaches to the antigen via the Fab region and acts as a bridge to complement via the Fc region. As a result, there is complement-mediated lysis as in hemolytic anemias, ABO transfusion reactions, or Rh hemolytic disease. In addition to causing lysis, complement activation attracts phagocytes to the site, with consequent release of enzymes that damage cell membranes.

Drugs (eg, penicillins, phenacetin, quinidine) can attach to surface proteins on red blood cells and initiate antibody formation. Such autoimmune antibodies (IgG) then interact with the cell surface and result in hemolysis. The direct antiglobulin (Coombs) test is typically positive (see Chapter 64). Other drugs (eg, quinine) can attach to platelets and induce autoantibodies that lyse them to produce thrombocytopenia with bleeding tendency. Others (eg, hydralazine) may modify host tissue and favor the production of autoantibodies directed at cell DNA, with results resembling those of systemic lupus erythematosus. Certain infections, eg, *Mycoplasma pneumoniae* infection, can induce antibodies that cross-react with red cell antigens, resulting in hemolytic anemia. In rheumatic fever, antibodies against the group A streptococci cross-react with cardiac tissue. In Goodpasture's syndrome, antibody to basement membranes of the kidneys and lungs form, resulting in severe damage to the membranes caused by enzymes released from leukocytes attracted to the site by complement component C5a (see p 378).

TYPE III: IMMUNE-COMPLEX HYPERSENSITIVITY   Arthus Reaction

Immune-complex hypersensitivity occurs when antigen-antibody complexes induce an inflammatory response in tissues (Fig 65–3). Normally, immune complexes are promptly removed by the reticuloendothelial system, but occasionally they persist and are **deposited in tissues,** resulting in several disorders. In persistent microbial or viral infections, immune complexes may be deposited in organs, eg, the kidneys, resulting in damage. In autoimmune disorders, "self" antigens may elicit antibodies that bind to organ antigens or deposit in organs as complexes, especially in joints (arthritis), kidneys (nephritis), or blood vessels (vasculitis).

Wherever immune complexes are deposited, they activate the complement system. Polymorphonuclear cells are attracted to the site, and inflammation and tissue injury occur. Two typical type III hypersensitivity reactions are the Arthus reaction and serum sickness.

Arthus Reaction   If animals are given an antigen repeatedly until they have high levels of IgG antibody* and that antigen is then injected subcutaneously or intradermally, intense edema and hem-

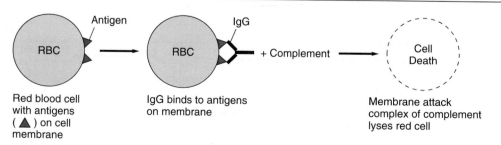

Figure 65–2. Cytotoxic hypersensitivity.

---

*Much more antibody is typically needed to elicit an Arthus reaction than an anaphylactic reaction.

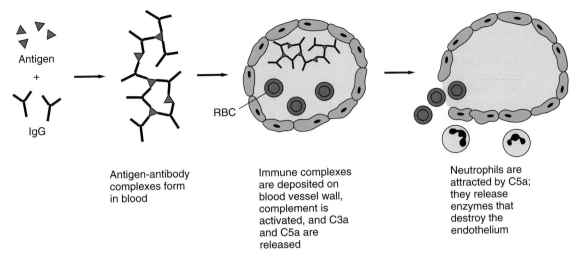

Figure 65–3. Immune complex hypersensitivity.

orrhage develop, reaching a peak in 3–6 hours. Antigen, antibody, and complement are deposited in vessel walls; polymorphonuclear cell infiltration and intravascular clumping of platelets then occur. These reactions can lead to vascular occlusion and necrosis. A clinical manifestation of the Arthus reaction is hypersensitivity pneumonitis (allergic alveolitis) associated with the inhalation of thermophilic actinomycetes ("farmer's lung").

Serum Sickness   Following the injection of foreign serum (or, more commonly these days, certain drugs), the antigen is excreted slowly. During this time, antibody production starts. The simultaneous presence of antigen and antibody leads to the formation of immune complexes, which may circulate or be deposited at various sites. Typical serum sickness results in fever, urticaria, arthralgia, lymphadenopathy, splenomegaly, and eosinophilia a few days to 2 weeks after injection of the foreign serum or drug. Although it takes several days for symptoms to appear, serum sickness is classed as an immediate reaction because symptoms occur promptly after immune complexes form. Symptoms improve as the immune system removes the antigen and subside when the antigen is eliminated. Nowadays, serum sickness is caused more commonly by drugs, eg, penicillin, than by foreign serum because foreign serum is used so infrequently.

Immune-Complex Diseases   Many clinical disorders associated with immune complexes have been described, although the antigen that initiates the disease is often in doubt. Several representative examples are described below.

A. Glomerulonephritis: Acute poststreptococcal glomerulonephritis is a well-accepted immune-complex disease. Its onset follows several weeks after a group A beta-hemolytic streptococcal infection, particularly of the skin, and often with nephritogenic serotypes of *Streptococcus pyogenes.* Typically, the complement level is low, suggesting an antigen-antibody reaction. Lumpy deposits of immunoglobulin and C3 are seen along glomerular basement membranes by immunofluorescence, suggesting the presence of antigen-antibody complexes. It is assumed that streptococcal antigen-antibody complexes, after being deposited on glomeruli, fix complement and attract neutrophils, which start the inflammatory process.

Similar lesions with "lumpy" deposits containing immunoglobulin and C3 occur in infective endocarditis, serum sickness, and certain viral infections, eg, hepatitis B and dengue hemorrhagic fever. Lesions containing immune complexes also occur in autoimmune diseases, eg, the nephritis of systemic lupus erythematosus, where the "lumpy" deposits contain DNA as the antigen (see below and p 377).

B. Rheumatoid Arthritis: Rheumatoid arthritis is a chronic inflammatory autoimmune disease of the joints seen commonly in young women. Serum and synovial fluid of patients contain "rheumatoid factor," ie, IgM and IgG antibodies that bind to the Fc fragment of normal human IgG. Deposits of immune complexes (containing the normal IgG and rheumatoid factor) on synovial membranes and in blood vessels activate complement and attract polymorphonuclear cells, causing inflammation. Patients have high titers of rheumatoid factor and low titers of complement in serum during active rheumatoid disease (see p 377).

C. Systemic Lupus Erythematosus: Systemic lupus erythematosus is a chronic inflammatory autoimmune disease that affects several organs, especially the skin of the face, the joints, and the kidneys. Antibodies are formed against DNA and other components of the nucleus of cells. These antibodies form immune complexes that activate complement. Complement activation produces C5a, which attracts neutrophils that release enzymes, thereby damaging tissue (see p 377).

TYPE IV: DELAYED (CELL-MEDIATED) HYPERSENSITIVITY

Delayed hypersensitivity is a function of **helper (CD4) T lymphocytes, not antibody** (Fig 65–4). It can be transferred by immunologically committed (sensitized) T cells, not by serum. The response is "delayed"; ie, it starts hours (or days) after contact with the antigen and often lasts for days. It consists mainly of mononuclear cell infiltration (macrophages and helper [CD4] T cells) and tissue induration, as typified by the tuberculin skin test.

Clinically Important Delayed Hypersensitivity Reactions

A. Contact Hypersensitivity: This manifestation of cell-mediated hypersensitivity occurs after sensitization with simple chemicals (eg, nickel, formaldehyde), plant materials (eg, poison ivy, poison oak), topically applied drugs (eg, sulfonamides, neomycin), some cosmetics, soaps, and other substances. In all cases, the small molecules acting as haptens enter the skin, attach to body proteins, and become complete antigens. Cell-mediated hypersensitivity is induced, particularly in the skin. Upon a later skin contact with the offending agent, the sensitized person develops erythema, itching, vesicles, eczema, or necrosis of skin within 12–48 hours. Patch testing on a small area of skin can sometimes identify the offending antigen. Subsequent avoidance of the material will prevent recurrences.

B. Tuberculin-Type Hypersensitivity: Delayed hypersensitivity to antigens of microorganisms occurs in many infectious diseases and has been used as an aid in diagnosis. It is typified by the tuberculin reaction. When a patient previously exposed to *Mycobacterium tuberculosis* is injected with a small amount of tuberculin (PPD) intradermally, there is little reaction in the first few hours. Gradually, however, induration and redness develop and reach a peak in 48–72 hours. A positive skin test indicates that the person **has been infected** with the agent, but it does *not* confirm the presence of current disease. However, if the skin test converts from negative to positive, it suggests that the patient has been recently infected. Infected persons do not always have a positive skin test, because overwhelming infection, disorders that suppress cell-mediated immunity (eg, uremia, measles,

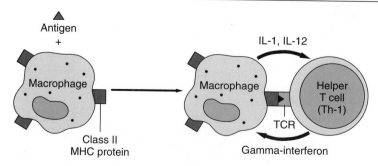

Figure 65–4. Delayed (cell-mediated) hypersensitivity. The macrophage ingests the antigen, processes it, and presents an epitope on its surface in association with class II MHC protein. The helper T (Th-1) cell is activated and produces gamma interferon, which activates macrophages. These two types of cells mediate delayed hypersensitivity.

sarcoidosis, lymphoma, and AIDS), or the administration of immunosuppressive drugs (eg, cortico-steroids, antineoplastics) may cause anergy.

A positive skin test response assists in diagnosis and provides support for chemoprophylaxis or chemotherapy. In leprosy, a positive lepromin test indicates the presence of tuberculoid leprosy with competent cell-mediated immunity whereas a negative lepromin test suggests the presence of lepromatous leprosy with impaired cell-mediated immunity. In systemic mycotic infections (eg, coccidioidomycosis and histoplasmosis), a positive skin test with the specific antigen indicates exposure to the organism. Cell-mediated hypersensitivity develops in many viral infections; however, serologic tests are more specific than skin tests both for diagnosis and for assessment of immunity. In protozoan and helminthic infections, skin tests may be positive, but they are generally not as useful as specific serologic tests.

Review Questions

1. What is the evidence that anaphylaxis is antibody-mediated rather than cell-mediated?
2. Describe the pathogenesis of anaphylaxis, including (a) the type of antibody, (b) the cells, and (c) the mediators.
3. What are some common atopic disorders and their allergens? What is the role of IgE in atopy?
4. What is the rationale behind desensitization to mitigate type I hypersensitivity reactions?
5. What are the similarities and differences between type II (cytotoxic) and type I (anaphylactic) hypersensitivity?
6. What is the pathogenesis of serum sickness? Nowadays, serum is not the main cause. What is?
7. What is the pathogenesis of poststreptococcal glomerulonephritis?
8. Why is cell-mediated hypersensitivity called "delayed"?
9. What is the pathogenesis of poison oak and poison ivy hypersensitivity?
10. Describe the immunologic process involved in a positive tuberculin skin test.

Tolerance & Autoimmune Disease 66

TOLERANCE

T cells can determine self from non-self.

Tolerance is specific immunologic **unresponsiveness;** ie, an immune response to a certain antigen (or epitope) does not occur, although the immune system is otherwise functioning normally. In general, antigens that are present during embryonic life are considered **"self"** and **do not stimulate** an immunologic response. The lack of an immune response is the result of the deletion of self-reactive T cell precursors in the thymus (Fig 66–1). On the other hand, antigens that are not present during the process of maturation, ie, that are encountered first when the body is immunologically mature, are considered "nonself" and usually elicit an immunologic response.

The main process by which T lymphocytes acquire the ability to distinguish self from nonself occurs in the fetal thymus (see Chapter 58). This process, called **clonal deletion,** involves the killing of T cells ("negative selection") that react against antigens (primarily self MHC proteins) present in the fetus at that time. (Note that exogenous substances injected into the fetus early in development are treated as self.) The cells die by a process of programmed cell death called **apoptosis.** Tolerance to self acquired within the thymus is called **central tolerance,** in contrast to tolerance acquired outside the thymus, which is called **peripheral tolerance.** The precise mechanism by which autoreactive T cells are recognized and killed in the thymus is uncertain. Furthermore, the process by which T cells become tolerant in adults after the thymus involutes is unknown.

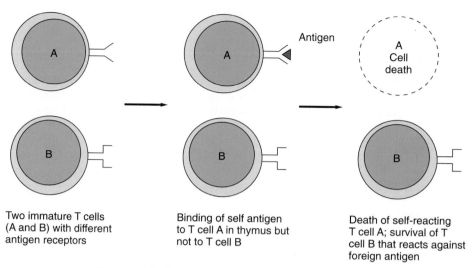

Figure 66–1. Production of T cell tolerance in the thymus.

Two immature T cells (A and B) with different antigen receptors

Binding of self antigen to T cell A in thymus but not to T cell B

Death of self-reacting T cell A; survival of T cell B that reacts against foreign antigen

Because some self-reactive T cells are not killed in the thymus, a mechanism to induce peripheral tolerance is also necessary. This is called **clonal anergy** and involves the functional inactivation of the surviving self-reactive T cells (Fig 66–2). Although anergic cells are nonfunctional, they can become functional and initiate an autoimmune disease if conditions change later in life. The mechanism of clonal anergy involves the inappropriate presentation of antigen, leading to a failure of interleukin-2 (IL-2) production. Inappropriate presentation is due to a failure of "costimulatory signals"; eg, sufficient amounts of IL-1 might not be made, or cell surface proteins, such as CD28 on the T cell and B7 on the B cell, might not interact properly, leading to a failure of signal transduction by *ras* proteins. Furthermore, B7 is an inducible protein, and failure to induce it in sufficient amounts can lead to anergy. In addition, the costimulatory proteins, CD40 on the B cell and CD40L on the helper T cell, may fail to interact properly.

B cells also become tolerant to self by two mechanisms: (1) clonal deletion, probably while the B cell precursors are in the bone marrow, and (2) clonal anergy of B cells in the periphery. However, tolerance in B cells is less complete than in T cells, an observation supported by the finding that most autoimmune diseases are mediated by antibodies.

Whether an antigen will induce tolerance rather than an immunologic response is largely determined by the following:

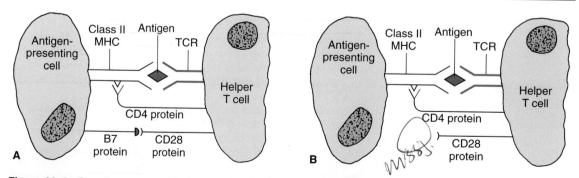

Figure 66–2. Clonal anergy outside the thymus. **A:** B7 protein on the antigen-presenting cell interacts with CD28 on the helper T cell, and full activation of the helper T cell occurs. **B:** B7 protein on the antigen-presenting cell is not produced, and so CD28 on the helper T cell does not give a costimulatory signal. Anergy of the helper T cell occurs despite interaction of the T cell receptor with the epitope.

(1) The immunologic **maturity** of the host; eg, neonatal animals are immunologically immature and do not respond too well to foreign antigens (for instance, neonates will accept allografts that would be rejected by mature animals).

(2) The **structure and dose** of the antigen; eg, a very simple molecule induces tolerance more readily than a complex one, and very high or very low doses of antigen may result in tolerance instead of an immune response. Purified polysaccharides or amino acid copolymers injected in very large doses result in "immune paralysis"—a lack of response.

Other aspects of the induction or maintenance of tolerance are as follows:

(1) T cells become tolerant more readily and remain tolerant longer than B cells.

(2) Administration of a cross-reacting antigen tends to terminate tolerance.

(3) Administration of immunosuppressive drugs enhances tolerance, eg, in transplants.

(4) Tolerance is maintained best if the antigen continues to be present.

AUTOIMMUNE DISEASES

The adult host usually exhibits tolerance to tissue antigens present during fetal life that are recognized as "self." However, in certain circumstances tolerance may be lost and immune reactions to host antigens may develop, resulting in autoimmune diseases. The most important step in the production of autoimmune disease is the **activation of self-reactive helper (CD4) T cells.** These self-reactive Th-1 or Th-2 cells can induce either cell-mediated or antibody-mediated autoimmune reactions, respectively. As described in Table 66–1, **most autoimmune diseases are antibody-mediated.**

Many autoimmune diseases exhibit a marked familial incidence, which suggests a **genetic predisposition** to these disorders. There is a strong association of some diseases with certain human leukocyte antigen (HLA) specificities, especially the class II genes. For example, rheumatoid arthritis occurs predominantly in individuals carrying the HLA-DR4 gene. Ankylosing spondylitis is 100 times more likely to occur in people who carry HLA-B27, a class I gene, than in those who do not carry that gene.

Table 66–1. Important autoimmune diseases.

Type of Immune Response	Autoimmune Disease	Target of the Immune Response
Antibody to receptors	Myasthenia gravis Graves' disease Insulin-resistant diabetes Lambert-Eaton myasthenia	Acetylcholine receptor TSH[1] receptor Insulin receptor Calcium channel receptor
Antibody to cell components other than receptors	Systemic lupus erythematosus Rheumatoid arthritis Rheumatic fever Hemolytic anemia Idiopathic thrombocytopenic purpura Goodpasture's syndrome Pernicious anemia Hashimoto's thyroiditis[2] Insulin-dependent diabetes mellitus[2] Addison's disease Acute glomerulonephritis Periarteritis nodosa Guillain-Barré syndrome	dsDNA, histones IgG in joints Heart and joint tissue RBC membrane Platelet membranes Basement membrane of kidney and lung Intrinsic factor and parietal cells Thyroglobulin Islet cells Adrenal cortex Glomerular basement membrane Small and medium-sized arteries Myelin protein
Cell-mediated (T cells and macrophages)	Allergic encephalomyelitis	Reaction to myelin protein causes brain demyelination

[1] TSH, thyroid-stimulating hormone.
[2] These diseases involve a significant cell-mediated as well as antibody-mediated response.

It should be noted, however, that whether a person develops an autoimmune disease or not is clearly multifactorial, because people with HLA genes known to predispose to certain autoimmune diseases nevertheless do not develop the disease; eg, many people carrying the HLA-DR4 gene do not develop rheumatoid arthritis. That is to say, HLA genes appear to be necessary but not sufficient to cause autoimmune diseases. In general, class II MHC-related diseases, eg, rheumatoid arthritis, Graves' disease (hyperthyroidism), and systemic lupus erythematosus, occur more commonly in women whereas class I MHC-related diseases, eg, ankylosing spondylitis and Reiter's syndrome, occur more commonly in men.

In summary, the current model is that autoimmune diseases occur in people (1) with a genetic predisposition that is determined by their MHC genes and (2) who are exposed to an environmental agent which triggers a cross-reacting immune response against some component of normal tissue. Furthermore, because autoimmune diseases increase in number with advancing age, another possible factor is a decline in the number of regulatory T cells, which allows any surviving autoreactive T cells to proliferate and cause disease.

Mechanisms   The following three main mechanisms for autoimmunity have been proposed.

A. Molecular Mimicry: Various bacteria and viruses are implicated as the source of cross-reacting antigens that trigger the activation of autoreactive T cells or B cells. For example, Reiter's syndrome occurs following *Shigella* or *Chlamydia* infections and Guillain-Barré syndrome occurs following *Campylobacter* infections. The concept of "molecular mimicry" is used to explain these phenomena; ie, the environmental trigger resembles (mimics) a component of the body sufficiently that an immune attack is directed against the cross-reacting body component. One of the best-characterized examples of molecular mimicry is the relationship between the M protein of *Streptococcus pyogenes* and the myosin of cardiac muscle. Antibodies against certain M proteins cross-react with cardiac myosin, leading to rheumatic fever.

B. Alteration of Normal Proteins: Drugs can bind to normal proteins and make them immunogenic. Procainamide-induced systemic lupus erythematosus is an example of this mechanism.

C. Release of Sequestered Antigens: Certain tissues, eg, sperm, central nervous system, and the lens and uveal tract of the eye, are sequestered so that their antigens are **not exposed** to the immune system. These are known as **immunologically privileged sites.** When such antigens enter the circulation accidentally, eg, after damage, they elicit both humoral and cellular responses, producing aspermatogenesis, encephalitis, or endophthalmitis, respectively. Sperm, in particular, must be in a sequestered, immunologically privileged site, because they develop after immunologic maturity has been reached and yet are normally not subject to immune attack.

Diseases   Table 66–1 describes several important autoimmune diseases according to the type of immune response causing the disease and the target affected by the autoimmune response. Some examples of autoimmune disease are described in more detail below.

A.   Diseases Involving Primarily One Type of Cell or Organ

1.   Allergic encephalitis—A clinically important example of allergic encephalitis occurs when people are injected with rabies vaccine made in rabbit brains. The immune response against the foreign myelin protein in the vaccine cross-reacts with human myelin, leading to inflammation of the brain. Although rare, this is a serious disease, and rabies vaccine made in rabbit brain is no longer used in the United States (see Chapter 39). Allergic encephalitis can also occur following certain viral infections, eg, measles or influenza, or following immunizations against these infections. These reactions are rare, and the basis for the autoimmune reaction is uncertain. Allergic encephalitis can be reproduced in the laboratory by injecting myelin basic protein into a rodent's brain, which initiates a cell-mediated response leading to demyelination.

2.   Chronic thyroiditis—When animals are injected with thyroid gland material, they develop humoral and cell-mediated immunity against thyroid antigens and a chronic thyroiditis. Humans with Hashimoto's chronic thyroiditis have antibodies to thyroglobulin, suggesting that these antibodies may provoke an inflammatory process that leads to fibrosis of the gland.

3. Hemolytic anemias, thrombocytopenias, and granulocytopenias—Various forms of these disorders have been attributed to the attachment of autoantibodies to cell surfaces and subsequent cell destruction. Pernicious anemia is caused by antibodies to intrinsic factor, a protein secreted by parietal cells of the stomach that facilitates the absorption of vitamin B_{12}. Idiopathic thrombocytopenic purpura is due to antibodies directed against platelets.

4. Diabetes, myasthenia gravis, and hyperthyroidism (Graves' disease)—In these diseases, antibodies to receptors play a pathogenic role. In extreme insulin resistance in diabetes, antibodies to insulin receptors have been demonstrated that interfere with insulin binding. In myasthenia gravis, which is characterized by severe muscular weakness, antibodies to acetylcholine receptors of neuromuscular junctions are found in the serum. Muscular weakness also occurs in Lambert-Eaton syndrome, in which antibodies form against the proteins in calcium channels. Some patients with Graves' disease have circulating antibodies to thyrotropin receptors, which, when they bind to the receptors, resemble thyrotropin in activity and stimulate the thyroid to produce more thyroxine.

5. Guillain-Barré Syndrome—This disease is the most common cause of acute paralysis in the United States. It follows a variety of infectious diseases such as viral illnesses (eg, upper respiratory infections, HIV infection, and mononucleosis caused by EBV and CMV), and diarrhea caused by *Campylobacter jejuni*. Antibodies against myelin protein are formed and result in a demyelinating polyneuropathy. The main symptoms are those of a rapidly progressing ascending paralysis. The treatment involves either intravenous immunoglobulins or plasmapheresis.

B. Diseases Involving Multiple Organs (Systemic Diseases)

1. Systemic lupus erythematosus (SLE)—In this disease, autoantibodies are formed against DNA, histones, nucleolar proteins, and other components of the cell nucleus. Antibodies against double-stranded DNA are the hallmark of SLE. It affects primarily women between the ages of 20 and 60 years. Individuals with HLA-DR2 or -DR3 genes are predisposed to SLE. The agent that induces these autoantibodies in most patients is unknown. However, two drugs, procainamide and hydralazine, are known to cause SLE.

Most of the clinical findings are caused by immune complexes that activate complement and, as a consequence, damage tissue. For example, the characteristic rash on the cheeks is the result of a vasculitis caused by immune complex deposition. The arthritis and glomerulonephritis commonly seen in SLE are also caused by immune complexes. However, the anemia, leukopenia, and thrombocytopenia are caused by cytotoxic antibodies rather than immune complexes.

The diagnosis of SLE is supported by detecting antinuclear antibodies (ANA) with fluorescent antibody tests and anti-double-stranded DNA antibodies with ELISA. Antibodies to several other nuclear components are also detected, as is a reduced level of complement. Treatment of SLE varies depending upon the severity of the disease and the organs affected. Aspirin, nonsterodial anti-inflammatory drugs, or corticosteroids are commonly used.

2. Rheumatoid arthritis (RA)—In this disease, autoantibodies are formed against IgG. These autoantibodies are called rheumatoid factors and are of the IgM class. RA affects primarily women between the ages of 30 and 50 years. People with HLA-DR4 genes are predisposed to RA. The agent that induces these autoantibodies is unknown.

The main clinical finding is inflammation of the small joints of the hands and feet. Other organs, such as the pleura, pericardium, and skin, can also be involved. Most of the clinical findings are caused by immune complexes that activate complement and, as a consequence, damage tissue. The diagnosis of RA is supported by detecting rheumatoid factors in the serum. Treatment of RA typically involves aspirin, nonsteroidal anti-inflammatory drugs, immunosuppressive drugs, or corticosteroids.

3. Rheumatic fever—Group A streptococcal infections regularly precede the development of rheumatic fever. Antibodies against the M protein of group A streptococci that cross-react with myosin in cardiac muscle and joint tissue are involved in the pathogenesis of rheumatic fever.

4. Reiter's syndrome—This syndrome is characterized by the triad of arthritis, conjunctivitis, and urethritis. Cultures of the affected areas do not reveal a causative agent. Infection by one of the intestinal pathogens, eg, *Shigella, Salmonella, Yersinia,* and *Campylobacter,* as well as other organisms such as *Chlamydia,* predisposes to the disease. Most patients are men who are HLA-B27-positive. The pathogenesis of the disease is unclear, but immune complexes may play a role.

5. Goodpasture's syndrome (GS)—In this syndrome, autoantibodies are formed against the collagen in basement membranes of the kidneys and lungs. GS affects primarily young men, and those with HLA-DR2 genes are at risk for this disease. The agent that induces these autoantibodies is unknown, but GS often follows a viral infection.

The main clinical findings are hematuria, proteinuria, and pulmonary hemorrhage. The clinical findings are caused by cytotoxic antibodies that activate complement. As a consequence, C5a is produced, neutrophils are attracted to the site, and enzymes are released by the neutrophils that damage the kidney and lung tissue. The diagnosis of GS is supported by detecting antibody and complement bound to basement membranes in fluorescent-antibody test. This is a rapidly progressive, often fatal disease, and so treatment, including plasma exchange to remove the antibodies and the use of immunosuppressive drugs, must be instituted promptly.

6. Other collagen vascular diseases—Other diseases in this category include ankylosing spondylitis, which is very common in people carrying the HLA-B27 gene, polymyositis-dermatomyositis, scleroderma, periarteritis nodosa, and Sjögren's syndrome.

Treatment   The conceptual basis for the treatment of autoimmune diseases is to reduce the patient's immune response sufficiently to eliminate the symptoms. Corticosteroids, such as prednisone, are the mainstay of treatment, to which antimetabolites, such as azathioprine and methotrexate, can be added. The latter are nucleoside analogues that inhibit DNA synthesis in the immune cells. Immunosuppressive therapy must be given cautiously because of the risk of opportunistic infections.

Review Questions

1. What are the factors that determine tolerance?
2. What are the hypotheses that may explain tolerance?
3. What are the suggested mechanisms for autoimmune diseases?
4. What is the immunopathogenesis of (a) rheumatic fever? (b) pernicious anemia? (c) myasthenia gravis? (d) Graves' disease? (e) systemic lupus erythematosus? (f) rheumatoid arthritis?

67

Tumor Immunity

TUMOR-ASSOCIATED ANTIGENS

Animals carrying a chemically or virally induced malignant tumor can develop resistance to that tumor and cause its **regression.** In the course of neoplastic transformation, **new antigens,** called **tumor-associated antigens (TAA),** develop at the cell surface and the host recognizes such cells as "nonself." In chemically induced tumors in experimental animals, TAAs are highly specific; ie, cells of one tumor will have different TAAs from those on cells of another tumor even when they arise within the same animal. In contrast, virally induced tumors possess TAAs that cross-react with one another if induced by the same virus. TAAs on tumor cells induced by different viruses do not cross-react.

MECHANISM OF TUMOR IMMUNITY

Cell-mediated reactions attack these "nonself" tumor cells and limit their proliferation. Such immune responses probably act as a **surveillance** system to detect and eliminate newly arising clones of neoplastic cells. In general, the immune response against tumor cells is weak and can be overcome experimentally by a large dose of tumor cells. Some tumor cells can escape surveillance by "modulation," ie, internalizing the surface antigen so that it no longer presents a target for immune attack.

The cell-mediated immune responses that affect tumor cells in vitro include natural killer (NK) cells, which act without antibody; killer (K) cells, which mediate antibody-dependent cytolysis (antibody-dependent cellular cytotoxicity); cytotoxic T cells; and activated macrophages. Whether these immune responses function to prevent or control tumors in vivo is unknown.

Tumor antigens can stimulate the development of specific antibodies as well. Some of these antibodies are cytotoxic, but others, called blocking antibodies, enhance tumor growth, perhaps by blocking recognition of tumor antigens by the host. Spontaneously arising human tumors may have new cell surface antigens against which the host develops both cytotoxic antibodies and cell-mediated immune responses. Enhancement of these responses can contain the growth of some tumors. For example, the administration of BCG vaccine (bacillus Calmette-Guérin, a bovine mycobacterium) into surface melanomas can lead to their partial regression. Immunomodulators, such as interleukins and interferons, are also being tested in such settings. One interleukin, tumor necrosis factor alpha (cachectin), is experimentally effective against a variety of solid tumors (see Chapter 58). In addition, lymphocytes activated by interleukin-2 (lymphokine-activated killer [LAK] cells) may be useful in cancer immunotherapy.

Another approach to cancer immunotherapy involves the use of tumor-infiltrating lymphocytes (TIL). The basis for this is the observation that some cancers are infiltrated by lymphocytes (NK cells and cytotoxic T cells) that seem likely to be trying to destroy the cancer cells. These lymphocytes are recovered from the surgically removed cancer, grown in cell culture until large numbers of cells are obtained, activated with interleukin-2, and returned to the patient in the expectation that the TIL will "home in" specifically on the cancer cells and kill them.

CARCINOEMBRYONIC ANTIGEN & ALPHA FETOPROTEIN

Some human tumors contain antigens that normally occur in fetal but not in adult human cells.

(1) Carcinoembryonic antigen circulates at elevated levels in the serum of many patients with carcinoma of the colon, pancreas, breast, or liver. It is found in fetal gut, liver, and pancreas and in very small amounts in normal sera. Detection of this antigen (by radioimmunoassay) is not helpful in diagnosis but may be helpful in management of such tumors. If the level declines after surgery, it suggests that the tumor is not spreading. Conversely, a rise in the level of carcinoembryonic antigen in patients with resected carcinoma of the colon suggests recurrence or spread of the tumor.

(2) Alpha-fetoprotein is present at elevated levels in the sera of hepatoma patients and is used as a marker for this disease. It is produced by fetal liver and is found in small amounts in some normal sera. It is, however, nonspecific; it occurs in several other malignant and nonmalignant diseases.

Monoclonal antibodies directed against new surface antigens on malignant cells (eg, B cell lymphomas) can be useful in diagnosis. Monoclonal antibodies coupled to toxins, such as diphtheria toxin or ricin, a product of the *Ricinus* plant, can kill tumor cells in vitro and someday may be useful for cancer therapy.

Review Questions

1. Describe immune surveillance against tumor cells from the point of view of (a) antigens and (b) host response.
2. Distinguish between carcinoembryonic antigen and alpha-fetoprotein.

68

Immunodeficiency

Immunodeficiency can occur in any of the four major components of the immune system: (1) B cells (antibody), (2) T cells, (3) complement, and (4) phagocytes. The deficiencies can be either congenital or acquired (Table 68–1). Clinically, recurrent or opportunistic infections are commonly seen. Recurrent infections with pyogenic bacteria, eg, staphylococci, indicate a B cell deficiency, whereas recurrent infections with certain fungi, viruses, or protozoa indicate a T cell deficiency.

CONGENITAL IMMUNODEFICIENCIES

B Cell Deficiencies

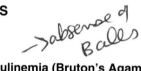 →absence of B cells.

A. X-Linked Hypogammaglobulinemia (Bruton's Agammaglobulinemia): Very low levels of all immunoglobulins (IgG, IgA, IgM, IgD, and IgE) and a virtual **absence of B cells** are found in young **boys;** female carriers are immunologically normal. Pre-B cells are present, but they fail to differentiate into B cells. This failure is caused by a mutation in the gene encoding tyrosine kinase, an important signal transduction protein. Cell-mediated immunity is relatively normal. Clinically, recurrent pyogenic bacterial infections, eg, otitis media, sinusitis, and pneumonia caused by *Streptococcus pneumoniae* and *Haemophilus influenzae,* occur in infants at about 6 months of age, when maternal antibody is no longer protective. Treatment with pooled gamma globulin reduces the number of infections.

B. Selective Immunoglobulin Deficiencies: IgA deficiency is the **most common** of these; IgG and IgM deficiencies are rarer. Patients with a deficiency of IgA typically have recurrent sinus and lung infections. (However, some individuals with IgA deficiency do not have frequent infections, possibly because their IgG and IgM levels confer protection.) The cause of IgA deficiency may be a failure of heavy-chain gene switching, since the amounts of IgG and IgM are normal. Patients with a deficiency of IgA should not be treated with gamma globulin preparations, because they may react against foreign IgA and, by cross-reaction, deplete their already low level of IgA.

Patients with selective IgM deficiency or deficiency of one or more of the IgG subclasses also have recurrent sinopulmonary infections caused by pyogenic bacteria such as *S pneumoniae, H influenzae,* or *S aureus.*

T Cell Deficiencies

A. Thymic Aplasia (DiGeorge's Syndrome): Severe viral, fungal, or protozoal infections occur in affected infants early in life as a result of a profound **deficit of T cells.** Both the thymus and the parathyroids fail to develop properly owing to a defect in the third and fourth pharyngeal pouches. The most common presenting symptom is tetany due to hypocalcemia caused by hypoparathyroidism. Other congenital abnormalities are common. Antibody production is either normal or decreased. A transplant of fetal thymus may reconstitute T cell immunity. A thymus from a child older than 14 weeks should not be used, because a graft-versus-host reaction may occur.

B. Chronic Mucocutaneous Candidiasis: In this disease, the skin and mucous membranes of children are infected with *Candida albicans,* which, in immunocompetent individuals, is a nonpathogenic member of the normal flora. These children have a T cell deficiency **specifically** for this organism; other T cell and B cell functions are normal. Treatment consists primarily of antifungal drugs.

C. Hyper-IgM Syndrome: In this syndrome, severe, recurrent pyogenic bacterial infections resembling those seen in X-linked hypogammaglobulinemia begin early in life. Patients have a high

Bone lymphocyte
→missing MHC
Classes I &II

Table 68–1. Important congenital immunodeficiencies.

Deficient Component and Name of Disease	Specific Deficiency	Molecular Defect	Clinical Features
B cell X-linked (Bruton's)	Absence of B cells; very low Ig levels.	Mutant tyrosine kinase.	Pyogenic infections.
Selective IgA	Very low IgA levels.	Failure of heavy-chain gene switching.	Sinus and lung infections.
T cell Thymic aplasia (DiGeorge's)	Absence of T cells.	Defective development of pharyngeal pouches; not a genetic disease.	Viral, fungal and protozoal infections; tetany.
Chronic mucocutaneous candidiasis	Deficient T cell response to *Candida*.	Unknown	Skin and mucous membrane infections with *Candida*.
Combined B and T cell Severe combined immunodeficiency (SCID)	Deficiency of both B cell and T cell function.	Either defective IL-2 receptor, absence of class II MHC proteins, or ADA or PNP deficiency	Bacterial, viral, fungal, and protozoal infections.
Complement Hereditary angioedema	Deficiency of C1 protease inhibitor.	Too much C3a, C4a, and C5a generated.	Edema, especially laryngeal edema.
C3b	Insufficient C3.	Unknown.	Pyogenic infections, especially with *S aureus*.
C6,7,8	Insufficient C6,7,8.	Unknown.	*Neisseria* infections.
Phagocytes Chronic granulomatous disease	Defective bactericidal activity because no oxidative burst.	Deficient NADPH oxidase activity.	Pyogenic infections, especially with *S aureus*.

concentration of IgM but very little IgG, IgA, and IgE. They have normal numbers of T cells and B cells. Although the main manifestations of this syndrome are alterations in antibodies, the mutation is in the gene encoding the CD40 ligand in the CD4-positive helper T cells. As a result, the helper T cells have a defect in the surface protein (CD40 ligand) that interacts with CD40 on the B cell surface. The failure to properly interact with CD40 results in an inability of the B cell to switch from the production of IgM to the other classes of antibodies. Treatment with pooled gamma globulin results in fewer infections.

Combined B Cell & T Cell Deficiencies

A. Severe Combined Immunodeficiency Disease (SCID): Recurrent infections caused by bacteria, viruses, fungi, and protozoa occur in early infancy (3 months of age), because **both B cells and T cells** are defective. In some children, the B and T cells are absent; in others, the number of cells is normal but they do not function properly. This is a group of inherited diseases, all of which are due to a defect in the differentiation of an early stem cell. There are two types: X-linked and autosomal. Some patients with X-linked SCID have a defect in the IL-2 receptor on T cells. Some patients with the autosomal form have a mutation in the gene encoding a tyrosine kinase called ZAP-70 that plays a role in signal transduction in T cells. Because immunity is so profoundly depressed, these children must be protected from exposure to microorganisms, usually by being enclosed in a plastic "bubble." Live, attenuated viral vaccines should *not* be given. Bone marrow transplant may restore immunity.

Patients with a hereditary absence of **adenosine deaminase (ADA) and purine nucleoside phosphorylase (PNP)** can have a severe deficiency of B cells and T cells, causing SCID, although some have only mild dysfunction. The absence of these enzymes results in an accumulation of dATP, an inhibitor of ribonucleotide reductase, and a consequent decrease in the deoxynucleoside triphosphate precursors of DNA. This severely affects bone marrow differentiation. Bone marrow transplantation can be helpful. Injections of ADA conjugated to polyethylene glycol reduce the number and severity of infections. Several patients with ADA deficiency have benefited from gene therapy. A retroviral vector carrying a normal copy of the ADA gene was allowed to infect the patient's bone marrow cells. The ADA gene functioned within some of these cells, and the patient's immune status improved.

Patient's with **bare lymphocyte syndrome** exhibit the signs and symptoms of a severe combined immunodeficiency and are especially susceptible to viral infections. These patients have defective class I or class II MHC proteins or both. Mutations in the gene encoding the TAP protein have been identified as one cause of the inability to display antigens on class I MHC proteins.

B. Wiskott-Aldrich Syndrome: Recurrent pyogenic infections, eczema, and bleeding due to thrombocytopenia during the first year of life characterize this syndrome. It is an X-linked disease and so occurs only in male infants. The most important defect is the inability to mount an IgM response to the capsular polysaccharides of bacteria, such as pneumococci. IgG levels and IgA levels are normal, but cell-mediated immunity is variable. The defect appears to be in the ability of T cells to provide help to B cells. The gene responsible for this syndrome has been identified, but the function of the protein has not been determined. Bone marrow transplantation may be helpful.

C. Ataxia-Telangiectasia: In this disease, ataxia (staggering), telangiectasia (enlarged small blood vessels of the conjunctivas and skin), and recurrent infections appear by two years of age. It is an autosomal recessive disease caused by mutations in the genes that encode DNA repair enzymes. Lymphopenia and IgA deficiency commonly occur. Treatment designed to correct the immunodeficiency has not been successful.

Complement Deficiencies

A. Hereditary Angioedema: This is an uncommon autosomal dominant disease due to a deficiency of C1 inhibitor. In the absence of inhibitor, C1 continues to act on C4 to generate C4a and subsequently additional vasoactive components such as C3a and C5a. This leads to capillary permeability and edema in several organs. Laryngeal edema can be fatal. Steroid drugs, such as oxymetholone and danazol, can be useful in increasing the concentration of C1 inhibitor.

B. Recurrent Infections: Patients with deficiencies in C1, C3, or C5 or the later components C6, C7, or C8 have an increased susceptibility to bacterial infections. Patients with C3 deficiency are particularly susceptible to sepsis with pyogenic bacteria such as *S aureus.* Those with reduced levels of C6, C7, or C8 are especially prone to bacteremia with *Neisseria meningitidis* or *N gonorrhoeae.*

C. Autoimmune Diseases: Patients with C2 and C4 deficiencies have diseases resembling systemic lupus erythematosus or other autoimmune diseases. C2 deficiency is the most common complement defect and is frequently asymptomatic.

D. Paroxysmal Nocturnal Hemoglobinuria: This rare disease is characterized by episodes of brownish urine (hemoglobinuria), particularly upon arising. The hemoglobinuria is due to complement-mediated hemolysis. This is caused by an acquired deficiency of decay-accelerating factor (DAF) on the surface of blood cell precursors, leading to an increased activation of complement (see Chapter 63). These patients have a defect in the gene for the molecules that anchor DAF and other proteins to the cell membrane. There is no specific treatment. Iron can be given for the anemia, and prednisone can be helpful.

Phagocyte Deficiencies

A. Chronic Granulomatous Disease (CGD): Patients with this disease have a marked susceptibility to opportunistic infections with certain bacteria and fungi, eg, *S aureus,* enteric gram-negative rods, and *Aspergillus fumigatus.* Viral and protozoal infections are not a major concern. In most cases, this is an X-linked disease that appears by the age of 2 years. (In some patients, the disease is autosomal.) It is due to a defect in the intracellular microbicidal activity of neutrophils as a result of a **lack of NADPH oxidase** activity (or similar enzymes). No oxidative burst occurs, because these enzymes are required for the generation of peroxides and superoxides that kill the organisms. B cell and T cell functions are usually normal. In the laboratory, diagnosis can be confirmed by the **nitroblue**

tetrazolium dye reduction test. Treatment is based on antimicrobial drugs. Gamma interferon significantly reduces the frequency of recurrent infections, probably because it increases phagocytosis by macrophages. White blood cell infusions may be helpful.

B. Chédiak-Higashi Syndrome: In this autosomal recessive disease, recurrent pyogenic infections, caused primarily by staphylococci and streptococci, occur. This is due to the failure of the **lysosomes** of neutrophils to empty their contents. Large granular inclusions composed of abnormal lysosomes are seen. Peroxide and superoxide formation is normal, as are B cell and T cell functions. Treatment involves antimicrobial drugs. There is no useful therapy for the phagocyte defect.

C. Job's Syndrome: Patients with this syndrome have recurrent "cold"* staphylococcal abscesses, eczema, and high levels of IgE. The main defect is a failure to produce gamma interferon by helper T cells. This leads to an increase in Th-2 cells and, as a consequence, a high IgE level. The increased IgE causes histamine release which blocks certain aspects of the inflammatory response, hence the "cold" abscesses. Histamine also inhibits neutrophil chemotaxis, another feature of this syndrome. Treatment consists of antimicrobial drugs.

D. Leukocyte Adhesion Deficiency Syndrome: Patients with this syndrome have severe pyogenic infections early in life because they have defective adhesion (LFA-1) proteins on the surface of their phagocytes. As a result, the phagocytes adhere poorly to the cells at the site of infection and phagocytosis of the bacteria is inadequate.

ACQUIRED IMMUNODEFICIENCIES

B Cell Deficiencies

A. Common Variable Hypogammaglobulinemia: Patients present with recurrent infections caused by pyogenic bacteria, eg, sinusitis and pneumonia caused by pyogenic bacteria such as *Streptococcus pneumoniae* and *Haemophilus influenzae*. The infections usually occur in persons between the ages of 15 and 35 years. The number of B cells is usually normal, but the ability to synthesize IgG (and other immunoglobulins) is greatly reduced. Cell-mediated immunity is usually normal. The cause of the failure to produce IgG is unknown but appears to be due to defective T cell signaling. Intravenous gamma globulin given monthly reduces the number of infections.

T Cell Deficiencies

A. Acquired Immunodeficiency Syndrome: Patients with acquired immunodeficiency syndrome (AIDS) present with opportunistic infections caused by certain bacteria, viruses, fungi, and protozoa (eg, *Mycobacterium avium-intracellulare,* herpesviruses, *C albicans,* and *Pneumocystis carinii*). This is due to greatly reduced helper T cell numbers caused by infection with the retrovirus human immunodeficiency virus (HIV; see Chapter 45). This virus specifically infects cells bearing the CD4 protein as a surface receptor. Markedly reduced numbers of CD4 cells occur, but elevated immunoglobulin levels are found. The response to specific immunizations is poor; this is attributed to the loss of helper T cell activity. AIDS patients also have a high incidence of tumors such as Kaposi's sarcoma and lymphomas, which may be due to a failure of immune surveillance. See Chapter 45 for information on treatment and prevention.

B. Measles: Patients with measles have a transient suppression of delayed hypersensitivity as manifested by a loss of PPD skin test reactivity. Quiescent tuberculosis can become active. In these patients, T cell function is altered but immunoglobulins are normal.

Chronic Fatigue Syndrome (Chronic Fatigue Immune Dysfunction Syndrome)
The predominant finding in patients with chronic fatigue syndrome (CFS) is persistent, debilitating fatigue that has lasted for at least 6 months and is not relieved by bed rest. Because fatigue is a nonspecific symptom, all other causes of fatigue, including physical (eg, cancer, autoimmune disease,

---

*"Cold" refers to the lack of inflammation with its associated redness and warmth.

and infection), and psychiatric (eg, depression and neurosis), as well as prolonged use of drugs (eg, tranquilizers), must be ruled out. The cause of CFS is unknown; attempts to isolate a causative organism from these patients have failed. A proposed relationship between CFS and chronic Epstein-Barr virus infection remains unsubstantiated.

There is a similarity between the symptoms of CFS and the symptoms that occur when alpha interferon or interleukin-2 is administered to patients. Abnormalities in various components of the immune system have been reported, eg, loss of delayed hypersensitivity reactivity in skin tests and increased levels of cytotoxic T cells, but no definitive findings have emerged. There is no specific laboratory test for CFS. The approach to therapy involves treating the symptoms. Studies with various antimicrobial drugs, such as acyclovir, ketoconazole, and gamma globulin, have revealed no effect.

Review Questions

1. X-linked hypogammaglobulinemia and selective IgA deficiency probably have different causes. What are they?
2. Contrast the types of infections that occur in children with X-linked hypogammaglobulinemia and thymic aplasia. Why are they different?
3. What is the most common clinical problem seen in patients with severe combined immunodeficiency disease? Why does this problem occur?
4. Which diseases are likely to occur in individuals with a deficiency of the late-acting complement components, ie, C6, C7, and C8?
5. What is the pathogenesis of chronic granulomatous disease? To which organisms are patients with this disease especially susceptible?
6. What is the immunodeficiency in AIDS? What are the consequences of this immunodeficiency?

Part VIII: Brief Summaries of Medically Important Organisms

Summaries of Medically Important Bacteria

GRAM-POSITIVE COCCI

Staphylococcus aureus

Diseases: Abscesses of many organs, endocarditis, gastroenteritis (food poisoning), toxic shock syndrome.

Characteristics: Gram-positive cocci in clusters. Coagulase-positive. Catalase-positive.

Habitat and Transmission: Habitat is the human skin and nose. Transmission is via the hands.

Pathogenesis: A variety of enzymes and toxins are made (see p 79). The two most important are coagulase and enterotoxin(s). Coagulase is the best correlate of pathogenicity. Enterotoxins cause food poisoning (one of these, TSST-1, causes toxic shock syndrome by stimulating many helper T cells to release large amounts of lymphokines, especially IL-2). Predisposing factors are breaks in the skin, foreign bodies such as sutures, neutrophil levels below 500/µL, intravenous drug abuse, and, for toxic shock syndrome, tampon use.

Laboratory Diagnosis: Gram-stained smear and culture. Yellow or gold colonies on blood agar. *Staphylococcus aureus* is coagulase-positive; *Staphylococcus epidermidis* is coagulase-negative. Serologic tests not useful.

Treatment: Penicillin G for sensitive isolates; β-lactamase-resistant penicillins such as nafcillin for resistant isolates; vancomycin for isolates resistant to nafcillin. About 85% are resistant to penicillin G. Plasmid-encoded β-lactamase mediates most resistance. Resistance to nafcillin may be due to changes in binding proteins. Some isolates are tolerant to penicillin.

Prevention: No vaccine or drug is available. Handwashing reduces spread.

Streptococcus pyogenes (Group A)

Diseases: Suppurative diseases, eg, pharyngitis and cellulitis; nonsuppurative diseases, eg, rheumatic fever and acute glomerulonephritis.

Characteristics: Gram-positive cocci in chains. Beta-hemolytic. Catalase-negative.

Habitat and Transmission: Habitat is the human throat and skin. Transmission is via respiratory droplets.

Pathogenesis: For suppurative infections, hyaluronidase ("spreading factor") mediates subcutaneous spread seen in cellulitis; erythrogenic toxin causes the rash of scarlet fever; M protein impedes phagocytosis. For nonsuppurative infections, rheumatic fever is caused by immunologic cross-reaction between bacterial antigen and human heart and joint tissue, and acute glomerulonephritis is caused by immune complexes bound to glomeruli.

Laboratory Diagnosis: Gram-stained smear and culture. Beta-hemolytic colonies on blood agar. (Hemolysis due to streptolysins O and S.) If isolate is sensitive to bacitracin, it is presumptively identified as *Streptococcus pyogenes*. Group determined by antiserum against cell wall C polysaccharide. Assay for antibody in patient's serum not done for suppurative infections. Patient's antistreptolysin O (ASO) antibody titer is tested to determine prior exposure to *S pyogenes* if rheumatic fever is suspected.

Treatment: Penicillin G (no significant resistance).

Prevention: Penicillin used in rheumatic fever patients to prevent recurrent *S pyogenes* pharyngitis.

Streptococcus agalactiae (Group B)

Diseases: Neonatal meningitis and sepsis.

Characteristics: Gram-positive cocci in chains. Beta-hemolytic. Catalase-negative.

Habitat and Transmission: Habitat is the human vagina. Transmission occurs during birth.

Pathogenesis: No toxins or virulence factors identified.

Laboratory Diagnosis: Gram-stained smear and culture. Beta-hemolytic colonies on blood agar. Organisms hydrolyze hippurate and are CAMP test-positive. Group determined by antiserum against cell wall polysaccharide.

Treatment: Penicillin G.

Prevention: No vaccine. Ampicillin prior to delivery may be useful if mother is culture-positive.

Streptococcus faecalis (Enterococcus; Group D)

Diseases: Urinary tract and biliary tract infections are most frequent.

Characteristics: Gram-positive cocci in chains. Catalase-negative.

Habitat and Transmission: Habitat is the human colon; urethra and female genital tract can be colonized. May enter bloodstream during gastrointestinal or genitourinary tract manipulations. May infect other sites, eg, endocarditis.

Pathogenesis: No toxins or virulence factors identified.

Laboratory Diagnosis: Gram-stained smear and culture. Alpha-, beta-, or nonhemolytic colonies on blood agar. Grows in 6.5% NaCl and hydrolyzes esculin in the presence of 40% bile. Serologic tests not useful.

Treatment: Penicillin plus an aminoglycoside such as gentamicin is synergistic. Organism is resistant to either drug given individually. Aminoglycoside resistance is due to an inability to penetrate. The penicillin weakens the cell wall, allowing the aminoglycoside to penetrate.

Prevention: Penicillin and gentamicin should be given to patients with damaged heart valves prior to intestinal or urinary tract procedures. No vaccine is available.

Streptococcus pneumoniae (Pneumococcus)

Diseases: The most common diseases are pneumonia and meningitis in adults and otitis media and sinusitis in children.

Characteristics: Gram-positive "lancet-shaped" cocci in pairs (diplococci) or short chains. Alpha-hemolytic. Catalase-negative.

Habitat and Transmission: Habitat is the human upper respiratory tract. Transmission is via respiratory droplets.

Pathogenesis: Induces inflammatory response. No known exotoxins. Polysaccharide capsule retards phagocytosis. Antipolysaccharide antibody opsonizes the organism and provides type-specific immunity. Viral respiratory infection predisposes to pneumococcal pneumonia by damaging mucociliary elevator; splenectomy predisposes to sepsis.

Laboratory Diagnosis: Gram-stained smear and culture. Alpha-hemolytic colonies on blood agar. Growth inhibited by bile and optochin. Quellung reaction occurs (swelling of capsule with type-specific antiserum). Serologic tests not useful. Latex agglutination test for capsular antigen in spinal fluid can be diagnostic.

Treatment: Penicillin G. Low-level and high-level resistance is caused by alterations in penicillin-binding proteins. No β-lactamase is made.

Prevention: Vaccine contains capsular polysaccharide of the 23 serotypes that cause bacteremia most frequently. Oral penicillin is used in immunocompromised children.

Viridans Group Streptococci (eg, *S sanguis, S mutans*)

Diseases: Endocarditis is the most important.

Characteristics: Gram-positive cocci in chains. Alpha-hemolytic. Catalase-negative.

Habitat and Transmission: Habitat is the human oropharynx. Organism enters bloodstream during dental procedures.

Pathogenesis: Bacteremia from dental procedures spreads organism to damaged heart valves. Organism is protected from host defenses within vegetations. No known toxins. Dextrans enhance adherence.

Laboratory Diagnosis: Gram-stained smear and culture. Alpha-hemolytic colonies on blood agar. Growth not inhibited by bile or optochin, in contrast to pneumococci. Many species are classified as viridans group streptococci. Serologic tests not useful.

Treatment: Penicillin G with or without an aminoglycoside.

Prevention: Penicillin for patients with damaged or prosthetic heart valves who undergo dental procedures.

GRAM-NEGATIVE COCCI

Neisseria meningitidis (Meningococcus)

Diseases: Meningitis and meningococcemia.

Characteristics: Gram-negative "kidney-bean" diplococci. Oxidase-positive. Large polysaccharide capsule.

Habitat and Transmission: Habitat is the human upper respiratory tract; transmission is via respiratory droplets.

Pathogenesis: After colonizing the upper respiratory tract, the organism reaches the meninges via the bloodstream. Endotoxin in cell wall causes symptoms of septic shock seen in meningococcemia. No known exotoxins; IgA protease produced. Capsule is antiphagocytic. Deficiency in late complement components predisposes to bacteremia.

Laboratory Diagnosis: Gram-stained smear and culture. Oxidase-positive colonies on chocolate agar. Ferments maltose in contrast to gonococci, which do not. Serologic tests not useful.

Treatment: Penicillin G (no significant resistance). Many isolates are resistant to sulfonamides because they contain plasmid-encoded enzymes that actively export the drug.

Prevention: Vaccine contains capsular polysaccharide of strains A, C, Y, and W-135. Rifampin given to close contacts to decrease oropharyngeal carriage.

Neisseria gonorrhoeae (Gonococcus)

Disease: Gonorrhea. Also neonatal conjunctivitis and pelvic inflammatory disease.

Characteristics: Gram-negative "kidney-bean" diplococci. Oxidase-positive. Insignificant capsule.

Habitat and Transmission: Habitat is the human genital tract. Transmission in adults is by sexual contact. Transmission to neonates is during birth.

Pathogenesis: Organism invades mucous membranes and causes inflammation. Endotoxin present. No exotoxins identified. IgA protease and pili are virulence factors.

Laboratory Diagnosis: Gram-stained smear and culture. Organism visible intracellularly within neutrophils in urethral exudate. Oxidase-positive colonies on Thayer-Martin medium. Gonococci do not ferment maltose, whereas meningococci do. Serologic tests not useful.

Treatment: Ceftriaxone for uncomplicated cases. If resistant, spectinomycin is used. Tetracycline added for urethritis due to *Chlamydia trachomatis.* High-level resistance to penicillin is caused by plasmid-encoded penicillinase especially prevalent in Southeast Asian strains. Low-level resistance to penicillin is caused by reduced permeability and altered binding proteins.

Prevention: No drug or vaccine. Condoms offer protection. Trace contacts and treat to interrupt transmission. Treat eyes of newborns with erythromycin ointment or silver nitrate to prevent conjunctivitis.

GRAM-POSITIVE RODS

Bacillus anthracis

Disease: Anthrax.

Characteristics: Large, gram-positive, spore-forming rods. Capsule composed of poly-D-glutamate. B anthracis is the only medically important organism that has a capsule composed of amino acids rather than polysaccharides.

Habitat and Transmission: Habitat is soil. Transmission is by contact with infected animals or inhalation of spores from animal hair and wool.

Pathogenesis: Anthrax toxin consists of three proteins: edema factor, which is an adenylate cyclase; protective antigen, which mediates the entry of the other two components into the cell; and lethal factor, whose mechanism of action is unknown. The capsule is antiphagocytic.

Laboratory Diagnosis: Gram-stained smear plus aerobic culture on blood agar. *Bacillus anthracis* is nonmotile, in contrast to other *Bacillus* species. Rise in antibody titer in indirect hemagglutination test is diagnostic.

Treatment: Penicillin G (no significant resistance).

Prevention: Vaccine consisting of protective antigen is given to individuals in high-risk occupations.

Clostridium tetani

Disease: Tetanus.

Characteristics: Anaerobic, gram-positive, spore-forming rods.

Habitat and Transmission: Habitat is the soil. Organism enters through traumatic breaks in the skin.

Pathogenesis: Spores germinate under anaerobic conditions in the wound. Organism produces exotoxin, which blocks release of inhibitory neurotransmitters (glycine and GABA). Excitatory neurons are unopposed, and extreme muscle spasm results.

Laboratory Diagnosis: Primarily a clinical diagnosis. Organism is rarely isolated. Serologic tests not useful.

Treatment: Hyperimmune human globulin to neutralize toxin. Also penicillin G and spasmolytic drugs (eg, valium). No significant resistance to penicillin.

Prevention: Toxoid vaccine (toxoid is formaldehyde-treated toxin). Usually given to children in combination with diphtheria toxoid and pertussis vaccine (DPT). If patient is injured and has not been immunized, give hyperimmune globulin plus toxoid. Debride wound.

Clostridium botulinum

Disease: Botulism.

Characteristics: Anaerobic, gram-positive, spore-forming rods.

Habitat and Transmission: Habitat is the soil. Organism and toxin transmitted in improperly preserved food.

Pathogenesis: Exotoxin inhibits the release of acetylcholine at the myoneural junction, causing flaccid paralysis. Failure to sterilize food during preservation allows spores to survive. Spores germinate in anaerobic environment and produce toxin. The toxin is heat-labile; therefore, foods eaten without proper cooking are usually implicated.

Laboratory Diagnosis: Presence of toxin in patient's serum or stool or in food. Detection of toxin involves either antitoxin in serologic tests or production of the disease in mice. Serologic tests for antibody in the patient are not useful.

Treatment: Antitoxin to types A, B, and E made in horses. Respiratory support may be required.

Prevention: Observing proper food preservation techniques, cooking all home-canned food, and discarding bulging cans.

Clostridium perfringens

Diseases: Gas gangrene (myonecrosis) and food poisoning.

Characteristics: Anaerobic, gram-positive, spore-forming rods.

Habitat and Transmission: Habitat is soil and human colon. Myonecrosis results from contamination of wound with soil or feces. Food poisoning is transmitted by ingestion of contaminated food.

Pathogenesis: Gas gangrene in wounds is caused by germination of spores under anaerobic conditions and the production of several cytotoxic factors, especially alpha toxin, a lecithinase that disrupts cell membranes. Food poisoning is caused by production of enterotoxin within the gut.

Laboratory Diagnosis: Gram-stained smear plus anaerobic culture. Spores not usually seen in clinical specimens; the organism is growing, and nutrients are not restricted. Production of lecithinase is detected on egg yolk agar and identified by enzyme inhibition with specific antiserum. Serologic tests not useful.

Treatment: Penicillin G plus debridement of the wound in gas gangrene (no significant resistance to penicillin). Only symptomatic treatment needed in food poisoning.

Prevention: Extensive debridement of the wound plus administration of penicillin decreases probability of gas gangrene. There is no vaccine.

Clostridium difficile

Disease: Pseudomembranous colitis.

Characteristics: Anaerobic, gram-positive, spore-forming rods.

Habitat and Transmission: Habitat is the human colon. Transmission is fecal-oral.

Pathogenesis: Enterotoxin causes watery diarrhea. Cytotoxin causes death of enterocytes, leading to pseudomembrane formation.

Laboratory Diagnosis: Cytotoxin in stool detected by cytopathic effect on cultured cells. Identified by neutralization of cytopathic effect with antibody.

Treatment: Metronidazole or vancomycin.

Prevention: No vaccine or drug is available.

Corynebacterium diphtheriae

Disease: Diphtheria.

Characteristics: Club-shaped gram-positive rods arranged in V or L shape. Granules stain metachromatically. Aerobic, non-spore-forming organism.

Habitat and Transmission: Habitat is the human throat. Transmission is via respiratory droplets.

Pathogenesis: Organism secretes an exotoxin that inhibits protein synthesis by adding ADP-ribose to EF-2. Toxin has two components: subunit A, which has the ADP-ribosylating activity, and subunit B, which binds the toxin to cell surface receptors.

Laboratory Diagnosis: Gram-stained smear and culture. Black colonies on tellurite plate. Document toxin production with precipitin test or by disease produced in laboratory animals. Serologic tests not useful.

Treatment: Antitoxin made in horses neutralizes the toxin. Penicillin G kills the organism. No significant resistance to penicillin.

Prevention: Toxoid vaccine (toxoid is formaldehyde-treated toxin), usually given to children in combination with tetanus toxoid and pertussis vaccine (DPT).

Listeria monocytogenes

Diseases: Meningitis and sepsis in newborns and immunocompromised adults.

Characteristics: Small gram-positive rods. Aerobic, non-spore-forming organism.

Habitat and Transmission: Organism colonizes the gastrointestinal and female genital tracts; in nature it is widespread in animals, plants, and soil. Transmission is across the placenta or by contact during delivery. Outbreaks of disease are related to unpasteurized milk products, eg, cheese.

Pathogenesis: No toxins identified. Immunosuppression and immunologic immaturity predispose to infection.

Laboratory Diagnosis: Gram-stained smear and culture. Small, beta-hemolytic colonies on blood agar. Tumbling motility. Serologic tests not useful.

Treatment: Ampicillin with or without gentamicin.

Prevention: No vaccine or drug is available.

GRAM-NEGATIVE RODS ASSOCIATED PRIMARILY WITH THE ENTERIC TRACT

Escherichia coli

Diseases: Urinary tract infection (UTI), sepsis, neonatal meningitis, and "traveler's diarrhea" are the most common.

Characteristics: Facultative gram-negative rods; ferment lactose.

Habitat and Transmission: Habitat is the human colon; it colonizes the vagina and urethra. From the urethra, it ascends and causes UTI. Acquired during birth in neonatal meningitis and by the fecal-oral route in diarrhea.

Pathogenesis: Endotoxin in cell wall causes septic shock. Two enterotoxins are produced. The heat-labile toxin (LT) stimulates adenylate cyclase by ADP-ribosylation. Increased cAMP causes outflow of chloride ions and water, resulting in diarrhea. The heat-stable toxin (ST) causes diarrhea, perhaps by stimulating guanylate cyclase. Virulence factors include pili for attachment to mucosal surfaces and a capsule that impedes phagocytosis. Verotoxin is an enterotoxin produced by *E coli* strains with the O157:H7 serotype. It causes bloody diarrhea associated with eating undercooked meat. Verotoxin inhibits protein synthesis by removing adenine from the 28S rRNA of human ribosomes.

Predisposing factors to UTI in women include the proximity of the anus to the vagina and urethra, as well as a short urethra. This leads to colonization of the urethra and vagina by the fecal flora. Abnormalities, eg, strictures, valves, and stones, predispose as well. Indwelling urinary catheters and intravenous lines predispose to UTI and sepsis, respectively. Colonization of the vagina leads to neonatal meningitis acquired during birth.

Laboratory Diagnosis: Gram-stained smear and culture. Lactose-fermenting colonies on EMB or MacConkey's agar. Green sheen on EMB agar. TSI agar shows acid slant and acid butt with gas. Differentiate from other lactose-positive organisms by biochemical reactions. For epidemiologic studies, type organism by O and H antigens by using known antisera. Serologic tests for antibodies in patient's serum not useful.

Treatment: Ampicillin or sulfonamides for urinary tract infections. Third-generation cephalosporins for meningitis and sepsis. Rehydration is effective in traveler's diarrhea; trimethoprim-sulfamethoxazole may shorten duration of symptoms. Antibiotic resistance mediated by plasmid-encoded enzymes, eg, β-lactamase and aminoglycoside-modifying enzymes.

392 / PART VIII

Prevention: Prevention of UTI involves limiting the frequency and duration of urinary catheterization. Prevention of sepsis involves promptly removing or switching sites of intravenous lines. Traveler's diarrhea is prevented by eating only cooked food and drinking boiled water in certain countries. Prophylactic doxycycline or Pepto-Bismol may prevent traveler's diarrhea.

Salmonella typhi

Disease: Typhoid fever.

Characteristics: Facultative gram-negative rods. Non-lactose-fermenting. Produces H_2S.

Habitat and Transmission: Habitat is the human colon only, in contrast to other salmonellae, which are found in the colons of animals as well. Transmission is by the fecal-oral route.

Pathogenesis: Invades the reticuloendothelial system. Endotoxin in cell wall causes fever. Capsule (Vi antigen) is a virulence factor. No exotoxins known. Decreased stomach acid resulting from ingestion of antacids or gastrectomy predisposes to *Salmonella* infections.

Laboratory Diagnosis: Gram-stained smear and culture. Non-lactose-fermenting colonies on EMB or MacConkey's agar. TSI agar shows alkaline slant and acid butt, with no gas and a small amount of H_2S. Biochemical and serologic reactions used to identify species. Identity can be determined by using known antisera against O, H, and Vi antigens in agglutination test. Widal test detects agglutinating antibodies to O and H antigens in patient's serum, but its use is limited.

Treatment: Most effective drug is ceftriaxone. Ampicillin and trimethoprim-sulfamethoxazole can be used in patients who are not severely ill. Resistance to chloramphenicol and ampicillin is mediated by plasmid-encoded acetylating enzymes and β-lactamase, respectively.

Prevention: Public health measures, eg, sewage disposal, chlorination of the water supply, stool cultures for food handlers, and hand washing prior to food handling. Both a killed vaccine and live, attenuated vaccine are available.

Salmonella enteritidis

Diseases: Enterocolitis. Sepsis with metastatic abscesses occasionally.

Characteristics: Facultative gram-negative rods. Non-lactose-fermenting. Produces H_2S. Motile, in contrast to *Shigella*. More than 1500 serotypes.

Habitat and Transmission: Habitat is the enteric tracts of humans and animals, eg, chickens and domestic livestock. Transmission is by the fecal-oral route.

Pathogenesis: Invades the mucosa of the small and large intestines. Can enter blood, causing sepsis. Infectious dose is at least 10^5 organisms, much greater than the infectious dose of *Shigella*. Endotoxin in cell wall; no exotoxin. Predisposing factors include lowered stomach acidity from either antacids or gastrectomy. Sickle cell disease predisposes to osteomyelitis.

Laboratory Diagnosis: Gram-stained smear and culture. Non-lactose-fermenting colonies on EMB or MacConkey's agar. TSI agar shows alkaline slant and acid butt, with gas and H_2S. Biochemical and serologic reactions used to identify species. Can identify the organism by using known antisera in agglutination assay. Widal test detects antibodies in patient's serum to the O and H antigens of the organism but is not widely used.

Treatment: Antibiotics usually not recommended for uncomplicated enterocolitis. Ceftriaxone or other drugs are used for sepsis depending on sensitivity tests. Resistance to ampicillin and chloramphenicol is mediated by plasmid-encoded β-lactamases and acetylating enzymes, respectively.

Prevention: Public health measures, eg, sewage disposal, chlorination of the water supply, stool cultures for food handlers, and hand washing prior to food handling. No vaccine is available.

Shigella species (eg, *S dysenteriae, S sonnei*)

Disease: Enterocolitis (dysentery).

Characteristics: Facultative gram-negative rods. Non-lactose-fermenting. Nonmotile, in contrast to *Salmonella.*

Habitat and Transmission: Habitat is the human colon only; unlike *Salmonella,* there are no animal carriers for *Shigella.* Transmission is by the fecal-oral route.

Pathogenesis: Invades the mucosa of the ileum and colon but does not penetrate farther, so sepsis is rare. Endotoxin in cell wall. Infectious dose is much lower (1–10 organisms) than that of *Salmonella.* Children in mental institutions and day-care centers experience outbreaks of shigellosis.

Laboratory Diagnosis: Gram-stained smear and culture. Non-lactose-fermenting colonies on EMB or MacConkey's agar. TSI agar shows an alkaline slant with an acid butt and no gas or H_2S. Identified by biochemical reactions or by serology with anti-O antibody in agglutination test. Serologic tests for antibodies in the patient's serum are not done.

Treatment: In most cases, fluid and electrolyte replacement only. In severe cases, ciprofloxacin. Resistance is mediated by plasmid-encoded enzymes, eg, β-lactamase, which degrades ampicillin, and a mutant pteroate synthetase, which reduces sensitivity to sulfonamides.

Prevention: Public health measures, eg, sewage disposal, chlorination of the water supply, stool cultures for food handlers, and hand washing prior to food handling. Prophylactic drugs not used. No vaccine is available.

Vibrio cholerae

Disease: Cholera.

Characteristics: Comma-shaped gram-negative rods. Oxidase-positive, which distinguishes them from Enterobacteriaceae.

Habitat and Transmission: Habitat is the human colon. Transmission is by the fecal-oral route.

Pathogenesis: Watery diarrhea caused by enterotoxin that activates adenylate cyclase by adding ADP-ribose to the stimulatory G protein. Increase in cAMP causes outflow of chloride ions and water. Toxin has two components: subunit A, which has the ADP-ribosylating activity; and subunit B, which binds the toxin to cell surface receptors. Organism produces mucinase, which enhances attachment to the intestinal mucosa. Role of endotoxin is unclear. Infectious dose is high (>10^7 organisms). Carrier state rare.

Laboratory Diagnosis: Gram-stained smear and culture. (During epidemics, cultures not necessary.) Agglutination of the isolate with known antisera confirms the identification.

Treatment: Treatment of choice is fluid and electrolyte replacement. Tetracycline is not necessary but shortens duration and reduces carriage.

Prevention: Public health measures, eg, sewage disposal, chlorination of the water supply, stool cultures for food handlers, and hand washing prior to food handling. Vaccine containing killed cells has limited effectiveness. Tetracycline used for close contacts.

Campylobacter jejuni

Disease: Enterocolitis.

Characteristics: Comma-shaped gram-negative rods. Microaerophilic. Grows well at 42 °C.

Habitat and Transmission: Habitat is human and animal feces. Transmission is by the fecal-oral route.

Pathogenesis: Invades mucosa of the colon but does not penetrate; therefore, sepsis rarely occurs. No enterotoxin known.

Laboratory Diagnosis: Gram-stained smear plus culture on special agar, eg, Skirrow's agar, at 42 °C in high-CO_2, low-O_2 atmosphere. Serologic tests not useful.

Treatment: Usually symptomatic treatment only; erythromycin for severe disease.

Prevention: Public health measures, eg, sewage disposal, chlorination of the water supply, stool cultures for food handlers, and hand washing prior to food handling. No preventive vaccine or drug is available.

Helicobacter pylori

Disease: Gastritis. Suspected cause of peptic ulcer.

Characteristics: Curved gram-negative rod.

Habitat and Transmission: Habitat is the human stomach. Transmission is by ingestion.

Pathogenesis: Organisms synthesize urease, which produces ammonia that damages gastric mucosa.

Laboratory Diagnosis: Gram stain and culture. Urease-positive. Serologic tests for antibody useful.

Treatment: Amoxicillin, metronidazole, and bismuth (Pepto-Bismol).

Prevention: No vaccine or drug is available.

Klebsiella pneumoniae

Diseases: Pneumonia, UTI, and sepsis.

Characteristics: Facultative gram-negative rods with large polysaccharide capsule.

Habitat and Transmission: Habitat is the human upper respiratory and enteric tracts. Organism is transmitted to the lungs by aspiration from upper respiratory tract and by inhalation of respiratory droplets. It is transmitted to the urinary tract by ascending spread of fecal flora.

Pathogenesis: Endotoxin causes fever and shock associated with sepsis. No exotoxin known. Organism has large capsule, which impedes phagocytosis. Chronic pulmonary disease predisposes to pneumonia; catheterization predisposes to UTI.

Laboratory Diagnosis: Gram-stained smear and culture. Characteristic mucoid colonies are a consequence of the organism's abundant polysaccharide capsule. Lactose-fermenting colonies on MacConkey's agar. Differentiated from *Enterobacter* and *Serratia* by biochemical reactions.

Treatment: Cephalosporins alone or with aminoglycosides, but antibiotic sensitivity testing must be done. Resistance is mediated by plasmid-encoded enzymes.

Prevention: No vaccine or drug is available. Urinary and intravenous catheters should be removed promptly.

Proteus species (eg, *P vulgaris, P mirabilis)*

Diseases: UTI and sepsis.

Characteristics: Facultative gram-negative rods. Non-lactose-fermenting. Highly motile. Produce urease. Antigens of OX strains of *P vulgaris* cross-react with many rickettsiae.

Habitat and Transmission: Habitat is the human colon and the environment (soil and water). Transmission to urinary tract is by ascending spread of fecal flora.

Pathogenesis: Endotoxin causes fever and shock associated with sepsis. No exotoxins known. Urease is a virulence factor because it degrades urea to produce ammonia, which raises the pH. This leads to stones, damage to epithelium, and infection. Organism is highly motile, which may facilitate entry into the bladder. Predisposing factors are colonization of the vagina, urinary catheters, and abnormalities of the urinary tract such as strictures, valves, and stones.

Laboratory Diagnosis: Gram-stained smear and culture. "Swarming" (spreading) effect over blood agar plate as a consequence of the organism's active motility. Non-lactose-fermenting colonies on EMB or MacConkey's agar. TSI agar shows an alkaline slant and acid butt with H_2S. Organism produces urease, whereas *Salmonella,* which can appear similar on TSI agar, does not. Serologic tests not useful.

Treatment: Ampicillin frequently used, but antibiotic sensitivities should be tested. Resistance is mediated by plasmid-encoded β-lactamase.

Prevention: No vaccine or drug is available. Prompt removal of urinary catheters helps prevent urinary tract infections.

Pseudomonas aeruginosa

Diseases: Wound infection, UTI, pneumonia, and sepsis. One of the most important causes of nosocomial infections especially in burn patients and those with cystic fibrosis.

Characteristics: Aerobic gram-negative rods. Non-lactose-fermenting. Pyocyanin (blue-green) pigment produced.

Habitat and Transmission: Habitat is environmental water sources, eg, in hospital respirators and humidifiers. Also inhabits the skin, upper respiratory tract, and colon of about 10% of people. Transmission is via water aerosols, aspiration, and fecal contamination.

Pathogenesis: Endotoxin is responsible for fever and shock associated with sepsis. Produces exotoxin A, which acts like diphtheria toxin (inactivates EF-2). Pili and capsule are virulence factors that mediate attachment and inhibit phagocytosis, respectively.

Laboratory Diagnosis: Gram-stained smear and culture. Non-lactose-fermenting colonies on EMB or MacConkey's agar. TSI agar shows an alkaline slant and an alkaline butt, because the sugars are not fermented. Oxidase-positive. Serologic tests not useful.

Treatment: Antibiotics must be chosen on the basis of antibiotic sensitivities, because resistance is common. Anti-pseudomonal penicillin and aminoglycoside are often used. Resistance is mediated by a variety of plasmid-encoded enzymes, eg, β-lactamases and acetylating enzymes.

Prevention: Disinfection of water-related equipment in the hospital, hand-washing, and prompt removal of urinary and intravenous catheters. There is no vaccine.

Bacteroides fragilis

Diseases: Sepsis, peritonitis, and abdominal abscess.

Characteristics: Anaerobic, gram-negative rods.

Habitat and Transmission: Habitat is the human colon, where it is the predominant anaerobe. Transmission occurs by spread from the colon to the blood or peritoneum.

Pathogenesis: Lipopolysaccharide in cell wall is chemically different from and less potent than typical endotoxin. No exotoxins known. Capsule is antiphagocytic. Predisposing factors to infection include bowel surgery and penetrating abdominal wounds.

Laboratory Diagnosis: Gram-stained smear plus anaerobic culture. Identification based on biochemical reactions and gas chromatography. Serologic tests not useful.

Treatment: Metronidazole, clindamycin, and cefoxitin are all effective. Abscesses should be surgically drained. Resistance to penicillin G, some cephalosporins, and aminoglycosides is common. Plasmid-encoded β-lactamase mediates resistance to penicillin.

Prevention: In bowel surgery, perioperative cefoxitin can reduce the frequency of postoperative infections. No vaccine is available.

GRAM-NEGATIVE RODS ASSOCIATED PRIMARILY WITH THE RESPIRATORY TRACT

Haemophilus influenzae

Diseases: Meningitis, otitis media, and pneumonia are common.

Characteristics: Small gram-negative (coccobacillary) rods. Type b capsule is polyribitol phosphate. Requires factors X (hemin) and V (NAD) for growth.

Habitat and Transmission: Habitat is the upper respiratory tract. Transmission is via respiratory droplets.

Pathogenesis: Polysaccharide capsule is the most important determinant of virulence; 95% of invasive disease is caused by capsular type b. IgA protease is produced. Most cases of meningitis occur in children under 2 years of age, because maternal antibody has waned and the immune response of the child can be inadequate. No exotoxins identified.

Laboratory Diagnosis: Gram-stained smear plus culture on chocolate agar. Growth requires both factors X and V. Determine serotype by using antiserum in various tests, eg, immunoelectrophoresis, or latex agglutination. Capsular antigen present in serum or cerebrospinal fluid. Serologic test not useful.

Treatment: Ceftriaxone is the treatment of choice for meningitis.

Prevention: Rifampin can prevent meningitis in close contacts. Vaccine containing the type b capsular polysaccharide conjugated to diphtheria toxoid or other protein is given between 2 and 18 months of age.

Legionella pneumophila

Disease: Legionnaires' disease ("atypical" pneumonia).

Characteristics: Gram-negative rods, but stain poorly with standard Gram's stain. Require increased iron and cysteine for growth in culture.

Habitat and Transmission: Habitat is environmental water sources. Transmission is via aerosol. Person-to-person transmission does not occur.

Pathogenesis: Aside from endotoxin, no toxins, enzymes, or virulence factors are known. Predisposing factors include being over age 55 years, smoking, and having a high alcohol intake. Immunosuppressed patients, eg, renal transplant recipients, are highly susceptible.

Laboratory Diagnosis: Microscopy with silver impregnation stain or fluorescent antibody. Culture on charcoal yeast extract agar containing increased amounts of iron and cysteine. Diagnosis usually made serologically.

Treatment: Erythromycin.

Prevention: No vaccine or prophylactic drug is available.

Bordetella pertussis

Disease: Whooping cough (pertussis).

Characteristics: Small gram-negative rods.

Habitat and Transmission: Habitat is the human respiratory tract. Transmission is via respiratory droplets.

Pathogenesis: Two toxins are produced. Pertussis toxin stimulates adenylate cyclase by adding ADP-ribose onto the inhibitory coupling protein. Toxin has two components: subunit A, which has the ADP-ribosylating activity, and subunit B, which binds the toxin to cell surface receptors. In addition, extracellular adenylate cyclase is produced, which can inhibit killing by phagocytes.

Laboratory Diagnosis: Gram-stained smear plus culture on Bordet-Gengou agar. Identified by biochemical reactions and slide agglutination with known antisera. Serologic tests not useful.

Treatment: Erythromycin.

Prevention: The acellular vaccine containing purified proteins is recommended rather than the killed vaccine, which contains whole organisms. Usually given to children in combination with diphtheria and tetanus toxoids.

GRAM-NEGATIVE RODS CAUSING ZOONOSES

Brucella species (eg, *B abortus, B suis, B melitensis*)

Disease: Brucellosis (undulant fever).

Characteristics: Small gram-negative rods.

Habitat and Transmission: Habitat is domestic livestock. Transmission is via unpasteurized milk and cheese, or direct contact with the infected animal.

Pathogenesis: Organisms localize in reticuloendothelial cells. Virulence associated with intracellular survival. Endotoxin necessary for pathogenesis. No exotoxin or capsule identified. Predisposing factors include consuming unpasteurized dairy products and working in an abattoir.

Laboratory Diagnosis: Gram-stained smear plus culture on blood agar plate. Identified by biochemical reactions and by agglutination with known antiserum. Diagnosis may be made serologically also.

Treatment: Tetracycline.

Prevention: Pasteurize milk; vaccinate cattle. No human vaccine is available.

Francisella tularensis

Disease: Tularemia.

Characteristics: Small gram-negative rods.

Habitat and Transmission: Habitat is many species of wild animals, especially rabbits, deer, and rodents. Transmission is by ticks (eg, *Dermacentor*), aerosols, contact, and ingestion.

Pathogenesis: Organisms localize in reticuloendothelial cells. Role of endotoxin is uncertain. No exotoxins known.

Laboratory Diagnosis: Culture is rarely done, because special media are required and there is a high risk of infection of laboratory personnel. Diagnosis is usually made by serologic tests.

Treatment: Streptomycin.

Prevention: Live, attenuated vaccine for persons in high-risk occupations. Protect against tick bites.

Pasteurella multocida

Disease: Wound infection, eg, cellulitis.

Characteristics: Small gram-negative rods.

Habitat and Transmission: Habitat is the mouths of many animals, especially cats and dogs. Transmission is by animal bites.

Pathogenesis: Spreads rapidly in skin and subcutaneous tissue. No exotoxins known.

Laboratory Diagnosis: Gram-stained smear and culture.

Treatment: Penicillin G.

Prevention: Ampicillin should be given to individuals with cat bites. There is no vaccine.

Yersinia pestis

Disease: Plague.

Characteristics: Small gram-negative rods with bipolar staining.

Habitat and Transmission: Habitat is wild rodents, eg, prairie dogs and squirrels. Transmission is by flea bite.

Pathogenesis: Dependent on several factors including endotoxin, an exotoxin, two antigens (V and W), and an envelope antigen that protects against phagocytosis.

Laboratory Diagnosis: Gram-stained smear. Other stains, eg, Wayson's, show typical "safety-pin" appearance more clearly. Cultures are hazardous and should be done only in specially equipped laboratories. Organism is identified by immunofluorescence. Diagnosis can be made by serologic tests.

Treatment: Streptomycin either alone or in combination with tetracycline. Strict quarantine for 72 hours.

Prevention: Control rodent population and avoid contact with dead rodents. Killed vaccine is available for persons in high-risk occupations. Close contacts should be given tetracycline.

MYCOBACTERIA & ACTINOMYCETES

Mycobacterium tuberculosis

Diseases: Tuberculosis.

Characteristics: Aerobic, acid-fast rods. High lipid content of cell wall. Lipids include mycolic acids and wax D. Grows very slowly.

Habitat and Transmission: Habitat is the human lungs. Transmission is via droplets produced by coughing.

Pathogenesis: Granulomas and caseation mediated by cellular immunity. Cord factor (trehalose mycolate) correlates with virulence. No exotoxins or endotoxin. Immunosuppression increases risk of reactivation.

Laboratory Diagnosis: Acid-fast rods seen with Ziehl-Neelsen (or Kinyoun) stain. Slow-growing (3–6 weeks) colony on Löwenstein-Jensen medium. Organisms produce niacin and are catalase-negative. No serologic tests. PPD skin test is positive if induration measuring 10 mm or more appears 48 hours after inoculation (delayed hypersensitivity). Positive skin test indicates exposure but not necessarily disease.

Treatment: Long-term therapy (6–9 months) with three drugs, isoniazid, rifampin, and pyrazin-amide. A fourth drug, ethambutol, is used in severe cases, eg, meningitis, and where the chance of isoniazid-resistant organisms is high, as in Southeast Asians.

Prevention: Isoniazid taken for 6–9 months can prevent reactivation tuberculosis in infected persons. BCG vaccine containing live, attenuated organisms may prevent or limit extent of disease but does not prevent infection. Vaccine used rarely in the United States but widely in parts of Europe and Asia.

Mycobacterium leprae

Disease: Leprosy.

Characteristics: Aerobic, acid-fast rods. Cannot be cultured in vitro. Optimal growth at less than body temperature.

Habitat and Transmission: Habitat is the human skin and nerves. Transmission is by prolonged contact. Patients with the lepromatous form are more likely to transmit than those with the tuberculoid form.

Pathogenesis: Lesions are usually situated in the cooler parts of the body, eg, skin and peripheral nerves. In tuberculoid leprosy, destructive lesions are due to the cell-mediated response to the organism. Damage to fingers is due to burns and other trauma, because nerve damage causes loss of sensation. In lepromatous leprosy, the cell-mediated response is lost and large numbers of organisms appear in the lesions and blood. No toxins or virulence factors are known.

Laboratory Diagnosis: Acid-fast rods are abundant in lepromatous leprosy, but few are found in the tuberculoid form. Cultures and serologic tests not done. Lepromin skin test is positive in the tuberculoid but not in the lepromatous form.

Treatment: Dapsone plus rifampin for the tuberculoid form. Clofazamine is added to that regimen for the lepromatous form or if the organism is resistant to dapsone. Treatment is for at least 2 years.

Prevention: Dapsone for close family contacts. No vaccine is available.

Actinomyces israelii

Disease: Actinomycosis (abscesses with draining sinus tracts).

Characteristics: Anaerobic, gram-positive branching rods.

Habitat and Transmission: Habitat is anaerobic crevices around the teeth. Transmission into tissues occurs during dental disease or trauma. Organism also aspirated into lungs.

Pathogenesis: No toxins or virulence factors known.

Laboratory Diagnosis: Gram-stained smear plus anaerobic culture on blood agar plate. "Sulfur granules" visible in the pus. No serologic tests.

Treatment: Penicillin G and surgical drainage.

Prevention: No vaccine or drug is available.

Nocardia asteroides

Disease: Nocardiosis (especially lung and brain abscesses).

Characteristics: Aerobic, gram-positive branching rods. Weakly acid-fast.

Habitat and Transmission: Habitat is the soil. Transmission is via airborne particles.

Pathogenesis: No toxins or virulence factors known. Immunosuppression and cancer predispose to infection.

Laboratory Diagnosis: Gram-stained smear and modified Ziehl-Neelsen stain. Aerobic culture on blood agar plate. No serologic tests.

Treatment: Sulfonamides.

Prevention: No vaccine or drug is available.

MYCOPLASMAS

Mycoplasma pneumoniae

Disease: "Atypical" pneumonia.

Characteristics: Smallest free-living organisms. Not seen on Gram-stained smear, because they have no cell wall. The only bacteria with cholesterol in cell membrane. Can be cultured in vitro.

Habitat and Transmission: Habitat is the human respiratory tract. Transmission is via respiratory droplets.

Pathogenesis: No exotoxins produced. No endotoxin because there is no cell wall. Produces hydrogen peroxide and cytolytic enzymes, which may damage the respiratory tract.

Laboratory Diagnosis: Microscopy not useful. Can be cultured on special bacteriologic media but takes at least 10 days to grow, which is too long to be clinically useful. Positive cold-agglutinin test is presumptive evidence. Complement fixation test for antibodies to *Mycoplasma pneumoniae* is more specific.

Treatment: Erythromycin.

Prevention: No vaccine or drug is available.

SPIROCHETES

Treponema pallidum

Disease: Syphilis.

Characteristics: Spirochetes. Not seen on Gram-stained smear. Not cultured in vitro.

Habitat and Transmission: Habitat is the human genital tract. Transmission is by sexual contact and from mother to fetus across the placenta.

Pathogenesis: Organism multiplies at site of inoculation and then spreads widely via the bloodstream. Many features of syphilis are attributed to blood vessel involvement. Primary and secondary lesions heal spontaneously. Tertiary lesions consist of gummas, aortitis, or central nervous system inflammation. No toxins or virulence factors known.

Laboratory Diagnosis: Seen by dark-field microscopy or immunofluorescence. Serologic tests important: VDRL (or RPR) is nontreponemal test used for screening; FTA-ABS is the most widely used specific test for *Treponema pallidum.*

Treatment: Penicillin is effective in the treatment of all stages of syphilis. There is no resistance.

Prevention: Benzathine penicillin given to contacts. No vaccine is available.

Borrelia burgdorferi

Disease: Lyme disease.

Characteristics: Spirochetes. Not seen on Gram-stained smear. Can be cultured in vitro.

Habitat and Transmission: The main reservoir is the white-footed mouse. Transmitted by the bite of ixodid ticks, especially in three areas in the United States: Northeast (eg, Connecticut), Midwest (eg, Wisconsin), and West Coast (eg, California).

Pathogenesis: Organism invades skin and spreads via the bloodstream to involve primarily the heart, joints, and central nervous system. No toxins or virulence factors identified.

Laboratory Diagnosis: Diagnosis usually made serologically, ie, by detecting IgM antibody.

Treatment: Doxycycline for early stages; penicillin G for late stages.

Prevention: Avoid tick bite. Can give doxycycline or amoxicillin to people who are bitten by a tick in endemic areas. There is no vaccine.

Leptospira interrogans

Disease: Leptospirosis.

Characteristics: Spirochetes that can be seen on dark-field microscopy but not light microscopy. Can be cultured in vitro.

Habitat and Transmission: Habitat is wild and domestic animals. Transmission is via animal urine (in the United States, transmission is chiefly via dog, livestock, and rat urine).

Pathogenesis: Two phases: an initial bacteremic phase and a subsequent immunopathologic phase with meningitis. No toxins or virulence factors known.

Laboratory Diagnosis: Dark-field microscopy and culture in vitro are available but not usually done. Diagnosis usually made by serologic testing.

Treatment: Penicillin G. There is no significant antibiotic resistance.

Prevention: Doxycycline effective for short-term exposure. Vaccination of domestic livestock and pets. Rat control.

CHLAMYDIAE

Chlamydia trachomatis

Diseases: Nongonococcal urethritis, cervicitis, inclusion conjunctivitis, lymphogranuloma venereum, and trachoma. Also pneumonia in infants.

Characteristics: Obligate intracellular parasites. Not seen on Gram-stained smear. Exists as inactive elementary body extracellularly and as metabolically active, dividing reticulate body intracellularly.

Habitat and Transmission: Habitat is the human genital tract and eyes. Transmission is by sexual contact and at birth. Transmission in trachoma is chiefly by hand-to-eye contact.

Pathogenesis: No toxins or virulence factors known.

Laboratory Diagnosis: Cytoplasmic inclusions seen on Giemsa- or fluorescent-antibody-stained smear. Glycogen-filled cytoplasmic inclusions can be visualized with iodine. Organism grows in cell culture and embryonated eggs.

Treatment: Tetracycline or erythromycin.

Prevention: Erythromycin effective in infected mother to prevent neonatal disease. No vaccine is available.

Chlamydia psittaci

Disease: Psittacosis.

Characteristics: Obligate intracellular parasites. Not seen on Gram-stained smear. Exists as inactive elementary body extracellularly and as metabolically active, dividing reticulate body intracellularly.

Habitat and Transmission: Habitat is birds, both psittacine and others. Transmission is via aerosol of dried bird feces.

Pathogenesis: No toxins or virulence factors known.

Laboratory Diagnosis: Cytoplasmic inclusion seen by Giemsa or fluorescent-antibody staining. Organism can be isolated from sputum, but this is rarely done. Diagnosis usually made serologically, eg, by complement fixation test.

Treatment: Tetracycline.

Prevention: No vaccine or drug is available.

RICKETTSIAE

Rickettsia rickettsii

Disease: Rocky Mountain spotted fever.

Characteristics: Obligate intracellular parasites. Not seen well on Gram-stained smear. Antigens cross-react with OX strains of *Proteus vulgaris* (Weil-Felix reaction).

Habitat and Transmission: *Dermacentor* ticks are the natural reservoir. Transmission is via tick bite.

Pathogenesis: Organism invades endothelial lining of capillaries, causing vasculitis. No toxins or virulence factors identified.

Laboratory Diagnosis: Stain and culture rarely done. Diagnosis usually made by complement fixation or Weil-Felix test.

Treatment: Tetracycline.

Prevention: Protective clothing and prompt removal of ticks. Tetracycline effective in exposed persons. No vaccine is available.

Coxiella burnetii

Disease: Q fever.

Characteristics: Obligate intracellular parasites. Not seen well on Gram-stained smear.

Habitat and Transmission: Habitat is domestic livestock. Transmission is by inhalation of aerosols of urine, feces, amniotic fluid, or placental tissue. The only rickettsia not transmitted to humans by an arthropod.

Pathogenesis: No toxins or virulence factors known.

Laboratory Diagnosis: Stain and culture rarely done. Diagnosis usually made by serologic tests. Weil-Felix test is negative.

Treatment: Tetracycline.

Prevention: Vaccine for high-risk occupations. No drug is available.

Summaries of Medically Important Viruses

DNA ENVELOPED VIRUSES

Herpes Simplex Virus Type 1

Diseases: Herpes labialis (fever blisters or cold sores), keratitis, encephalitis.

Characteristics: Enveloped virus with icosahedral nucleocapsid and linear double-stranded DNA. No virion polymerase. One serotype; cross-reaction with HSV-2 occurs. No herpes group-specific antigen.

Transmission: By saliva or direct contact with virus from the vesicle.

Pathogenesis: Initial vesicular lesions occur in the mouth or on the face. The virus then travels up the axon and becomes latent in sensory (trigeminal) ganglia. Recurrences occur in skin innervated by affected sensory nerve and are induced by fever, sunlight, stress, etc. Dissemination occurs in patients with depressed cell-mediated immunity.

Laboratory Diagnosis: Virus causes cytopathic effect (CPE) in cell culture. It is identified by antibody neutralization or fluorescent-antibody test. Tzanck smear reveals multinucleated giant cells. This implicates a herpesvirus but is not specific for HSV-1. A rise in antibody titer can be used to diagnose a primary infection but not recurrences. Intranuclear inclusions seen in infected cells.

Treatment: Acyclovir for encephalitis and disseminated disease. Acyclovir has no effect on the latent state of the virus. Trifluorothymidine for keratitis. Primary infections and localized recurrences are self-limited. A variety of over-the-counter drying agents can be used to promote healing.

Prevention: Recurrences can be prevented by avoiding the specific inciting agent such as intense sunlight. Acyclovir can reduce recurrences. No vaccine is available.

Herpes Simplex Virus Type 2

Diseases: Herpes genitalis, aseptic meningitis, and neonatal infection.

Characteristics: Enveloped virus with icosahedral nucleocapsid and linear double-stranded DNA. No virion polymerase. One serotype; cross-reaction with HSV-1 occurs. No herpes group-specific antigen.

Transmission: Sexual contact in adults and during passage through the birth canal in neonates.

Pathogenesis: Initial vesicular lesions occur on genitals. The virus then travels up the axon and becomes latent in sensory (lumbar or sacral) ganglion cells. Recurrences may be induced by stress.

Laboratory Diagnosis: Virus causes CPE in cell culture. Identify by antibody neutralization or fluorescent-antibody test. Tzanck smear reveals multinucleated giant cells but is not specific for HSV-2. A rise in antibody titer can be used to diagnose a primary infection but not recurrences.

Treatment: Acyclovir is useful in the treatment of both primary and recurrent disease. It has no effect on the latent state.

Prevention: Primary disease can be prevented by protection from exposure to vesicular lesions. Recurrences can be reduced by the long-term use of oral acyclovir. There is no vaccine.

Varicella-Zoster Virus

Diseases: Varicella (chickenpox) in children and zoster (shingles) in adults.

Characteristics: Enveloped virus with icosahedral nucleocapsid and linear double-stranded DNA. No virion polymerase. One serotype.

Transmission: Varicella is transmitted primarily by respiratory droplets. Zoster is not transmitted; it is caused by a reactivation of latent virus.

Pathogenesis: Initial infection is in the respiratory tract. It spreads via the blood to the internal organs such as the liver and then to the skin. After the acute episode of varicella, the virus remains latent in the sensory ganglia and can reactivate to cause zoster years later, especially in older and immunocompromised individuals.

Laboratory Diagnosis: Virus causes CPE in cell culture and can be identified by fluorescent-antibody test. Multinucleated giant cells seen in smears from the base of the vesicle. Intranuclear inclusions seen in infected cells. A 4-fold rise in antibody titer in convalescent-phase serum is diagnostic.

Treatment: No antiviral therapy is indicated for varicella or zoster in the immunocompetent patient. In the immunocompromised patient, acyclovir can prevent dissemination.

Prevention: Vaccine contains live, attenuated virus. Immunocompromised patients exposed to the virus should receive passive immunization with varicella-zoster immune globulin (VZIG) and acyclovir to prevent disseminated disease.

Cytomegalovirus

Diseases: Cytomegalic inclusion body disease in infants. Mononucleosis in transfusion recipients. Pneumonia and hepatitis in immunocompromised patients.

Characteristics: Enveloped virus with icosahedral nucleocapsid and linear double-stranded DNA. No virion polymerase. One serotype.

Transmission: Virus is found in many human body fluids including blood, saliva, semen, cervical mucus, breast milk, and urine. It is transmitted via these fluids, across the placenta, or by organ transplantation.

Pathogenesis: Initial infection usually in the oropharynx. In fetal infections, the virus spreads to many organs, eg, central nervous system and kidneys. In adults, lymphocytes are frequently involved. A latent state occurs in leukocytes. Disseminated infection in immunocompromised patients can result from either a primary infection or reactivation of a latent infection.

Laboratory Diagnosis: The virus causes CPE in cell culture and can be identified by fluorescent-antibody test. "Owl's eye" nuclear inclusions are seen. A 4-fold rise in antibody titer in convalescent-phase serum is diagnostic.

Treatment: Ganciclovir is beneficial in treating pneumonia and retinitis. Acyclovir is ineffective.

Prevention: No vaccine is available. Ganciclovir suppresses retinitis. Do not transfuse CMV antibody-positive blood into newborns or antibody-negative immunocompromised patients.

Epstein-Barr Virus

Diseases: Infectious mononucleosis; associated with Burkitt's lymphoma in east African children.

Characteristics: Enveloped virus with icosahedral nucleocapsid and linear double-stranded DNA. No virion polymerase. One serotype.

Transmission: Virus found in human oropharynx and B lymphocytes. It is transmitted primarily by saliva.

Pathogenesis: Infection begins in the pharyngeal epithelium, spreads to the cervical lymph nodes, then travels via the blood to the liver and spleen.

Laboratory Diagnosis: The virus is rarely isolated. Lymphocytosis, including atypical lymphocytes, occurs. Heterophil antibody is typically positive (Monospot test). A significant rise in EBV-specific antibody to viral capsid antigen is diagnostic.

Treatment: No effective drug is available.

Prevention: There is no drug or vaccine.

Hepatitis B Virus

Diseases: Hepatitis B; associated with hepatocellular carcinoma.

Characteristics: Enveloped virus with incomplete circular double-stranded DNA; ie, one strand has about one-third missing and the other strand is "nicked" (not covalently bonded). DNA polymerase in virion. There are three important antigens: the surface antigen, the core antigen, and the e antigen, which is located in the core. In patient's serum, long rods and spherical forms composed solely of HBsAg predominate. HBV has one serotype based on the surface antigen.

Transmission: Transmitted by blood, during birth, and by sexual intercourse.

Pathogenesis: Hepatocellular injury due to immune attack by cytotoxic (CD8) T cells. Antigen-antibody complexes cause arthritis, rash, and glomerulonephritis. Chronic hepatitis and cirrhosis can occur. Hepatocellular carcinoma may be related to the integration of part of the viral DNA into hepatocyte DNA.

Laboratory Diagnosis: HBV has not been grown in cell culture. Three serologic tests are commonly used: surface antigen (HBsAg), surface antibody (HBsAb), and core antibody (HBcAb). See Chapter 41 for a discussion of the results of these tests.

Treatment: No specific treatment.

Prevention: There are three main approaches: (1) vaccine that contains HBsAg as the immunogen; (2) hyperimmune serum globulins obtained from donors with high titers of HBsAb; and (3) education of chronic carriers regarding precautions.

Smallpox Virus

Disease: Smallpox (eradicated in 1977).

Characteristics: Poxviruses are the largest viruses. Enveloped virus with linear double-stranded DNA. DNA-dependent RNA polymerase in virion. One serologic type.

Transmission: By respiratory droplets or direct contact with the virus from skin lesions.

Pathogenesis: The virus infects the mucosal cells of the upper respiratory tract, then spreads to the local lymph nodes and by viremia to the liver and spleen and later the skin. Skin lesions progress in the following order: macule, papule, vesicle, pustule, crust.

Laboratory Diagnosis: Virus identified by CPE in cell culture or "pocks" on chorioallantoic membrane. Electron microscopy reveals typical particles; cytoplasmic inclusions seen in light microscopy. Viral antigens in the vesicle fluid can be detected by precipitin tests. A 4-fold or greater rise in antibody titer in the convalescent-phase serum is diagnostic.

Treatment: None.

Prevention: Vaccine contains live attenuated vaccinia virus. Vaccine is no longer used except by the military, because the disease has been eradicated.

DNA NONENVELOPED VIRUS

Adenovirus

Diseases: Upper and lower tract respiratory disease, especially pharyngitis and pneumonia. Enteric strains cause diarrhea. Some strains cause sarcomas in certain animals but not humans.

Characteristics: Nonenveloped virus with icosahedral nucleocapsid and linear double-stranded DNA. No virion polymerase. There are 34 serotypes, some associated with specific diseases.

Transmission: Respiratory droplet primarily; iatrogenic transmission in eye disease.

Pathogenesis: Virus preferentially infects epithelium of respiratory tract and eyes. After acute infection, persistent, low-grade virus production without symptoms can occur in the pharynx.

Laboratory Diagnosis: Virus causes CPE in cell culture and can be identified by fluorescent-antibody or complement fixation test. Antibody titer rise in convalescent-phase serum is diagnostic.

Treatment: None.

Prevention: Live vaccine against types 3, 4, and 7 is used in the military to prevent pneumonia.

Papillomavirus

Diseases: Papillomas (warts); condylomata acuminata; associated with carcinoma of the cervix and penis.

Characteristics: Nonenveloped virus with icosahedral nucleocapsid and circular double-stranded DNA. No virion polymerase. There are at least 60 types which are determined by DNA sequence not by antigenicity. Many types infect the epithelium and cause papillomas at specific body sites.

Transmission: Direct contact of skin or genital lesions.

Pathogenesis: Two early viral genes, E6 and E7, encode proteins that inhibit the activity of proteins encoded by tumor suppressor genes, eg, the p53 gene and the retinoblastoma gene, respectively.

Laboratory Diagnosis: Diagnosis is made clinically by finding koilocytes in the lesions. DNA hybridization tests are available. Virus isolation and serologic tests are not done.

Treatment: Podophyllin or liquid nitrogen are most commonly used. Alpha interferon is also available.

Prevention: There is no drug or vaccine.

RNA ENVELOPED VIRUSES

Influenza Virus

Disease: Influenza.

Characteristics: Enveloped virus with a helical nucleocapsid and segmented, single-stranded RNA of negative polarity. RNA polymerase in virion. The two major antigens are the hemagglutinin and the neuraminidase on separate surface spikes. Antigenic shift in these proteins as a result of reassortment of RNA segments accounts for the epidemics of influenza. Antigenic drift due to mutations also contributes. The virus has many serotypes because of these antigenic shifts and drifts. The antigenicity of the internal capsid protein determines whether the virus is an A, B, or C influenza virus.

Transmission: Respiratory droplets.

Pathogenesis: Infection is limited primarily to the epithelium of the respiratory tract.

Laboratory Diagnosis: Virus grows in cell culture and embryonated eggs and can be detected by hemadsorption or hemagglutination. It is identified by hemagglutination inhibition or complement fixation. Antibody titer rise in convalescent-phase serum is diagnostic.

Treatment: Amantadine is available but infrequently used.

Prevention: Vaccine contains inactivated strains of A and B virus currently causing disease. The vaccine is not a good immunogen and must be given annually. Recommended for people over age 65 years and for those with chronic diseases, especially of the heart and lungs. Amantadine provides good prophylaxis in unvaccinated people who have been exposed.

Measles Virus

Disease: Measles. Subacute sclerosing panencephalitis is a rare late complication.

Characteristics: Enveloped virus with a helical nucleocapsid and one piece of single-stranded, negative-polarity RNA. RNA polymerase in virion. It has a single serotype.

Transmission: Respiratory droplets.

Pathogenesis: Initial site of infection is the upper respiratory tract. Virus spreads to local lymph nodes and then via the blood to other organs including the skin. Giant cell pneumonia and encephalitis can occur. The maculopapular rash is due to cell-mediated immune attack by cytotoxic T cells on virus-infected vascular endothelial cells in the skin.

Laboratory Diagnosis: The virus is rarely isolated. Serologic tests are used if necessary.

Treatment: No antiviral therapy is available.

Prevention: Vaccine contains live attenuated virus. Usually given in combination with mumps and rubella vaccines.

Mumps Virus

Disease: Mumps. Sterility due to bilateral orchitis is a rare complication.

Characteristics: Enveloped virus with a helical nucleocapsid and one piece of single-stranded, negative-polarity RNA. RNA polymerase in virion. It has a single serotype.

Transmission: Respiratory droplets.

Pathogenesis: The initial site of infection is the upper respiratory tract. The virus spreads to local lymph nodes and then via the bloodstream to other organs, especially the parotid glands, testes, ovaries, meninges, and pancreas.

Laboratory Diagnosis: The virus can be isolated in cell culture and detected by hemadsorption. Diagnosis can also be made serologically.

Treatment: No antiviral therapy is available.

Prevention: Vaccine contains live attenuated virus. Usually given in combination with measles and rubella vaccines.

Rubella Virus

Disease: Rubella. Congenital rubella syndrome is characterized by developmental malformations, especially cardiovascular and neurologic, and by prolonged virus excretion.

Characteristics: Enveloped virus with an icosahedral nucleocapsid and one piece of single-stranded positive-polarity RNA. No polymerase in virion. It has a single serotype.

Transmission: Respiratory droplets.

Pathogenesis: The initial site of infection is the nasopharynx, from which it spreads to local lymph nodes. It then disseminates to the skin via the bloodstream. The rash is attributed to both viral replication and immune injury. During maternal infection, the virus replicates in the placenta and then spreads to fetal tissue. If infection occurs during the first trimester, a high frequency of congenital malformations occurs.

Laboratory Diagnosis: Virus growth in cell culture is detected by interference with plaque formation by coxsackievirus; rubella virus does not cause CPE. To determine whether an adult woman is immune, a single serum specimen to detect IgG antibody in the hemagglutination inhibition test is used. To detect whether recent infection has occurred, either a single serum specimen for IgM antibody or a set of acute- and convalescent-phase sera for IgA antibody can be used.

Treatment: No antiviral therapy is available.

Prevention: Vaccine contains live attenuated virus. Usually given in combination with measles and mumps vaccine.

Parainfluenza Virus

Disease: Bronchiolitis in infants, croup in young children, and the common cold in adults.

Characteristics: Enveloped virus with helical nucleocapsid and one piece of single-stranded, negative-polarity RNA. RNA polymerase in virion. Unlike influenza viruses, the antigenicity of its hemagglutinin and neuraminidase is stable. There are four serotypes.

Transmission: Respiratory droplets.

Pathogenesis: Infection and death of respiratory epithelium without systemic spread of the virus. Multinucleated giant cells caused by the viral fusion protein are a hallmark.

Laboratory Diagnosis: Isolation of the virus in cell culture is detected by hemadsorption. Immunofluorescence is used for identification. A 4-fold or greater rise in antibody titer is diagnostic in primary infections, but the heterotypic response limits its usefulness in repeated infections.

Treatment: None.

Prevention: No vaccine or drug is available.

Respiratory Syncytial Virus

Diseases: Bronchiolitis and pneumonia in infants.

Characteristics: Enveloped virus with a helical nucleocapsid and one piece of single-stranded, negative-polarity RNA. RNA polymerase in virion. Unlike other paramyxoviruses, it has only a fusion protein in its surface spikes. It has no hemagglutinin. It has a single serotype.

Transmission: Respiratory droplets.

Pathogenesis: Infection involves primarily the lower respiratory tract in infants without systemic spread. Immune response probably contributes to pathogenesis.

Laboratory Diagnosis: Isolation in cell culture. Multinucleated giant cells visible. Immunofluorescence is used for identification. Serology is not useful for diagnosis in infants.

Treatment: Aerosolized ribavirin for sick infants.

Prevention: No vaccine or prophylactic drug is available.

Rabies Virus

Disease: Rabies.

Characteristics: Bullet-shaped enveloped virus with a helical nucleocapsid and one piece of single-stranded, negative-polarity RNA. RNA polymerase in virion. The virus has a single serotype.

Transmission: Animal bite, usually by wild animals such as skunks, raccoons, and bats. In the United States, dogs are infrequently involved. Transmitted rarely by inhalation of bat guano.

Pathogenesis: Viral receptor is the acetylcholine receptor on the neuron. Replication of virus at the site of the bite, followed by ascension up the nerve to the central nervous system. After replicating in the brain, the virus migrates peripherally to the salivary glands, where it enters the saliva.

When the animal is in the agitated state as a result of encephalitis, virus in the saliva can be transmitted via a bite.

Laboratory Diagnosis: Tissue can be stained with fluorescent antibody or with various dyes to detect inclusions called Negri bodies. The virus can be isolated in newborn mice, but because this takes 1 or 2 weeks, it cannot be used to determine whether a person should receive the vaccine. Serologic testing is useful only to make the diagnosis in the clinically ill patient; it does not help the person who has been bitten. It is also used to evaluate the antibody response to the vaccine given before exposure to those in high-risk occupations.

Treatment: No antiviral therapy is available.

Prevention: Preexposure prevention of rabies consists of the vaccine only. Postexposure prevention consists of (1) washing the wound; (2) giving immune serum, mostly into the wound; and (3) giving the inactivated vaccine made in human cell culture. The decision to give the immune serum and the vaccine depends on the circumstances. Prevention of rabies in dogs and cats by using a live attenuated vaccine has reduced human rabies significantly.

Human Immunodeficiency Virus

Disease: Acquired immunodeficiency syndrome (AIDS).

Characteristics: Enveloped virus with two copies (diploid) of a single-stranded, positive-polarity RNA genome. RNA-dependent DNA polymerase (reverse transcriptase) makes a DNA copy of the genome which integrates into host cell DNA. The *tat* gene encodes a protein that activates viral transcription. It is a type D retrovirus (lentivirus). Antigenicity of the gp120 protein changes rapidly; therefore, there are many serotypes.

Transmission: Transfer of body fluids, eg, blood and semen. Also transplacental.

Pathogenesis: Receptor is CD4 protein found primarily on helper T cells. Infects and kills helper T cells, which predisposes to opportunistic infections. Other cells bearing CD4 proteins on the surface, eg, astrocytes, are infected also.

Laboratory Diagnosis: Virus can be isolated from blood or semen, but this procedure is not routinely available. Diagnosis is usually made by detecting antibody with ELISA as screening test and Western blot as confirmatory test.

Treatment: Azidothymidine (AZT), ddI, and ddC inhibit HIV replication by inhibiting reverse transcriptase. Protease inhibitors, eg, indinavir, prevent cleavage of precursor polypeptides. Clinical improvement occurs, but the virus persists. Treatment of the opportunistic infection depends on the organism.

Prevention: Screening of blood prior to transfusion for the presence of antibody. "Safe sex," including the use of condoms. AZT can be given to HIV-infected mothers and their newborns. There is no vaccine.

Hepatitis C Virus

Disease: Hepatitis C; associated with hepatocellular carcinoma.

Characteristics: Enveloped virus with one piece of single-stranded, positive-polarity RNA. No polymerase in virion. HCV has multiple serotypes.

Transmission: Transmitted by blood, sexually, and from mother to child.

Pathogenesis: Hepatocellular injury probably caused by cytotoxic T cells. HCV does not cause a cytopathic effect. Chronic hepatitis and chronic carrier state occur. Strong predisposition to hepatocellular carcinoma.

Laboratory Diagnosis: Serologic testing detects antibody to HCV.

Treatment: Alpha interferon mitigates chronic hepatitis but does not eradicate the carrier state.

Prevention: Posttransfusion hepatitis can be prevented by detection of antibodies in donated blood. There is no vaccine, and hyperimmune globulins are not available.

Hepatitis D Virus

Disease: Hepatitis D (delta).

Characteristics: Defective virus that uses hepatitis B surface antigen as its protein coat. HDV can replicate only in cells already infected with HBV; ie, HBV is a helper virus for HDV. Genome is one piece of single-stranded, negative-polarity, circular RNA. No polymerase in virion. HDV has one serotype.

Transmission: Transmitted by blood, sexually, and from mother to child.

Pathogenesis: Hepatocellular injury probably caused by cytotoxic T cells. Chronic hepatitis and chronic carrier state occur.

Laboratory Diagnosis: Serologic testing detects either delta antigen or antibody to delta antigen.

Treatment: Alpha interferon mitigates symptoms but does not eradicate the carrier state.

Prevention: Prevention of HBV infection by using the HBV vaccine and the hyperimmune globulins will prevent HDV infection also.

RNA NONENVELOPED VIRUSES

Poliovirus

Diseases: Paralytic poliomyelitis and aseptic meningitis.

Characteristics: Naked nucleocapsid with single-stranded, positive-polarity RNA. No virion polymerase. There are three serotypes.

Transmission: Fecal-oral route.

Pathogenesis: The virus replicates in the pharynx and the gastrointestinal tract. It can spread to the local lymph nodes and then through the bloodstream to the central nervous system. Most infections are asymptomatic or very mild. Aseptic meningitis is more frequent than paralytic polio. Paralysis is the result of death of motor neurons, especially anterior horn cells in the spinal cord. Pathogenesis of postpolio syndrome is unknown.

Laboratory Diagnosis: Recovery of the virus from spinal fluid indicates infection of the central nervous system. Isolation of the virus from stools indicates infection but not necessarily disease. It can be found in the gastrointestinal tracts of asymptomatic carriers. The virus can be detected in cell culture by CPE and identified by neutralization with type-specific antiserum. A significant rise in antibody titer in convalescent-phase serum is also diagnostic.

Treatment: No antiviral therapy is available.

Prevention: Disease can be prevented by both the inactivated (Salk) vaccine and the attenuated (Sabin) vaccine; both induce humoral antibody that neutralizes the virus in the bloodstream. The oral Sabin vaccine is used for routine childhood immunizations, because it (1) induces IgA immunity in the gut, thereby interfering with transmission; (2) induces immunity of longer duration; and (3) is administered orally. Immune globulins are available but rarely used.

Coxsackieviruses

Diseases: Aseptic meningitis, herpangina, pleurodynia, myocarditis, and pericarditis are the most important diseases.

Characteristics: Naked nucleocapsid with single-stranded, positive-polarity RNA. No virion polymerase. Group A and B viruses are defined by their different pathogenicity in mice. There are multiple serotypes in each group.

Transmission: Fecal-oral route.

Pathogenesis: The initial site of infection is the oropharynx, but the main site is the gastrointestinal tract. The virus spreads through the bloodstream to various organs.

Laboratory Diagnosis: The virus can be detected by CPE in cell culture and identified by neutralization. A significant rise in antibody titer in convalescent-phase serum is diagnostic.

Treatment: No antiviral therapy is available.

Prevention: No vaccine is available.

Hepatitis A Virus

Disease: Hepatitis A.

Characteristics: Naked nucleocapsid virus with a single-stranded, positive-polarity RNA. No virion polymerase. Virus has a single serotype.

Transmission: Fecal-oral route.

Pathogenesis: The virus replicates in the gastrointestinal tract and then spreads to the liver during a brief viremic period. The virus is not cytopathic for the hepatocyte. Hepatocellular injury is probably caused by immune attack by cytotoxic T cells.

Laboratory Diagnosis: The most useful test is IgM antibody. Isolation of the virus from clinical specimens is not done.

Treatment: No antiviral drug is available.

Prevention: Vaccine contains killed virus. Administration of immune globulin during the incubation period can mitigate the disease.

Reoviruses (Especially Rotavirus)

Disease: The most important reovirus is rotavirus, which causes gastroenteritis (diarrhea), especially in young children.

Characteristics: Naked double-layered capsid with 10 or 11 segments of double-stranded RNA. RNA polymerase in virion. Rotavirus is resistant to stomach acid and hence can reach the gastrointestinal tract. There are at least six serotypes.

Transmission: Reoviruses are transmitted either by respiratory droplet or by the fecal-oral route. Human rotaviruses are found only in humans and are transmitted by the fecal-oral route.

Pathogenesis: Rotavirus infection is limited to the gastrointestinal tract, especially the small intestine.

Laboratory Diagnosis: Detection of rotavirus in the stool by ELISA. A significant rise in antibody titer in convalescent-phase serum is useful. Isolation of the virus is not done from clinical specimens.

Treatment: No antiviral drug is available.

Prevention: No vaccine is available.

Rhinoviruses

Disease: Common cold.

Characteristics: Naked nucleocapsid viruses with single-stranded, positive-polarity RNA. No virion polymerase. There are more than 100 serotypes. Rhinoviruses are destroyed by stomach acid and do not replicate in the gastrointestinal tract, in contrast to other picornaviruses such as poliovirus, coxsackievirus, and echovirus, which are resistant to stomach acid.

Transmission: Aerosol droplets and hand-to-nose contact.

Pathogenesis: Infection is limited to the mucosa of the upper respiratory tract and conjunctiva. The virus replicates best at the low temperatures of the nose and less well at 37 °C, accounting for its failure to infect the lower respiratory tract.

Laboratory Diagnosis: Laboratory tests are rarely used clinically. The virus can be recovered from nose or throat washings by growth in cell culture. Serologic tests are not useful.

Treatment: No antiviral therapy is available.

Prevention: No vaccine is available because there are too many serotypes.

Summaries of Medically Important Fungi

FUNGI CAUSING CUTANEOUS & SUBCUTANEOUS INFECTIONS

Dermatophytes (eg, *Trichophyton, Microsporum, Epidermophyton* species)

Diseases: Dermatophytoses, eg, tinea capitis, tinea cruris, and tinea pedis.

Characteristics: These fungi are molds that use keratin as a nutritional source. Not dimorphic. Habitat of most dermatophytes that cause human disease is human skin, with the exception of *Microsporum canis,* which inhabits the skin of dogs and cats.

Transmission: Skin scales.

Pathogenesis: These fungi grow only in the superficial keratinized layer of the skin. They do not invade underlying tissue. The lesions are due to the inflammatory response to the fungi. Frequency of infection is enhanced by moisture and warmth. An important host defense is provided by the fatty acids produced by sebaceous glands. The "id" reaction is a hypersensitivity response in one skin location, eg, fingers, to the presence of the organism in another, eg, feet.

Laboratory Diagnosis: Skin scales should be examined microscopically in a KOH preparation for the presence of hyphae. The organism is identified by the appearance of its mycelium and its asexual spores on Sabouraud's agar. Serologic tests are not useful.

Skin test: Trichophytin antigen can be used to determine the competence of a patient's cell-mediated immunity. Not used for diagnosis of tinea.

Treatment: Topical agents, such as miconazole, clotrimazole, or tolnaftate, are used. Undecylenic acid is effective against tinea pedis. Griseofulvin is the treatment of choice for tinea unguium and tinea capitis.

Prevention: Skin should be kept dry and cool.

Sporothrix schenckii

Disease: Sporotrichosis.

Characteristics: Thermally dimorphic. Habitat is soil or vegetation.

Transmission: Traumatic penetration of skin.

Pathogenesis: Local abscess or ulcer with nodules in draining lymphatics.

Laboratory Diagnosis: Cigar-shaped budding cells visible in pus. Culture on Sabouraud's agar shows typical morphology.

Skin Test: None.

Treatment: Potassium iodide, ketoconazole.

Prevention: Skin should be protected when gardening.

FUNGI CAUSING SYSTEMIC INFECTIONS

Histoplasma capsulatum

Disease: Histoplasmosis.

Characteristics: Thermally dimorphic, ie, a yeast at body temperature and a mold in the soil at ambient temperature. The mold form produces tuberculate chlamydospores (asexual spores). The mold grows preferentially in soil enriched with bird droppings. Endemic in Ohio and Mississippi River valley areas.

Transmission: Inhalation of airborne asexual spores (microconidia).

Pathogenesis: Microconidia enter the lung and differentiate into yeast cells. The yeast cells are ingested by alveolar macrophages and multiply within them. An immune response is mounted, and granulomas form. Most infections are contained at this level, but suppression of cell-mediated immunity can lead to disseminated disease.

Laboratory Diagnosis: Sputum or tissue can be examined microscopically and cultured on Sabouraud's agar. Yeasts visible within macrophages. The presence of tuberculate chlamydospores in culture at 25 °C is diagnostic. A rise in antibody titer is useful for diagnosis, but cross-reaction with other fungi (eg, *Coccidioides*) occurs.

Skin Test: Histoplasmin, a mycelial extract, is the antigen. Useful for epidemiologic purposes to determine the incidence of infection. A positive result indicates only that infection has occurred; it cannot be used to diagnose active disease. Skin testing can induce antibodies, so serologic tests must be done first.

Treatment: Amphotericin B for disseminated disease; itraconazole for pulmonary disease. No treatment is indicated for primary histoplasmosis.

Prevention: Endemic areas should be avoided. No vaccine or prophylactic drug is available.

Coccidioides immitis

Disease: Coccidioidomycosis.

Characteristics: Thermally dimorphic. At 37 °C in the body, it forms spherules containing endospores. At 25 °C, it grows as a mold. The cells at the tip of the hyphae differentiate into asexual spores (arthrospores). Natural habitat is the soil of arid regions, eg, San Joaquin valley in California.

Transmission: Inhalation of airborne arthrospores.

Pathogenesis: Arthrospores differentiate into spherules in the lungs. Spherules rupture, releasing endospores that form new spherules, thereby disseminating the infection within the body. A cell-mediated immune response contains the infection in most people, but those who are immunocompromised are at high risk for disseminated disease.

Laboratory Diagnosis: Sputum or tissue should be examined microscopically for spherules and cultured on Sabouraud's agar. A rise in IgM precipitin antibodies indicates recent infection. A rising titer of complement-fixing IgG antibodies indicates dissemination; a decreasing titer indicates a response to therapy.

Skin Test: Either coccidioidin, a mycelial extract, or spherulin, an extract of spherules, is the antigen. Useful in determining whether the patient has been infected. A positive test indicates prior infection but not necessarily active disease.

Treatment: Amphotericin B for disseminated disease; ketoconazole for limited pulmonary disease. No treatment is indicated for primary coccidioidomycosis.

Prevention: Endemic areas should be avoided. No vaccine or prophylactic drug is available.

Blastomyces dermatitidis

Disease: Blastomycosis.

Characteristics: Thermally dimorphic. The yeast form has a single, broad-based bud and a thick, refractile wall. Natural habitat is rich soil (eg, near beaver dams).

Transmission: Inhalation of airborne asexual spores.

Pathogenesis: Inhaled conidia differentiate into yeasts, which initially cause abscesses followed by formation of granulomas. Dissemination is rare, but when it occurs, skin and bone are most commonly involved.

Laboratory Diagnosis: Sputum or skin lesions examined microscopically for yeasts with a broad-based bud. Culture on Sabouraud's agar also. Serologic tests are not useful.

Skin Test: Little value.

Treatment: Itraconazole is the drug of choice.

Prevention: No vaccine or prophylactic drug is available.

Paracoccidioides brasiliensis

Disease: Paracoccidioidomycosis.

Characteristics: Thermally dimorphic. The yeast form has multiple buds (resembles the steering wheel of a ship).

Transmission: Inhalation of airborne conidia.

Pathogenesis: Inhaled conidia differentiate to the yeast form in lungs. Can disseminate to many organs.

Laboratory Diagnosis: Yeasts with multiple buds visible in pus or tissues. Culture on Sabouraud's agar shows typical morphology.

Skin Test: Not useful.

Treatment: Itraconazole.

Prevention: No vaccine or prophylactic drug is available.

FUNGI CAUSING OPPORTUNISTIC INFECTIONS

Aspergillus fumigatus

Diseases: Invasive aspergillosis is the major disease. Allergic bronchopulmonary aspergillosis is important also.

Characteristics: Mold with septate hyphae that branch at a V-shaped angle. Not dimorphic. Habitat is the soil.

Transmission: Inhalation of airborne condidia.

Pathogenesis: Opportunistic pathogen. In immunocompromised patients, invasive disease occurs. The organism invades blood vessels, causing thrombosis and infarction. In a person with a lung cavity, a "fungus ball" (aspergilloma) can develop. An allergic person can develop allergic bronchopulmonary aspergillosis.

Laboratory Diagnosis: Septate hyphae invading tissue are visible microscopically. Invasion distinguishes disease from colonization. Forms characteristic mycelium when cultured on Sabouraud's agar. Serologic tests detect IgG precipitins in patients with aspergillomas and IgE antibodies in patients with allergic bronchopulmonary aspergillosis.

Skin Test: None available.

Treatment: Amphotericin B for invasive aspergillosis. Some lesions can be surgically removed. Steroid therapy is recommended for allergic bronchopulmonary aspergillosis.

Prevention: No vaccine or prophylactic drug is available.

Candida albicans

Diseases: Thrush, disseminated candidiasis, and chronic mucocutaneous candidiasis.

Characteristics: *Candida albicans* is a yeast when part of the normal flora of mucous membranes but forms pseudohyphae and hyphae when it invades tissue. The yeast form produces germ tubes when incubated in serum at 37 °C. Not thermally dimorphic.

Transmission: Part of the normal flora of skin, mucous membranes, and gastrointestinal tract. No person-to-person transmission.

Pathogenesis: Opportunistic pathogen. Predisposing factors include depressed immune system, altered skin and mucous membrane, suppression of normal flora, and presence of foreign bodies. Thrush is most common in infants, immunosuppressed patients, and persons on antibiotic therapy. Skin lesions occur frequently on moisture-damaged skin. Disseminated infection occurs in immunosuppressed patients and intravenous drug abusers. Chronic mucocutaneous candidiasis occurs in children with a T cell defect in immunity to *Candida*.

Laboratory Diagnosis: Microscopic examination of tissue reveals yeasts and pseudohyphae. If only yeasts are found, colonization is suggested. The yeast is gram-positive. Forms colonies of yeasts on Sabouraud's agar. Germ tube formation and production of chlamydospores distinguish *C albicans* from virtually all other species of *Candida*. Serologic tests not useful.

Skin Test: Used to determine competency of cell-mediated immunity rather than to diagnose candidal disease.

Treatment: Skin and mucous membrane disease can be treated with oral or topical antifungal agents such as nystatin or miconazole. Disseminated disease requires amphotericin B. Chronic mucocutaneous candidiasis is treatable with ketoconazole.

Prevention: Predisposing factors should be reduced or eliminated. Oral thrush can be prevented by using clotrimazole troches or nystatin "swish and swallow." There is no vaccine.

Cryptococcus neoformans

Disease: Cryptococcosis, especially cryptococcal meningitis.

Characteristics: Heavily encapsulated yeast. Not dimorphic. Habitat is soil, especially where enriched by pigeon droppings.

Transmission: Inhalation of airborne yeast cells.

Pathogenesis: Organisms cause influenzalike syndrome or pneumonia. They spread via the bloodstream to the meninges. Reduced cell-mediated immunity predisposes to severe disease, but some cases of cryptococcal meningitis occur in immunocompetent people.

Laboratory Diagnosis: Visualization of the encapsulated yeast in India ink preparations of spinal fluid. Culture of sputum or spinal fluid on Sabouraud's agar produces colonies of yeasts. Latex agglutination test detects polysaccharide capsular antigen in spinal fluid.

Skin Test: Not available.

Treatment: Amphotericin B plus flucytosine for meningitis.

Prevention: Cryptococcal meningitis can be prevented in AIDS patients by using oral fluconazole. There is no vaccine.

Mucor & *Rhizopus* species

Disease: Mucormycosis.

Characteristics: Molds with nonseptate hyphae. Not dimorphic. Habitat is the soil.

Transmission: Inhalation of airborne sporangiospores.

Pathogenesis: Opportunistic pathogens. They cause disease primarily in ketoacidotic diabetic and leukemic patients. The nose and sinuses are typically involved. Hyphae invade the mucosa and progress into underlying tissue and vessels, leading to necrosis and infarction.

Laboratory Diagnosis: Microscopic examination of tissue for the presence of invasive hyphae. Forms characteristic mycelium when cultured on Sabouraud's agar. Serologic tests are not available.

Skin Test: None.

Treatment: Amphotericin B and surgical debridement.

Prevention: No vaccine or prophylactic drug is available. Control of underlying disease, eg, diabetes, tends to prevent mucormycosis.

Summaries of Medically Important Parasites

PROTOZOA

1. Intestinal & Urogenital Infections

Entamoeba histolytica

Diseases: Amebic dysentery and liver abscess.

Characteristics: Intestinal protozoan. Motile ameba (trophozoite); forms cysts with four nuclei. Life cycle: Humans ingest cysts, which form trophozoites in small intestine. Trophozoites pass to the colon and multiply. Cysts form in the colon.

Transmission and Epidemiology: Fecal-oral transmission of cysts. Human reservoir. Occurs worldwide, especially in tropics.

Pathogenesis: Trophozoites invade colon epithelium and produce "teardrop" ulcer. Can spread to liver and cause abscess.

Laboratory Diagnosis: Trophozoites or cysts visible in stool. Serologic testing (indirect hemagglutination test) positive with invasive disease.

Treatment: Metronidazole plus iodoquinol.

Prevention: Proper disposal of human waste. Water purification. Hand-washing.

Giardia lamblia

Disease: Giardiasis, especially diarrhea.

Characteristics: Intestinal protozoan. Pear-shaped, flagellated trophozoite, forms cyst with four nuclei. Life cycle: Humans ingest cysts, which form trophozoites in duodenum. Trophozoites encyst and are passed in feces.

Transmission and Epidemiology: Fecal-oral transmission of cysts. Human and animal reservoir. Occurs worldwide.

Pathogenesis: Trophozoites attach to wall but do not invade. They interfere with absorption of fat and protein.

Laboratory Diagnosis: Trophozoites or cysts visible in stool. String test used if necessary.

Treatment: Metronidazole.

Prevention: Water purification. Hand-washing.

Cryptosporidium parvum

Disease: Cryptosporidiosis, especially diarrhea.

Characteristics: Intestinal protozoan. Life cycle: Oocysts release sporozoites; they form trophozoites. After schizonts and merozoites form, microgametes and macrogametes are produced; they unite to form a zygote and then an oocyst.

Transmission and Epidemiology: Fecal-oral transmission of cysts. Human and animal reservoir. Occurs worldwide.

Pathogenesis: Trophozoites attach to wall of small intestine but do not invade.

Laboratory Diagnosis: Oocysts visible in stool with acid-fast stain.

Treatment: None.

Prevention: None.

Trichomonas vaginalis

Disease: Trichomoniasis.

Characteristics: Urogenital protozoan. Pear-shaped, flagellated trophozoites. No cysts or other forms.

Transmission and Epidemiology: Transmitted sexually. Human reservoir. Occurs worldwide.

Pathogenesis: Trophozoites attach to wall of vagina and cause inflammation and discharge.

Laboratory Diagnosis: Trophozoites visible in secretions.

Treatment: Metronidazole for both sexual partners.

Prevention: Condoms limit transmission.

2. Blood & Tissue Infections

Plasmodium species (*P vivax, P ovale, P malariae, & P falciparum*)

Disease: Malaria.

Characteristics: Blood and tissue protozoan. Life cycle: Sexual cycle consists of gametogony in humans and sporogony in mosquitoes; asexual cycle (schizogony) occurs in humans. Sporozoites in saliva of female *Anopheles* mosquito enter the human bloodstream and rapidly invade hepatocytes (exoerythrocytic phase). There they multiply and form merozoites (*Plasmodium vivax* and *Plasmodium ovale* also form hypnozoites, a latent form). Merozoites leave the hepatocytes and infect red cells (erythrocytic phase). There they form schizonts that release more merozoites, which infect other red cells in a synchronous pattern (3 days for *Plasmodium malariae;* 2 days for the others). Some merozoites become male and female gametocytes, which, when ingested by female *Anopheles,* release male and female gametes. These unite to produce a zygote, which forms an oocyst containing many sporozoites. These are released and migrate to salivary glands.

Transmission and Epidemiology: Transmitted by female *Anopheles* mosquitoes. Occurs primarily in the tropical areas of Asia, Africa, and Latin America.

Pathogenesis: Merozoites destroy red cells. Cyclic fever pattern is due to periodic release of merozoites. *Plasmodium falciparum* can infect red cells of all ages and cause aggregates of red cells that occlude capillaries. This can cause tissue anoxia, especially in the brain (cerebral malaria) and the kidney (blackwater fever). Hypnozoites can cause relapses.

Laboratory Diagnosis: Organisms visible in blood smear.

Treatment: Chloroquine if sensitive. For chloroquine-resistant *P falciparum,* use mefloquine or quinine plus Fansidar (sulfadoxine and pyrimethamine). Primaquine for hypnozoites of *P vivax* and *P ovale.*

Prevention: Chloroquine. Primaquine to prevent relapses. For those in areas with a high risk of chloroquine resistance, mefloquine or chloroquine plus Fansidar. Protection from bites. Control mosquitoes by using insecticides and by draining water from breeding areas.

Pneumocystis carinii

Disease: Pneumonia.

Characteristics: Respiratory pathogen (? protozoan). Reclassified in 1988 as a yeast. Life cycle: uncertain.

Transmission and Epidemiology: Transmitted by inhalation. Humans are reservoir. Occurs worldwide. Most infections asymptomatic.

Pathogenesis: Organisms in alveoli cause inflammation. Immunosuppression predisposes to disease.

Laboratory Diagnosis: Organisms visible in silver stain of lung tissue or lavage fluid.

Treatment: Trimethoprim-sulfamethoxazole, pentamidine.

Prevention: Trimethoprim-sulfamethoxazole or aerosolized pentamidine in immunosuppressed individuals.

Toxoplasma gondii

Disease: Toxoplasmosis.

Characteristics: Tissue protozoan. Life cycle: Cysts in cat feces or in meat are ingested by humans and differentiate in the gut into forms that invade the gut wall. They infect macrophages and form trophozoites (tachyzoites) that multiply rapidly, kill cells, and infect other cells. Cysts containing bradyzoites form later. Cat ingests cysts in raw meat, and bradyzoites excyst, multiply, and form male and female gametocytes. These fuse to form oocysts in cat gut, which are excreted in cat feces.

Transmission and Epidemiology: Transmitted by ingestion of cysts and transplacentally from mother to fetus. Cat is definitive host; humans and other mammals are intermediate hosts. Occurs worldwide.

Pathogenesis: Trophozoites infect many organs, especially brain, eyes, and liver. Cysts persist in tissue.

Laboratory Diagnosis: Serologic tests for IgM and IgG antibodies are usually used. Trophozoites or cysts visible in tissue.

Treatment: Sulfonamide and pyrimethamine for congenital or disseminated disease.

Prevention: Meat should be cooked. Pregnant women should not handle cats, litter boxes, or raw meat.

Trypanosoma cruzi

Disease: Chagas' disease.

Characteristics: Blood and tissue protozoan. Life cycle: Trypomastigotes in blood of reservoir host are ingested by reduviid bug and form epimastigotes and then trypomastigotes in the gut. When the bug bites, it defecates and feces containing trypomastigotes contaminate the wound. Organisms enter the blood and form amastigotes within cells; these then become trypomastigotes.

Transmission and Epidemiology: Transmitted by reduviid bugs. Humans and many animals are reservoirs. Occurs in rural Latin America.

Pathogenesis: Amastigotes kill cells, especially cardiac muscle.

Laboratory Diagnosis: Trypomastigotes visible in blood, but bone marrow biopsy, culture in vitro, xenodiagnosis, or serologic tests may be required.

Treatment: Nifurtimox for acute disease. No effective drug for chronic disease.

Prevention: Protection from bite. Insect control.

Trypanosoma gambiense & Trypanosoma rhodesiense

Disease: Sleeping sickness (African trypanosomiasis).

Characteristics: Blood and tissue protozoan. Life cycle: Trypomastigotes in blood of human or animal reservoir are ingested by tsetse fly. They differentiate in the gut to form epimastigotes and then metacyclic trypomastigotes in salivary glands. When fly bites, trypomastigotes enter the blood. Repeated variation of surface antigen occurs, which allows the organism to evade the immune response.

Transmission and Epidemiology: Transmitted by tsetse flies. *Trypanosoma gambiense* has a human reservoir and occurs primarily in west Africa. *Trypanosoma rhodesiense* has an animal reservoir (especially wild antelope) and occurs primarily in east Africa.

Pathogenesis: Trypomastigotes infect brain, causing encephalitis.

Laboratory Diagnosis: Trypomastigotes visible in blood in early stages and in cerebrospinal fluid in late stages. Serologic tests useful.

Treatment: Suramin in early disease. Suramin plus melarsoprol if central nervous system symptoms exist.

Prevention: Protection from bite. Insect control.

Leishmania donovani

Disease: Kala-azar (visceral leishmaniasis).

Characteristics: Blood and tissue protozoan. Life cycle: Human macrophages containing amastigotes are ingested by sandfly. Amastigotes differentiate in fly gut to promastigotes, which migrate to pharynx. When fly bites, promastigotes enter blood macrophages and form amastigotes. These can infect other reticuloendothelial cells, especially in spleen and liver.

Transmission and Epidemiology: Transmitted by sandflies (*Phlebotomus* or *Lutzomyia*). Animal reservoir (chiefly dogs, small carnivores, and rodents) in Africa, Middle East, and parts of China. Human reservoir in India.

Pathogenesis: Amastigotes kill reticuloendothelial cells, especially in liver, spleen, and bone marrow.

Laboratory Diagnosis: Amastigotes visible in bone marrow smear. Serologic tests useful. Skin test indicates prior infection.

Treatment: Sodium stibogluconate.

Prevention: Protection from bite. Insect control.

CESTODES

Diphyllobothrium latum

Disease: Diphyllobothriasis.

Characteristics: Cestode (fish tapeworm). Scolex has two elongated sucking grooves; no circular suckers or hooks. Gravid uterus forms a rosette. Oval eggs have an operculum at one end. Life cycle: Humans ingest undercooked fish containing sparganum larvae. Larvae attach to gut wall and become adults containing gravid proglottids. Eggs are passed in feces. In fresh water, eggs hatch and the embryos are eaten by copepods. When these are eaten by freshwater fish, larvae form in the fish muscle.

Transmission and Epidemiology: Transmitted by eating raw or undercooked freshwater fish. Humans are definitive hosts; copepods are the first and fish the second intermediate hosts, respectively. Occurs worldwide but endemic in Scandinavia, Japan, and north-central United States.

Pathogenesis: Tapeworm in gut causes little damage.

Laboratory Diagnosis: Eggs visible in stool.

Treatment: Praziquantel.

Prevention: Adequate cooking of fish. Proper disposal of human waste.

Echinococcus granulosus

Disease: Hydatid cyst disease.

Characteristics: Cestode (dog tapeworm). Scolex has four suckers and a double circle of hooks. Adult worm has only three proglottids. Life cycle: Dogs are infected when they ingest the entrails of sheep, eg, liver, containing hydatid cysts. The adult worms develop in the gut, and eggs are passed in the feces. Eggs are ingested by sheep (and humans) and hatch hexacanth larvae in the gut that migrate in the blood to various organs, especially the liver and brain. Larvae form large, unilocular hydatid cysts containing many protoscoleces and daughter cysts.

Transmission and Epidemiology: Transmitted by ingestion of eggs in food contaminated with dog feces. Dogs are main definitive hosts; sheep are intermediate hosts; humans are dead-end hosts. Endemic in sheep-raising areas, eg, Mediterranean, Middle East, some western states of the United States.

Pathogenesis: Hydatid cyst is a space-occupying lesion. Also, if cyst ruptures, antigens in fluid can cause anaphylaxis.

Laboratory Diagnosis: Serologic tests, eg, indirect hemagglutination. Pathologic examination of excised cyst.

Treatment: Albendazole or surgical removal of cyst.

Prevention: Sheep entrails should not be fed to dogs.

Taenia saginata

Disease: Taeniasis.

Characteristics: Cestode (beef tapeworm). Scolex has four suckers but no hooks. Gravid proglottids have 15–20 uterine branches. Life cycle: Humans ingest undercooked beef containing cysticerci. Larvae attach to gut wall and become adult worms with gravid proglottids. Terminal proglottids detach, pass in feces, and are eaten by cattle. In the gut, oncosphere embryos hatch, burrow into blood vessels, and migrate to skeletal muscles, where they develop into cysticerci.

Transmission and Epidemiology: Transmitted by eating raw or undercooked beef. Humans are definitive hosts; cattle are intermediate hosts. Occurs worldwide but endemic in areas of Asia, Latin America, and eastern Europe.

Pathogenesis: Tapeworm in gut causes little damage. In contrast to *Taenia solium,* cysticercosis does not occur.

Laboratory Diagnosis: Gravid proglottids visible in stool. Eggs seen less frequently.

Treatment: Praziquantel.

Prevention: Adequate cooking of beef. Proper disposal of human waste.

Taenia solium

Diseases: Taeniasis and cysticercosis.

Characteristics: Cestode (pork tapeworm). Scolex has four suckers and a circle of hooks. Gravid proglottids have 5–10 uterine branches. Life cycle: Humans ingest undercooked pork containing cysticerci. Larvae attach to gut wall and develop into adult worms with gravid proglottids. Terminal proglottids detach, pass in feces, and are eaten by pigs. In gut, oncosphere (hexacanth) embryos burrow into blood vessels and migrate to skeletal muscle, where they develop into cysticerci. If humans eat *T solium* eggs in food contaminated with human feces, the oncospheres burrow into blood vessels and disseminate to organs (eg, brain, eyes) where they encyst to form cysticerci.

Transmission and Epidemiology: Taeniasis acquired by eating raw or undercooked pork. Cysticercosis acquired only by ingesting eggs in fecally contaminated food or water. Humans are definitive hosts; pigs or humans are intermediate hosts. Occurs worldwide but endemic in areas of Asia, Latin America, and southern Europe.

Pathogenesis: Tapeworm in gut causes little damage. Cysticerci can expand and cause symptoms of mass lesions, especially in brain.

Laboratory Diagnosis: Gravid proglottids visible in stool. Eggs seen less frequently.

Treatment: Praziquantel for intestinal worms and for cerebral cysticercosis.

Prevention: Adequate cooking of pork. Proper disposal of human waste.

TREMATODES

Clonorchis sinensis

Disease: Clonorchiasis.

Characteristics: Trematode (liver fluke). Life cycle: Humans ingest undercooked fish containing encysted larvae (metacercariae). In duodenum, immature flukes enter biliary duct, become adults, and release eggs that are passed in feces. Eggs are eaten by snails; the eggs hatch and form miracidia. These multiply through generations (rediae) and then produce many free-swimming cercariae, which encyst under scales of fish and are eaten by humans.

Transmission and Epidemiology: Transmitted by eating raw or undercooked freshwater fish. Humans are definitive hosts; snails and fish are first and second intermediate hosts, respectively. Endemic in the Orient.

Pathogenesis: Inflammation of biliary tract.

Laboratory Diagnosis: Eggs visible in feces.

Treatment: Praziquantel.

Prevention: Adequate cooking of fish. Proper disposal of human waste.

Paragonimus westermani

Disease: Paragonimiasis.

Characteristics: Trematode (lung fluke). Life cycle: Humans ingest undercooked freshwater crab meat containing encysted larvae (metacercariae). In gut, immature flukes enter peritoneal cavity, burrow through diaphragm into lung parenchyma, and become adults. Eggs enter bronchioles and are coughed up or swallowed. In fresh water, eggs hatch, releasing miracidia that enter snails, multiply through generations (rediae), and then form many cercariae that infect and encyst in crabs.

Transmission and Epidemiology: Transmitted by eating raw or undercooked crab meat. Humans are definitive hosts; snails and crabs are first and second intermediate hosts, respectively. Endemic in the Orient and India.

Pathogenesis: Inflammation and secondary bacterial infection of lung.

Laboratory Diagnosis: Eggs visible in sputum or feces.

Treatment: Praziquantel.

Prevention: Adequate cooking of crabs. Proper disposal of human waste.

Schistosoma (S mansoni, S japonicum, & S haematobium)

Disease: Schistosomiasis.

Characteristics: Trematode (blood fluke). Adults exist as two sexes but are attached to each other. Eggs are distinguished by spines: *Schistosoma mansoni* has large lateral spine; *Schistosoma japonicum* has small lateral spine; *Schistosoma haematobium* has terminal spine. Life cycle: Humans are infected by cercariae penetrating skin. Cercariae form larvae that penetrate blood vessels and are carried to the liver, where they become adults. The flukes migrate retrograde in the portal vein to reach the mesenteric venules (*S mansoni* and *S japonicum*) or urinary bladder venules (*S haematobium*). Eggs penetrate the gut or bladder wall, are excreted, and hatch in fresh water. The ciliated larvae (miracidia) penetrate snails and multiply through generations to produce many free-swimming cercariae.

Transmission and Epidemiology: Transmitted by penetration of skin by cercariae. Humans are definitive hosts; snails are intermediate hosts. Endemic in tropical areas: *S mansoni* in Africa and Latin America, *S haematobium* in Africa and Middle East, *S japonicum* in the Orient.

Pathogenesis: Eggs in tissue induce inflammation, granulomas, fibrosis, and obstruction, especially in liver and spleen. *S mansoni* damages the colon (inferior mesenteric venules), *S japonicum* damages the small intestine (superior mesenteric venules), and *S haematobium* damages the bladder. Bladder damage predisposes to carcinoma.

Laboratory Diagnosis: Eggs visible in feces or urine. Eosinophilia occurs.

Treatment: Praziquantel.

Prevention: Proper disposal of human waste. Swimming in endemic areas should be avoided.

NEMATODES

1.   Intestinal Infection

Ancylostoma duodenale & Necator americanus

Disease: Hookworm.

Characteristics: Intestinal nematode. Life cycle: Larvae penetrate skin, enter the blood, and migrate to the lungs. They enter alveoli, pass up the trachea, then are swallowed. They become adults in small intestine and attach to walls via teeth (*Ancylostoma*) or cutting plates (*Necator*). Eggs are passed in feces and form noninfectious rhabditiform larvae and then infectious filariform larvae.

Transmission and Epidemiology: Filariform larvae in soil penetrate skin of feet. Humans are the only hosts. Endemic in the tropics.

Pathogenesis: Anemia due to blood loss from gastrointestinal tract.

Laboratory Diagnosis: Eggs visible in feces. Eosinophilia occurs.

Treatment: Mebendazole or pyrantel pamoate.

Prevention: Use of footwear. Proper disposal of human waste.

Ascaris lumbricoides

Disease: Ascariasis.

Characteristics: Intestinal nematode. Life cycle: Humans ingest eggs, which form larvae in gut. Larvae migrate through the blood to the lungs, where they enter the alveoli, pass up the trachea, and are swallowed. In the gut, they become adults and lay eggs that are passed in the feces. They embryonate, ie, become infective in soil.

Transmission and Epidemiology: Transmitted by food contaminated with soil containing eggs. Humans are the only hosts. Endemic in the tropics.

Pathogenesis: Larvae in lung can cause pneumonia. Heavy worm burden can cause intestinal obstruction or malnutrition.

Laboratory Diagnosis: Eggs visible in feces. Eosinophilia occurs.

Treatment: Mebendazole or pyrantel pamoate.

Prevention: Proper disposal of human waste.

Enterobius vermicularis

Disease: Pinworm infection.

Characteristics: Intestinal nematode. Life cycle: Humans ingest eggs, which develop into adults in gut. At night, females migrate from the anus and lay many eggs on skin and in environment. Embryo within egg becomes an infective larva within 4–6 hours. Reinfection is common.

Transmission and Epidemiology: Transmitted by ingesting eggs. Humans are the only hosts. Occurs worldwide.

Pathogenesis: Worms and eggs cause perianal pruritus.

Laboratory Diagnosis: Eggs visible by "Scotch tape" technique. Adult worms found in diapers.

Treatment: Mebendazole or pyrantel pamoate.

Prevention: None.

Strongyloides stercoralis

Disease: Strongyloidiasis.

Characteristics: Intestinal nematode. Life cycle: Larvae penetrate skin, enter the blood, and migrate to the lungs. They move into alveoli and up the trachea and are swallowed. They become adults and enter the mucosa, where females produce eggs that hatch in the colon into noninfectious, rhabditiform larvae that are usually passed in feces. Occasionally, rhabditiform larvae molt in the gut to form infectious, filariform larvae that can enter the blood and migrate to the lung (autoinfection). The noninfectious larvae passed in feces form infectious filariform larvae in the soil. These larvae can either penetrate the skin or form adults. Adults in soil can undergo several entire life cycles there. This free-living cycle can be interrupted when filariform larvae contact the skin.

Transmission and Epidemiology: Filariform larvae in soil penetrate skin. Endemic in the tropics.

Pathogenesis: Little effect in immunocompetent persons. In immunocompromised persons, massive superinfection can occur accompanied by secondary bacterial infections.

Laboratory Diagnosis: Larvae visible in stool. Eosinophilia occurs.

Treatment: Thiabendazole.

Prevention: Proper disposal of human waste.

Trichinella spiralis

Disease: Trichinosis.

Characteristics: Intestinal nematode that encysts in tissue. Life cycle: Humans ingest undercooked meat containing encysted larvae, which mature into adults in small intestine. Female worms release larvae that enter blood and migrate to skeletal muscle or brain, where they encyst.

Transmission and Epidemiology: Transmitted by ingestion of raw or undercooked meat, usually pork. Reservoir hosts are primarily pigs and rats. Humans are dead-end hosts. Occurs worldwide but endemic in eastern Europe and west Africa.

Pathogenesis: Inflammation of muscle.

Laboratory Diagnosis: Encysted larvae visible in muscle biopsy. Eosinophilia occurs. Serologic tests positive.

Treatment: Thiabendazole effective early against adults. None for established disease.

Prevention: Adequate cooking of pork.

Trichuris trichiura

Disease: Whipworm infection.

Characteristics: Intestinal nematode. Life cycle: Humans ingest eggs, which develop into adults in gut. Eggs are passed in feces into soil, where they embryonate, ie, become infectious.

Transmission and Epidemiology: Transmitted by food or water contaminated with soil containing eggs. Humans are the only hosts. Occurs worldwide, especially in the tropics.

Pathogenesis: Worm in gut usually causes little damage.

Laboratory Diagnosis: Eggs visible in feces.

Treatment: Mebendazole.

Prevention: Proper disposal of human waste.

2. Tissue Infection

Dracunculus medinensis

Disease: Dracunculiasis.

Characteristics: Tissue nematode. Life cycle: Humans ingest copepods containing infective larvae in drinking water. Larvae are released in gut, migrate to body cavity, mature, and mate. Fertilized female migrates to subcutaneous tissue and forms a papule, which ulcerates. Motile larvae are released into water, where they are eaten by copepods and form infective larvae.

Transmission and Epidemiology: Transmitted by copepods in drinking water. Humans are major definitive hosts. Many domestic animals are reservoir hosts. Endemic in tropical Africa, Middle East, and India.

Pathogenesis: Adult worms in skin cause inflammation and ulceration.

Laboratory Diagnosis: Not useful.

Treatment: Niridazole. Extraction of worm from skin ulcer.

Prevention: Purification of drinking water.

Loa loa

Disease: Loiasis.

Characteristics: Tissue nematode. Life cycle: Bite of deer fly (mango fly) deposits infective larvae, which crawl into the skin and develop into adults that migrate subcutaneously. Females produce microfilariae, which enter the blood. These are ingested by deer flies, in which the infective larvae are formed.

Transmission and Epidemiology: Transmitted by deer flies. Humans are the only definitive hosts. No animal reservoir. Endemic in central and west Africa.

Pathogenesis: Hypersensitivity to adult worms causes "swelling" in skin. Adult worm seen crawling across conjunctivas.

Laboratory Diagnosis: Microfilariae visible on blood smear.

Treatment: Diethylcarbamazine.

Prevention: Deer fly control.

Onchocerca volvulus

Disease: Onchocerciasis (river blindness).

Characteristics: Tissue nematodes. Life cycle: Bite of female blackfly deposits infective larvae, which mature in body cavity. Worms enter subcutaneous tissue, where they mature within skin nodules. Females produce microfilariae, which migrate in interstitial fluids and are ingested by blackflies, in which the infective larvae are formed.

Transmission and Epidemiology: Transmitted by female blackflies. Humans are the only definitive hosts. No animal reservoir. Endemic along rivers of tropical Africa and Central America.

Pathogenesis: Microfilariae in eye ultimately can cause blindness. Adults induce inflammatory nodules in skin.

Laboratory Diagnosis: Microfilariae visible in skin biopsy, not in blood.

Treatment: Ivermectin affects microfilariae, not adult worms. Suramin for adult worms.

Prevention: Blackfly control and ivermectin.

Toxocara canis

Disease: Visceral larva migrans.

Characteristics: Nematode larvae cause disease. Life cycle in humans: *Toxocara* eggs are passed in dog feces and ingested by humans. They hatch into larvae in small intestine; larvae enter the blood and migrate to organs, especially liver, brain, and eyes, where they are trapped and die.

Transmission and Epidemiology: Transmitted by ingestion of eggs in food or water contaminated with dog feces. Dogs are definitive hosts. Humans are dead-end hosts.

Pathogenesis: Granulomas form around dead larvae. Granulomas in the retina can cause blindness.

Laboratory Diagnosis: Larvae visible in tissue. Serologic tests useful.

Treatment: Diethylcarbamazine.

Prevention: Dogs should be dewormed.

Wuchereria bancrofti

Disease: Filariasis.

Characteristics: Tissue nematodes. Life cycle: Bite of female mosquito deposits infective larvae that penetrate bite wound, form adults, and produce microfilariae. These circulate in the blood, chiefly at night, and are ingested by mosquitoes, in which the infective larvae are formed.

Transmission and Epidemiology: Transmitted by female mosquitoes of several genera, especially *Anopheles* and *Culex,* depending on geography. Humans are the only definitive hosts. Endemic in many tropical areas.

Pathogenesis: Adult worms cause inflammation that blocks lymphatic vessels (elephantiasis). Chronic, repeated infection required for symptoms to occur.

Laboratory Diagnosis: Microfilariae visible on blood smear.

Treatment: Diethylcarbamazine affects microfilariae. No treatment for adult worms.

Prevention: Mosquito control.

Part IX: Clinical Cases

These 10 cases illustrate the importance of microbiology to the practice of medicine. In each case, questions are asked at a specific point to stimulate your thinking. Answers to the questions are provided at the end of each case.

CASE 1

Chief Complaint
A 21-year-old man in shock with a temperature of 41 °C.

History
The patient was well until 3 days ago, when mild frontal headaches began. On the morning of admission he felt very hot and had a shaking chill. That afternoon he became confused and fainted, at which time he was brought to the hospital.

Physical Exam
T 41 °C, BP 70/30, P 140, R 24. The patient was intermittently alert.
Pertinent findings include:
Skin: Several ecchymoses on the trunk and bleeding from the nose and mouth.
Neck: Supple. No signs of meningeal irritation.
Lungs: Clear.
Heart: No murmur.
Abdomen: Negative except for surgical scar in left upper quadrant, indicating a splenectomy.
Neurologic: No localizing signs.

Laboratory
Blood: Hematocrit 22%; WBC 2800; differential 15% bands, 60% polys, 22% lymphs, 3% eos; platelets 20,000.
Urine: 2+ protein, occasional WBC and RBC.
Chest x-ray: Lungs and heart normal.

Course
Four hours after admission, the patient became comatose and his blood pressure continued to fall despite antibiotics, transfusions, and blood pressure support with dopamine. Cardiac arrest occurred 2 hours later, cardiopulmonary resuscitation efforts failed, and the patient died. No autopsy was performed.

Comment
This is a case of septic shock, a medical emergency. It is typified by the abrupt onset of fever and hypotension. The shaking chill suggests bacteremia. The rapid downhill course is compatible with bacterial infection, especially by "encapsulated pyogens" (see below) or enteric gram-negative rods.

Questions
1. What is the most important specimen to obtain to make a microbiologic diagnosis?
2. Which three organisms are most likely to cause sepsis in this patient?
3. How would you distinguish among these three in the laboratory?
4. What is the main predisposing factor to infection in this patient?

Laboratory Results
Gram-positive, lancet-shaped diplococci were seen in the blood culture. Subculture to blood agar revealed small, translucent, alpha-hemolytic colonies that were bile-soluble and inhibited by optochin.

A quellung test with Omni-serum, which contains antibodies against 83 types of pneumococci, was positive.

Diagnosis

Sepsis due to *Streptococcus pneumoniae*.

Questions

5. What is the source of the patient's bacteremia?
6. Why was the patient bleeding into the skin (ecchymoses) and from the nose and mouth?
7. How could this infection have been prevented?
8. Which drugs would you have given this patient shortly after his arrival at the hospital?
9. Is drug resistance a problem with *S pneumoniae?*
10. What is the mode of action of the drugs you would use?
11. What are the serious side effects of these drugs?

Answers to Questions

1. Blood culture. One should be obtained before empirical therapy is started. Three blood cultures are recommended to ensure a 95% probability of isolating the organism.
2. The three major encapsulated pyogens cause 75% of septic shock cases in asplenic patients, ie, pneumococci (50%), meningococci (15%), and *Haemophilus influenzae* (10%). (*H influenzae* sepsis occurs primarily in children.) Other important agents include *Escherichia coli* and *Staphylococcus aureus.*
3. **(a)** Gram stain: Pneumococci are gram-positive, lancet-shaped diplococci; meningococci are gram-negative, kidney bean-shaped diplococci, and *H influenzae* are small, coccobacillary gram-negative rods.
   (b) Culture: *H influenzae* requires X and V factors; meningococci are oxidase-positive, whereas pneumococci are inhibited by bile and optochin.
   (c) Quellung reaction: Antibody causes the capsules of pneumococci and meningococci to swell. The organism can be identified with specific antibody, and the serotype can be determined.
4. Splenectomy increases the risk of septic shock 100-fold. The spleen is an important filter for bacteria in the blood as well as a source of antibody. The patient's spleen was removed 10 years before as treatment for his hereditary spherocytosis.
5. Pneumococci are commonly part of the normal flora of the nasopharynx. From there they can enter the bloodstream. Pneumonia can be a source of pneumococcal bacteremia, but this patient's lungs were clear and the chest x-ray was normal. Pneumococci are acquired by respiratory aerosol, and they colonize the nasopharynx.
6. Disseminated intravascular coagulation (DIC) can accompany septic shock. DIC consumes clotting factors, and bleeding results. DIC is usually associated with endotoxin, ie, with gram-negative organisms. Teichoic acids of gram-positive organisms also can activate complement, leading to platelet aggregation and leaky capillaries.
7. Pneumococcal vaccine should be given to all patients who have had a splenectomy. It contains the capsular polysaccharide of the 23 types that most commonly cause bacteremia. Meningococcal vaccine, which contains the capsular polysaccharides of four common types, can also be given. A vaccine against *H influenzae* type b is available as well. In splenectomized children, daily oral penicillin is used to prevent pneumococcal infection.
8. In view of the severity of the patient's illness, bactericidal drugs given intravenously were indicated. The choice of drugs was governed by the organisms most likely to be involved. He was treated with ampicillin, gentamicin, chloramphenicol, and nafcillin. Pneumococci and meningococci are susceptible to penicillins. Many enteric gram-negative rods are susceptible to aminoglycosides, and enterococci are killed by a combination of penicillin and aminoglycosides. Chloramphenicol affects many organisms, including ampicillin-resistant *H influenzae*. Nafcillin was added to cover *S aureus*. (*Note:* Other regimens are also useful. A combination of penicillin, cefuroxime, and gentamicin is another common choice.)
9. Most pneumococci are susceptible to penicillin G. There is low-level resistance in some strains, but these are easily treatable with high doses of penicillin. Highly resistant strains are uncommon; ie, they are about 1% of all isolates in United States. Vancomycin is the drug of choice for these strains. Meningococci are also susceptible to penicillin G. About 25% of *H influenzae* isolates are resistant to ampicillin because they carry plasmid-mediated β-lactamase. Almost all of these isolates are susceptible to chloramphenicol.

10. Penicillins prevent cell wall synthesis by inhibiting transpeptidation. Aminoglycosides inhibit protein synthesis by binding to the 30S ribosomal subunit and preventing the formation of polysomes; ie, monosomes accumulate. Chloramphenicol blocks protein synthesis by inhibiting peptidyltransferase.
11. Penicillins cause anaphylaxis and serum sickness. Aminoglycosides affect the kidneys. Chloramphenicol depresses the bone marrow and, rarely, causes aplastic anemia.

CASE 2

Chief Complaint
A 4-year-old boy with diarrhea for 2 days.

History
His mother said he was well until 2 days ago, when he stopped eating and felt feverish. He then developed abdominal pain and nonbloody diarrhea, which became progressively more severe. No vomiting or shaking chills occurred. There was no history of recent antibiotic use or travel outside San Francisco. No one else in the family was ill.

Physical Exam
T 38 °C, BP 120/70, P 100, R 16. The patient was an acutely ill child, appearing flushed and dehydrated. The only abnormal finding was diffuse abdominal tenderness without rebound.

Laboratory
Blood: Hematocrit 38%; WBC 10,000 with normal differential.
Urine: Normal.

Comment
Diarrhea typically is due either to enterotoxins or to bacterial invasion of the bowel wall. It is important to determine which mechanism is occurring, because that information is helpful in determining the diagnosis and treatment.

Questions
1. Which test should be done on the stool immediately that can provide evidence of whether the diarrhea is toxigenic or invasive (inflammatory)?
2. What are the possible organisms that can cause diarrhea in this patient?
3. If this had occurred in a developing country rather than in the United States, which other important bacterium should be considered?
4. Do the organisms you thought of in answer to questions 2 and 3 cause toxigenic or inflammatory diarrhea?
5. What is the most important specimen to obtain to make a microbiologic diagnosis?

Course
A stain for fecal leukocytes revealed many polymorphonuclear leukocytes (PMNs). The stool was positive for occult blood.

Question
6. In view of these findings, which three organisms are most likely to be the cause of this child's diarrhea?

Course
At this point, a clinical assessment should be made to determine the empirical treatment, ie, what to do until the results of the cultures are known. The mainstay of treatment is fluid replacement, eg, with a solution containing sodium, potassium, and glucose. Antimotility agents are best avoided, because they reduce the natural purgative effect and tend to prolong the excretion of organisms.

A rectal swab was taken for culture; the patient's mother was given advice regarding oral hydration, and the patient was sent home.

Culture of the stool revealed lactose-negative colonies on eosin-methylene blue (EMB) agar. Triple sugar iron agar showed an alkaline slant, acid butt, and no H_2S. The urease test was negative.

Question

7. On the basis of these findings, which genus of organisms has most probably been isolated?

Course

An agglutination test with antiserum to the O antigen of *Shigella* and *Salmonella* was performed to identify the organism. Agglutination was observed with *Shigella* group B antiserum, indicating that the organism was *Shigella flexneri*. The identification was confirmed by using an API strip, which contains 20 biochemical reactions.

The patient's mother was contacted, and the results of the culture were discussed with her. She reported that her child's diarrhea was almost gone and he was feeling well.

Questions

8. What is the natural habitat of the organism?
9. As the family was well, where was the organism likely to have come from?
10. If treatment were indicated, which drugs would you give?
11. Is there a prolonged carrier state associated with this infection?
12. Can shigellosis be prevented?

Answers to Questions

1. Stain for fecal leukocytes. Test for occult blood also.
2. Likely organisms: *Escherichia coli, Clostridium perfringens, Bacillus cereus, Staphylococcus aureus* (but less likely in this case since no vomiting occurred), *Shigella, Salmonella, Campylobacter.* Less likely: *Yersinia enterocolitica, Vibrio parahaemolyticus;* viruses such as rotavirus and Norwalk virus; parasites such as *Entamoeba histolytica* and *Giardia lamblia.*
3. *Vibrio cholerae.*
4. Known toxin producers: *V cholerae, S aureus, B cereus, C perfringens,* strains of *E coli.* Known inflammatory agents: *Shigella, Salmonella, Campylobacter,* strains of *E coli, Y enterocolitica.* Uncertain: *E histolytica, G lamblia, V parahaemolyticus.*
5. Stool culture. A blood culture would not be done, because there were no signs of sepsis, eg, no shaking chill, normal blood pressure. An examination for ova and parasites would not be done at this stage unless there were a specific indication, eg, travel.
6. *Shigella, Salmonella,* and *Campylobacter.*
7. *Shigella.*
8. Human gastrointestinal tract. There is no animal reservoir for shigellae, in contrast to many *Salmonella* species.
9. His playmates, perhaps at the day-care center.
10. Either trimethoprim-sulfamethoxazole or ampicillin can be given. Because strains can be resistant, sensitivity test should be done.
11. Shigellosis is typically a self-limited disease with few or no sequelae. There is no prolonged carrier state, unlike for some *Salmonella* infections, eg, *Salmonella typhi* infections.
12. Shigellosis can be prevented by public health measures, eg, hand-washing prior to food handling, and by treatment of sewage. However, prevention is difficult in young children because their personal cleanliness and bowel habits are less than perfect. There is no vaccine. Prophylactic antibiotics are not used.

CASE 3

Chief Complaint

A 10-year-old girl with leukemia who has had a fever for 2 days.

History

The patient was well until 1 year ago, when the diagnosis of acute leukemia was made. She was treated with chemotherapy, and remission occurred. One month prior to admission, increasing fatigue and weight loss were noted and a bone marrow revealed 50% blast forms. Chemotherapy, including steroids, was instituted. Two days ago her temperature rose to 39 °C without specific localizing symptoms.

Physical Exam

T 39 °C, BP 100/60, P 100, R 20. The patient appeared thin and chronically ill.

Pertinent findings include:

Skin: Pale with several ecchymoses. No petechiae or jaundice.

Head and neck: Normal

Lungs: Clear.

Heart: No murmurs.

Abdomen: No tenderness, masses, or organomegaly.

Lymph nodes: Not enlarged.

Neurologic: Normal.

Laboratory

Blood: Hematocrit 20%; WBC 600; differential 10% bands, 30% polys, 55% lymphs, 5% monos; platelets 26,000.

Urine: Normal.

Chest x-ray: Normal.

Comment

Fever in an immunocompromised (neutropenic) host is commonly caused by infection. Because infection is the leading cause of death in these patients, it is important that treatment be instituted immediately, before the culture results are ready. Immunocompromised patients with infections frequently have muted signs and symptoms because they are less capable of mounting an inflammatory response.

Questions

1. What are the common bacteria, viruses, and fungi to cause infection in a neutropenic patient?
2. What empirical therapy would you start prior to receipt of the culture results?
3. Which specimens would you obtain for culture?

Course

The patient was treated with ticarcillin, nafcillin, and tobramycin intravenously. She remained febrile during the next 48 hours, and all cultures showed no growth. The following day, the patient complained of pain in her left eye and blurred vision. Funduscopy revealed a white, cottony lesion in the perimacular region. She also complained of a sore throat, and inspection revealed several whitish, adherent plaques on the posterior pharynx.

Question

4. In view of these findings, what is the likely genus of the pathogen?

Course

Amphotericin B was started. On day 4, the blood cultures revealed oval, gram-positive organisms without capsules. They were 2–3 times larger than staphylococci. Some of the cells were budding.

Questions

5. Which genus of organism was recovered from the blood culture?
6. How would you distinguish among various species of organisms in this genus?
7. What is the natural habitat of this organism?
8. What is the mode of action of amphotericin B?
9. What is the major site of toxicity with amphotericin B?
10. Could this infection have been prevented?

Course

Two days later, the patient developed a right hemiparesis; she died the following day. Autopsy revealed a massive cerebral infarct and invasive *Candida* esophagitis. The esophageal site was thought to be the origin of the fungemia.

Answers to Questions

1. The opportunistic pathogens commonly seen in neutropenic patients are as follows:
   (a) Bacteria: Staphylococci, eg, *Staphylococcus aureus* and *Staphylococcus epidermidis;* gram-negative rods, eg, *Escherichia coli, Klebsiella pneumoniae,* and *Pseudomonas aeruginosa.*

(b) Viruses: Herpesviruses, eg, herpes simplex virus type 1, cytomegalovirus, and varicella-zoster virus.

(c) Fungi: *Candida albicans, Aspergillus fumigatus,* and *Mucor* and *Rhizopus* species.

2. Combination therapy of bactericidal drugs is commonly used, eg, ticarcillin and tobramycin, which are effective against many of the common bacterial pathogens. Nafcillin can be added for the β-lactamase-producing *S aureus.* Trimethoprim-sulfamethoxazole is also used to cover several types of bacteria and *Pneumocystis.* Because of the toxic side effects of amphotericin B, antifungal therapy is not typically part of the initial empirical therapy.

3. Blood, urine, and stool plus specific sites of symptoms, if any. Cultures should be taken before antibiotics are started.

4. *Candida* species, such as *C albicans* and *C tropicalis,* since (a) there was no response to antibiotics, (b) no bacteria grew on culture, (c) cottony exudates in the retina are typical of *Candida,* and (d) the throat lesions resemble thrush.

5. The description best fits a species of *Candida.*

6. *C albicans* produces germ tubes, whereas almost all other *Candida* species do not. Biochemical tests, eg, sugar assimilation tests, can also be used.

7. *C albicans* is part of the normal human flora on the skin and in the mouth, gastrointestinal tract, and vagina.

8. It disrupts fungal cell membranes. Its selective toxicity is based on its binding to ergosterol in the fungal membranes but not to the cholesterol in human cell membranes.

9. The kidneys. Serum creatinine levels should be monitored.

10. No preventive measures for candidal infections have been shown to be effective. Trimethoprim-sulfamethoxazole is given to patients with defective cell-mediated immunity to prevent *Pneumocystis* pneumonia.

CASE 4

Chief Complaint

A 26-year-old woman with lower abdominal pain for 3 days.

History

The patient was well until 3 days ago, when malaise, anorexia, and mild, crampy, left-lower-quadrant pain began. The symptoms intensified during the last 24 hours. She now feels feverish and has vomited twice, and her pain is moderately severe. No shaking chill, diarrhea, dysuria, or hematuria has occurred. She has noticed an increased amount of yellowish vaginal discharge. The discharge is non-bloody and has no odor. Her last menstrual period ended 3 days ago.

Physical Exam

T 39 °C, BP 120/80, P 96, R 14.
  Pertinent physical findings include:
  Abdomen: Left-lower-quadrant tenderness without rebound. No masses or organomegaly. Bowel sounds normal. No costovertebral-angle tenderness.
  Pelvis: Introitus and vagina: Normal.
  Cervix: Inflamed with a small amount of purulent discharge at os; motion tenderness elicited.
  Uterus: Normal size; no tenderness or masses.
  Adnexae: Very tender on left. No masses felt.

Laboratory

  Blood: Hematocrit 40%; WBC 17,400; differential 12% bands, 65% polys, 20% lymphs, 3% monos.
  Urine: Normal.
  Abdominal x-ray: No distended bowel loops.

Comment

This is a case of pelvic inflammatory disease (acute salpingitis and cervicitis). Because infertility can result, prompt and appropriate treatment is important. A clinical judgment must be made whether to hospitalize patients with pelvic inflammatory disease; this depends on, eg, the severity of the illness and the reliability of the patient to follow an outpatient regimen. This patient was hospitalized.

Questions
1. Which organisms are most likely to cause this infection?
2. Which specimen(s) would you obtain for culture?
3. Knowing the organisms that might be involved, what empirical antibiotic therapy would you suggest? (There are several alternatives.)

Course
Culdocentesis yielded 20 mL of bloody, foul-smelling, purulent fluid, which was sent for aerobic and anaerobic culture. Gram stain of the fluid revealed gram-negative diplococci and gram-negative rods.

The patient was started on cefoxitin and doxycycline intravenously. Within 24 hours, her pain was significantly diminished and her temperature dropped to 37.5 °C.

Aerobic cultures revealed oxidase-positive colonies on Thayer-Martin medium that were gram-negative diplococci microscopically. Anaerobic cultures grew numerous, similar-appearing colonies consisting of gram-negative rods.

Questions
4. What is the most likely organism isolated in the aerobic cultures?
5. Which genus of anaerobic organisms seems likely?

Course
Subsequent laboratory tests confirmed the presence of two organisms, *Neisseria gonorrhoeae* and *Bacteroides fragilis*. The patient's signs and symptoms resolved by 48 hours, and both antibiotics were continued for an additional 48 hours. She was discharged to continue taking doxycycline orally for the next 10 days.

Questions
6. Since syphilis can be acquired at the same time as gonorrhea, how would you test for this disease?
7. How would you prevent gonorrhea from spreading to others?
8. What is the mode of action of cefoxitin and of doxycycline?
9. Is antibiotic resistance a clinical concern with *N gonorrhoeae* and *B fragilis*?

Answers to Questions
1. *N gonorrhoeae* is the most common cause. Mixed infections, with or without gonococci, are frequent. Other organisms isolated include *Escherichia coli,* enterococci, and various anaerobes, eg, peptostreptococci and *B fragilis. Chlamydia trachomatis* can also be involved.
2. Culture of pus from the cervix should be done. In addition, culdocentesis (aspiration of fluid from the "cul-de-sac" behind the cervix) is an important diagnostic procedure. If fluid is obtained, it should be cultured.
3. One suggested regimen for hospitalized patients includes cefoxitin (a cephalosporin effective against gonococci, including penicillinase-producing strains, and against anaerobes) and doxycycline (a tetracycline effective against *C trachomatis* and various enteric gram-negative rods, eg, *E coli*). For other regimens, see the *Sexually Transmitted Disease Guidelines* published by the Centers for Disease Control and Prevention or an infectious-disease text.
4. *N gonorrhoeae.*
5. *Bacteroides* species, eg, *B fragilis,* or *Fusobacterium* species.
6. VDRL. The VDRL test is nonspecific. Therefore, if it is positive, it should be confirmed with a specific treponemal test, eg, the fluorescent treponemal antibody-absorption (FTA-ABS) test. If VDRL is negative, consider repeating it in 2 weeks.
7. Sexual contacts should be traced and treated. Also, cultures from the patient should be performed, either upon discharge from the hospital or a few days thereafter.
8. Cefoxitin, a cephalosporin, inhibits peptidoglycan synthesis by blocking transpeptidation. Doxycycline, a tetracycline, inhibits protein synthesis at the level of the 30S ribosomal subunit.
9. Some strains of gonococci produce penicillinase, which renders many penicillins ineffective. Some strains of *B fragilis* produce penicillinase also. Antibiotic susceptibility testing should be performed with both organisms.

CASE 5

Chief Complaint
A 52-year-old man with a cough for the past 3 days.

History
The patient was in his usual state of health until 3 days ago, when fever and a cough began abruptly, accompanied by anorexia and a severe frontal headache. The cough is productive of a small amount of whitish, nonbloody sputum. No chest pain or myalgias occurred. A shaking chill accompanied by sweating occurred yesterday. Mild, nonbloody diarrhea without nausea or vomiting began yesterday also.

The patient is a clerk at a supermarket. His medical history is significant for a kidney transplant 2 years ago. To prevent rejection, he takes azathioprine and prednisone. His smoking and drinking habits include two packs of cigarettes and a six-pack of beer per day—more on weekends. His wife and children are well. He has no pets and no history of recent travel.

Physical Exam
T 40 °C, BP 130/70, P 96, R 24. The patient was an acutely ill man, appearing flushed and short of breath.
Pertinent findings include:
Eyes, ears, and throat: Normal. No sinus tenderness.
Neck: Supple.
Lungs: Inspiratory rales heard over left posterior lung. No dullness to percussion.
Heart: Normal
Abdomen: Normal.
Neurologic: Normal.

Laboratory
Blood: Hematocrit 46%; WBC 18,000; differential 9% bands, 77% polys, 12% lymph, 2% eos.
Urine: No sugar, 1+ protein, 10 RBC/HPF,* 2 WBC/HPF.
Chest x-ray: Segmental infiltrate in left lower lobe.

Questions
1. What are the two important specimens to obtain to make a microbiologic diagnosis?
2. Which procedure should you do with one of the specimens as soon as possible that might provide information regarding the cause of this disease?

Course
A sputum specimen was obtained for Gram stain and culture. The Gram stain revealed many polys but no predominant organism. Few gram-positive and gram-negative cocci were seen. A blood culture was taken.

Comment
The clinical presentation suggests atypical pneumonia; there is scant, nonpurulent sputum, and a Gram stain shows polys but no organisms.

Questions
3. What are some of the causes of atypical pneumonia?
4. Patients who take azathioprine and prednisone have reduced immunity. Which organisms typically cause pneumonia in immunocompromised adults?

Comment
The following findings are in accord with a diagnosis of *Legionella* pneumonia: (1) a middle-aged man who smokes and drinks; (2) an immunocompromised patient; (3) multisystem involvement as indicated by headache, diarrhea, and microscopic hematuria; and (4) no predominant organism on Gram stain.

---

* HPF = high-power field.

Course

In view of the suggestive findings described above, examination of the sputum with fluorescent antibody to *Legionella pneumophila* was performed and was positive.

Questions

5. What is the treatment of choice for *Legionella* pneumonia?
6. What is the mechanism of action of this drug?
7. What is the natural habitat of this organism?
8. Can the organism be cultured in the laboratory?
9. In addition to fluorescent-antibody staining of sputum and culturing on special agar, what is another method for making the diagnosis of *Legionella* pneumonia?
10. Why was the organism not seen in the Gram-stained smear?

Course

The patient was treated with erythromycin intravenously for 7 days and then with oral erythromycin for an additional 2 weeks. He rapidly defervesced within 24 hours, and his cough resolved gradually during the following week.

Answers to Questions

1. Sputum and blood.
2. Gram-stained smear of sputum.
3. *Mycoplasma pneumoniae* is the most common cause. However, *Legionella pneumophila*, *Chlamydia pneumoniae*, *Chlamydia psittaci* (psittacosis), and viruses, eg, influenza virus, also cause this clinical picture.
4. **(a)** Bacteria: Most are gram-negative rods, eg, *Klebsiella, Pseudomonas,* and *Legionella. Staphylococcus aureus* is important also.
   (b) Viruses: Cytomegalovirus, herpes simplex virus type 1, varicella-zoster virus.
   (c) Fungi: *Candida, Aspergillus.*
   (d) Parasites: *Pneumocystis, Strongyloides.*
5. Erythromycin.
6. It inhibits bacterial protein synthesis at the level of the 50S ribosomal subunit.
7. Environmental water sources, eg, air-conditioning units, hospital water taps, and bodies of water such as lakes.
8. Yes, on special agar high in iron and cysteine, but cultures are not commonly done.
9. A greater than 4-fold rise in antibody titer to *Legionella* between the acute- and convalescent-phase sera detected by indirect immunofluorescence.
10. Although it has a gram-negative cell wall, it stains poorly by the standard Gram stain procedure. The reason for this is unknown.

CASE 6

Chief Complaint

A 30-year-old woman with nausea and vomiting for 3 days.

History

The patient was well until 1 week ago, when she noted some stiffness and swelling in the fingers of both hands; this lasted a few days. Four days ago, malaise, fatigue, and anorexia began, followed the next day by nausea and vomiting, which have continued to the present. No hematemesis or diarrhea has occurred. Upper abdominal aching began yesterday. The smell of food induces nausea. She noticed that her urine was darker than usual today.

She is a waitress who smokes two packs of cigarettes and drinks a six-pack of beer per day. She has had five sex partners in the last 3 months. No recent travel, transfusions, or intravenous drug abuse. No one else she knows has similar symptoms.

Physical Exam

T 37 °C, BP 130/80, P 80, R 12.
   Pertinent findings include:
   Skin: No jaundice, petechiae, or spider angiomas.

Eyes: Sclerae were icteric.
Abdomen: Punch tenderness elicited in right upper quadrant. Tender liver edge palpable 4 cm below costal margin. Spleen not palpable. No masses. Abdomen not distended. Bowel sounds normal.
Pelvic: Within normal limits.
Rectal: Stool light color. Occult blood negative.

Laboratory

Blood: Hematocrit 40%; WBC 8200; differential 50% polys, 45% lymphs, 5% monos.
Urine: Normal, except that bilirubin test was positive.
Chemistry: Total bilirubin 4 mg (direct 3 mg; indirect 1 mg); alanine aminotransferase 600 mg%; alkaline phosphatase 100 mg%; electrolytes within normal limits.
Abdominal x-ray: Within normal limits.

Comment

This case is typical of viral hepatitis. Many viruses can infect the liver. It is important to determine the specific cause, because there are both personal and public health implications with some agents, eg, hepatitis B virus.

Questions

1. Which viruses should be considered possible causes of this patient's disease?
2. Which tests would you order to determine the virus that caused this disease?

Course

The results of the serologic tests were as follows: IgM HAV antibody, negative; HBV surface antigen, positive; IgM HBV core antibody, positive; HBV surface antibody, negative.

Questions

3. In view of these results, which disease does the patient have?
4. If a different jaundiced patient's test results were IgM HAV antibody negative, HBV surface antigen negative, IgM HBV core antibody positive, and HBV surface antibody negative, what would your interpretation be?
5. If a different jaundiced patient's test results were IgM HAV antibody negative, HBV surface antigen negative, IgM HBV core antibody negative, and HBV surface antibody positive, what would your interpretation be?
6. What is your explanation for the arthralgias described at the beginning of the history?
7. What specific antiviral therapy, if any, is available for hepatitis B?
8. How did she acquire this disease?

Course

The patient's symptoms intensified during the next 3 days and then gradually resolved over the next 2 weeks; the serum bilirubin declined to normal. However, the patient's HBV surface antigen remained positive at 3, 6, and 12 months after discharge and no HBV surface antibody was detectable.

Questions

9. What is your interpretation of these HBV surface antigen results?
10. What is the best laboratory test to determine whether she is likely to transmit HBV to others?
11. What would you advise this patient regarding (a) donating blood, (b) dental surgery and other operations, (c) protecting her newborn child if she becomes pregnant, (d) sharing a toothbrush, (e) sexual activity, (f) problems with chronic liver disease, (g) possibility of carcinoma of the liver, and (h) effect of infection with hepatitis delta virus?

Answers to Questions

1. Hepatitis A and B viruses; non-A, non-B (NANB) viruses, especially hepatitis C and hepatitis D (delta) viruses. Also Epstein-Barr virus and cytomegalovirus. Yellow fever virus can infect the liver, but this patient had not traveled to an endemic area.
2. Four serologic tests are typically ordered: (a) IgM antibody to HAV, (b) IgM antibody to HBV core antigen, (c) HBV surface antigen, and (d) HBV surface antibody. At this stage, the test for antibody to HCV would not be ordered because there is no test for IgM antibody and IgG is detectable only several months after infection.

3. Acute hepatitis B.
4. Acute hepatitis B. During the "window" phase, the surface antigen and surface antibody are negative; only the core antibody is positive. The positive IgM result indicates recent infection.
5. This patient had hepatitis B in the past and is now immune. The patient is not a chronic carrier; surface antigen is negative. Because neither hepatitis A nor hepatitis B was demonstrated by the serologic tests, it is likely that the patient has NANB hepatitis (or some other viral hepatitis). A test for antibody to HCV should be done.
6. Arthralgias are common during the prodromal period of hepatitis B. They are probably due to HBV-antibody immune complexes deposited in the joints.
7. There are no antiviral drugs for hepatitis B. Only supportive therapy is available. Immune globulins are not used for treatment, only for prevention.
8. Because she has no history of either blood transfusions or intravenous drug abuse, it is probable that the virus was acquired sexually.
9. The patient is a chronic carrier of HBV.
10. Serologic test for e antigen. This is the best indicator of the presence of infectious HBV in the blood. No direct assay for infectious virus is presently available.
11. (a) Do not donate blood.
    (b) Advise your dentist and all medical personnel that you are HBV surface antigen-positive.
    (c) The newborn should be actively immunized with the hepatitis B vaccine and passively immunized with hepatitis B immune globulins.
    (d) Do not share toothbrushes or other personal articles that may contact blood, eg, razors.
    (e) Sex partners should be immunized with hepatitis B vaccine.
    (f) Chronic active hepatitis may result.
    (g) A higher incidence of carcinoma of the liver occurs in chronic carriers.
    (h) Patients infected with HBV who are superinfected with hepatitis delta virus can experience a severe form of hepatitis.

CASE 7

Chief Complaint
A 20-year-old man with a cough of several weeks' duration.

History
The patient is a recent immigrant from Southeast Asia who noted the gradual onset of tiredness and loss of appetite about 1 month ago. A week or so later, he felt feverish and the cough began. At first the cough was nonproductive, but for the past week he has brought up several tablespoons per day of greenish sputum that is streaked with blood. He has lost 10 lb during the past month. He is a nonsmoker and has had no exposure to industrial respiratory pollutants.

Physical Exam
T 38 °C, BP 124/70, P 80, R 16. The patient did not appear acutely ill.
Pertinent findings include:
Lungs: Rales heard in right upper lobe. No dullness to percussion.
Heart: Normal.
Abdomen: Normal.
Lymph nodes: Not enlarged.

Laboratory
Blood: Hematocrit 38; WBC 11,000; Differential 3% bands, 63% polys, 30% lymphs, 4% monos.
Urine: Normal.
Chest x-ray: Infiltrate in posterior segment of right upper lobe with suggestion of a cavity.

Question
1. Which two procedures should you do with the sputum that could provide immediate information regarding the organism causing the illness?

Course
Gram stain of the sputum revealed mixed flora with no predominant organism. The acid-fast stain showed numerous long, slender, pink rods. A sputum specimen was sent for culture.

Questions

2. In view of these results, what is the most likely diagnosis?
3. What is the treatment of choice for this disease?
4. Is antibiotic resistance a problem?
5. Approximately how long after the start of treatment is the patient considered to be infectious for others?
6. How is the organism transmitted?
7. What is the natural habitat of the organism?
8. Why is the organism acid-fast?
9. Can the organism be cultured in the laboratory?
10. What is the role of serologic tests in making the diagnosis of tuberculosis?
11. What should be done for the members of his family?
12. What is the immunologic basis for a positive skin test?
13. Can atypical mycobacteria, eg, *Mycobacterium kansasii* and *Mycobacterium avium-intracellulare,* cause a similar clinical picture?

Course

The patient was hospitalized because there was doubt about whether he would reliably take the antitubercular drugs. He was treated with isoniazid (INH), rifampin, pyrazinamide, and ethambutol, and his symptoms abated. Routine sputum cultures were negative. After 2 weeks, he was discharged to return to the clinic for follow-up cultures and chest x-rays 1 month later. Four weeks after they were taken, his cultures were reported positive for *Mycobacterium tuberculosis.* Drug susceptibility tests subsequently reported the isolate to be sensitive to INH. After 2 months of treatment, pyrazinamide and ethambutol were discontinued. INH and rifampin were continued for a total of 6 months. Follow-up cultures were negative, and chest x-rays showed resolution of the lesions.

Answers to Questions

1. Gram stain and acid-fast stain.
2. Tuberculosis.
3. Multiple-drug therapy for 6–9 months is the accepted mode of treatment. Isoniazid (INH) is bactericidal and is the mainstay of treatment. It is frequently combined with rifampin and either pyrazinamide or ethambutol or both.
4. Southeast Asians have a high rate of infection with INH-resistant strains of *M tuberculosis.* Therapy with four drugs, ie, INH, rifampin, pyrazinamide, and ethambutol, should be used if INH resistance is suspected.
5. Approximately 2–3 weeks, but treatment must continue for at least 6–9 months to avoid recurrences.
6. Transmitted by inhalation of aerosolized organisms from expectorated sputum.
7. Human lungs.
8. The high concentration of lipid makes mycobacteria acid-fast. These lipids prevent the dyes used in the Gram stain from penetrating; hence, they stain poorly on a Gram-stained smear.
9. Yes, on special media, eg, Löwenstein-Jensen medium. It is very slow-growing, so cultures should be held for at least 6 weeks. It will not grow on blood agar.
10. There are no serologic tests for tuberculosis.
11. If they are asymptomatic, they should be skin-tested with PPD. If positive, they should be given INH. If they are symptomatic, they should be investigated for tuberculosis by sputum cultures.
12. Cell-mediated immune response to the *M tuberculosis* proteins in PPD. This response forms an indurated area at least 10 mm in diameter in the skin.
13. Yes. The clinical picture can be indistinguishable, so cultures must be done. Atypical mycobacteria are frequently more resistant to drugs than is *M tuberculosis.*

CASE 8

Chief Complaint

An 18-year-old woman with a sore throat for the last 3 days.

History

The patient was well until 3 days ago, when she experienced the gradual onset of malaise, anorexia, and mild sore throat. The symptoms have intensified, and she now feels that her throat is "on fire."

At present she is feverish, has a frontal headache, and has completely lost her interest in food. She received DPT vaccine as a child.

Physical Exam
T 39 °C, BP 126/70, P 92, R 18. The patient appeared acutely ill.
  Pertinent findings include:
  Skin: No rash or jaundice.
  Throat: Intensely red and swollen; yellowish exudate on left tonsil. No adherent membrane on pharynx.
  Neck: Several tender, enlarged lymph nodes. No signs of meningeal irritation.
  Chest: Clear.
  Heart: Normal.
  Abdomen: Not distended. No tenderness. Tender liver edge felt 2 cm below costal margin. Spleen tip palpable. Bowel sounds normal.
  Neurologic: Normal.

Laboratory
  Blood: Hematocrit 39%; WBC 14,000; Differential: 52% polys, 45% lymphs, 3% monos; platelets 100,000.
  Urine: Normal.
  Chest x-ray: Normal.

Questions
  1. What is your differential diagnosis?
  2. Which laboratory tests would you order to make a microbiologic diagnosis?

Course
She was admitted to the college infirmary. The following day, a throat culture revealed alpha-hemolytic streptococci. A Monospot test was negative. Transaminases were elevated to twice normal levels. Bilirubin and alkaline phosphatase were normal. WBC 16,000. Differential: 48% polys, 50% lymphs (3% are atypical), 2% monos.

Questions
  3. In view of these laboratory findings, what is your diagnostic impression?
  4. In view of your diagnostic impression, what treatment would you prescribe?

Course
Aspirin and warm salt-water gargles were given. However, during the next 2 days her throat remained sore, swallowing was difficult, and only liquids were taken. The throat remained inflamed, and the liver and spleen were still palpable. The following day the temperature, which had reached 40 °C, dropped to 38 °C and the patient began to feel somewhat better. A repeat blood count showed WBC 15,000 with 45% polys, 53% lymphs (15% are atypical), and 2% monos. The Monospot test was positive.

Comment
This is a typical case of infectious mononucleosis with the cardinal findings of fever, pharyngitis, and cervical lymphadenopathy. Hepatosplenomegaly is common. Laboratory findings include a lymphocytosis with atypical cells and a positive heterophil antibody test. Both the atypical cells and heterophil antibody can appear several days after the patient presents.

Questions
  5. How is this infection transmitted?
  6. Is EBV infection common in the United States?
  7. In which age group is infectious mononucleosis common?
  8. What are heterophil antibodies?
  9. Should you try to make the diagnosis of infectious mononucleosis by recovering EBV in cell culture?
  10. Can infectious mononucleosis be contracted more than once?
  11. Is there a vaccine or drug for the prevention of infectious mononucleosis?

Answers to Questions

1. This clinical picture is typical of infectious mononucleosis caused by Epstein-Barr virus (EBV). However, other viruses, such as herpes simplex virus, coxsackieviruses, and adenoviruses, also cause pharyngitis, as do certain bacteria, eg, *Streptococcus pyogenes* and *Neisseria gonorrhoeae.* Cytomegalovirus and *Toxoplasma gondii* can cause a mononucleosislike picture but typically without a prominent pharyngitis. Viral hepatitis also can manifest with many of this patient's features but is not associated with pharyngitis. Diphtheria is highly unlikely, because the patient was immunized and this disease is rare in the United States.

2. Throat culture for *S pyogenes* and a heterophil antibody test (Monospot test).

3. Streptococcal pharyngitis can be ruled out; only alpha-hemolytic colonies were found on throat culture. The heterophil test can be negative early in infectious mononucleosis. The liver function tests and the finding of several atypical lymphs support the diagnosis of infectious mononucleosis.

4. The treatment for infectious mononucleosis is supportive. There is no antiviral therapy. Acyclovir, which is effective against certain other herpesviruses, namely herpes simplex virus types 1 and 2 and varicella-zoster virus, is not effective against EBV.

5. EBV is present in saliva. Transmission between young adults is primarily by kissing. EBV infects oropharyngeal cells, causing the pharyngitis.

6. Yes. Over 90% of adults in the United States have antibodies to EBV.

7. Infectious mononucleosis occurs primarily in young adults. EBV infection in children either is asymptomatic or results in an undifferentiated viral pharyngitis without the other concomitant symptoms of infectious mononucleosis.

8. Heterophil antibodies are agglutinins for sheep or horse red blood cells formed during EBV infection. These antibodies are not directed against any EBV antigens; they may be formed against some cellular component modified by EBV infection. Because heterophil antibodies are nonspecific, EBV infections should be confirmed by IgM antibody to viral capsid antigen in difficult-to-diagnose cases.

9. Isolation of EBV in cell culture is not used for clinical diagnosis. EBV can be cultured in the laboratory, but this test is not routinely available.

10. EBV-induced infectious mononucleosis can be contracted only once. Lifelong immunity is not due to heterophil agglutinins; those usually disappear within a few years. Antibody to viral capsid antigen persists for life, but it is unclear whether this antibody, other antibodies, or the cell-mediated response provides this immunity. Recurrences of "mononucleosis" may be due to other causes, eg, cytomegalovirus or *Toxoplasma.*

11. No vaccine or drug is available that prevents infectious mononucleosis.

CASE 9

Chief Complaint

A 1-year-old girl who had a seizure about 20 minutes ago.

History

She was well except for an upper respiratory tract infection during the past 2 days. Last night she felt feverish and became very sleepy. She was difficult to arouse this morning and then had a generalized convulsion. Her mother brought her to the emergency room immediately. Immunizations: oral polio and DPT vaccines given at 2, 4, and 6 months.

Physical Exam

T 40 °C, BP 100/70, P 120, R 16. A somnolent child who was irritable when examined.
Pertinent findings include:
Skin: No petechiae or ecchymoses.
Eyes: Pupils regular and equal. No papilledema.
Ears: Normal.
Throat: Mild inflammation. No exudate.
Neck: Marked rigidity.
Lungs: Clear.
Heart: Normal.

Abdomen: Normal.
Neurologic: Deep-tendon reflexes normal. Remainder of the exam deferred because the patient was too irritable to cooperate.

Laboratory
Blood: Hematocrit 40%; WBC 21,000; differential 16% bands, 80% polys, 4% monos.
Urine: Normal.
Chest x-ray: Normal.

Questions
1. What are the two most important specimens to obtain to make a microbiologic diagnosis?
2. Which laboratory test should be done immediately on one of the specimens that may provide information regarding the cause of this infection?
3. What is the most likely organism to cause this infection? What are two other possibilities?
4. How would you distinguish among these three organisms on Gram's stain?

Comment
This case is typical of acute bacterial meningitis, a life-threatening emergency. It demands immediate empirical therapy, which is guided by the physician's impression of what is likely to be the causative organism. The main criteria used to formulate this impression are the age of the patient; preexisting medical conditions, eg, immunocompromised state; and analysis of the spinal fluid including a Gram-stained smear, the number of white cells, and whether they are polys or lymphocytes. Spinal fluid protein and glucose are also important, but those values may take time to obtain and therapy should be initiated as soon as possible.

Course
A lumbar puncture was performed. The spinal fluid appeared cloudy, and the opening pressure was 300 mm of water. There were 2800 cells/mm^3, of which 88% were polys. The Gram stain revealed very short gram-negative rods. Specimens of spinal fluid were sent for glucose, protein, and culture. A blood culture was done, and at the same time an intravenous infusion was started and antibiotic therapy begun.

Questions
5. Which antibiotics would you begin as your empirical therapy?
6. Which immunologic test can be done on the spinal fluid that might identify the organism?

Course
Treatment with ampicillin and chloramphenicol was begun, and the patient was admitted to the hospital. The latex agglutination test on the spinal fluid was positive for *Haemophilus influenzae*. The spinal fluid protein and glucose values were 300 and 15 mg%, respectively. The following day, her temperature dropped to 38.5 °C and she was more responsive.

The microbiology laboratory reported growth of a small gram-negative rod resembling *H influenzae* in the blood culture. Spinal fluid cultures on chocolate agar (with IsoVitaleX) grew many colonies of a small gram-negative rod. There was no growth on the blood agar plate.

Questions
7. What are the growth requirements of *H influenzae* that can be used to identify the organism in the clinical laboratory?
8. Most (90%) *H influenzae* isolates causing invasive disease, eg, bacteremia and meningitis, are type b. What determines the type?

Course
The isolate from both the blood and spinal fluid cultures was identified as *H influenzae*. The disk test for β-lactamase production by the isolate was negative, and susceptibility tests showed that the organism was sensitive to ampicillin. Chloramphenicol was discontinued.

The patient continued to improve and was afebrile by 48 hours. Ampicillin was continued for 14 days. A lumbar puncture performed prior to discharge revealed almost normal values.

Questions

9. What is the natural habitat of this organism, and how is it acquired?
10. What is the role of the organism's capsular polysaccharide in causing disease?
11. Do exotoxins play a role in pathogenesis by *H influenzae?* Does the organism contain endotoxin?
12. How can *H influenzae* meningitis be prevented?

Answers to Questions

1. Blood culture and spinal fluid.
2. Gram stain of the spinal fluid.
3. *H influenzae* used to be by far the most frequent cause of meningitis in children between the ages of 6 months and 6 years. *Streptococcus pneumoniae* and *Neisseria meningitidis* are now more frequent causes at this age.
4. *H influenzae* is a short "coccobacillary" gram-negative rod. *S pneumoniae* is a gram-positive coccus in pairs or short chains. *N meningitidis* is a kidney-bean-shaped gram-negative coccus.
5. Combination therapy of ampicillin and chloramphenicol was commonly used when this case occurred. Ampicillin is effective against *H influenzae* meningitis, but approximately 25% of isolates are ampicillin-resistant as a result of β-lactamase. Chloramphenicol is added to cover these resistant organisms. When the results of susceptibility tests are known, one drug is discontinued. Ceftriaxone is now the treatment of choice.
6. Latex agglutination test for capsular polysaccharide of *H influenzae, S pneumoniae, N meningitidis,* and other encapsulated bacteria is rapid, accurate, and inexpensive. Counterimmunoelectrophoresis for capsular polysaccharide in the spinal fluid can also be done, but it takes longer and may not be readily available.
7. *H influenzae* requires both X (heme) and V (NAD) factors.
8. The antigenicity of the capsular polysaccharide.
9. It colonizes the human nasopharynx and is transmitted by respiratory tract secretions.
10. It retards phagocytosis of the organism.
11. Exotoxins are not known to be involved. Like all gram-negative organisms, *H influenzae* contains endotoxin.
12. (a) The vaccine containing the capsular polysaccharide of type b *H influenzae* coupled to diphtheria toxoid or another protein should be given to all children between 2 and 18 months of age.
    (b) Rifampin should be given to close household contacts of the patient and to the patient to eradicate nasopharyngeal carriage. If the patient attends a day-care center, contacts there should be given rifampin.

CASE 10

Chief Complaint
A 32-year-old man with diarrhea for the past 3 weeks.

History
The patient was well until 6 months ago, when fever, shortness of breath, and cough began. Chest x-ray followed by bronchoscopy resulted in the diagnosis of *Pneumocystis* pneumonia. He was treated with trimethoprim-sulfamethoxazole and recovered. His HIV antibody test was positive. Studies of his peripheral lymphocytes showed a CD4 count of 50/mm³.

For the past 3 weeks he has had frequent loose, watery bowel movements. There were no bloody or tarry stools. Stools were not fatty or foul-smelling. Crampy lower abdominal pain was associated with each movement. No nausea, vomiting, or fever has occurred. He has lost about 7 lb. There was no recent antibiotic use. The diarrhea has not responded to over-the-counter antidiarrheal drugs.

Physical Exam
T 37 °C, BP 130/70, P 84, R 12. Patient was not in acute distress.
Pertinent findings include:
Skin: Moderately dehydrated. No jaundice.
Lungs: Normal.

164. The ability of a virus to produce disease can result from a variety of mechanisms. Which one of the following mechanisms is LEAST likely?
(A) Cytopathic effect in infected cells
(B) Malignant transformation of infected cells
(C) Immune response to virus-induced antigens on the surface of infected cells
(D) Production of an exotoxin that activates adenylate cyclase

165. Which one of the following forms of immunity to viruses would be LEAST likely to be lifelong?
(A) Passive immunity
(B) Passive-active immunity
(C) Active immunity
(D) Cell-mediated immunity

166. Which one of the following statements concerning interferons is LEAST accurate?
(A) Interferons are proteins that influence host defenses in many ways, one of which is the induction of an antiviral state
(B) Interferons are synthesized only by virus-infected cells
(C) Interferons inhibit a broad range of viruses, not just the virus that induced the interferon
(D) Synthesis of several host enzymes is induced by interferon in target cells

167. You have isolated a virus from the stool of a patient with diarrhea and shown that its genome is composed of multiple pieces of double-stranded RNA. Which one of the following is UNLIKELY to be true?
(A) Each piece of RNA encodes a different protein
(B) The virus encodes an RNA-directed RNA polymerase
(C) The virion contains an RNA polymerase
(D) The genome integrates into the host chromosome

168. A temperate bacteriophage has been induced from a new pathogenic strain of *Escherichia coli* that produces a toxin. Which one of the following is the MOST convincing way to show that the phage encodes the toxin?
(A) Carry out conjugation of the pathogenic strain with a nonpathogenic strain
(B) Infect an experimental animal with the phage
(C) Lysogenize a nonpathogenic strain with the phage
(D) Look for transposable elements in the phage DNA

169. Each of the following statements concerning retroviruses is correct EXCEPT:
(A) The virus particle carries an RNA-directed DNA polymerase encoded by the viral genome

(B) The viral genome consists of three segments of double-stranded RNA
(C) The virion is enveloped and enters cells via an interaction with specific receptors on the host cell
(D) During infection, the virus synthesizes a DNA copy of its RNA, and this DNA becomes covalently integrated into host cell DNA

170. A stock of virus particles has been found by electron microscopy to contain 10^8 particles/mL, but a plaque assay reveals only 10^5 plaque-forming units/mL. The BEST interpretation of these results is that
(A) only one particle in 1000 is infectious
(B) a nonpermissive cell line was used for the plaque assay
(C) several kinds of viruses were present in the stock
(D) the virus is a temperature-sensitive mutant

171. Reasonable mechanisms for viral persistence in infected individuals include all of the following EXCEPT:
(A) generation of defective-interfering particles
(B) virus-mediated inhibition of host DNA synthesis
(C) integration of a provirus into the genome of the host
(D) host tolerance to viral antigens

172. Each of the following statements concerning viral surface proteins is correct EXCEPT:
(A) They elicit antibody that neutralizes infectivity of the virus
(B) They determine the species specificity of the virus-cell interaction
(C) They participate in active transport of nutrients across the viral envelope membrane
(D) They protect the genetic material against nucleases

173. Each of the following statements concerning viral vaccines is correct EXCEPT:
(A) In live, attenuated vaccines, the virus has lost its ability to cause disease but has retained its ability to induce neutralizing antibody
(B) In live, attenuated vaccines, the possibility of reversion to virulence is of concern
(C) With inactivated vaccines, IgA mucosal immunity is usually induced
(D) With inactivated vaccines, protective immunity is due mainly to the production of IgG

174. The major barrier to the control of rhinovirus upper respiratory infections by immunization is
(A) the poor local and systemic immune response to these viruses
(B) the number and antigenic diversity of the viruses

462 / PART X

(C) the side effects of the vaccine

(D) the inability to grow the viruses in cell culture

175. The feature of the influenza virus genome that contributes MOST to the antigenic variation of the virus is

(A) a high G + C content, which augments binding to nucleoproteins

(B) inverted repeat regions, which create "sticky ends"

(C) segmented nucleic acid

(D) unique methylated bases

176. What is the BEST explanation for the selective action of acyclovir (acycloguanosine) in herpes simplex virus-infected cells?

(A) Acyclovir binds specifically to herpesvirus receptors on the infected cell surface

(B) Viral phosphokinase phosphorylates acyclovir more effectively than does the host cell phosphokinase

(C) Acyclovir inhibits the RNA polymerase in the virus particle

(D) Acyclovir blocks the matrix protein of the virus, thereby preventing release by budding

177. Each of the following statements concerning interferon is correct EXCEPT:

(A) Interferon inhibits the growth of both DNA and RNA viruses

(B) Interferon is induced by double-stranded RNA

(C) Interferon made by cells of one species acts more effectively in the cells of that species than in the cells of other species

(D) Interferon acts by preventing viruses from entering the cell

178. Each of the following statements concerning the viruses that infect humans is correct EXCEPT:

(A) The ratio of physical particles to infectious particles is less than 1

(B) The purified nucleic acid of some viruses is infectious, but at a lower efficiency than the intact virions

(C) Some viruses contain lipoprotein envelopes derived from the plasma membrane of the host cell

(D) The nucleic acid of some viruses is single-stranded DNA and that of others is double-stranded RNA

179. Which one of the following statements about virion structure and assembly is CORRECT?

(A) Most viruses acquire surface glycoproteins by budding through the nuclear membrane

(B) Helical nucleocapsids are found primarily in DNA viruses

(C) The symmetry of virus particles prevents inclusion of any nonstructural proteins, such as enzymes

(D) Enveloped viruses use a matrix protein to mediate interactions between viral glycoproteins in the plasma membrane and structural proteins in the nucleocapsid

180. Each of the following statements concerning viruses is correct EXCEPT:

(A) Viruses can reproduce only within cells

(B) The proteins on the surface of the virus mediate the entry of the virus into host cells

(C) Neutralizing antibody is directed against proteins on the surface of the virus

(D) Viruses replicate by binary fission

181. Viruses are obligate intracellular parasites. Each of the following statements concerning this fact is correct EXCEPT:

(A) Viruses cannot generate energy outside of cells

(B) Viruses cannot synthesize proteins outside of cells

(C) Viruses must degrade host cell DNA in order to obtain nucleotides

(D) Enveloped viruses require host cell membranes to obtain their envelopes

182. Each of the following statements concerning lysogeny is correct EXCEPT:

(A) Viral genes replicate independently of bacterial genes

(B) Viral genes responsible for lysis are repressed

(C) Viral DNA is integrated into bacterial DNA

(D) Some lysogenic bacteriophage encode toxins that cause human disease

183. Each of the following viruses possesses an outer envelope of lipoprotein EXCEPT:

(A) varicella-zoster virus

(B) papillomavirus

(C) influenza virus

(D) human immunodeficiency virus

184. Which one of the following viruses possesses a genome of single-stranded RNA that is infectious when purified?

(A) Influenza virus

(B) Rotavirus

(C) Measles virus

(D) Poliovirus

185. Each of the following viruses possesses an RNA polymerase in the virion EXCEPT:

(A) hepatitis A virus

(B) smallpox virus

(C) mumps virus

(D) rotavirus

186. Each of the following viruses possesses a DNA polymerase in the virion EXCEPT:

(A) human immunodeficiency virus

(B) human T cell leukemia virus

(C) Epstein-Barr virus

(D) hepatitis B virus

187. Each of the following viruses possesses double-stranded nucleic acid as its genome EXCEPT:
(A) coxsackievirus
(B) herpes simplex virus
(C) rotavirus
(D) adenovirus

188. Viroids
(A) are defective viruses that are missing the DNA coding for the matrix protein
(B) consist of RNA without a protein or lipoprotein outer coat
(C) cause tumors in experimental animals
(D) require an RNA polymerase in the particle for replication to occur

189. Each of the following statements about both measles virus and rubella virus is correct EXCEPT:
(A) They are RNA enveloped viruses
(B) Their virions contain an RNA polymerase
(C) They have a single antigenic type
(D) They are transmitted by respiratory aerosol

190. Each of the following statements about both influenza virus and rabies virus is correct EXCEPT:
(A) They are enveloped RNA viruses
(B) Their virions contain an RNA polymerase
(C) A killed vaccine is available for both viruses
(D) They each have a single antigenic type

191. Each of the following statements about both poliovirus and rhinoviruses is correct EXCEPT:
(A) They are nonenveloped RNA viruses
(B) They have multiple antigenic types
(C) Their virions contain an RNA polymerase
(D) They do not integrate their genome into host cell DNA

192. Each of the following statements about human immunodeficiency virus (HIV) is correct EXCEPT:
(A) HIV is an enveloped RNA virus
(B) The virion contains an RNA-dependent DNA polymerase
(C) A DNA copy of the HIV genome integrates into host cell DNA
(D) Acyclovir inhibits HIV replication

Answers (Questions 159–192):

159 (B)	166 (B)	173 (C)	180 (D)	187 (A)
160 (D)	167 (D)	174 (B)	181 (C)	188 (B)
161 (C)	168 (C)	175 (C)	182 (A)	189 (B)
162 (B)	169 (B)	176 (B)	183 (B)	190 (D)
163 (D)	170 (A)	177 (D)	184 (D)	191 (C)
164 (D)	171 (B)	178 (A)	185 (A)	192 (D)
165 (A)	172 (C)	179 (D)	186 (C)	

Directions (Questions 193–211): Select the one lettered option that is MOST CLOSELY associated with the numbered items. Each lettered option may be selected once, more than once, or not at all.

Questions 193–196
(A) DNA enveloped virus
(B) DNA nonenveloped virus
(C) RNA enveloped virus
(D) RNA nonenveloped virus
(E) Viroid

193. Herpes simplex virus
194. Human T cell leukemia virus
195. Human papillomavirus
196. Rotavirus

Questions 197–201
(A) Attachment and penetration of virion
(B) Viral mRNA synthesis
(C) Viral protein synthesis
(D) Viral genome DNA synthesis
(E) Assembly and release of progeny virus

197. Main site of action of acyclovir
198. Main site of action of amantadine
199. Function of virion polymerase of influenza virus
200. Main site of action of antiviral antibody
201. Step at which budding occurs

Questions 202–206
(A) Poliovirus
(B) Epstein-Barr virus
(C) Agent of scrapie and kuru
(D) Hepatitis B virus
(E) Respiratory syncytial virus

202. Part of the genome DNA is synthesized by the virion polymerase
203. The translation product of viral mRNA is a polyprotein that is cleaved to form virion structural proteins
204. It is remarkably resistant to ultraviolet light
205. It causes latent infection of B cells
206. It carries a fusion protein on the surface of the virion envelope

Questions 207–211
(A) Hepatitis A virus
(B) Hepatitis B virus
(C) Hepatitis C virus
(D) Hepatitis D virus

207. Enveloped DNA virus that is transmitted by blood
208. Enveloped RNA virus that has the surface antigen of another virus

209. Enveloped RNA virus that is the most common cause of non-A, non-B hepatitis

210. Nonenveloped RNA virus that is transmitted by the fecal-oral route

211. Purified surface protein of this virus is the immunogen in a vaccine

Answers (Questions 193–211):

193 (A)	197 (D)	201 (E)	205 (B)	209 (C)
194 (C)	198 (A)	202 (D)	206 (E)	210 (A)
195 (B)	199 (B)	203 (A)	207 (B)	211 (B)
196 (D)	200 (A)	204 (C)	208 (D)	

Clinical Virology

Directions (Questions 212–275): Select the ONE lettered answer that is BEST in each question.

212. Which one of the following outcomes is MOST common following a primary herpes simplex virus infection?
(A) Complete eradication of virus and virus-infected cells
(B) Persistent asymptomatic viremia
(C) Establishment of latent infection
(D) Persistent cytopathic effect in infected cells

213. Each of the following pathogens is likely to establish chronic or latent infection EXCEPT:
(A) cytomegalovirus
(B) hepatitis A virus
(C) hepatitis B virus
(D) herpes simplex virus

214. Each of the following statements regarding poliovirus and its vaccine is correct EXCEPT:
(A) Poliovirus is transmitted by the fecal-oral route
(B) Pathogenesis by poliovirus primarily involves the death of sensory neurons
(C) The live, attenuated vaccine, which contains three serotypes, is recommended for use in children
(D) An unimmunized adult traveling to underdeveloped countries should receive the inactivated vaccine

215. Which one of the following strategies is MOST likely to induce lasting intestinal mucosal immunity to poliovirus?
(A) Parenteral (intramuscular) vaccination with inactivated vaccine
(B) Oral administration of poliovirus immune globulin
(C) Parenteral vaccination with live vaccine
(D) Oral vaccination with live vaccine

216. Each of the following clinical syndromes is associated with infection by picornaviruses EXCEPT:
(A) myocarditis/pericarditis
(B) hepatitis
(C) mononucleosis
(D) meningitis

217. Each of the following statements concerning rubella vaccine is correct EXCEPT:
(A) The vaccine prevents reinfection, thereby limiting the spread of virulent virus
(B) The immunogen in the vaccine is killed rubella virus
(C) The vaccine induces antibodies that prevent dissemination of the virus by neutralizing it during the viremic stage
(D) The incidence of both childhood rubella and congenital rubella syndrome has decreased significantly since the advent of the vaccine

218. Each of the following statements concerning the rabies vaccine for use in humans is correct EXCEPT:
(A) The vaccine contains live, attenuated rabies virus
(B) If your patient is bitten by a wild animal, eg, a skunk, the rabies vaccine should be given
(C) When the vaccine is used for postexposure prophylaxis, rabies immune globulin should also be given
(D) The virus in the vaccine is grown in human cell cultures, thus decreasing the risk of allergic encephalomyelitis

219. Each of the following statements concerning influenza is correct EXCEPT:

(A) Major epidemics of the disease are caused by influenza A viruses rather than influenza B and C viruses

(B) Likely sources of new antigens for influenza A viruses are the viruses that cause influenza in animals

(C) Major antigenic changes (shifts) of viral surface proteins are seen primarily in influenza A viruses rather than in influenza B and C viruses

(D) The antigenic changes that occur with antigenic drift are due to reassortment of the multiple pieces of the influenza virus genome

220. Each of the following statements concerning the prevention and treatment of influenza is correct EXCEPT:

(A) As with all live vaccines, the influenza vaccine should not be given to pregnant women

(B) Booster doses of the vaccine are recommended since the duration of immunity is only a year

(C) Amantadine is an effective prophylactic drug only against influenza A viruses

(D) The major antigen in the vaccine is the hemagglutinin

221. A 6-month-old child develops a persistent cough and a fever. Physical examination and chest x-ray suggest pneumonia. Which one of the following organisms is LEAST likely to cause this infection?

(A) Respiratory syncytial virus

(B) Adenovirus

(C) Parainfluenza virus

(D) Rotavirus

222. A 45-year-old man was attacked by a bobcat and bitten repeatedly about the face and neck. The animal was shot by a companion and brought back to the public health authorities. Once you decide to immunize against rabies virus, how would you proceed?

(A) Use hyperimmune serum only

(B) Use active immunization only

(C) Use hyperimmune serum and active immunization

(D) Use active immunization and follow this with hyperimmune serum if adequate antibody titers are not obtained in the patient's serum

223. Each of the following statements concerning mumps is correct EXCEPT:

(A) Mumps virus is a paramyxovirus and hence has a single-stranded RNA genome

(B) Meningitis is a recognized complication of mumps

(C) Mumps orchitis in children prior to puberty often causes sterility

(D) During mumps, the virus spreads through the bloodstream (viremia) to various internal organs

224. Each of the following statements concerning respiratory syncytial virus (RSV) is correct EXCEPT:

(A) RSV has a single-stranded RNA genome

(B) RSV induces the formation of multinucleated giant cells

(C) RSV causes pneumonia primarily in children

(D) RSV infections can be effectively treated with acyclovir

225. The principal reservoir for the antigenic shift variants of influenza virus appears to be

(A) people in isolated communities such as the Arctic

(B) animals, specifically pigs, horses, and fowl

(C) soil, especially in the tropics

(D) sewage

226. The role of an infectious agent in the pathogenesis of kuru was BEST demonstrated by which one of the following observations?

(A) A 16-fold rise in antibody titer to the agent was observed

(B) The viral genome was isolated from infected neurons

(C) Electron micrographs of the brains of infected individuals demonstrated intracellular structures resembling paramyxovirus nucleocapsids

(D) The disease was serially transmitted to experimental animals

227. A 64-year-old man with chronic lymphatic leukemia develops progressive deterioration of mental and neuromuscular function. At autopsy the brain shows enlarged oligodendrocytes whose nuclei contain naked, icosahedral virus particles. The MOST likely diagnosis is

(A) herpes encephalitis

(B) Creutzfeldt-Jakob disease

(C) subacute sclerosing panencephalitis

(D) progressive multifocal leukocephalopathy

(E) rabies

228. A 20-year-old man, who for many years had received daily injections of growth hormone prepared from human pituitary glands, develops ataxia, slurred speech, and dementia. At autopsy the brain shows widespread neuronal degeneration, a spongy appearance due to many vacuoles between the cells, no inflammation, and no evidence of virus particles. Mice injected with homogenized brain tissue develop a similar disease after 6 months. The MOST likely diagnosis is

(A) herpes encephalitis

(B) Creutzfeldt-Jakob disease

(C) subacute sclerosing panencephalitis

(D) progressive multifocal leukoencephalopathy

(E) rabies

229. A 24-year-old woman has had fever and a sore throat for the past week. Moderately severe pharyngitis and bilateral cervical lymphadenopathy are seen on physical examination. Which one of the following viruses is LEAST likely to cause this picture?
(A) Varicella-zoster virus
(B) Adenovirus
(C) Coxsackievirus
(D) Epstein-Barr virus

230. Scrapie and kuru possess all of the following characteristics EXCEPT:
(A) a histologic picture of spongiform encephalopathy
(B) transmissibility to animals associated with a long incubation period
(C) slowly progressive deterioration of brain function
(D) prominent intranuclear inclusions in oligo-dendrocytes

231. Each of the following statements concerning subacute sclerosing panencephalitis is correct EXCEPT:
(A) Immunosuppression is a frequent predisposing factor
(B) Aggregates of helical nucleocapsids are found in infected cells
(C) High titers of measles antibody are found in cerebrospinal fluid
(D) Slowly progressive deterioration of brain function occurs

232. The slow virus disease that MOST clearly has immunosuppression as an important factor in its pathogenesis is
(A) progressive multifocal leukoencephalopathy
(B) subacute sclerosing panencephalitis
(C) Creutzfeldt-Jakob disease
(D) scrapie

233. A 30-year-old man develops fever and jaundice. He consults a physician, who finds that blood tests for HBs antigen and anti-HBs antibody are negative. Which one of the following additional tests is MOST useful to establish that the hepatitis was indeed due to hepatitis B virus?
(A) HBe antigen
(B) Anti-HBc antibody
(C) Anti-HBe antibody
(D) Delta antigen

234. Which one of the following is the MOST reasonable explanation for the ability of hepatitis B virus to cause chronic infection?
(A) Infection does not elicit the production of antibody
(B) The liver is an "immunologically sheltered" site

(C) Viral DNA can persist within the host cell
(D) Many humans are immunologically tolerant to HBs antigen

235. The routine screening of transfused blood for HBs antigen has not eliminated the problem of posttransfusion hepatitis. For which one of the following viruses has screening eliminated a large number of cases of post-transfusion hepatitis?
(A) Hepatitis A virus
(B) Hepatitis C virus
(C) Cytomegalovirus
(D) Epstein-Barr virus

236. A 35-year-old man addicted to intravenous drugs has been a carrier of HBs antigen for 10 years. He suddenly develops acute fulminant hepatitis and dies within 10 days. Which one of the following laboratory tests would contribute MOST to a diagnosis?
(A) Anti-HBs antibody
(B) HBe antigen
(C) Anti-HBc antibody
(D) Anti-delta virus antibody

237. Which one of the following is the BEST evidence on which to base a decisive diagnosis of acute mumps disease?
(A) A positive skin test
(B) A 4-fold rise in antibody titer to mumps surface antigen
(C) A history of exposure to a child with mumps
(D) Orchitis in young adult male

238. Varicella-zoster virus and herpes simplex virus share many characteristics. Which one of the following characteristics is NOT shared?
(A) Inapparent disease, manifested only by virus shedding
(B) Persistence of latent virus after recovery from acute disease
(C) Vesicular rash
(D) Linear, double-stranded DNA genome

239. Herpes simplex virus and cytomegalovirus share many features. Which one of the following features is LEAST likely to be shared?
(A) Important cause of morbidity and mortality in the newborn
(B) Congenital abnormalities due to transplacental passage
(C) Important cause of serious disease in immunosuppressed individuals
(D) Mild or inapparent infection

240. The eradication of smallpox was facilitated by several features of the virus. Which one of the following contributed LEAST to eradication?
(A) It has one antigenic type
(B) Inapparent infection is rare
(C) Administration of live vaccine reliably induces immunity

(D) It multiplies in the cytoplasm of infected cells

241. Which one of the following statements concerning infectious mononucleosis is the MOST accurate?

(A) Multinucleated giant cells are found in the skin lesions

(B) Infected T lymphocytes are abundant in peripheral blood

(C) Isolation of virus is necessary to confirm the diagnosis

(D) Infectious mononucleosis is transmitted by virus in saliva

242. Which one of the following statements about genital herpes is LEAST accurate?

(A) Acyclovir reduces the number of recurrent disease episodes by eradicating latently infected cells

(B) Genital herpes can be transmitted in the absence of apparent lesions

(C) Multinucleated giant cells with intranuclear inclusions are found in the lesions

(D) Initial disease episodes are generally more severe than recurrent episodes

243. The influenza vaccine currently in use in the United States is

(A) an inactivated vaccine consisting of formaldehyde-treated influenza virions, which primarily induce antibody to hemagglutinin

(B) a live, attenuated vaccine prepared from a variant of equine influenza virus

(C) a vaccine consisting of purified peptide fragments of the hemagglutinin and neuraminidase glycoproteins

(D) a live, attenuated vaccine composed of the current influenza A, B, and C isolates

244. Which of the following is the MOST common lower respiratory pathogen in infants?

(A) Respiratory syncytial virus

(B) Adenovirus

(C) Rhinovirus

(D) Coxsackievirus

245. Which of the following conditions is LEAST likely to be caused by adenoviruses?

(A) Conjunctivitis

(B) Pneumonia

(C) Pharyngitis

(D) Glomerulonephritis

246. Regarding the serologic diagnosis of infectious mononucleosis, which one of the following is CORRECT?

(A) A heterophil antibody is formed that reacts with a capsid protein of Epstein-Barr virus

(B) A heterophil antibody is formed that agglutinates sheep or horse red blood cells

(C) A heterophil antigen occurs that cross-reacts with *Proteus* OX19 strains

(D) A heterophil antigen occurs following infection with cytomegalovirus

247. Herpes simplex virus type 1 (HSV-1) is distinct from HSV-2 in several different ways. Which one of the following is the LEAST accurate statement?

(A) HSV-1 causes lesions above the umbilicus more frequently than HSV-2 does

(B) Infection by HSV-1 is not associated with any tumors in humans

(C) Antiserum to HSV-1 neutralizes HSV-1 much more effectively than HSV-2

(D) HSV-1 causes frequent recurrences, whereas HSV-2 infection rarely recurs

248. Which one of the following statements about the *src* gene and *src* protein of Rous sarcoma virus is INCORRECT?

(A) The *src* gene encodes a protein with epidermal growth factor activity

(B) The *src* protein catalyzes phosphotransfer from ATP to tyrosine residues in protein

(C) The *src* protein is required to maintain neoplastic transformation of infected cells

(D) The viral *src* gene is derived from a cellular gene found in all vertebrate species

249. Each of the following statements supports the idea that cellular proto-oncogenes participate in human carcinogenesis EXCEPT:

(A) The c-*abl* gene is rearranged on the Philadelphia chromosome in myeloid leukemias and encodes a protein with heightened tyrosine kinase activity

(B) The N-*myc* gene is amplified as much as 100-fold in many advanced cases of neuroblastoma

(C) The receptor for platelet-derived growth factor is a transmembrane protein that exhibits tyrosine kinase activity

(D) The c-Ha-*ras* gene is mutated at specific codons in several types of human cancer

250. Each of the following statements concerning human immunodeficiency virus (HIV) is correct EXCEPT:

(A) Screening tests for antibodies are useful to prevent transmission of HIV through transfused blood

(B) The opportunistic infections seen in AIDS are primarily the result of a loss of cell-mediated immunity

(C) Zidovudine (azidothymidine) inhibits the RNA-dependent DNA polymerase

(D) The presence of circulating antibodies that neutralize HIV is evidence that an individual is protected against HIV-induced disease

251. Which one of the following statements concerning viral meningitis and viral encephalitis is CORRECT?

(A) Herpes simplex virus type 2 is the leading cause of viral meningitis

(B) Herpes simplex virus type 1 is an important cause of viral encephalitis

(C) The spinal fluid protein is usually decreased in viral meningitis

(D) The diagnosis of viral meningitis can be made by using the India ink stain on a sample of spinal fluid

252. Each of the following statements is correct EXCEPT:

(A) Coxsackieviruses are enteroviruses and can replicate in both the respiratory and gastrointestinal tracts

(B) Influenza viruses have multiple serotypes based on hemagglutinin and neuraminidase proteins located on the envelope surface

(C) Flaviviruses are RNA enveloped viruses that replicate in animals as well as humans

(D) Adenoviruses are RNA enveloped viruses that are an important cause of sexually transmitted disease

253. Which one of the following statements concerning the prevention of viral disease is CORRECT?

(A) Adenovirus vaccine contains purified penton fibers and is usually given to children in conjunction with polio vaccine

(B) Coxsackievirus vaccine contains live virus that induces IgA, which prevents reinfection by homologous serotypes

(C) Flavivirus immunization consists of hyperimmune serum plus a vaccine consisting of subunits containing the surface glycoprotein

(D) Influenza virus vaccine contains killed virus that induces neutralizing antibody directed against the hemagglutinin

254. Each of the following statements concerning hepatitis C virus (HCV) and hepatitis D virus (HDV) is correct EXCEPT:

(A) HCV is an important cause of posttransfusion hepatitis

(B) Delta virus is a defective virus with an RNA genome and a capsid composed of hepatitis B surface antigen

(C) HDV is transmitted primarily by the fecal-oral route

(D) People infected with HCV commonly become chronic carriers of HCV and are predisposed to hepatocellular carcinoma

255. Each of the following statements concerning measles virus is correct EXCEPT:

(A) Measles virus is an enveloped virus with a single-stranded RNA genome

(B) One of the important complications of measles is encephalitis

(C) The initial site of measles virus replication is the upper respiratory tract, from which it spreads via the blood to the skin

(D) Latent infection by measles virus can be explained by the integration of provirus into the host cell DNA

256. Each of the following statements concerning measles vaccine is correct EXCEPT:

(A) The vaccine contains live, attenuated virus

(B) The vaccine should not be given in conjunction with other viral vaccines since interference can occur

(C) Virus in the vaccine contains only one serotype

(D) The vaccine should not be given prior to 15 months of age since maternal antibodies can prevent an immune response

257. Each of the following statements concerning rubella is correct EXCEPT:

(A) Congenital abnormalities occur primarily when a pregnant woman is infected during the first trimester

(B) Women who say that they have never had rubella can, nevertheless, have neutralizing antibody in their serum

(C) In a 6-year-old child, rubella is a mild, self-limited disease with few complications

(D) Acyclovir is effective in the treatment of congenital rubella syndrome

258. Each of the following statements concerning rabies and rabies virus is correct EXCEPT:

(A) The virus has a lipoprotein envelope and single-stranded RNA as its genome

(B) The virus has a single antigenic type (serotype)

(C) In the United States, dogs are the most common reservoir

(D) The incubation period is usually long (several weeks) rather than short (several days)

259. Each of the following statements concerning arboviruses is correct EXCEPT:

(A) The pathogenesis of dengue hemorrhagic shock syndrome is associated with the heterotypic anamnestic response

(B) Wild birds are the reservoir for encephalitis viruses but not for yellow fever virus

(C) Ticks are the main mode of transmission for both encephalitis viruses and yellow fever virus

(D) There is a live, attenuated vaccine that effectively prevents yellow fever

260. Each of the following statements concerning rhinoviruses is correct EXCEPT:

(A) Rhinoviruses are picornaviruses, ie, small, nonenveloped viruses with an RNA genome

(B) Rhinoviruses are an important cause of lower respiratory tract infections, especially in patients with chronic obstructive pulmonary disease

(C) Rhinoviruses do not infect the gastrointestinal tract because they are inactivated by the acid pH in the stomach

(D) There is no vaccine against rhinoviruses because they have too many antigenic types

261. Each of the following statements concerning herpes simplex virus type 2 (HSV-2) is correct EXCEPT:

(A) Natural infection with HSV-2 confers only partial immunity against a second primary infection

(B) HSV-2 causes vesicular lesions, typically in the genital area

(C) HSV-2 can cause virus-specific alterations of the cell membrane, leading to cell fusion and the formation of multinucleated giant cells

(D) Recurrent disease episodes due to reactivation of latent HSV-2 are usually more severe than the primary episode

262. Each of the following statements concerning Epstein-Barr virus is correct EXCEPT:

(A) Many infections are mild or inapparent

(B) The earlier in life primary infection is acquired, the more likely the typical picture of infectious mononucleosis will be manifest

(C) Latently infected lymphocytes regularly persist following an acute episode of infection

(D) Infection confers immunity against second episodes of infectious mononucleosis

263. Each of the following statements regarding rotaviruses is correct EXCEPT:

(A) A live, attenuated vaccine against rotaviruses is available

(B) Rotaviruses are a leading cause of diarrhea in young children

(C) Rotaviruses are transmitted primarily by the fecal-oral route

(D) Rotaviruses belong to the reovirus family, which have a double-stranded, segmented RNA genome

264. Each of the following statements concerning the antigenicity of influenza A virus is correct EXCEPT:

(A) Antigenic shifts, which represent major changes in antigenicity, occur infrequently and are due to the recombination (reassortment) of segments of the viral genome

(B) Antigenic shifts affect both the hemagglutinin and the neuraminidase

(C) The worldwide epidemics caused by influenza A virus are due to antigenic shifts

(D) The protein involved in antigenic drift is primarily the internal ribonucleoprotein

265. Each of the following statements concerning adenoviruses is correct EXCEPT:

(A) Adenoviruses are composed of a double-stranded DNA genome and a capsid without an envelope

(B) Adenoviruses cause both sore throat and pneumonia

(C) Adenoviruses have only one serologic type

(D) Adenoviruses are implicated as a cause of tumors in animals but not humans

266. Each of the following statements concerning the prevention of viral respiratory tract disease is correct EXCEPT:

(A) To prevent disease caused by adenoviruses, a live enteric-coated vaccine that causes asymptomatic enteric infection is used in the military

(B) To prevent disease caused by influenza A virus, an inactivated vaccine is available for the civilian population

(C) There is no vaccine available against respiratory syncytial virus

(D) To prevent disease caused by rhinoviruses, a vaccine containing purified capsid proteins is used

267. Each of the following statements concerning herpesvirus latency is correct EXCEPT:

(A) Exogenous stimuli can cause reactivation of latent infection, with induction of symptomatic disease

(B) During latency, antiviral antibody is not demonstrable in the sera of infected individuals

(C) Episodes of herpesvirus reactivation are more frequent and more severe in patients with impaired cell-mediated immunity

(D) Virus can be recovered from latently infected cells by cocultivation with susceptible cells

268. Each of the following statements concerning rhinoviruses is correct EXCEPT:

(A) Rhinoviruses are one of the most frequent causes of the common cold

(B) Rhinoviruses grow better at 33 than at 37 °C; hence, they tend to cause disease in the upper respiratory tract rather than the lower respiratory tract

(C) Rhinoviruses are members of the picornaviruses family and hence resemble poliovirus in their structure and replication

(D) The immunity provided by the rhinovirus vaccine is excellent since there is only one serotype

269. Which one of the following statements concerning poliovirus infection is CORRECT?

(A) Congenital infection of the fetus is an important complication

(B) The virus replicates extensively in the gastrointestinal tract

(C) A skin test is available to determine prior exposure to the virus

(D) Amantadine is an effective preventive agent

270. Each of the following statements concerning yellow fever is correct EXCEPT:
   (A) Yellow fever virus is transmitted by the *Aedes aegypti* mosquito in the urban form of yellow fever
   (B) Infection by yellow fever virus causes significant damage to hepatocytes
   (C) Nonhuman primates in the jungle are a major reservoir of yellow fever virus
   (D) Acyclovir is an effective treatment for yellow fever

271. Which one of the following statements concerning mumps is CORRECT?
   (A) Although the salivary glands are the most obvious sites of infection, the testes, ovaries, and pancreas can be involved as well
   (B) Since there is no vaccine against mumps, passive immunization is the only means of preventing the disease
   (C) The diagnosis of mumps is made on clinical grounds since the virus cannot be grown in cell culture and serologic tests are inaccurate
   (D) Second episodes of mumps can occur since there are two serotypes of the virus and protection is type-specific

272. Many of the oncogenic retroviruses carry oncogenes closely related to normal cellular genes, called proto-oncogenes. Which one of the following statements concerning proto-oncogenes is INCORRECT?
   (A) Several proto-oncogenes have been found in mutant form in human cancers that lack evidence for viral etiology
   (B) Several viral oncogenes and their progenitor proto-oncogenes encode protein kinases specific for tyrosine
   (C) Some proto-oncogenes encode cellular growth factors and receptors for growth factors
   (D) Proto-oncogenes are closely related to transposons found in bacteria

273. Each of the following statements concerning human immunodeficiency virus is correct EXCEPT:
   (A) The CD4 protein on the T cell surface is the receptor for the virus
   (B) There is appreciable antigenic diversity in the envelope glycoprotein of the virus

(C) One of the viral genes codes for a protein that augments the activity of the viral transcriptional promoter
(D) A major problem with testing for antibody to the virus is its cross-reactivity with human T cell leukemia virus type I

274. Each of the following statements concerning human immunodeficiency virus is correct EXCEPT:
   (A) Patients infected with HIV typically form antibodies against both the envelope glycoproteins (gp120 and gp41) and the internal group-specific antigen (p24)
   (B) HIV probably arose as an endogenous virus of humans since HIV proviral DNA is found in the DNA of certain normal human cells
   (C) Transmission of HIV occurs primarily by the transfer of blood or semen in adults, but neonates are primarily infected transplacentally
   (D) The Western blot test is more specific for HIV infection than the ELISA is

275. Each of the following statements concerning hepatitis A virus is correct EXCEPT:
   (A) The initial site of viral replication is the gastrointestinal tract
   (B) Hepatitis A virus commonly causes asymptomatic infection in children
   (C) The diagnosis is usually made by isolating the virus in cell culture
   (D) Gamma globulin is used to prevent the disease in exposed persons

Answers (Questions 212–275):

212 (C)	225 (B)	238 (A)	251 (B)	264 (D)
213 (B)	226 (D)	239 (B)	252 (D)	265 (C)
214 (B)	227 (D)	240 (D)	253 (D)	266 (D)
215 (D)	228 (B)	241 (D)	254 (C)	267 (B)
216 (C)	229 (A)	242 (A)	255 (D)	268 (D)
217 (B)	230 (D)	243 (A)	256 (B)	269 (B)
218 (A)	231 (A)	244 (A)	257 (D)	270 (D)
219 (D)	232 (A)	245 (D)	258 (C)	271 (A)
220 (A)	233 (B)	246 (B)	259 (C)	272 (D)
221 (D)	234 (C)	247 (D)	260 (B)	273 (D)
222 (C)	235 (B)	248 (A)	261 (D)	274 (B)
223 (C)	236 (D)	249 (C)	262 (B)	275 (C)
224 (D)	237 (B)	250 (D)	263 (A)	

Directions (Questions 276–294): Select the ONE lettered option that is MOST closely associated with the numbered items. Each lettered option may be selected once, more than once, or not at all.

Questions 276–279
  (A) Yellow fever virus
  (B) Rabies virus
  (C) Rotavirus
  (D) Rubella virus
  (E) Rhinovirus
276. Diarrhea
277. Jaundice
278. Congenital abnormalities
279. Encephalitis

Questions 280–284
  (A) Bronchiolitis
  (B) Meningitis
  (C) Pharyngitis
  (D) Shingles
  (E) Subacute sclerosing panencephalitis
280. Adenovirus
281. Measles virus
282. Respiratory syncytial virus
283. Coxsackievirus
284. Varicella-zoster virus

Questions 285–289
  (A) Adenovirus
  (B) Parainfluenza virus
  (C) Rhinovirus
  (D) Coxsackievirus
  (E) Epstein-Barr virus

285. Causes myocarditis and pleurodynia
286. Grows better at 33 than 37 °C
287. Causes tumors in laboratory rodents
288. Causes croup in young children
289. Causes infectious mononucleosis

Questions 290–294
  (A) Hepatitis C virus
  (B) Cytomegalovirus
  (C) Human papillomavirus
  (D) Dengue virus
  (E) St. Louis encephalitis virus
290. It is implicated as the cause of carcinoma of the cervix
291. Wild birds are an important reservoir
292. It is an important cause of pneumonia in immunocompromised patients
293. Donated blood containing antibody to this RNA virus should not be used for transfusion
294. It causes a hemorrhagic fever that can be life-threatening

Answers (Questions 276–294):

276 (C)	280 (C)	284 (D)	288 (B)	292 (B)
277 (A)	281 (E)	285 (D)	289 (E)	293 (A)
278 (D)	282 (A)	286 (C)	290 (C)	294 (D)
279 (B)	283 (B)	287 (A)	291 (E)	

Mycology

Directions (Questions 295–317): Select the ONE lettered answer that is BEST in each question.

295. Which one of the following fungi is MOST likely to be found within reticuloendothelial cells?
  (A) *Histoplasma capsulatum*
  (B) *Candida albicans*
  (C) *Cryptococcus neoformans*
  (D) *Sporothrix schenckii*

296. Your patient is a woman with a vaginal discharge. You suspect, on clinical grounds, that it may be due to *Candida albicans*. Which one of the following statements is LEAST accurate or appropriate?
  (A) A Gram stain of the discharge should reveal budding yeasts
  (B) Culture of the discharge on Sabouraud's agar should produce a white mycelium with aerial conidia

(C) To identify the organism, you should determine whether germ tubes are produced

(D) You should ask her whether she is taking antibiotics

297. You have made a clinical diagnosis of meningitis in a 50-year-old immunocompromised woman. A latex agglutination test on the spinal fluid for capsular polysaccharide antigen is positive. Of the following organisms, which one is the MOST likely cause?
(A) *Histoplasma capsulatum*
(B) *Cryptococcus neoformans*
(C) *Aspergillus fumigatus*
(D) *Candida albicans*

298. Fungi often colonize lesions due to other causes. Which one of the following is LEAST likely to be present as a colonizer?
(A) *Aspergillus*
(B) *Mucor*
(C) *Sporothrix*
(D) *Candida*

299. Your patient complains of an "itching rash" on her abdomen. On examination, you find that the lesions are red, circular, with a vesiculated border and a healing central area. You suspect tinea corporis. Of the following choices, the MOST appropriate laboratory procedure to make the diagnosis is a
(A) potassium hydroxide mount of skin scrapings
(B) Giemsa stain for multinucleated giant cells
(C) fluorescent-antibody stain of the vesicle fluid
(D) 4-fold rise in antibody titer against the organism

300. Each of the following statements concerning *Cryptococcus neoformans* is correct EXCEPT:
(A) Its natural habitat is the soil, especially associated with pigeon feces
(B) Pathogenesis is related primarily to the production of exotoxin A
(C) Budding yeasts are found in the lesions
(D) The initial site of infection is usually the lung

301. A woman who pricked her finger while pruning some rose bushes develops a local pustule that progresses to an ulcer. Several nodules then develop along the local lymphatic drainage. The MOST likely agent is
(A) *Cryptococcus neoformans*
(B) *Candida albicans*
(C) *Sporothrix schenckii*
(D) *Aspergillus fumigatus*

302. Several fungi are associated with disease in immunocompromised patients. Which one of the following is the LEAST frequently associated?

(A) *Cryptococcus neoformans*
(B) *Aspergillus fumigatus*
(C) *Malassezia furfur*
(D) *Mucor* species

303. Fungal cells that reproduce by budding are seen in the infected tissues of patients with
(A) candidiasis, cryptococcosis, and sporotrichosis
(B) mycetoma, candidiasis, and mucormycosis
(C) tinea corporis, tinea unguium, and tinea versicolor
(D) sporotrichosis, mycetoma, and aspergillosis

304. Infection by a dermatophyte is MOST often associated with
(A) intravenous drug abuse
(B) inhalation of the organism from contaminated bird feces
(C) adherence of the organism to perspiration-moist skin
(D) fecal-oral transmission

305. Aspergillosis is recognized in tissue by the presence of
(A) budding cells
(B) septate hyphae
(C) metachromatic granules
(D) pseudohyphae

306. Which one of the following is NOT a characteristic of histoplasmosis?
(A) Person-to-person transmission
(B) Specific geographic distribution
(C) Yeasts in the tissue
(D) Mycelial phase in the soil

307. Each of the following statements concerning mucormycosis is correct EXCEPT:
(A) The fungi that cause mucormycosis are transmitted by airborne asexual spores
(B) Tissue sections from a patient with mucormycosis show budding yeasts
(C) Hyphae typically grow in blood vessels and cause necrosis of tissue
(D) Ketoacidosis in diabetic patients is a predisposing factor to mucormycosis

308. Each of the following statements concerning fungi is correct EXCEPT:
(A) Yeasts are fungi that reproduce by budding
(B) Molds are fungi that have elongated filaments called hyphae
(C) Thermally dimorphic fungi exist as yeasts at 37 °C and as molds at 25 °C
(D) Both yeasts and molds have a cell wall made of peptidoglycan

309. Each of the following statements concerning yeasts is correct EXCEPT:
(A) Yeasts have chitin in their cell walls and ergosterol in their cell membranes
(B) Yeasts form ascospores when they invade tissue

(C) Yeasts have eukaryotic nuclei and contain mitochondria in their cytoplasm

(D) Yeasts produce neither endotoxin nor exotoxins

310. Each of the following statements concerning fungi and protozoa is correct EXCEPT:

(A) Both fungi and protozoa are eukaryotic organisms

(B) Fungi possess a cell wall, whereas protozoa do not

(C) Both fungi and protozoa use flagella as their organ of motility

(D) Both fungi and protozoa generate energy in mitochondria

311. You suspect that your patient's disease may be caused by *Cryptococcus neoformans*. Which one of the following findings would be MOST useful in establishing the diagnosis?

(A) A positive heterophil agglutination test for the presence of antigen

(B) A history of recent travel in the Mississippi River valley area

(C) The finding of encapsulated budding cells in spinal fluid

(D) Recovery of an acid-fast organism from the patient's sputum

312. Each of the following statements concerning *Candida albicans* is correct EXCEPT:

(A) *C albicans* is a budding yeast that forms pseudohyphae when it invades tissue

(B) *C albicans* is transmitted primarily by respiratory aerosol

(C) *C albicans* causes thrush

(D) Impaired cell-mediated immunity is an important predisposing factor to disease

313. Each of the following statements concerning *Coccidioides immitis* is correct EXCEPT:

(A) The mycelial phase of the organism grows primarily in the soil, which is its natural habitat

(B) In the body, spherules containing endospores are formed

(C) A rising titer of complement-fixing antibody indicates disseminated disease

(D) Most infections are symptomatic and require treatment with amphotericin B

314. Each of the following statements concerning *Histoplasma capsulatum* is correct EXCEPT:

(A) The natural habitat of *H capsulatum* is the soil, where it grows as a mold

(B) *H capsulatum* is transmitted by airborne conidia, and its initial site of infection is the lung

(C) Within the body, *H capsulatum* grows primarily intracellularly within macrophages

(D) Infection does not elicit a cell-mediated immune response, and no skin test is available

315. Each of the following statements concerning infection caused by *Coccidioides immitis* is correct EXCEPT:

(A) *C immitis* is a dimorphic fungus

(B) *C immitis* is acquired by inhalation of arthrospores

(C) Resistance to amphotericin B is plasmid-mediated

(D) Infection occurs primarily in the southwestern states and California

316. Each of the following statements concerning *Blastomyces dermatitidis* is correct EXCEPT:

(A) *B dermatitidis* grows as a mold in the soil in North America

(B) *B dermatitidis* is a dimorphic fungus that forms yeast cells in tissue

(C) *B dermatitidis* infection is commonly diagnosed by serologic tests since it does not grow in culture

(D) *B dermatitidis* causes granulomatous skin lesions

317. *Aspergillus fumigatus* can be involved in a variety of clinical conditions. Which one of the following is LEAST likely to occur?

(A) Tissue invasion in immunocompromised host

(B) Allergy following inhalation of airborne particles of the fungus

(C) Colonization of tuberculous cavities in the lung

(D) Thrush

Answers (Questions 295–317):

295 (A)	300 (B)	305 (B)	310 (C)	315 (C)
296 (B)	301 (C)	306 (A)	311 (C)	316 (C)
297 (B)	302 (C)	307 (B)	312 (B)	317 (D)
298 (C)	303 (A)	308 (D)	313 (D)	
299 (A)	304 (C)	309 (B)	314 (D)	

Directions (Questions 318–325): Select the ONE lettered option that is MOST closely associated with the numbered items. Each lettered option may be selected once, more than once, or not at all.

Questions 318–321

(A) *Histoplasma capsulatum*

(B) *Candida albicans*

(C) *Aspergillus fumigatus*

(D) *Sporothrix schenckii*

318. A budding yeast that is a member of the normal flora of the vagina

319. A dimorphic organism that is transmitted by trauma to the skin

320. A dimorphic fungus that typically is acquired by inhalation of asexual spores

321. A mold that causes pneumonia in immunocompromised patients

Questions 322–325

(A) *Coccidioides immitis*
(B) *Rhizopus nigricans*
(C) *Blastomyces dermatitidis*
(D) *Cryptococcus neoformans*

322. A yeast acquired by inhalation that causes meningitis primarily in immunocompromised patients

323. A mold that invades blood vessels primarily in patients with diabetic ketoacidosis

324. A dimorphic fungus that is acquired by inhalation by people living in certain areas of the southwestern states in the United States

325. A dimorphic fungus that causes granulomatous skin lesions in people living throughout North America

Answers (Questions 318–325):

318 (B) 321 (C) 324 (A)
319 (D) 322 (D) 325 (C)
320 (A) 323 (B)

Parasitology

Directions (Questions 326–352): Select the ONE lettered answer that is BEST in each question.

326. Children at day-care centers in the United States have a high rate of infections with which one of the following?
(A) *Ascaris lumbricoides*
(B) *Entamoeba histolytica*
(C) *Enterobius vermicularis*
(D) *Necator americanus*

327. The anatomic location of inflammation caused by *Schistosoma mansoni* is primarily
(A) lung alveoli
(B) intestinal venules
(C) renal tubules
(D) bone marrow

328. In malaria, the form of plasmodia that is transmitted from mosquito to human is the
(A) sporozoite
(B) gametocyte
(C) merozoite
(D) hypnozoite

329. Which one of the following protozoa primarily infects macrophages?
(A) *Plasmodium vivax*
(B) *Leishmania donovani*
(C) *Trypanosoma cruzi*
(D) *Trichomonas vaginalis*

330. Each of the following parasites has an intermediate host as part of its life cycle EXCEPT:
(A) *Trichomonas vaginalis*
(B) *Taenia solium*
(C) *Echinococcus granulosus*
(D) *Toxoplasma gondii*

331. Each of the following parasites passes through the lung during human infection EXCEPT:
(A) *Strongyloides stercoralis*
(B) *Necator americanus*
(C) *Wuchereria bancrofti*
(D) *Ascaris lumbricoides*

332. Each of the following parasites is transmitted by flies EXCEPT:
(A) *Schistosoma mansoni*
(B) *Onchocerca volvulus*
(C) *Trypanosoma gambiense*
(D) *Loa loa*

333. Each of the following parasites is transmitted by mosquitoes EXCEPT:
(A) *Leishmania donovani*
(B) *Wuchereria bancrofti*
(C) *Plasmodium vivax*
(D) *Plasmodium falciparum*

334. Pigs or dogs are the source of human infection by each of the following parasites EXCEPT:
(A) *Echinococcus granulosus*
(B) *Taenia solium*
(C) *Ascaris lumbricoides*
(D) *Trichinella spiralis*

335. Each of the following parasites is transmitted by eating inadequately cooked fish or seafood EXCEPT:
(A) *Diphyllobothrium latum*
(B) *Ancylostoma duodenale*
(C) *Paragonimus westermani*
(D) *Clonorchis sinensis*

336. Laboratory diagnosis of a patient with a suspected liver abscess due to *Entamoeba histolytica* should include
(A) stool examination and indirect hemagglutination test
(B) stool examination and blood smear
(C) indirect hemagglutination test and skin test
(D) xenodiagnosis and string test

337. Each of the following statements concerning *Toxoplasma gondii* is correct EXCEPT:
(A) *T gondii* can be transmitted across the placenta to the fetus
(B) *T gondii* can be transmitted by cat feces
(C) *T gondii* can cause encephalitis in immunocompromised patients
(D) *T gondii* can be diagnosed by finding trophozoites in the stool

338. Each of the following statements concerning *Giardia lamblia* is correct EXCEPT:
(A) *G lamblia* has both a trophozoite and a cyst stage in its life cycle
(B) *G lamblia* is transmitted by the fecal-oral route from both human and animal sources
(C) *G lamblia* causes hemolytic anemia
(D) *G lamblia* can be diagnosed by the string test

339. Each of the following statements concerning malaria is correct EXCEPT:
(A) The female *Anopheles* mosquito is the vector
(B) Early in infection, sporozoites enter hepatocytes
(C) Release of merozoites from red blood cells causes periodic fever and chills
(D) The principal site of gametocyte formation is the human gastrointestinal tract

340. Each of the following statements concerning *Trichomonas vaginalis* is correct EXCEPT:
(A) *T vaginalis* is transmitted sexually
(B) *T vaginalis* can be diagnosed by visualizing the trophozoite
(C) *T vaginalis* can be treated effectively with metronidazole
(D) *T vaginalis* causes bloody diarrhea

341. Which one of the following agents is used to prevent malaria?
(A) Mebendazole
(B) Chloroquine
(C) Inactivated vaccine
(D) Praziquantel

342. Each of the following statements concerning *Pneumocystis carinii* is correct EXCEPT:

(A) *P carinii* infections primarily involve the respiratory tract
(B) *P carinii* can be diagnosed by seeing cysts in tissue
(C) *P carinii* infections are symptomatic primarily in immunocompromised patients
(D) *P carinii* symptomatic infections can be prevented by administering penicillin orally

343. Each of the following statements concerning *Trypanosoma cruzi* is correct EXCEPT:
(A) *T cruzi* is transmitted by the reduviid bug
(B) *T cruzi* occurs primarily in tropical Africa
(C) *T cruzi* can be diagnosed by seeing trypomastigotes in a blood smear
(D) *T cruzi* typically affects heart muscle, leading to cardiac failure

344. Each of the following statements concerning sleeping sickness is correct EXCEPT:
(A) Sleeping sickness is caused by a trypanosome
(B) Sleeping sickness is transmitted by tsetse flies
(C) Sleeping sickness can be diagnosed by finding eggs in the stool
(D) Sleeping sickness occurs primarily in tropical Africa

345. Each of the following statements concerning kala-azar is correct EXCEPT:
(A) Kala-azar is caused by *Leishmania donovani*
(B) Kala-azar is transmitted by the bite of sandflies
(C) Kala-azar occurs primarily in rural Latin America
(D) Kala-azar can be diagnosed by finding amastigotes in bone marrow

346. Each of the following statements concerning *Diphyllobothrium latum* is correct EXCEPT:
(A) *D latum* is transmitted by undercooked fish
(B) *D latum* has operculated eggs
(C) Crustaceans (copepods) are intermediate hosts for *D latum*
(D) *D latum* has a scolex with a circle of hooks

347. Each of the following statements concerning hydatid cyst disease is correct EXCEPT:
(A) The disease is caused by *Echinococcus granulosus*
(B) The cysts occur primarily in the liver
(C) The disease is caused by a parasite whose adult form lives in dogs' intestines
(D) The disease occurs primarily in tropical Africa

348. Each of the following statements concerning *Schistosoma haematobium* is correct EXCEPT:
(A) *S haematobium* is acquired by humans when cercariae penetrate the skin
(B) Snails are intermediate hosts of *S haematobium*

(C) *S haematobium* eggs have no spine

(D) *S haematobium* infection predisposes to bladder carcinoma

349. Each of the following statements concerning hookworm infection is correct EXCEPT:

(A) Hookworm infection can cause anemia

(B) Hookworm infection is acquired by humans when filariform larvae penetrate the skin

(C) Hookworm infection is caused by *Necator americanus*

(D) Hookworm infection can be diagnosed by finding the trophozoite in the stool

350. Each of the following statements concerning *Ascaris lumbricoides* is correct EXCEPT:

(A) *A lumbricoides* is one of the largest nematodes

(B) *A lumbricoides* is transmitted by ingestion of eggs

(C) Both dogs and cats are intermediate hosts of *A lumbricoides*

(D) *A lumbricoides* can cause pneumonia

351. Each of the following statements concerning *Strongyloides stercoralis* is correct EXCEPT:

(A) *S stercoralis* is acquired by ingestion of eggs

(B) *S stercoralis* undergoes a free-living life cycle in soil

(C) *S stercoralis* causes a marked eosinophilia

(D) *S stercoralis* produces filariform larvae

352. Each of the following statements concerning trichinosis is correct EXCEPT:

(A) Trichinosis is acquired by eating undercooked pork

(B) Trichinosis is caused by a protozoan that has both a trophozoite and a cyst stage in its life cycle

(C) Trichinosis can be diagnosed by seeing cysts in muscle biopsy specimens

(D) Eosinophilia is a prominent finding

Answers (Questions 326–352):

326 (C)	332 (A)	338 (C)	344 (C)	350 (C)
327 (B)	333 (A)	339 (D)	345 (C)	351 (A)
328 (A)	334 (C)	340 (D)	346 (D)	352 (B)
329 (B)	335 (B)	341 (B)	347 (D)	
330 (A)	336 (A)	342 (D)	348 (C)	
331 (C)	337 (D)	343 (B)	349 (D)	

Directions (Questions 353–386): Select the ONE lettered option that is MOST closely associated with the numbered items. Each lettered option may be selected once, more than once, or not at all.

Questions 353–360

(A) *Dracunculus medinensis*

(B) *Loa loa*

(C) *Onchocerca volvulus*

(D) *Wuchereria bancrofti*

(E) *Toxocara canis*

353. Causes river blindness

354. Transmitted by mosquito

355. Acquired by drinking contaminated water

356. Treated by extracting worm from skin ulcer

357. Transmitted by deer fly or mango fly

358. Causes visceral larva migrans

359. Causes filariasis

360. Acquired by ingestion of worm eggs

Questions 361–372

(A) *Giardia lamblia*

(B) *Plasmodium vivax*

(C) *Taenia saginata*

(D) *Clonorchis sinensis*

(E) *Enterobius vermicularis*

361. A trematode (fluke) acquired by eating undercooked fish

362. A cestode (tapeworm) acquired by eating undercooked beef

363. A nematode (roundworm) transmitted primarily from child to child

364. A protozoan transmitted by mosquito

365. A protozoan transmitted by the fecal-oral route

366. Primarily affects the biliary ducts

367. Causes diarrhea as the most prominent symptom

368. Causes perianal itching as the most prominent symptom

369. Causes fever, chills, and anemia

370. Can be treated with metronidazole

371. Can be treated with mebendazole or pyrantel pamoate

372. Can be treated with chloroquine and primaquine

Questions 373–386

(A) *Entamoeba histolytica*

(B) *Plasmodium falciparum*

(C) *Taenia solium*

(D) *Paragonimus westermani*

(E) *Strongyloides stercoralis*

373. A cestode (tapeworm) acquired by eating undercooked pork

374. A nematode (roundworm) acquired when filariform larvae penetrate the skin

375. A protozoan transmitted by the fecal-oral route

376. A trematode (fluke) acquired by eating undercooked crab meat

377. A protozoan that infects red blood cells

378. Laboratory diagnosis based on finding eggs in sputum

379. Causes cysticercosis in humans

380. Chloroquine-resistant strains occur

381. Autoinfection within humans, especially in immunocompromised patients
382. Causes blackwater fever
383. Causes bloody diarrhea and liver abscesses
384. Produces "banana-shaped" gametocytes
385. Produces cysts with four nuclei
386. Has a scolex with suckers and a circle of hooks

Answers (Questions 353–386):

353 (C)	360 (E)	367 (A)	374 (E)	381 (E)
354 (D)	361 (D)	368 (E)	375 (A)	382 (B)
355 (A)	362 (C)	369 (B)	376 (D)	383 (A)
356 (A)	363 (E)	370 (A)	377 (B)	384 (B)
357 (B)	364 (B)	371 (E)	378 (D)	385 (A)
358 (E)	365 (A)	372 (B)	379 (C)	386 (C)
359 (D)	366 (D)	373 (C)	380 (B)	

Immunology

Directions (Questions 387–474): Select the ONE lettered answer that is BEST in each question.

387. Which category of hypersensitivity BEST describes hemolytic disease of the newborn caused by Rh incompatibility?
(A) Atopic or anaphylactic
(B) Cytotoxic
(C) Immune complex
(D) Delayed
388. The principal difference between cytotoxic (type II) and immune complex (type III) hypersensitivity is
(A) the class (isotype) of antibody
(B) the site where antigen-antibody complexes are formed
(C) the participation of complement
(D) the participation of T cells
389. A child stung by a bee experiences respiratory distress within minutes and lapses into unconsciousness. This reaction is probably mediated by
(A) IgE antibody
(B) IgG antibody
(C) sensitized T cells
(D) complement
(E) IgM antibody
390. A patient with rheumatic fever develops a sore throat from which beta-hemolytic streptococci are cultured. The patient is started on treatment with penicillin, and the sore throat resolves within several days. However, 7 days after initiation of penicillin therapy the patient develops a fever of 103 °F, a generalized rash, and proteinuria. This MOST probably resulted from
(A) recurrence of the rheumatic fever
(B) a different infectious disease

(C) an IgE response to penicillin
(D) an IgG-IgM response to penicillin
(E) a delayed hypersensitivity reaction to penicillin
391. A kidney biopsy specimen taken from a patient with acute glomerulonephritis and stained with fluorescein-conjugated anti-human IgG antibody would probably show
(A) no fluorescence
(B) uniform fluorescence of the glomerular basement membrane
(C) patchy, irregular fluorescence of the glomerular basement membrane
(D) fluorescent B cells
(E) fluorescent macrophages
392. A patient with severe asthma gets no relief from antihistamines. The symptoms are MOST likely to be caused by
(A) interleukin-2
(B) slow-reacting substance A (leukotrienes)
(C) serotonin
(D) bradykinin
393. Hypersensitivity to penicillin and hypersensitivity to poison oak are both
(A) mediated by IgE antibody
(B) mediated by IgG and IgM antibody
(C) initiated by haptens
(D) initiated by Th-2 cells
394. A recipient of a 2-haplotype MHC-matched kidney from a relative still needs immunosuppression to prevent graft rejection because
(A) graft-versus-host disease is a problem
(B) class II MHC antigens will not be matched
(C) minor histocompatibility antigens will not be matched
(D) complement components will not be matched

395. Bone marrow transplantation in immunocompromised patients presents which major problem?
    (A) Potentially lethal graft-versus-host disease
    (B) High risk of T cell leukemia
    (C) Inability to use a live donor
    (D) Delayed hypersensitivity

396. What is the role of class II MHC proteins on donor cells in graft rejection?
    (A) They are the receptors for interleukin-2, which is produced by macrophages when they attack the donor cells
    (B) They are recognized by helper T cells, which then activate cytotoxic T cells to kill the donor cells
    (C) They induce the production of blocking antibodies that protect the graft
    (D) They induce IgE which mediates graft rejection

397. Grafts between genetically identical individuals (ie, identical twins)
    (A) are rejected slowly as a result of minor histocompatibility antigens
    (B) are subject to hyperacute rejection
    (C) are not rejected, even without immunosuppression
    (D) are not rejected if a kidney is grafted, but skin grafts are rejected

398. Penicillin is a hapten in both humans and mice. To explore the hapten-carrier relationship, a mouse was injected with penicillin covalently bound to bovine serum albumin and, at the same time, with egg albumin to which no penicillin was bound. Of the following, which one will induce a secondary response to penicillin when injected into the mouse 1 month later?
    (A) Penicillin
    (B) Penicillin bound to egg albumin
    (C) Egg albumin
    (D) Bovine serum albumin

399. AIDS is caused by a human retrovirus that kills
    (A) B lymphocytes
    (B) lymphocyte stem cells
    (C) CD4-positive T lymphocytes
    (D) CD8-positive T lymphocytes

400. Chemically induced tumors have tumor-associated transplantation antigens that
    (A) are always the same for a given carcinogen
    (B) are different for two tumors of different histologic type even if induced by the same carcinogen
    (C) are very strong antigens
    (D) do not induce an immune response

401. Polyomavirus (a DNA virus) causes tumors in "nude mice" (nude mice do not have a thymus, because of a genetic defect) but not in normal mice. The BEST interpretation is that
    (A) macrophages are required to reject polyomavirus-induced tumors
    (B) natural killer cells can reject polyomavirus-induced tumors without help from T lymphocytes
    (C) T lymphocytes play an important role in the rejection of polyomavirus-induced tumors
    (D) B lymphocytes play no role in rejection of polyomavirus-induced tumors

402. C3 is cleaved to form C3a and C3b by C3 convertase. C3b is involved in all of the following EXCEPT:
    (A) altering vascular permeability
    (B) promoting phagocytosis
    (C) forming alternative-pathway C3 convertase
    (D) forming C5 convertase

403. After binding to its specific antigen, a B lymphocyte may switch its
    (A) immunoglobulin light-chain isotype
    (B) immunoglobulin heavy-chain class
    (C) variable region of the immunoglobulin heavy chain
    (D) constant region of the immunoglobulin light chain

404. Diversity is an important feature of the immune system. Which one of the following statements about it is INCORRECT?
    (A) Humans can make antibodies with about 10^8 different $V_H \times V_L$ combinations
    (B) A single cell can synthesize IgM antibody then switch to IgA antibody
    (C) The hematopoietic stem cell carries the genetic potential to create more than 10^4 immunoglobulin genes
    (D) A single B lymphocyte can produce antibodies of many different specificities, but a plasma cell is monospecific

405. C3a and C5a can cause
    (A) bacterial lysis
    (B) vascular pemeability
    (C) phagocytosis of IgE-coated bacteria
    (D) aggregation of C4 and C2

406. Neutrophils are attracted to an infected area by
    (A) IgM
    (B) C1
    (C) C5a
    (D) C8

407. Complement fixation refers to
    (A) the ingestion of C3b-coated bacteria by macrophages
    (B) the destruction of complement in serum by heating at 56 °C for 30 minutes
    (C) the binding of complement components by antigen-antibody complexes
    (D) the interaction of C3b with mast cells

408. The classic complement pathway is initiated by interaction of C1 with
    (A) antigen
    (B) factor B
    (C) antigen-IgG complexes
    (D) bacterial lipopolysaccharides

409. Patients with severely reduced C3 levels tend to have
  (A) increased numbers of severe viral infections
  (B) increased numbers of severe bacterial infections
  (C) low gamma globulin levels
  (D) frequent episodes of hemolytic anemia

410. Individuals with a genetic deficiency of C6 have
  (A) decreased resistance to viral infections
  (B) increased hypersensitivity reactions
  (C) increased frequency of cancer
  (D) decreased resistance to *Neisseria* bacteremia

411. Natural killer cells are
  (A) B cells that can kill without complement
  (B) cytotoxic T cells
  (C) increased by immunization
  (D) able to kill virus-infected cells without prior sensitization

412. A positive tuberculin skin test (a delayed hypersensitivity reaction) indicates that
  (A) a humoral immune response has occurred
  (B) a cell-mediated immune response has occurred
  (C) both the T and B cell systems are functional
  (D) only the B cell system is functional

413. Reaction to poison ivy or poison oak is
  (A) an IgG-mediated response
  (B) an IgE-mediated response
  (C) a cell-mediated response
  (D) an Arthus reaction

414. A child disturbs a wasp nest, is stung repeatedly, and goes into shock within minutes, manifesting respiratory failure and vascular collapse. This is MOST likely to be due to
  (A) systemic anaphylaxis
  (B) serum sickness
  (C) an Arthus reaction
  (D) cytotoxic hypersensitivity

415. "Isotype switching" of immunoglobulin classes by B cells involves
  (A) simultaneous insertion of V_H genes adjacent to each C_H gene
  (B) successive insertion of a single V_H gene adjacent to different C_H genes
  (C) activation of homologous genes on chromosome 6
  (D) switching of light-chain types (kappa and lambda)

416. Which one of the following pairs of genes is linked on a single chromosome?
  (A) V gene for lambda chain and C gene for kappa chain
  (B) C gene for gamma chain and C gene for kappa chain
  (C) V gene for lambda chain and V gene for heavy chain
  (D) C gene for gamma chain and C gene for alpha chain

417. Idiotypic determinants are located within
  (A) hypervariable regions of heavy and light chains
  (B) constant regions of light chains
  (C) constant regions of heavy chains
  (D) the hinge region

418. A primary immune response in an adult human requires approximately how much time to produce detectable antibody levels in the blood?
  (A) 12 hours
  (B) 3 days
  (C) 1 week
  (D) 3 weeks

419. The membrane IgM and IgD on the surface of an individual B cell
  (A) have identical heavy chains but different light chains
  (B) are identical except for their C_H regions
  (C) are identical except for their V_H regions
  (D) have different V_H and V_L regions

420. During the maturation of a B lymphocyte, the first immunoglobulin heavy chain synthesized is the
  (A) mu chain
  (B) gamma chain
  (C) epsilon chain
  (D) alpha chain

421. In the immune response to a hapten-protein conjugate, in order to get anti-hapten antibodies it is essential that
  (A) the hapten be recognized by helper T cells
  (B) the protein be recognized by helper T cells
  (C) the protein be recognized by B cells
  (D) the hapten be recognized by suppressor T cells

422. In the determination of serum insulin levels by radioimmunoassay, which one of the following is NOT needed?
  (A) Isotope-labeled insulin
  (B) Anti-insulin antibody made in goats
  (C) Anti-goat gamma globulin made in rabbits
  (D) Isotope-labeled anti-insulin antibody made in goats

423. Which one of the following sequences is appropriate for testing a patient for antibody against the AIDS virus with the ELISA procedure? (The assay is carried out in a plastic plate with an incubation and a wash step after each addition except the final one.)
  (A) Patient's serum/enzyme substrate/HIV antigen/enzyme-labeled antibody against HIV
  (B) HIV antigen/patient's serum/enzyme-labeled antibody against human gamma globulin/ enzyme substrate
  (C) enzyme-labeled antibody against human gamma globulin/patient's serum/HIV antigen/enzyme substrate

(D) enzyme-labeled antibody against HIV/HIV antigen/patient's serum/enzyme substrate

424. The BEST method to demonstrate IgG on the glomerular basement membrane in a kidney tissue section is the
- **(A)** precipitin test
- **(B)** complement fixation test
- **(C)** agglutination test
- **(D)** indirect fluorescent-antibody test

425. A woman had a high fever, hypotension, and a diffuse macular rash. When all cultures showed no bacterial growth, a diagnosis of toxic shock syndrome was made. Regarding the mechanism by which the toxin causes this disease, which one of the following is LEAST accurate?
- **(A)** The toxin is not processed within the macrophage
- **(B)** The toxin binds to both the class II MHC protein and the T cell receptor
- **(C)** The toxin activates many CD4-positive T cells, and large amounts of interleukins are released
- **(D)** The toxin has an A-B subunit structure—the B subunit binds to a receptor, and the A subunit enters the cells and activates them.

426. A patient with a central nervous system disorder is maintained on the drug methyldopa. Hemolytic anemia develops, which resolves shortly after the drug is withdrawn. This is MOST probably an example of
- **(A)** atopic hypersensitivity
- **(B)** cytotoxic hypersensitivity
- **(C)** immune-complex hypersensitivity
- **(D)** cell-mediated hypersensitivity

427. Which one of the following substances is NOT released by activated helper T cells?
- **(A)** Alpha interferon
- **(B)** Gamma interferon
- **(C)** Interleukin-2
- **(D)** Interleukin-4

428. A delayed hypersensitivity reaction is characterized by
- **(A)** edema without a cellular infiltrate
- **(B)** an infiltrate composed of neutrophils
- **(C)** an infiltrate composed of helper T cells and macrophages
- **(D)** an infiltrate composed of eosinophils

429. Two dissimilar inbred strains of mice, A and B, are crossed to yield an F_1 hybrid strain, AB. If a large dose of spleen cells from an adult A mouse is injected into an adult AB mouse, which one of the following is MOST likely to occur?
- **(A)** The spleen cells will be destroyed
- **(B)** The spleen cells will survive and will have no effect in the recipient
- **(C)** The spleen cells will induce a graft-versus-host reaction in the recipient
- **(D)** The spleen cells will survive and induce tolerance of strain A grafts in the recipient

430. This question is based on the same strains of mice described in the previous question. If adult AB spleen cells are injected into a newborn B mouse, which one of the following is MOST likely to occur?
- **(A)** The spleen cells will be destroyed
- **(B)** The spleen cells will survive without any effect on the recipient
- **(C)** The spleen cells will induce a graft-versus-host reaction in the recipient
- **(D)** The spleen cells will survive and induce tolerance of strain A grafts in the recipient

431. The minor histocompatibility antigens on cells
- **(A)** are detected by reaction with antibodies and complement
- **(B)** are controlled by several genes in the major histocompatibility complex
- **(C)** are unimportant in human transplantation
- **(D)** induce reactions that can cumulatively lead to a strong rejection response

432. Which one of the following is NOT true of class I MHC antigens?
- **(A)** They can be assayed by a cytotoxic test that uses antibody and complement
- **(B)** They can usually be identified in the laboratory in a few hours
- **(C)** They are controlled by at least three gene loci in the major histocompatibility complex
- **(D)** They are found mainly on B cells, macrophages, and activated T cells

433. An antigen found in relatively high concentration in the plasma of normal fetuses and a high proportion of patients with progressive carcinoma of the colon is
- **(A)** viral antigen
- **(B)** carcinoembryonic antigen
- **(C)** alpha-fetoprotein
- **(D)** heterophil antigen

434. An antibody directed against the idiotypic determinants of a human IgG antibody would react with
- **(A)** the Fc part of the IgG
- **(B)** an IgM antibody produced by the same plasma cell that produced the IgG
- **(C)** all human kappa chains
- **(D)** all human gamma chains

435. Which one of the following is NOT true of the gene segments that combine to make up a heavy-chain gene?
- **(A)** Many V region segments are available
- **(B)** Several J segments and several D segments are available
- **(C)** V, D, and J segments combine to encode the antigen-binding site
- **(D)** A V segment and a J segment are pre-selected by an antigen to make up the variable-region portion of the gene

436. When immune complexes from the serum are deposited on glomerular basement membrane, damage to the membrane is caused mainly by
(A) gamma interferon
(B) phagocytosis
(C) cytotoxic T cells
(D) enzymes released by polymorphonuclear cells

437. If an individual was genetically unable to make J chains, which immunoglobulin(s) would be affected?
(A) IgG
(B) IgM
(C) IgA
(D) IgG and IgM
(E) IgM and IgA

438. The antibody-binding site is formed primarily by
(A) the constant regions of H and L chains
(B) the hypervariable regions of H and L chains
(C) the hypervariable regions of H chains
(D) the variable regions of H chains
(E) the variable regions of L chains

439. The class of immunoglobulin present in highest concentration in the blood of a human newborn is
(A) IgG
(B) IgM
(C) IgA
(D) IgD
(E) IgE

440. Individuals of blood group type AB
(A) are Rh(D)-negative
(B) are "universal recipients" of transfusions
(C) have circulating anti-A and anti-B antibodies
(D) have the same haplotype

441. Cytotoxic T cells induced by infection with virus A will kill target cells
(A) from the same host infected with any virus
(B) infected by virus A and identical at class I MHC loci of the cytotoxic T cells
(C) infected by virus A and identical at class II MHC loci of the cytotoxic T cells
(D) infected with a different virus and identical at class I MHC loci of the cytotoxic cells
(E) infected with a different virus and identical at class II MHC loci of the cytotoxic cells

442. Antigen-presenting cells that activate helper T cells must express which one of the following on their surfaces?
(A) IgE
(B) Gamma interferon
(C) Class I MHC antigens
(D) Class II MHC antigens

443. Which one of the following does NOT contain C3b?

(A) Classic-pathway C5 convertase
(B) Alternative-pathway C5 convertase
(C) Classic-pathway C3 convertase
(D) Alternative-pathway C3 convertase

444. Which one of the following is NOT true regarding the alternative complement pathway?
(A) It can be triggered by infectious agents in absence of antibody
(B) It does not require C1, C2, or C4
(C) It cannot be initiated unless C3b fragments are already present
(D) It has the same terminal sequence of events as the classic pathway

445. In setting up a complement fixation test for antibody, the reactants should be added in what sequence? (Ag = antigen; Ab = antibody; C = complement; EA = antibody-coated indicator erythrocytes.)
(A) Ag + EA + C/wait/ + patient's serum
(B) C + patient's serum + EA/wait/ + Ag
(C) Ag + patient's serum + EA/wait/ + C
(D) Ag + patient's serum + C/wait/ + EA

446. Proteins from two samples of animal blood, A and B, were tested by the double-diffusion (Ouchterlony) test in agar against antibody to bovine albumin. Which sample(s) contain horse blood? An explanation of the answer to this question is given on p 486.

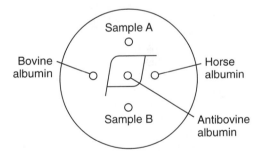

(A) Sample A
(B) Sample B
(C) Both samples
(D) Neither sample

447. Complement lyses cells by
(A) enzymatic digestion of the cell membrane
(B) activation of adenylate cyclase
(C) insertion of complement proteins into the cell membrane
(D) inhibition of elongation factor 2

448. Graft and tumor rejection are mediated primarily by
(A) non-complement-fixing antibodies
(B) phagocytic cells
(C) helper T cells
(D) cytotoxic T cells

449. Which one of the following properties of antibodies is NOT dependent on the structure of the heavy-chain constant region?
  (A) Ability to cross the placenta
  (B) Isotype (class)
  (C) Ability to fix complement
  (D) Affinity for antigen

450. In which one of the following situations would a graft-versus-host reaction be MOST likely to occur? (Mouse strains A and B are highly inbred; AB is an F_1 hybrid between strain A and strain B.)
  (A) Newborn strain A spleen cells injected into a strain B adult
  (B) X-irradiated adult strain A spleen cells injected into a strain B adult
  (C) Adult strain A spleen cells injected into an x-irradiated strain AB adult
  (D) Adult strain AB spleen cells injected into a strain A newborn

451. In a mixed-lymphocyte culture, lymphocytes from person X, who is homozygous for the HLA-Dw7 allele, are irradiated and then cultured with lymphocytes from person Z. It is found that DNA synthesis is NOT stimulated. The proper conclusion to be drawn is that
  (A) person Z is homozygous for HLA-Dw7
  (B) person Z is homozygous or heterozygous for HLA-Dw7
  (C) person Z is heterozygous for HLA-Dw7
  (D) person Z does not carry the HLA-Dw7 allele

452. A patient skin-tested with purified protein derivative (PPD) to determine previous exposure to *Mycobacterium tuberculosis* develops induration at the skin test site 48 hours later. Histologically, the reaction site would MOST probably show
  (A) Eosinophils
  (B) Neutrophils
  (C) Helper T cells and macrophages
  (D) B cells

453. Hemolytic disease of the newborn caused by Rh blood group incompatibility requires maternal antibody to enter the fetal bloodstream. Therefore, the mediator of this disease is
  (A) IgE antibody
  (B) IgG antibody
  (C) IgM antibody
  (D) IgA antibody

454. An Rh-negative woman married to a heterozygous Rh-positive man has three children. The probability that all three of their children are Rh-positive is
  (A) 1:2
  (B) 1:4
  (C) 1:8
  (D) zero

455. Which one of the following statements BEST explains the relationship between inflammation of the heart (carditis) and infection with group A beta-hemolytic streptococci?
  (A) Streptococcal antigens induce antibodies cross-reactive with heart tissue
  (B) Streptococci are polyclonal activators of B cells
  (C) Streptococcal antigens bind to IgE on the surface of heart tissue and histamine is released
  (D) Streptococci are ingested by neutrophils that release proteases that damage heart tissue

456. Your patient became ill 10 days ago with a viral disease. Laboratory examination reveals that the patient's antibodies against this virus have a high ratio of IgM to IgG. What is your conclusion?
  (A) It is unlikely that the patient has encountered this organism previously
  (B) The patient is predisposed to IgE-mediated hypersensitivity reactions
  (C) The information given is irrelevant to previous antigen exposure
  (D) It is likely that the patient has an autoimmune disease

457. If you measure the ability of cytotoxic T cells from an HLA-B27 person to kill virus X-infected target cells, which one of the following statements is CORRECT?
  (A) Any virus X-infected target cell will be killed
  (B) Only virus X-infected cells of HLA-B27 type will be killed
  (C) Any HLA-B27 cell will be killed
  (D) No HLA-B27 cell will be killed

458. You have a patient who makes autoantibodies against his own red blood cells, leading to hemolysis. Which one of the following mechanisms is MOST likely to explain the hemolysis?
  (A) Perforins from cytotoxic T cells lyse the red cells
  (B) Neutrophils release proteases that lyse the red cells
  (C) Interleukin-2 binds to its receptor on the red cells, which results in lysis of the red cells
  (D) Complement is activated, and membrane attack complexes lyse the red cells

459. Your patient is a child who has no detectable T or B cells. This immunodeficiency is most probably the result of a defect in
  (A) the thymus
  (B) the bursal equivalent
  (C) T cell-B cell interaction
  (D) stem cells originating in the bone marrow

460. The role of the macrophage during an antibody response is to

(A) make antibody
(B) lyse virus-infected target cells
(C) activate cytotoxic T cells
(D) process antigen and present it

461. The structural basis of blood group A and B antigen specificity is
(A) a single terminal sugar residue
(B) a single terminal amino acid
(C) multiple differences in the carbohydrate portion
(D) multiple differences in the protein portion

462. Complement can enhance phagocytosis because of the presence on macrophages and neutrophils of receptors for
(A) factor D
(B) C3b
(C) C6
(D) properdin

463. The main advantage of passive immunization over active immunization is that
(A) it can be administered orally
(B) it provides antibody more rapidly
(C) antibody persists for a longer period
(D) it contains primarily IgM

464. On January 15, a patient developed an illness suggestive of influenza, which lasted 1 week. On February 20, she had a similar illness. She had no influenza immunization during this period. Her hemagglutination inhibition titer to influenza A virus was 10 on January 18, 40 on January 30, and 320 on February 20. Which one of the following is the MOST appropriate interpretation?
(A) The patient was ill with influenza A on January 15
(B) The patient was ill with influenza A on February 20
(C) The patient was not infected with influenza virus
(D) The patient has an autoimmune disease

465. An individual who is heterozygous for Gm allotypes contains two allelic forms of IgG in serum, but individual lymphocytes produce only one of the two forms. This phenomenon, known as "allelic exclusion," is consistent with
(A) a rearrangement of a heavy-chain gene on only one chromosome in a lymphocyte
(B) rearrangements of heavy-chain genes on both chromosomes in a lymphocyte
(C) a rearrangement of a light-chain gene on only one chromosome in a lymphocyte
(D) rearrangements of light-chain genes on both chromosomes in a lymphocyte

466. Each of the following statements concerning class I MHC proteins is correct EXCEPT:
(A) They are cell surface proteins on virtually all cells
(B) They are recognition elements for cytotoxic T cells
(C) They are codominantly expressed

(D) They are important in the skin test response to *Mycobacterium tuberculosis*

467. Which one of the following is the BEST method of reducing the effect of graft-versus-host disease in a bone marrow recipient?
(A) Matching the complement components of donor and recipient
(B) Administering alpha interferon
(C) Removing mature T cells from the graft
(D) Removing pre-B cells from the graft

468. Regarding Th-1 and Th-2 cells, which one of the following is LEAST accurate?
(A) Th-1 cells produce gamma interferon and promote cell-mediated immunity
(B) Th-2 cells produce interleukin-4 and -5 and promote antibody-mediated immunity
(C) Both Th-1 and Th-2 cells have both CD3 and CD4 proteins on their outer cell membrane
(D) Before naive Th cells differentiate into Th-1 or Th-2 cells, they are double-positives; ie, they produce both gamma interferon and interleukin-4

469. Each of the following statements concerning the variable regions of heavy chains and the variable regions of light chains in a given antibody molecule is correct EXCEPT:
(A) They have the same amino acid sequence
(B) They define the specificity for antigen
(C) They are encoded on different chromosomes
(D) They contain the hypervariable regions

470. Each of the following statements concerning class II MHC proteins is correct EXCEPT:
(A) They are found on the surface of both B and T cells
(B) They have a high degree of polymorphism
(C) They are involved in the presentation of antigen by macrophages
(D) They have a binding site for CD4 proteins

471. Which one of the following statements concerning immunoglobulin allotypes is CORRECT?
(A) Allotypes are found only on heavy chains
(B) Allotypes are determined by class I MHC genes
(C) Allotypes are confined to the variable regions
(D) Allotypes are due to genetic polymorphism within a species

472. Each of the following statements concerning immunologic tolerance is correct EXCEPT:
(A) Tolerance is not antigen-specific; ie, paralysis of the immune cells results in a failure to produce a response against many antigens
(B) Tolerance is more easily induced in T cells than in B cells
(C) Tolerance is more easily induced in neonates than in adults
(D) Tolerance is more easily induced by simple molecules than by complex ones

473. Each of the following statements concerning a hybridoma cell is correct EXCEPT:

(A) The spleen cell component provides the ability to form antibody

(B) The myeloma cell component provides the ability to grow indefinitely

(C) The antibody produced by a hybridoma cell is IgM, because heavy-chain switching does not occur

(D) The antibody produced by a hybridoma cell is homogeneous; ie, it is directed against a single epitope

474. Each of the following statements concerning haptens is correct EXCEPT:

(A) A hapten can combine with (bind to) an antibody

(B) A hapten cannot induce an antibody by itself; rather, it must be bound to a carrier protein to be able to induce antibody

(C) In both penicillin-induced anaphylaxis and poison ivy, the allergens are haptens

(D) Haptens must be processed by CD8+ cells to become immunogenic

Answers (Questions 387–474):

387 (B)	405 (B)	423 (B)	441 (B)	459 (D)
388 (B)	406 (C)	424 (D)	442 (D)	460 (D)
389 (A)	407 (C)	425 (D)	443 (C)	461 (A)
390 (D)	408 (C)	426 (B)	444 (C)	462 (B)
391 (C)	409 (B)	427 (A)	445 (D)	463 (B)
392 (B)	410 (D)	428 (C)	446 (B)	464 (A)
393 (C)	411 (D)	429 (C)	447 (C)	465 (A)
394 (C)	412 (B)	430 (D)	448 (D)	466 (D)
395 (A)	413 (C)	431 (D)	449 (D)	467 (C)
396 (B)	414 (A)	432 (D)	450 (C)	468 (D)
397 (C)	415 (B)	433 (B)	451 (B)	469 (A)
398 (D)	416 (D)	434 (B)	452 (C)	470 (A)
399 (C)	417 (A)	435 (D)	453 (B)	471 (D)
400 (B)	418 (C)	436 (D)	454 (C)	472 (A)
401 (C)	419 (B)	437 (E)	455 (A)	473 (C)
402 (A)	420 (A)	438 (B)	456 (A)	474 (D)
403 (B)	421 (B)	439 (A)	457 (B)	
404 (D)	422 (D)	440 (B)	458 (D)	

Directions (Questions 475–535): Select the ONE lettered option that is MOST closely associated with the numbered items. Each lettered option may be selected once, more than once, or not at all.

Questions 475–480

(A) T cells

(B) B cells

(C) Macrophages

(D) B cells and macrophages

(E) T cells, B cells, and macrophages

475. Major source of interleukin-1

476. Acted on by interleukin-1

477. Major source of interleukin-2

478. Express class I MHC markers

479. Express class II MHC markers

480. Express surface immunoglobulin

Questions 481–484

(A) Primary antibody response

(B) Secondary antibody response

481. Appears more quickly and persists longer

482. Relatively richer in IgG

483. Relatively richer in IgM

484. Typically takes 7–10 days for antibody to appear

Questions 485–488

(A) Blood group A

(B) Blood group O

(C) Blood groups A and O

(D) Blood group AB

485. People with this type have circulating anti-A antibodies

486. People with this type have circulating anti-B antibodies

487. People with this type are called "universal donors"

488. People with this type are called "universal recipients"

Questions 489–494

(A) Variable region of light chain

(B) Variable region of heavy chain

(C) Variable regions of light and heavy chains

(D) Constant region of heavy chain

(E) Constant regions of light and heavy chains

489. Determines immunoglobulin class

490. Determines allotypes

491. Determines idiotypes

492. Binding of IgG to macrophages

493. Fixation of complement by IgG

494. Antigen-binding site

Questions 495–498

The following double-immunodiffusion plate contains antibody prepared against whole human serum in the center well. Identify the contents of each peripheral well from the following list (each well to be used once). An explanation of the answer to this question is given on p 486.

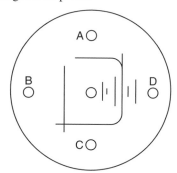

495. Whole human serum
496. Human IgG
497. Baboon IgG
498. Human transferrin

Questions 499–501

(**A**) Immediate hypersensitivity
(**B**) Cytotoxic hypersensitivity
(**C**) Immune-complex hypersensitivity
(**D**) Delayed hypersensitivity
499. Irregular deposition of IgG along glomerular basement membrane
500. Involves mast cells and basophils
501. Mediated by lymphokines

Questions 502–505

(**A**) IgM
(**B**) IgG
(**C**) IgA
(**D**) IgE
502. Crosses the placenta
503. Can contain a polypeptide chain not synthesized by a B lymphocyte
504. Found in the milk of lactating women
505. Binds firmly to mast cells and triggers anaphylaxis

Questions 506–509

(**A**) Agglutination
(**B**) Precipitin test
(**C**) Immunofluorescence
(**D**) Enzyme immunoassay
506. Concentration of IgG in serum
507. Surface IgM on cells in a bone marrow smear
508. Growth hormone in serum
509. Type A blood group antigen on erythrocytes

Questions 510–513

(**A**) IgA
(**B**) IgE
(**C**) IgG
(**D**) IgM
510. Present in highest concentration in serum
511. Present in highest concentration in secretions
512. Present in lowest concentration in serum
513. Contains 10 heavy and 10 light chains

Questions 514–517

In this double-diffusion (Ouchterlony) assay, the center well contains antibody against whole human serum. The peripheral (numbered) wells each contain one of the following proteins:

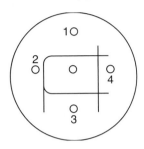

(**A**) Human serum albumin at low concentration
(**B**) Human serum albumin at high concentration
(**C**) Human serum transferrin
(**D**) Sheep serum albumin
514. Which protein is present in well no. 1?
515. Which protein is present in well no. 2?
516. Which protein is present in well no. 3?
517. Which protein is present in well no. 4?
An explanation of the answer to this question is given on p 486.

Questions 518–521

(**A**) Class I MHC proteins
(**B**) Class II MHC proteins
518. Involved in the presentation of antigen to CD4 positive cells
519. Involved in the presentation of antigen to CD8 positive cells
520. Involved in antibody responses to T-dependent antigens
521. Involved in target cell recognition by cytotoxic T cells

Questions 522–525

(**A**) Fab fragment of IgG
(**B**) Fc fragment of IgG
522. Contains an antigen-combining site
523. Contains hypervariable regions
524. Contains a complement-binding site
525. Is crystallizable

Questions 526–530

(**A**) Severe combined immunodeficiency disease (SCID)
(**B**) X-linked hypogammaglobulinemia
(**C**) Thymic aplasia
(**D**) Chronic granulomatous disease
(**E**) Hereditary angioedema
526. Caused by a defect in the ability of neutrophils to kill microorganisms

527. Caused by a development defect that results in a profound loss of T cells
528. Caused by a deficiency in an inhibitor of the C1 component of complement
529. Caused by a marked deficiency of B cells
530. Caused by a virtual absence of both B and T cells

Questions 531–535

(A) Systemic lupus erythematosus
(B) Rheumatoid arthritis
(C) Rheumatic fever
(D) Graves' disease
(E) Myasthenia gravis

531. Associated with antibody to the thyroid-stimulating hormone (TSH) receptor
532. Associated with antibody to IgG
533. Associated with antibody to the acetylcholine receptor
534. Associated with antibody to DNA
535. Associated with antibody to streptococci

Answers (Questions 475–535):

475 (C)	488 (D)	500 (A)	512 (B)	524 (B)
476 (A)	489 (D)	501 (D)	513 (D)	525 (B)
477 (A)	490 (E)	502 (B)	514 (B)	526 (D)
478 (E)	491 (C)	503 (C)	515 (A)	527 (C)
479 (D)	492 (D)	504 (C)	516 (D)	528 (E)
480 (B)	493 (D)	505 (D)	517 (C)	529 (B)
481 (B)	494 (C)	506 (D)	518 (B)	530 (A)
482 (B)	495 (D)	507 (C)	519 (A)	531 (D)
483 (A)	496 (C)	508 (D)	520 (B)	532 (B)
484 (A)	497 (A)	509 (A)	521 (A)	533 (E)
485 (B)	498 (B)	510 (C)	522 (A)	534 (A)
486 (C)	499 (C)	511 (A)	523 (A)	535 (C)
487 (B)				

Explanation of question 446: There is a line of identity between sample A and bovine albumin, therefore sample A is bovine albumin. There is a line of identity between sample B and horse albumin, therefore sample B is horse albumin. The answer to the question is therefore (B). Note that there is a spur formed between the wells containing sample A and horse albumin and between the wells containing sample B and bovine albumin. The spur indicates partial identity between the two proteins. Partial identity means that there are epitopes shared between the two albumins but that, because they are from different species, there are epitopes unique to each protein, also. A spur is formed by the interaction of the subset of antibodies in the anti-bovine serum with the **unique** epitopes in bovine albumin. The other lines are formed by the interaction of the subset of antibodies in the anti-bovine serum with the epitopes **shared** by the two albumins.

Explanation of questions 495–498: The center well contains antibody against whole human serum; therefore, well D must contain whole human serum because there are multiple lines representing some of the many proteins in whole human serum. There is a line of identity between well C and a protein in whole human serum and a line of partial identity with that same protein and well A. This indicates that well C contains human IgG and well A contains baboon IgG. The concept of partial identity is explained above in the discussion of question 446. There is a line of nonidentity between wells B and C; therefore, well B contains human transferrin, a protein immunologically distinct from human IgG.

Explanation of questions 514–517: There is a line of identity between wells 1 and 2; therefore, they contain human serum albumin (HSA). Note that the line of immunoprecipitate is very close to well 2. This line would not form if well 2 contained the high concentration of HSA because it would be a zone of antigen excess and the line only forms in a zone of equivalence. Therefore, well 2 contains the low concentration and well 1 contains the high concentration of HSA. There is a line of partial identity between well 2 and 3, therefore well 3 contains sheep serum albumin (SSA). There is a line of nonidentity between wells 1 and 4 and wells 3 and 4, therefore well 4 contains human transferrin which is immunologically distinct from HSA and SSA.

Extended Matching Questions

Directions (Questions 536–593): Each set of matching questions in this section consists of a list of lettered options followed by several numbered items. For each numbered item, select the ONE lettered option that is MOST closely associated with it. Each lettered option may be selected once, more than once, or not at all.

(A) Capsule
(B) Periplasmic space
(C) Peptidoglycan
(D) Lipid A
(E) 30S ribosomal subunit
(F) G protein
(G) Pilus
(H) ADP-ribosylating enzyme
(I) Mesosome
(J) Flagellum
(K) Transposon

536. Is the site of action of lysozyme
537. Mediates adherence of bacteria to mucous membranes
538. Is the toxic component of endotoxin

(A) Skin
(B) Colon
(C) Nose
(D) Stomach
(E) Vagina
(F) Mouth
(G) Outer third of urethra
(H) Gingival crevice
(I) Pharynx

539. Anatomic location where *Bacteroides fragilis* is most commonly found
540. Anatomic location where *Actinomyces israelii* is most commonly found

(A) Toxic shock syndrome toxin
(B) Tetanus toxin
(C) Diphtheria toxin
(D) Cholera toxin
(E) Coagulase
(F) Botulinum toxin
(G) Alpha toxin of *C perfringens*
(H) M protein
(I) Endotoxin
(J) Verotoxin

541. Blocks release of acetylcholine
542. Its lipid component causes fever and shock by inducing TNF

543. Causes fever and shock by binding to the T cell receptor
544. Inhibits protein synthesis by ADP-ribosylation of elongation factor 2
545. Increases cyclic AMP by ADP-ribosylation of a G protein

(A) Ampicillin
(B) Nafcillin
(C) Clindamycin
(D) Gentamicin
(E) Tetracycline
(F) Amphotericin B
(G) Ciprofloxacin
(H) Rifampin
(I) Sulfonamide
(J) Erythromycin
(K) Metronidazole
(L) Isoniazid

546. Inhibits protein synthesis by blocking formation of the initiation complex so that no polysomes form
547. Inhibits DNA gyrase
548. Inhibits folic acid synthesis; analogue of para-aminobenzoic acid
549. Inhibits peptidoglycan synthesis; resistant to β-lactamase
550. Inhibits RNA polymerase

(A) *Streptococcus pneumoniae*
(B) *Streptococcus pyogenes*
(C) *Haemophilus influenzae*
(D) *Salmonella typhi*
(E) *Staphylococcus aureus*
(F) *Enterococcus faecalis*
(G) *Clostridium tetani*
(H) *Bordetella pertussis*
(I) *Escherichia coli*
(J) *Streptococcus agalactiae*
(K) *Staphylococcus epidermidis*
(L) *Streptococcus mutans*

551. Immunogen in the vaccine is capsular polysaccharide coupled to a protein carrier
552. Immunogen in the vaccine is a toxoid
553. Causes acute glomerulonephritis; is beta-hemolytic
554. Causes urinary tract infections; grows in 6.5% NaCl
555. Causes neonatal meningitis; is bacitracin-resistant
556. Causes meningitis in adults; is alpha-hemolytic and optochin-sensitive
557. Causes food poisoning; is coagulase-positive

(A) *Escherichia coli*
(B) *Shigella sonnei*
(C) *Salmonella typhi*
(D) *Salmonella enteritidis*
(E) *Proteus mirabilis*
(F) *Pseudomonas aeruginosa*
(G) *Vibrio cholerae*
(H) *Campylobacter jejuni*
(I) *Helicobacter pylori*
(J) *Bacteroides fragilis*

558. Causes of gastritis and peptic ulcer; produces urease
559. Causes bloody diarrhea; does not ferment lactose and does not produce H_2S
560. Causes peritonitis; is an obligate anaerobe
561. Causes wound infections with blue-green pus; is oxidase-positive
562. Comma-shaped rod; causes high-volume watery diarrhea

(A) *Legionella pneumophila*
(B) *Yersinia pestis*
(C) *Haemophilus influenzae*
(D) *Corynebacterium diphtheriae*
(E) *Pasteurella multocida*
(F) *Bordetella pertussis*
(G) *Brucella melitensis*
(H) *Listeria monocytogenes*
(I) *Clostridium perfringens*
(J) *Neisseria gonorrhoeae*

563. Gram-positive spore-forming rod that causes myonecrosis
564. Gram-negative rod that is transmitted by cat bite
565. Gram-negative rod that causes cough and lymphocytosis

(A) *Mycobacterium tuberculosis*
(B) *Borrelia burgdorferi*
(C) *Nocardia asteroides*
(D) *Treponema pallidum*
(E) *Coxiella burnetii*
(F) *Mycoplasma pneumoniae*
(G) *Mycobacterium leprae*
(H) *Chlamydia trachomatis*
(I) *Rickettsia rickettsii*
(J) *Leptospira interrogans*

566. Spirochete that does not have an animal reservoir
567. Obligate intracellular parasite that forms elementary bodies
568. Respiratory pathogen without a cell wall

(A) Influenza virus
(B) Adenovirus
(C) Hepatitis A virus
(D) Hepatitis B virus
(E) Herpes simplex virus
(F) Measles virus
(G) Human immunodeficiency virus
(H) Rabies virus
(I) Reovirus

569. Nonenveloped virus with single-stranded, positive-polarity RNA
570. Enveloped virus with two identical strands of positive-polarity RNA
571. Enveloped virus with double-stranded DNA and DNA polymerase in the virion
572. Enveloped virus with segmented, negative-polarity, single-stranded RNA
573. Nonenveloped virus with segmented double-stranded RNA

(A) Herpes simplex virus type 1
(B) Rabies virus
(C) Varicella-zoster virus
(D) Measles virus
(E) Epstein-Barr virus
(F) Influenza virus
(G) Rubella virus
(H) Herpes simplex virus type 2
(I) Mumps virus
(J) Cytomegalovirus
(K) Parainfluenza virus
(L) Respiratory syncytial virus

574. Leading cause of congenital malformations; no vaccine available
575. Causes a painful vesicular rash along the course of a thoracic nerve
576. Causes encephalitis; killed vaccine available
577. Causes pharyngitis, lymphadenopathy, and a positive heterophil test
578. Causes retinitis and pneumonia in patients deficient in helper T cells
579. Causes encephalitis, especially in the temporal lobe
580. Causes pneumonia primarily in infants; induces giant cells
581. Causes orchitis that can result in sterility

(A) Human papillomavirus
(B) Hepatitis A virus
(C) Rotavirus
(D) Adenovirus
(E) Hepatitis delta virus
(F) Parvovirus B19
(G) Human immunodeficiency virus
(H) Hepatitis B virus
(I) Muerto Canyon virus
(J) Human T cell leukemia virus
(K) Prion
(L) Hepatitis C virus

582. Most important cause of diarrhea in infants
583. A vaccine containing purified viral protein is available
584. Defective virus with an RNA genome

(A) *Coccidioides immitis*
(B) *Cryptococcus neoformans*
(C) *Blastomyces dermatitidis*
(D) *Sporothrix schenckii*
(E) *Aspergillus fumigatus*
(F) *Candida albicans*
(G) *Histoplasma capsulatum*
(H) *Mucor* species
(I) *Microsporum canis*

585. Dimorphic fungus that enters the body through puncture wounds in the skin

586. Nonseptate mold that invades tissue, especially in acidotic patients

587. Yeast that forms pseudohyphae when it invades tissue

(A) *Giardia lamblia*
(B) *Plasmodium vivax*
(C) *Leishmania donovani*
(D) *Entamoeba histolytica*
(E) *Toxoplasma gondii*
(F) *Trypanosoma cruzi*
(G) *Pneumocystis carinii*
(H) *Plasmodium falciparum*
(I) *Naegleria* species
(J) *Trichomonas vaginalis*

588. Acquired while swimming; causes meningitis

589. Transmitted by reduviid bug and invades cardiac muscle

590. Amastigotes found within macrophages

(A) *Echinococcus granulosus*
(B) *Clonorchis sinensis*
(C) *Strongyloides stercoralis*
(D) *Taenia solium*
(E) *Necator americanus*
(F) *Enterobius vermicularis*
(G) *Schistosoma haematobium*
(H) *Wuchereria bancrofti*
(I) *Trichinella spiralis*
(J) *Taenia saginata*

591. Infection predisposes to bladder carcinoma

592. Ingestion of larvae can cause cysticercosis

593. Acquired by penetration of feet by larvae; causes anemia

Answers (Questions 536–593):

536 (C)	548 (I)	560 (J)	572 (A)	584 (E)
537 (G)	549 (B)	561 (F)	573 (I)	585 (D)
538 (D)	550 (H)	562 (G)	574 (J)	586 (H)
539 (B)	551 (C)	563 (I)	575 (C)	587 (F)
540 (H)	552 (G)	564 (E)	576 (B)	588 (I)
541 (F)	553 (B)	565 (F)	577 (E)	589 (F)
542 (I)	554 (F)	566 (D)	578 (J)	590 (C)
543 (A)	555 (J)	567 (H)	579 (A)	591 (G)
544 (C)	556 (A)	568 (F)	580 (L)	592 (D)
545 (D)	557 (E)	569 (C)	581 (I)	593 (E)
546 (D)	558 (I)	570 (G)	582 (C)	
547 (G)	559 (B)	571 (D)	583 (H)	

Clinical Case Questions

Directions (Questions 594–654): Select the ONE lettered answer that is BEST in each question.

CASE 1. Your patient is a 20-year-old woman with the sudden onset of fever to 104 °F and a severe headache. Physical examination reveals nuchal rigidity. You suspect meningitis and do a spinal tap. Gram stain of the spinal fluid reveals many neutrophils and many gram-negative diplococci.

594. Of the following bacteria, which one is MOST likely to be the cause?
(A) *Haemophilus influenzae*
(B) *Neisseria meningitidis*
(C) *Streptococcus pneumoniae*
(D) *Pseudomonas aeruginosa*

595. Additional history reveals that she has had several serious infections with this organism previously. On the basis of this, which one of the following is the MOST likely predisposing factor?
(A) She is HIV antibody-positive
(B) She is deficient in CD8-positive T cells
(C) She is deficient in one of the late-acting complement components
(D) She is deficient in antigen presentation by her macrophages

CASE 2. Your patient is a 70-year-old man with a long history of smoking who now has a fever and a cough productive of greenish sputum. You suspect pneumonia, and a chest x-ray confirms your suspicion.

596. If a Gram stain of the sputum reveals very small gram-negative rods and there is no growth on a blood agar but colonies do grow on chocolate agar supplemented with NAD and heme, which one of the following bacteria is the MOST likely cause?
    (A) *Chlamydia pneumoniae*
    (B) *Legionella pneumophila*
    (C) *Mycoplasma pneumoniae*
    (D) *Haemophilus influenzae*

CASE 3. Your patient is a 50-year-old woman who returned yesterday from a vacation in Peru, where there is an epidemic of cholera. She now has multiple episodes of diarrhea.

597. Of the following, which one is MOST compatible with cholera?
    (A) Watery diarrhea without blood, no polys in the stool, and growth of curved gram-negative rods in the blood culture
    (B) Watery diarrhea without blood, no polys in the stool, and no organisms in the blood culture
    (C) Bloody diarrhea, polys in the stool, and growth of curved gram-negative rods in the blood culture
    (D) Bloody diarrhea, polys in the stool, and no organisms in the blood culture

CASE 4. Your patient is a 55-year-old man who is coughing up greenish blood-streaked sputum. For the past 2 weeks, he has had fever and night sweats. He thinks he has lost about 10 pounds. On physical examination, there are crackles in the apex of the right lung, and a chest x-ray shows a cavity in that location.

598. Of the following, which one is the LEAST likely finding?
    (A) Gram stain of the sputum shows no predominant organism
    (B) Culture of the sputum on blood agar shows no predominant organism
    (C) Culture of the sputum on Lowenstein-Jensen medium shows tan colonies after incubation for 4 weeks
    (D) Rapid plasma reagin test reveals the causative organism

CASE 5. Your patient is a 5-year-old girl with bloody diarrhea and no vomiting. There is no history of travel outside of San Francisco. Stool culture grows both lactose-positive and lactose-negative colonies on EMB agar.

599. Of the following organisms, which one is MOST likely to be the cause?
    (A) *Shigella sonnei*
    (B) *Salmonella typhi*

    (C) *Campylobacter jejuni*
    (D) *Helicobacter pylori*

CASE 6. Your patient is a 25-year-old woman with acute onset of pain in her left lower quadrant. On pelvic examination, there is a cervical exudate and tenderness in the left adnexa. You conclude that she has pelvic inflammatory disease (PID) and order laboratory tests.

600. Of the following, which one is the LEAST informative laboratory result?
    (A) Gram stain of the cervical exudate shows gram-negative diplococci within polys
    (B) Culture of the cervical exudate on Thayer-Martin agar shows oxidase-positive colonies
    (C) Fluorescent-antibody test shows cytoplasmic inclusions
    (D) Complement fixation test shows a rise in antibody titer

CASE 7. Your patient is a 22-year-old man with fever, fatigue, and a new diastolic murmur. You suspect endocarditis and do a blood culture.

601. Which of the following statements is LEAST accurate?
    (A) If he had dental surgery recently, one of the most likely organisms to grow would be a viridans group streptococcus
    (B) If he is an intravenous drug user, one of the most likely organisms to grow would be *Candida albicans*
    (C) If he had colon surgery recently, one of the most likely organisms to grow would be *Enterococcus faecalis*
    (D) If he has a prosthetic aortic valve, one of the most likely organisms to grow would be *Streptococcus agalactiae*

In fact, none of the above organisms grew in the blood culture. What did grow was a gram-positive coccus arranged in clusters. When subcultured on blood agar, the colonies were surrounded by a zone of clear hemolysis, and a coagulase test was positive.

602. In view of this, which one of the following is MOST accurate?
    (A) He is probably an intravenous drug user
    (B) He probably lives on a farm and has had contact with pregnant sheep
    (C) He probably has a common sexually transmitted disease
    (D) He probably has been camping and was bitten by a tick

CASE 8. Your patient is a 70-year-old woman who had a hysterectomy for carcinoma of the uterus 3 days ago. She has an indwelling urinary catheter in place and now has a fever to 39°C, and the urine in the collection bottle is cloudy. A Gram stain of the urine specimen shows many neutrophils and gram-positive cocci in chains. You also do a urine culture.

603. Which one of the following is the MOST likely set of findings on the urine culture?
  (A) Beta-hemolytic colonies that are bacitracin-sensitive
  (B) Alpha-hemolytic colonies that are optochin-sensitive
  (C) Nonhemolytic colonies that grow in 6.5% sodium chloride
  (D) Nonhemolytic colonies that grow only anaerobically

CASE 9. Your patient is a 27-year-old woman who was treated with oral ampicillin for cellulitis caused by *Streptococcus pyogenes.* Several days later, she developed bloody diarrhea. You suspect that she may have pseudomembranous colitis.

604. Regarding the causative organism of pseudomembranous colitis, which one of the following is the MOST accurate?
  (A) It is an anaerobic gram-positive rod that produces exotoxins
  (B) It is a comma-shaped gram-negative rod that grows best at 41 °C
  (C) It is an obligate intracellular parasite that grows in cell culture but not on blood agar
  (D) It is a yeast that forms germ tubes when incubated in human serum at 37 °C

CASE 10. Your patient is a 10-year-old girl who has had pain in her left arm for the past 5 days. On physical examination, her temperature is 38 °C and there is tenderness of the humerus near her deltoid. On x-ray of the humerus, an area of raised periosteum and erosion of bone is seen. You do a blood culture.

605. Which one of the following is the MOST likely set of findings?
  (A) Gram-negative rods that grow on EMB agar, forming purple colonies and a green sheen
  (B) Gram-positive cocci that grow on blood agar, causing a clear zone of hemolysis, and are coagulase-positive
  (C) Gram-positive rods that grow only anaerobically and form a double zone of hemolysis on blood agar
  (D) Gram-negative diplococci that grow on blood agar, are oxidase-positive, and ferment maltose

CASE 11. Your patient is a 30-year-old man who is HIV antibody-positive and has a history of *Pneumocystis* pneumonia 2 years ago. He now has an ulcerating lesion on the side of his tongue. A Giemsa stain of the biopsy specimen reveals budding yeasts within macrophages. A culture of the specimen

grows an organism that is a budding yeast at 37 °C but produces hyphae at 25 °C.

606. Of the following, which one is the MOST likely organism to cause this infection?
  (A) *Coccidioides immitis*
  (B) *Aspergillus fumigatus*
  (C) *Histoplasma capsulatum*
  (D) *Cryptococcus neoformans*

CASE 12. Your patient is a 10-year-old boy who is receiving chemotherapy for acute leukemia. He develops fever, headache, and a stiff neck, and you make a presumptive diagnosis of meningitis and do a lumbar puncture. A Gram stain reveals a small gram-positive rod, and culture of the spinal fluid grows a beta-hemolytic colony on blood agar.

607. Regarding this organism, which one of the following is MOST accurate?
  (A) It has more than 100 serologic types
  (B) It produces an exotoxin that inhibits elongation factor 2
  (C) It is commonly acquired by eating unpasteurized dairy products
  (D) There is a toxoid vaccine available against this organism

CASE 13. Mrs. Jones calls to say that she, her husband, and their child have had nausea and vomiting for the past hour or so. Also, they have had some nonbloody diarrhea. You ask when their last meal together was, and she says they had a picnic lunch in the park about 3 hours ago. They have no fever.

608. Which one of the following is the MOST likely finding?
  (A) Gram stain of the leftover food would show many gram-positive cocci in clusters
  (B) Gram stain of the stool would show many gram-negative diplococci
  (C) KOH prep of the leftover food would show many budding yeasts
  (D) Acid-fast stain of the stool would show many acid-fast rods

CASE 14. Your patient is a 9-year-old boy who was sent home from school because his teacher thought he was acting strangely. This morning, he had a seizure and was rushed to the hospital. On physical examination, his temperature is 40 °C and he has no nuchal rigidity. A CT scan is normal. A lumbar puncture is done, and the spinal fluid protein and glucose are normal. A Gram stain of the spinal fluid reveals no organisms and no polys. He is treated with various antibiotics but becomes comatose and dies 2 days later. The blood culture and spinal fluid culture grow no bacteria or fungi. On autopsy of the brain, eosinophilic inclusion bodies are seen in the cytoplasm of neurons.

609. Of the following, which one is the MOST likely cause?
- **(A)** Prions
- **(B)** JC virus
- **(C)** Rabies virus
- **(D)** Herpes simplex virus type 1

CASE 15. Your patient is a 20-year-old man who was in a fist fight and suffered a broken jaw and lost two teeth. Several weeks later, he developed an abscess at the site of the trauma that drained to the surface of the skin, and yellowish granules were seen in the pus.

610. Regarding this disease, which one of the following is MOST accurate?
- **(A)** The causative organism is a gram-positive rod that forms long filaments
- **(B)** The causative organism is a comma-shaped gram-negative rod that produces an exotoxin which increases cyclic AMP
- **(C)** The causative organism cannot be seen in the Gram stain but can be seen in an acid-fast stain
- **(D)** A combination of gram-negative cocci and spirochetes cause this disease

CASE 16. Your patient is a 25-year-old man who is HIV antibody-positive and a CD4 count of 120 cells (normal, 1000–1500). He has had a mild headache for the past week and vomited once yesterday. On physical examination, he has a temperature of 38 °C and mild nuchal rigidity but no papilledema. The rest of the physical examination is negative.

611. Of the following, which one is the MOST likely to be found on examination of the spinal fluid?
- **(A)** Lymphs and gram-positive cocci resembling *Stretococcus pneumoniae*
- **(B)** Lymphs and budding yeasts resembling *Cryptococcus neoformans*
- **(C)** Polys and anaerobic gram-negative rods resembling *Bacteroides fragilis*
- **(D)** Polys and septate hyphae resembling *Aspergillus fumigatus*

CASE 17. Your patient is a 25-year-old woman with a sore throat since yesterday. On physical examination, her throat is red but no exudate is seen. Two enlarged, tender cervical lymph nodes are palpable. Her temperature is 101 °F. A throat culture reveals no beta-hemolytic colonies. After receiving this result, you do another physical examination, which reveals an enlarged spleen. A heterophil antibody test finds that sheep red blood cells are agglutinated by the patient's serum.

612. Which one of the following is the MOST likely cause of this disease?
- **(A)** *Steptococcus pyogenes*
- **(B)** *Corynebacterium diphtheriae*
- **(C)** Epstein-Barr virus
- **(D)** Influenza virus

CASE 18. Your patient is a 15-year-old boy with migratory polyarthritis, fever, and a new, loud cardiac murmur. You make a clinical diagnosis of rheumatic fever.

613. Which one of the following laboratory results is MOST compatible with this diagnosis?
- **(A)** A blood culture is positive for *Streptococcus pyogenes* at this time
- **(B)** A throat culture is positive for *Streptococcus pyogenes* at this time
- **(C)** A Gram stain of the joint fluid shows gram-positive cocci in chains at this time
- **(D)** An anti-streptolysin O assay is positive at this time

614. Which one of the following modes of pathogenesis is MOST compatible with this diagnosis?
- **(A)** Bacteria attach to joint and heart tissue via pili, invade, and cause inflammation
- **(B)** Bacteria secrete exotoxins that circulate via the blood to the joints and heart
- **(C)** Bacterial antigens induce antibodies that cross-react with joint and heart tissue
- **(D)** Bacterial endotoxin induces interleukin-1 and tumor necrosis factor, which cause inflammation in joint and heart tissue

615. Which one of the following approaches is MOST likely to prevent endocarditis in patients with rheumatic fever?
- **(A)** They should take the streptococcal polysaccharide vaccine
- **(B)** They should take penicillin if they have dental surgery
- **(C)** They should take the toxoid vaccine every 5 years
- **(D)** They should take rifampin if they have abdominal surgery

CASE 19. Your patient is a 10-year-old girl who has leukemia and is receiving chemotherapy through an indwelling venous catheter. She now has a fever of 39 °C but is otherwise asymptomatic. You do a blood culture, and the laboratory reports growth of *Staphylococcus epidermidis*.

616. Which one of the following results is LEAST likely to be found by the clinical laboratory?
- **(A)** Gram-positive cocci in clusters were seen on Gram stain of the blood culture
- **(B)** Subculture of the blood culture onto blood agar revealed nonhemolytic colonies
- **(C)** A coagulase test on the colonies was negative
- **(D)** A catalase test on the colonies was negative

CASE 20. Your patient is a 25-year-old woman with several purpuric areas indicative of bleeding into the skin. Her vital signs are as follows: temperature, 38 °C; blood pressure, 70/40; pulse, 140; respiratory rate, 24. You think she has septic shock and do a blood culture.

617. Which one of the following organisms is LEAST likely to be the cause of her septic shock?
  (A) *Corynebacterium diphtheriae*
  (B) *Neisseria meningitidis*
  (C) *Clostridium perfringens*
  (D) *Escherichia coli*

618. Of the following mechanisms, which one is LEAST likely to be involved with the pathogenesis of her septic shock?
  (A) Increased amount of interleukin-1
  (B) Activation of the alternate pathway of complement
  (C) Increased amount of tumor necrosis factor
  (D) Increased amount of antigen-antibody complexes

CASE 21. Your patient is a 55-year-old man with severe cellulitis of the right leg, high fever, and a teeth-chattering chill. He is a fisherman who was working on his boat in the waters off the Texas coast yesterday.

619. Which one of the following organisms is MOST likely to be the cause of his disease?
  (A) *Yersinia pestis*
  (B) *Vibrio vulnificus*
  (C) *Pasteurella multocida*
  (D) *Brucella melitensis*

CASE 22. Your patient is a 30-year-old woman with facial nerve paralysis. She also has fever and headache but does not have a stiff neck. On physical examination, she has a circular, erythematous, macular rash on the back of her thigh. You suspect that she has Lyme disease.

620. Of the following tests, which one is the MOST appropriate to order to confirm a diagnosis of Lyme disease?
  (A) Blood culture to grow the organism
  (B) Stain for inclusion bodies within cells involved in the rash
  (C) Test for serum antibody against the organism
  (D) Dark-field microscopy

CASE 23. Your patient is a 60-year-old man with confusion for 2 months. He has no history of fever or stiff neck. On physical examination, he was ataxic and his coordination was abnormal. A diagnosis of tertiary syphilis was made by the laboratory.

621. Of the following tests, which one is the MOST appropriate to make a diagnosis of tertiary syphilis?
  (A) Spinal fluid culture to grow the organism
  (B) Stain for inclusion bodies in the lymphocytes in the spinal fluid
  (C) Test for antibody in the spinal fluid that reacts with cardiolipin
  (D) ELISA for the antigen in the spinal fluid

CASE 24. Your patient is a 65-year-old man who had an adenocarcinoma of the pancreas that was surgically removed. Several blood transfusions were given, and he did well until 2 weeks later, when fever, vomiting, and diarrhea began. Blood and stool cultures were negative, and the tests for *Clostridium difficile* and hepatitis B surface antigen were negative. A liver biopsy revealed intranuclear inclusion bodies.

622. Of the following, which one is the MOST likely cause?
  (A) Adenovirus
  (B) Cytomegalovirus
  (C) Hepatitis A virus
  (D) Rotavirus

CASE 25. Your patient is a 3-year-old girl with fever and pain in her right ear. On physical examination, the drum is found to be perforated and a bloody exudate is seen. A Gram stain of the exudate reveals gram-positive diplococci.

623. Of the following, which one is the MOST likely cause?
  (A) *Streptococcus pyogenes*
  (B) *Staphylococcus aureus*
  (C) *Corynebacterium diphtheriae*
  (D) *Streptococcus pneumoniae*

CASE 26. Your patient is a 70-year-old man with a fever of 40 °C and a very painful cellulitis of the right buttock. The skin appears necrotic, and there are several fluid-filled bullae. Crepitus can be felt, indicating gas in the tissue. A Gram stain of the exudate reveals large gram-positive rods.

624. Of the following, which one is the MOST likely cause?
  (A) *Clostridium perfringens*
  (B) *Bacillus anthracis*
  (C) *Corynebacterium diphtheriae*
  (D) *Actinomyces israelii*

CASE 27. Your patient is a 45-year-old woman with a cadaveric renal transplant that is being rejected despite immunosuppressive therapy. She is now in renal failure with a blood pH of 7.32. This morning, she awoke with a pain near her right eye. On physical examination, her temperature is 38 °C and the skin near her eye is necrotic. A biopsy specimen of the lesion contains nonseptate hyphae invading the blood vessels.

625. Of the following, which one is the MOST likely cause?
  (A) *Histoplasma capsulatum*
  (B) *Aspergillus fumigatus*
  (C) *Cryptococcus neoformans*
  (D) *Mucor* species

CASE 28. Your patient is a 35-year-old man who is HIV antibody-positive and has a CD4 count of 85 cells. He recently had a seizure, and an MRI scan indicates a lesion in the temporal lobe. A brain biopsy specimen reveals multinucleated giant cells with intranuclear inclusions.

626. Of the following, which one is the MOST likely cause?
    (A) Herpes simplex virus
    (B) Parvovirus B19
    (C) Coxsackievirus
    (D) Western equine encephalitis virus

CASE 29. Your patient is a 40-year-old woman with a severe attack of diarrhea that began on the airplane while she was returning from a vacation in the Middle East. She had had multiple episodes of watery, nonbloody diarrhea and little vomiting. She is afebrile. A stool culture reveals only lactose-fermenting colonies on EMB agar.

627. Of the following, which one is the MOST likely cause?
    (A) *Shigella sonnei*
    (B) *Helicobacter pylori*
    (C) *Escherichia coli*
    (D) *Pseudomonas aeruginosa*

CASE 30. Your patient is a 20-year-old man with a sore throat for the past 3 days. On physical examination, his temperature is 38 °C, the pharynx is red, and several tender submaxillary nodes are palpable.

628. Of the following, which one is the MOST likely organism to cause this infection?
    (A) *Streptococcus agalactiae* (group B streptococcus)
    (B) *Streptococcus sanguis* (a viridans group streptococcus)
    (C) Parvovirus B19
    (D) Epstein-Barr virus

You do a throat culture, and many small, translucent colonies that are beta-hemolytic grow on blood agar. Gram stain of one of these colonies reveals gram-positive cocci in chains.

629. Of the following, which one is the MOST likely organism to cause this infection?
    (A) *Streptococcus pneumoniae*
    (B) *Streptococcus pyogenes*
    (C) *Streptococcus agalactiae* (group B streptococcus)
    (D) *Peptostreptococcus* species

CASE 31. Your patient is a 55-year-old woman with a lymphoma, who is receiving chemotherapy via intravenous catheter. She suddenly develops fever, shaking chills, and hypotension.

630. Of the following, which one is the LEAST likely organism to cause this infection?
    (A) *Streptococcus pneumoniae*
    (B) *Klebsiella pneumoniae*
    (C) *Mycoplasma pneumoniae*
    (D) *Proteus mirabilis*

631. If a blood culture grows a gram-negative rod, which one of the following is the LEAST likely organism to cause this infection?
    (A) *Bordetella pertussis*
    (B) *Escherichia coli*
    (C) *Pseudomonas aeruginosa*
    (D) *Serratia marcescens*

632. Of the following virulence factors, which one is the MOST likely to cause the fever and hypotension?
    (A) Pilus
    (B) Capsule
    (C) Lecithinase
    (D) Lipopolysaccharide

CASE 32. Your patient is a 30-year-old woman who was part of a tour group visiting a Central American country. The day before leaving, several members of the group developed fever, abdominal cramps, and bloody diarrhea.

633. Of the following, which one is the LEAST likely organism to cause this infection?
    (A) *Shigella dysenteriae*
    (B) *Salmonella enteritidis*
    (C) *Vibrio cholerae*
    (D) *Campylobacter jejuni*

A stool culture reveals no lactose-negative colonies on the EMB agar.

634. Which one of the following is the MOST likely organism to cause this infection?
    (A) *Shigella dysenteriae*
    (B) *Salmonella enteritidis*
    (C) *Vibrio cholerae*
    (D) *Campylobacter jejuni*

CASE 33. Your patient is a 78-year-old man who had an episode of acute urinary retention and had to be catheterized. He then underwent cystoscopy to determine the cause of the retention. Two days later, he developed fever and suprapubic pain. Urinalysis revealed 50 WBC and 10 RBC per high-power field. Culture of the urine revealed a thin film of bacterial growth over the entire blood agar plate, and the urease test was positive.

635. Which one of the following is the MOST likely organism to cause this infection?
    (A) *Escherichia coli*
    (B) *Proteus mirabilis*
    (C) *Streptococcus faecalis*
    (D) *Branhamella* (*Moraxella*) *catarrhalis*

CASE 34. Your patient is a 40-year-old man with a depigmented lesion on his chest that appeared about a month ago. The skin of the lesion is thickened and has lost sensation. He has lived most of his life in rural Louisiana.

636. Of the following tests, which one is the MOST appropriate to do to reveal the cause of this disease?
- **(A)** Perform a biopsy of the lesion and do an acid-fast stain
- **(B)** Culture on Sabouraud's agar and look for germ tubes
- **(C)** Culture on blood agar anaerobically and do a Gram stain
- **(D)** Obtain serum for a Weil-Felix agglutination test

CASE 35. Your patient is a 28-year-old man with third-degree burns over a large area of his back and left leg. This morning, he spiked a fever to 40 °C and had two teeth-chattering chills. A blood culture grows a gram-negative rod that is oxidase-positive and produces a blue-green pigment.

637. Of the following, which one is the MOST likely organism to cause this infection?
- **(A)** *Bacteroides melaninogenicus*
- **(B)** *Pseudomonas aeruginosa*
- **(C)** *Proteus mirabilis*
- **(D)** *Haemophilus influenzae*

CASE 36. Your patient is a 32-year-old moving-van driver who lives in St. Louis. He arrived in San Francisco about 10 days ago after picking up furniture in Little Rock, Dallas, Albuquerque, and Phoenix. He now has a persistent cough and fever to 101 °F, and he feels poorly. On physical examination, crackles are heard in the left lower lobe, and chest x-ray reveals an infiltrate in that area.

638. Of the following, which one is the LEAST accurate statement?
- **(A)** He probably has spherules containing endospores in his lung
- **(B)** If dissemination to the bone occurs, this indicates a failure of his cell-mediated immunity
- **(C)** He probably acquired this disease by inhaling arthrospores
- **(D)** The causative organism of this disease exists as a yeast in the soil

CASE 37. Your patient is a 25-year-old man with an ulcerated lesion on his penis that is not painful. You suspect that it may be a chancre.

639. Of the following, which one of the following tests is the MOST appropriate to do with the material from the lesion?
- **(A)** Dark-field microscopy
- **(B)** Gram stain
- **(C)** Acid-fast stain
- **(D)** Culture on Thayer-Martin agar

640. Which one of the following tests is the MOST appropriate to do with the patient's blood?
- **(A)** Culture on blood agar
- **(B)** Assay for antibodies that react with cardiolipin
- **(C)** Assay for neutralizing antibody in human cell culture
- **(D)** Heterophil antibody test

CASE 38. Your patient is a 6-year-old boy with papular and pustular skin lesions on his face. A serous, "honey-colored" fluid exudes from the lesions. You suspect impetigo. A Gram stain of the pus reveals many neutrophils and gram-positive cocci in chains.

641. If you cultured the pus on blood agar, which one of the following would you be MOST likely to see?
- **(A)** Small beta-hemolytic colonies containing bacteria that are bacitracin-sensitive
- **(B)** Small alpha-hemolytic colonies containing bacteria that are resistant to optochin
- **(C)** Large nonhemolytic colonies containing bacteria that are oxidase-positive
- **(D)** Small nonhemolytic colonies containing bacteria that grow in 6.5% NaCl

CASE 39. Your patient is a 66-year-old woman being treated with chemotherapy for lymphoma. She develops fever to 38 °C and a nonproductive cough. A chest x-ray reveals an infiltrate. You treat her empirically with an appropriate antibiotic. The following day, several vesicles appear on her chest.

642. Which one of the following viruses is the MOST likely cause of her disease?
- **(A)** Measles virus
- **(B)** Respiratory syncytial virus
- **(C)** Varicella-zoster virus
- **(D)** Rubella virus

CASE 40. Your patient is a 40-year-old woman with systemic lupus erythematosus who is being treated with high-dose prednisone during a flare of her disease. She develops a fever to 38 °C and a cough productive of a small amount of greenish sputum. On physical examination, you hear coarse breath sounds in the left lower lobe. Chest x-ray reveals an infiltrate in that region. Gram stain of the sputum reveals long filaments of gram-positive rods.

643. Which one of the following organisms is the MOST likely cause of this disease?
- **(A)** *Mycobacterium kansasii*
- **(B)** *Listeria monocytogenes*
- **(C)** *Nocardia asteroides*
- **(D)** *Mycoplasma pneumoniae*

CASE 41. Your patient is a 10-year-old girl with acute leukemia who responded well to her first round of chemotherapy but not to the most recent one. In view of this, she had a bone marrow transplant and is on an immunosuppressive regimen. She is markedly granulocytopenic. Ten days after the transplant, she spikes a fever and coughs up bloody, purulent sputum. Chest x-ray shows pneumonia. A wet mount of the sputum shows septate hyphae with dichotomous (Y-shape) branching.

644. Which one of the following organisms is the MOST likely cause of this disase?

(A) *Histoplasma capsulatum*
(B) *Aspergillus fumigatus*
(C) *Rhizopus nigricans*
(D) *Candida albicans*

CASE 42. Your patient is a 30-year-old man with acute onset of fever to 40 °C and a swollen, very tender right femoral node. His blood pressure is 90/50, and his pulse is 110. As you examine him, he has a teeth-chattering shaking chill. He returned from a camping trip in the Southern California desert 2 days ago.

645. Regarding this disease, which one of the following is MOST accurate?

(A) An aspirate of the node will reveal a small gram-negative rod
(B) The organism was probably acquired by eating food contaminated with rodent excrement
(C) The aspirate of the node should be cultured on Lowenstein-Jensen agar and an acid-fast stain performed
(D) The organism causes disease primarily in people with impaired cell-mediated immunity

CASE 43. Your patient is a 62-year-old woman with a history of carcinoma of the sigmoid colon that was removed 5 days ago. The surgery was complicated by the escape of bowel contents into the peritoneal cavity. She now has fever and pain in the perineum and left buttock. On physical examination, her temperature is 39 °C and myonecrosis with a foul-smelling discharge is found. A gram stain of the exudate reveals gram-negative rods.

646. Of the following, which one is the MOST likely organism to cause this infection?

(A) *Helicobacter pylori*
(B) *Bacteroides fragilis*
(C) *Salmonella typhi*
(D) *Vibrio parahemolyticus*

CASE 44. Your patient is an 18-year-old woman with a swollen left ankle. Two days ago, when the ankle began to swell, she thought she had twisted it playing soccer. However, today she has a fever to 38 °C and the ankle has become noticeably more swollen, warm, and red. Her other joints are asymptomatic. You aspirate fluid from the joint.

647. Using the joint fluid, which one of the following procedures is MOST likely to provide diagnostic information?

(A) Acid-fast stain and culture on Lowenstein-Jensen medium
(B) Gram stain and culture on chocolate agar
(C) Darkfield microscopy and the VDRL test
(D) India ink stain and culture on Sabouraud's agar

CASE 45. Your patient is a 6-year-old boy with a history of several episodes of pneumonia. A sweat test revealed an increased amount of chloride, indicating that he has cystic fibrosis. He now has a fever and is coughing up a thick, greenish sputum. A Gram stain of the sputum reveals gram-negative rods.

648. Of the following, which one is the MOST likely organism to cause this infection?

(A) *Pseudomonas aeruginosa*
(B) *Haemophilus influenzae*
(C) *Legionella pneumophila*
(D) *Bordetella pertussis*

CASE 46. Your patient is a 7-year-old boy with fever, two episodes of vomiting, and a severe headache that began this morning. He has no diarrhea. On physical examination, his temperature is 39 °C and nuchal rigidity is found. Examination of the spinal fluid revealed a white cell count of 800, of which 90% were lymphs, and a normal concentration of both protein and glucose. A Gram stain of the spinal fluid revealed no bacteria.

649. Of the following, which one is the MOST likely to cause this infection?

(A) *Chlamydia trachomatis*
(B) *Mycobacterium avium-intracellulare*
(C) Coxsackievirus
(D) Adenovirus

CASE 47. Your patient is a 22-year-old man who has been on a low-budget trip to India, where he ate many of the local foods. He has had a low-grade fever, anorexia, and mild abdominal pain for about a month. You suspect that he may have typhoid fever.

650. If he does have typhoid fever, which one of the following is the LEAST likely laboratory finding?

(A) Culture of the blood reveals gram-negative rods
(B) Culture of the stool grows lactose-negative colonies in EMB agar
(C) His serum contains antibodies that agglutinate *Salmonella typhi*
(D) His serum contains antibodies that cause a positive Weil-Felix reaction

CASE 48. Your patient is a 30-year-old man who is HIV antibody-positive and has had two episodes of *Pneumocystis* pneumonia. He now complains of pain in his mouth and difficulty swallowing. On physical examination, you find several whitish plaques on his oropharyngeal mucosa.

651. Regarding the most likely causative organism, which one of the following statements is MOST accurate?

(A) It is a filamentous gram-positive rod that is part of the normal flora in the mouth

(B) It is an anaerobic gram-negative rod that is part of the normal flora in the colon

(C) It is a yeast that forms pseudohyphae when it invades tissue

(D) It is a spirochete that grows only in cell culture

CASE 49. Your patient is a 20-year-old woman with a rash that began this morning. She has been feeling feverish and anorexic for the past few days. On physical examination, there is a papular rash bilaterally over the chest, abdomen, and upper extremities including the hands. There are no vesicles. Cervical and axillary lymph nodes were palpable. Her temperature was 38 °C. White blood count was 9000 with a normal differential.

652. Of the following organisms, which one is the MOST likely cause of her disease?

(A) *Histoplasma capsulatum*

(B) *Coxiella burnetii*

(C) *Neisseria meningitidis*

(D) *Treponema pallidum*

CASE 50. Your patient is a 10-year-old boy who fell, abraded the skin of his thigh, and developed cellulitis; ie, the skin was red, hot, and tender. Several days later, the infection was treated with a

topical antibiotic ointment and the cellulitis gradually healed. However, 2 weeks later, he told his mother that his urine was cloudy and reddish, and she noted that his face was swollen. You suspect acute glomerulonephritis.

653. Regarding the causative organism, what is the MOST likely appearance of a Gram stain of the exudate from the skin infection?

(A) Gram-positive cocci in grapelike clusters

(B) Gram-positive cocci in chains

(C) Gram-positive diplococci

(D) Gram-negative diplococci

654. What is the pathogenesis of the cloudy urine and facial swelling?

(A) Toxin mediated

(B) Direct invasion by the bacteria

(C) Immune-complex mediated

(D) Cell-mediated immunity (delayed hypersensitivity)

Answers (Questions 594–654)

594 (B)	607 (C)	619 (B)	631 (A)	643 (C)
595 (C)	608 (A)	620 (C)	632 (D)	644 (B)
596 (D)	609 (C)	621 (C)	633 (C)	645 (A)
597 (B)	610 (A)	622 (B)	634 (D)	646 (B)
598 (D)	611 (B)	623 (D)	635 (B)	647 (B)
599 (A)	612 (C)	624 (A)	636 (A)	648 (A)
600 (D)	613 (D)	625 (D)	637 (B)	649 (C)
601 (D)	614 (C)	626 (A)	638 (D)	650 (D)
602 (A)	615 (B)	627 (C)	639 (A)	651 (C)
603 (C)	616 (D)	628 (D)	640 (B)	652 (D)
604 (A)	617 (A)	629 (B)	641 (A)	653 (B)
605 (B)	618 (D)	630 (C)	642 (C)	654 (C)
606 (C)				

Part XI: USMLE (National Board) Practice Examination

This practice examination consists of 160 microbiology and immunology questions. You should be able to complete it in 1 hour and 40 minutes. The answer key is located at the end of the examination.

In an attempt to resemble the actual USMLE Step 1, the questions in this practice examination are randomly assorted; ie, they are not grouped according to subject matter, unlike Part X of this book. The coverage of subject areas on this practice examination is approximately the same as on the USMLE. Note that many of the "one-best-answer" questions are written in the "except" or "least-accurate" format. This provides you with three correct answers, which will enhance your learning from these questions.

Questions

Directions (Questions 1–136): Select the ONE lettered answer that is BEST in each question.

1. One of the first steps in the process of many infections is adherence of bacteria to mucous membranes. The bacterial structure that mediates adherence is the
   (A) pilus
   (B) peptidoglycan
   (C) flagellum
   (D) endotoxin

2. Some viruses typically infect white blood cells as an important part of their pathogenesis. Which one of the following is LEAST likely to do this?
   (A) Cytomegalovirus
   (B) Human immunodeficiency virus
   (C) Rabies virus
   (D) Epstein-Barr virus

3. A 10-year-old child with acute myeloblastic leukemia was treated with chemotherapy but developed fever on the ninth neutropenic day despite prophylaxis with antimicrobial drugs. Skin lesions appeared, and biopsy specimens contained budding yeasts and pseudohyphae. Which one of the following organisms is the MOST likely cause?
   (A) *Aspergillus fumigatus*
   (B) *Candida albicans*

   (C) *Histoplasma capsulatum*
   (D) *Sporothrix schenckii*

4. Regarding macrophages, which one of the following is MOST accurate?
   (A) They typically have IgG on their surface
   (B) They have antigen-specific receptors on their surface
   (C) They must pass through the thymus in order to be effective in antigen presentation
   (D) They typically produce interleukin-1 in conjunction with antigen presentation

5. One of the most important procedures in microbiology is the Gram stain. Regarding this stain, which one of the following is LEAST accurate?
   (A) Both gram-positive and gram-negative bacteria stain blue with crystal violet
   (B) Exposure of the bacteria to ethanol or acetone fixes the crystal violet to the bacterial peptidoglycan
   (C) Gram-positive bacteria retain the crystal violet, whereas gram-negative bacteria do not
   (D) Some bacteria, eg, *Mycoplasma,* lack a cell wall and do not stain with the Gram stain

6. Regarding the nature of medically important viruses, which one of the following statements is LEAST accurate?
  (A) Poliovirus is a nonenveloped virus with RNA as its genome
  (B) Epstein-Barr virus is a nonenveloped virus with RNA as its genome
  (C) Hepatitis B virus is an enveloped virus with DNA as its genome
  (D) Influenza virus is an enveloped virus with RNA as its genome

7. In the table below, three recipient mice are labeled A, B, and C. The three mice are X-irradiated to destroy their own T and B cells; they then receive either B cells, T cells, or both. Each mouse is then immunized with antigen X, and the presence of antibodies against X is determined 7 days later.

Mouse	Received B Cells Only	Received T Cells Only	Received both B Cells and T Cells
A	+	−	−
B	−	+	−
C	−	−	+

Which one of the following statements is the MOST accurate?
  (A) Mouse A will produce the highest antibody titer
  (B) Mouse B will produce the highest antibody titer
  (C) Mouse C will produce the highest antibody titer
  (D) Mice B and C will have equal titers

8. Each of the following statements regarding the capsules of bacteria is correct EXCEPT:
  (A) Most bacterial capsules are polysaccharides and serve to protect the bacteria by inhibiting phagocytosis
  (B) Bacterial capsules can vary antigenically, and as a result, some bacteria have many serologic types
  (C) Bacterial capsules can be purified and used in vaccines against certain bacteria, eg, the pneumococcus
  (D) Most gram-positive bacteria have capsules, whereas gram-negative bacteria rarely do

9. Each of the following statements regarding polymerases in virions is correct EXCEPT:
  (A) Influenza virus requires a virion polymerase because the genome is negative-polarity single-stranded RNA
  (B) Rabies virus requires a virion polymerase because the genome is negative-polarity single-stranded RNA
  (C) Hepatitis A virus requires a virion polymerase because the genome is double-stranded DNA

  (D) Rotavirus requires a virion polymerase because the genome is double-stranded RNA

10. Each of the following statements regarding *Coccidioides immitis* is correct EXCEPT:
  (A) It is a dimorphic fungus that grows as a mold in the soil and as spherules in the body
  (B) Infection usually results from the inhalation of asexual spores (arthroconida); hence, the primary site of infection is the lung
  (C) When cultured in the laboratory, the organism forms budding yeasts
  (D) The most important host defense against this organism is cell-mediated immunity

11. A mouse with MHC haplotype A was infected with virus X. Seven days later, cytotoxic T lymphocytes were obtained from the mouse and mixed with virus X-infected target cells of two haplotypes: MHC A and MHC B. In which of the following cells is lysis MOST likely to occur?
  (A) MHC A cells only
  (B) MHC B cells only
  (C) Both MHC A and MHC B cells
  (D) Neither MHC A nor MHC B cells

12. Each of the following statements regarding herpes simplex virus type 2 is correct EXCEPT:
  (A) Painful vesicular lesions occur on the genitals of both men and women
  (B) It is an important cause of encephalitis in adults
  (C) Acyclovir can be used to treat primary lesions in an immunocompetent host
  (D) It is an important cause of neonatal infection

13. Each of the following statements regarding bacterial exotoxins is correct EXCEPT:
  (A) They are an integral part of the cell wall
  (B) They are produced by both *Staphylococcus aureus* and *Escherichia coli*
  (C) They are polypeptides consisting of two functional regions: one that binds to cell receptors and one that has the toxic activity
  (D) Treatment of some exotoxins with formaldehyde yields a toxoid, which is used as the immunogen in certain vaccines

14. Some viruses exist as single serotypes, whereas others have multiple serotypes. Which one of the following has a SINGLE serotype?
  (A) Influenza virus
  (B) Coxsackievirus
  (C) Varicella-zoster virus
  (D) Adenovirus

15. Each of the following statements regarding bacterial endotoxin is correct EXCEPT:
  (A) Both gram-negative rods and gram-negative cocci have endotoxin

(B) Endotoxin is a lipopolysaccharide, the lipid portion of which mediates the toxicity

(C) Endotoxin causes hypotension by catalyzing the addition of ADP-ribose to the alpha chain of T cell receptors

(D) Endotoxin causes fever by inducing interleukin-1 production by macrophages

16. Each of the following statements regarding the C3 component of the complement cascade is correct EXCEPT:

(A) It is involved in both the classic and the alternative pathways

(B) Its C3a fragment can cause anaphylaxis by releasing histamine from mast cells

(C) Its C3b fragment binds to both IgG and surface receptors on neutrophils

(D) Its C3b fragment is part of the complex that causes lysis of gram-negative bacteria such as *Neisseria*

17. Regarding the prevention of bacterial diseases by vaccines, which one of the following is LEAST accurate?

(A) Tetanus toxoid is produced by treating tetanus toxin with formalin, which inactivates its ability to cause disease but leaves its antigenicity intact

(B) Diphtheria vaccine contains diphtheria toxoid and produces few side effects when given to children

(C) Both the pertussis vaccine and the *Haemophilus influenzae* vaccine contain inactivated whole bacteria and produce significant side effects in children

(D) The pneumococcal vaccine contains the capsular polysaccharide of many serotypes and is recommended primarily for older people

18. When certain viruses infect cells they cause characteristic changes in the cells called cytopathic effect (CPE). Regarding CPE, which one of the following is LEAST accurate?

(A) Herpes simplex virus causes multinucleated giant cells with intranuclear inclusions in the skin

(B) Rabies virus causes cytoplasmic inclusions in the brain

(C) Respiratory syncytial virus causes multinucleated giant cells in the lungs

(D) Poliovirus causes intranuclear inclusions in neutrophils

19. Each of the following statements regarding the organisms of the normal flora is correct EXCEPT:

(A) The predominant organisms on the skin are coagulase-negative staphylococci

(B) The predominant organisms in the nose are acid-fast rods

(C) The predominant organisms in the throat are gram-positive cocci in chains that form alpha-hemolytic colonies on blood agar

(D) The predominant organisms in the colon are strict (obligate) anaerobes

20. Usually we are tolerant to our own tissues, yet autoimmune diseases occur. Which one of the following is LEAST likely to be involved in autoimmunity?

(A) Release of sequestered antigens

(B) Loss of clonal anergy by B cells

(C) Increased production of interleukin-2

(D) Reduced class II MHC protein production

21. Each of the following statements regarding the mode of action of antimicrobial drugs is correct EXCEPT:

(A) Both penicillins and cephalosporins inhibit cell wall synthesis

(B) Both penicillins and cephalosporins are bactericidal drugs

(C) Penicillins act primarily by preventing the synthesis of muramic acid

(D) Cephalosporins act primarily by inhibiting transpeptidation

22. Several viruses infect the intestinal tract as their initial site of infection. Which one of the following is LEAST likely to do this?

(A) Hepatitis A virus

(B) Poliovirus

(C) Rotavirus

(D) Mumps virus

23. Penicillins are very effective antibacterial drugs, but their use is limited by allergic reactions. In these allergies, penicillins act as haptens. Which one of the following is MOST accurate?

(A) Penicillins bind to receptors on B cells and stimulate an antibody response; ie, they are T-independent antigens

(B) Penicillins interact with T cell receptors on CD4-positive T cells and activate them

(C) Penicillins bind to carrier proteins, then the penicillin interacts with the B cell receptor and the carrier protein epitope is presented to the helper T cell

(D) Penicillins interact with the early complement components (C1, C4, C2, and C3) to release inflammatory mediators

24. Regarding both *Histoplasma capsulatum* and *Blastomyces dermatitidis,* which one of the following is LEAST accurate?

(A) Both organisms are dimorphic

(B) Humoral immunity is the main host defense against both organisms

(C) Both organisms are acquired by inhalation of asexual spores

(D) Both organisms exist as yeasts in the patient

25. Your patient has several attacks of sneezing, runny nose, and itchy eyes every spring, which you suspect is due to an allergy to some plant pollen. You refer the patient to an allergist, who does skin tests with various allergens and gets a wheal-and-flare reaction with several pollens. Which one of the following is the MOST likely sequence of events that produced the wheal-and-flare reaction?
    (A) Allergen binds to IgM in the plasma, which activates complement to produce C3b
    (B) Allergen binds to IgM on the surface of B cells, and interleukin-1 is released
    (C) Allergen binds to IgE on the surface of mast cells, and histamine is released
    (D) Allergen binds to IgE in the plasma, the allergen-IgE complex binds to the mast cell, and interleukin-1 is released

26. Your patient is a drug addict who has the symptoms of septicemia. You do a blood culture, which reveals *Staphylococcus aureus*. Unfortunately, the laboratory reports that the organism is penicillin-resistant. Which one of the following is LEAST accurate?
    (A) The organism may produce β-lactamase
    (B) The organism may have altered penicillin-binding proteins
    (C) Resistance may be due to inability of the penicillin to penetrate inside the organism
    (D) Resistance may be due to the production of catalase by the organism

27. Each of the following statements regarding the host defenses against viral infection is correct EXCEPT:
    (A) Interleukin-2 can protect uninfected cells from viral infection by inhibiting the release of virus from cells
    (B) Secretory IgA can prevent viral infection of the mucosal cells of the oropharynx
    (C) Interferon can protect uninfected cells from viral infection by inhibiting viral replication within cells
    (D) Serum IgG can prevent viral infection by inhibiting the entry of virus into cells

28. Each of the following statements regarding streptococci is correct EXCEPT:
    (A) Streptococci are gram-positive cocci that typically form chains
    (B) Group A and group B streptococci are in different groups because they have different polysaccharides in their cell wall
    (C) Beta-hemolysis (clear hemolysis) is caused by certain streptococci because they produce enzymes (hemolysins) that lyse red cells
    (D) Streptococci are classified primarily by the antigenic differences in their flagella

29. Each of the following statements regarding infectious mononucleosis is correct EXCEPT:
    (A) The causative agent is usually transmitted by the fecal-oral route
    (B) Infection by the causative agent is widespread; ie, more than half of the persons in the United States have antibodies against the virus
    (C) Atypical lymphocytes are commonly seen in blood smears
    (D) The heterophil antibody test is usually positive; ie, the patient's serum contains antibodies that agglutinate horse red blood cells

30. An 8-year-old boy with acute leukemia was treated with chemotherapy and has been in remission for the past year. However, a few weeks ago, symptoms returned, and a bone marrow transplant is now being considered.

    The following HLA typing results were obtained:

Patient	A2,3	B7,44	C2,5
Father	A3,11	B7,18	C3,5
Mother	A2,23	B13,44	C2,7
Sister	A2,11	B18,44	C2,3
Brother	A11,23	B13,18	C3,7

    Mixed-lymphocyte culture results using irradiated patient cells and responding cells from the four family members and the patient were as follows:

Source of the Responding Cells	Counts per Minute of Tritiated Thymidine Incorporated
Patient	200
Father	800
Mother	600
Sister	300
Brother	1600

    Who is the BEST bone marrow donor?
    (A) Father
    (B) Mother
    (C) Sister
    (D) Brother

31. Each of the following statements regarding poststreptococcal nonsuppurative complications is correct EXCEPT:
    (A) Both acute rheumatic fever and acute glomerulonephritis are preceded by *Streptococcus pyogenes* infection
    (B) Rheumatic fever occurs when an immune response against streptococcal antigens cross-reacts with cardiac muscle and with joint cartilage

(C) Glomerulonephritis occurs when streptococci infect the nephrons and release catalase, which causes disruption of the glomerular membrane and loss of protein in the urine

(D) Patients with rheumatic fever typically have a high titer of antibody to streptolysin O (a hemolysin)

32. Regarding *Aspergillus* and *Mucor,* which one of the following is LEAST accurate?

(A) Both organisms are dimorphic; they are molds in the body and yeasts in the soil

(B) Both organisms are opportunistic pathogens; ie, they cause disease primarily in immunocompromised patients

(C) In biopsy specimens, *Aspergillus* can be distinguished from *Mucor* because *Aspergillus* has septate hyphae whereas *Mucor* does not

(D) Skin tests are rarely used to determine whether a patient has been infected with these organisms

33. Each of the following statements regarding *Streptococcus pneumoniae* is correct EXCEPT:

(A) Pneumococci are gram-positive diplococci that form alpha-hemolytic colonies on blood agar

(B) Pneumococci are distinguished from viridans streptococci by their appearance on a blood agar plate

(C) There are at least 80 serotypes of pneumococci, which are distinguished on the basis of their capsular polysaccharides

(D) The major site of colonization of pneumococci is the human oropharynx; there is no animal reservoir

34. Each of the following statements regarding antiviral drugs is correct EXCEPT:

(A) Amantadine prevents influenza A virus from replicating by inhibiting penetration of the virus into the infected cell

(B) Acyclovir prevents herpes simplex virus type 1 from replicating by inhibiting the viral DNA polymerase

(C) Ganciclovir prevents the replication of cytomegalovirus

(D) Azidothymidine (AZT) prevents human immunodeficiency virus from replicating by inhibiting the binding of the virus to the cell surface receptor

35. Each of the following statements regarding *Corynebacterium diphtheriae* and the disease diphtheria is correct EXCEPT:

(A) A Gram stain of the exudate from a lesion reveals gram-positive rods

(B) Diphtheria toxin blocks protein synthesis in human cells by inhibiting elongation factor 2

(C) The natural habitat of the organism is the soil, where it forms spores

(D) The antigen in the vaccine is diphtheria toxoid

36. Your patient is a 44-year-old man with a B cell lymphoma. Which one of the following findings is MOST likely in this patient?

(A) Chromosomal rearrangements that put an oncogene next to an immunoglobulin gene

(B) A monoclonal peak of IgE

(C) Antibodies to hepatitis B virus

(D) Immature CD4-positive T cells producing large amounts of interleukin-1

37. Each of the following statements regarding herpes simplex virus type 1 is correct EXCEPT:

(A) It typically causes vesicular skin lesions

(B) It can become latent in the neurons of sensory ganglia

(C) Lesions typically occur on the face

(D) It is transmitted most often by sexual contact

38. Each of the following statements regarding *Haemophilus influenzae* is correct EXCEPT:

(A) It is a very small, coccobacillary gram-negative rod

(B) It is found only in humans; ie, there is no animal reservoir

(C) Bacteremia is caused by encapsulated strains, but strains without capsules cause disease also

(D) Prevention of invasive disease primarily involves personal measures such as hand-washing, since there is no vaccine

39. Each of the following statements regarding papillomaviruses is correct EXCEPT:

(A) They are DNA viruses that do not have an envelope

(B) Genital warts are one of the most common sexually transmitted diseases

(C) Neutralization tests to detect a rise in antibody titer are the most common diagnostic method

(D) They encode a protein that binds to the retinoblastoma gene protein, which may explain the ability of the virus to cause cancer

40. Each of the following statements regarding bacterial spores is correct EXCEPT:

(A) They are formed primarily when the organism has inadequate nutrients

(B) They are formed primarily by gram-negative cocci such as *Neisseria*

(C) They require temperatures above boiling in order to be killed

(D) Most bacterial spores can survive in the soil for long periods (years)

41. Each of the following statements regarding hepatitis A virus is correct EXCEPT:

(A) It is transmitted by the fecal-oral route

(B) Most childhood disease is mild or inapparent

(C) Immunity after infection is typically life-long

(D) The live, attenuated vaccine is recommended for individuals traveling to endemic areas

42. Each of the following statements regarding the mode of action of antimicrobial drugs is correct EXCEPT:

(A) Both aminoglycosides and tetracyclines act by inhibiting protein synthesis

(B) The reason why sulfonamides selectively inhibit the growth of bacteria more than human cells is that bacteria must synthesize folic acids, whereas human cells do not

(C) Amphotericin B inhibits certain fungi but is ineffective against most bacteria because it binds much more efficiently to fungal ribosomal proteins than to those in bacteria

(D) Quinolones, eg, ciprofloxacin, inhibit bacterial DNA synthesis by inhibiting the gyrase that unwinds DNA

43. Each of the following statements regarding activated helper (CD4) T cells is correct EXCEPT:

(A) They secrete growth and differentiation factors for B cells

(B) They express IgM on their surface

(C) They express receptors for interleukin-2

(D) They secrete interleukin-2

44. Each of the following statements regarding varicella-zoster virus is correct EXCEPT:

(A) In primary infections, it causes varicella (chickenpox), which is characterized by vesicular skin lesions

(B) In recurrent infections, it causes zoster (shingles), which is characterized by vesicular skin lesions

(C) It rarely causes disseminated disease in immunocompromised patients

(D) Multinucleated giant cells are seen in the lesions

45. Your patient is a 1-year-old child with a high fever who had two episodes of vomiting followed by a generalized seizure. You suspect meningitis and do a lumbar puncture. A Gram stain and culture of the spinal fluid is MOST likely to reveal which one of the following?

(A) Gram-negative coccobacillary rods that require both X (hemin) and V (NAD) factors to grow

(B) Gram-positive cocci in clusters that are coagulase-positive

(C) Gram-positive diplococci that are optochin-sensitive

(D) Large gram-negative rods that grow on blood agar and ferment lactose

46. Each of the following statements regarding hepatitis A and B viruses is correct EXCEPT:

(A) In certain patients, hepatitis B virus causes persistent infections and infectious virus is present in the blood

(B) Hepatitis B surface antigen (HBsAg) is the component in the hepatitis B vaccine that induces protective antibody

(C) The presence of hepatitis e antigen (HBeAg) in certain patients' blood indicates that the blood is likely to be infectious

(D) Certain patients have antibody to hepatitis A virus in their blood, indicating that a chronic carrier state is present

47. Your patient has septicemia caused by a gram-negative rod. You administer an aminoglycoside (gentamicin), to which the patient initially responds, but now is getting worse. The laboratory reports that the organism isolated from the most recent blood culture is resistant to gentamicin, whereas it was formerly sensitive. Regarding the most recent isolate, which one of the following is the LEAST accurate?

(A) It may have acquired a plasmid by conjugation with another gram-negative rod

(B) It may have a mutation in the gene that codes for a ribosomal protein

(C) It may have an altered cell membrane so the drug cannot penetrate

(D) It may have a dihydrofolate reductase with a reduced binding affinity

48. Which one of the following statements provides the BEST evidence implicating human T cell leukemia virus (HTLV-I) as a causative agent of human cancer?

(A) There is a high frequency of infection among adults born in Kyushu, Japan

(B) HTLV-I proviral DNA is found in tumor cells in many cases of adult T cell leukemia

(C) HTLV-I was isolated from a T cell lymphoma in the United States

(D) HTLV-I is a retrovirus

49. Which one of the following organisms is MOST likely to produce food poisoning within 3 hours of ingestion?

(A) *Staphylococcus aureus*

(B) *Salmonella enteritidis*

(C) Enterotoxigenic *Escherichia coli*

(D) *Enterococcus faecalis*

50. As a clinical virologist investigating an epidemic of pneumonia in a remote part of the world, you have isolated a virus from the pulmonary washings of a patient with the disease. Which one of the following would be the LEAST helpful in your attempts to show that the virus was the specific cause of the disease?

(A) Demonstration of a rise in antiviral antibodies in the patient from whom you isolated the virus

(B) Isolation of the same virus from many other patients with the same disease but not from healthy controls

(C) Production of cytopathic effect (plaques) by infection of cultured cells

(D) Induction by the virus of a similar disease in primates

51. Regarding the virus you isolated in the previous question, you study it and find that it consists of a helical nucleocapsid within an envelope and contains single-stranded RNA of negative polarity. Which one of the following statements about the virus is LEAST accurate?

(A) The virus particle also contains an RNA-directed RNA polymerase

(B) The purified viral genome is infectious

(C) The virus is very sensitive to inactivation by detergents and heat

(D) The virus assembles at the plasma membrane and is released by budding through the membrane

52. Regarding various gram-negative rods, which one of the following is the LEAST accurate?

(A) The cell wall of gram-negative rods contains endotoxin which is a lipopolysaccharide whose toxic component is lipid A

(B) E coli, which is part of the normal flora of the colon, can be distinguished from Salmonella and Shigella, which are two important enteric pathogens, by lactose fermentation; ie, E coli ferments lactose whereas the others do not

(C) Klebsiella, Enterobacter, and Serratia, which are part of the normal flora of the colon, cause nosocomial (hospital) outbreaks of pneumonia and urinary tract infections

(D) The O antigens of E coli and Klebsiella are enterotoxins that cause diarrhea

53. Each of the following statements regarding cytotoxic (CD8) T cells is correct EXCEPT:

(A) For activation, they require interleukin-2 provided by helper T cells

(B) They require complement to kill cells

(C) They recognize antigen only when it is presented in association with class I MHC proteins

(D) They are important in killing virus-infected cells

54. Each of the following statements regarding cytomegalovirus is correct EXCEPT:

(A) It is an important cause of congenital abnormalities

(B) It is transmitted by both saliva and blood

(C) Patients receiving transplants are at risk for severe disseminated disease

(D) Recurrent disease is characterized by vesicular skin lesions

55. Several fungal diseases are acquired by inhalation and cause primary infection in the lungs. Which one of the following organisms is LEAST likely to follow this pattern of pathogenesis?

(A) Candida albicans

(B) Coccidioides immitis

(C) Cryptococcus neoformans

(D) Histoplasma capsulatum

56. Regarding Shigella and Campylobacter, which one of the following is LEAST accurate?

(A) Both are gram-negative rods

(B) Both typically cause white blood cells to appear in the stool

(C) Both have an animal reservoir that acts as a source of infection for humans

(D) Both can be cultured on bacteriologic media in the clinical laboratory

57. A secondary immune response is more rapid and intense than a primary response. The MOST likely explanation of this observation is that

(A) antigen persists longer in the secondary response

(B) antigen presentation is more rapid in the secondary response

(C) a pool of cells with specific class I MHC proteins is generated during the primary response

(D) a pool of both memory B cells and memory T cells is generated during the primary response

58. Measles virus and rubella virus share several features. Which one of the following is LEAST accurate?

(A) They are both enveloped RNA viruses

(B) They are both transmitted by respiratory aerosol and cause diseases characterized by a skin rash

(C) They both induce lifelong immunity following natural infection

(D) They are both a significant cause of congenital abnormalities

59. Each of the following statements regarding Borrelia burgdorferi is correct EXCEPT:

(A) It is a gram-negative rod that is divided into four serotypes on the basis of its capsular polysaccharide

(B) It is the causative agent of Lyme disease

(C) It is transmitted from the animal reservoir to humans by tick bite

(D) Because it does not grow well on bacteriologic media, infections are typically diagnosed serologically

60. Human immunodeficiency virus (HIV) is classified as a retrovirus. The rationale for the term "retrovirus" is that

(A) pieces of the genome RNA are spliced into a single strand before translation

(B) the genome RNA is transcribed into DNA

(C) it reverses its morphology from type D to type C when it enters the cell

(D) the promoter region of the genome RNA is in the reverse position

61. Each of the following statements regarding chlamydiae is correct EXCEPT:

(A) They can replicate only within cells because they cannot synthesize sufficient energy for independent growth

(B) They replicate in the cytoplasm of infected cells, where they form inclusions that are useful diagnostically

(C) Their life cycle consists of a metabolically inactive particle in the extracellular phase

(D) They produce an exotoxin that inhibits elongation factor 2

62. Each of the following statements regarding IgA is correct EXCEPT:

(A) Secretory IgA in the gastrointestinal tract limits the attachment of bacteria to the gut mucosa

(B) People with an IgA deficiency have an increased number of respiratory tract infections

(C) IgA fixes complement, thereby enhancing phagocytosis by neutrophils

(D) IgA is the main immunoglobulin in mother's milk

63. Each of the following statements regarding influenza virus is correct EXCEPT:

(A) Influenza A virus causes more epidemics and more serious disease than influenza B and C viruses do

(B) Influenza viruses cannot be grown in cell culture; hence, the diagnosis can only be made serologically

(C) Influenza A virus undergoes major antigenic changes in its hemagglutinin (antigenic shift), which allow the virus to evade existing immunity

(D) Influenza viruses are transmitted primarily by aerosol and primarily affect the lower respiratory tract

64. Each of the following statements regarding Q fever is correct EXCEPT:

(A) It is caused by *Coxiella burnetii*

(B) It is contracted by inhalation of aerosolized organisms

(C) The natural habitat of the causative agent is small rodents

(D) The diagnosis is made primarily by using serologic tests

65. Each of the following statements regarding hepatitis C and D viruses is correct EXCEPT:

(A) Both are transmitted by blood

(B) Both are RNA viruses

(C) Both require prior infection with hepatitis B virus to complete their replicative cycle

(D) Both are known to cause infection and disease in the United States

66. Each of the following statements regarding syphilis is correct EXCEPT:

(A) In congenital syphilis, no antibody is formed against *Treponema pallidum* because the fetus is tolerant to the organism

(B) The characteristic lesion of primary syphilis is a painless ulcer

(C) In secondary syphilis, both the rapid plasma reagin (RPR) and the fluorescent treponemal antibody-absorbed (FTA-ABS) tests are usually positive

(D) In tertiary syphilis, lesions commonly appear in the brain and spinal cord, but there are only a few organisms in these lesions

67. In the body, some fungi are yeasts whereas others are molds. To make a diagnosis microscopically, it is important to know what to look for. Which one of the following genera is a YEAST in the body?

(A) *Aspergillus*

(B) *Cryptococcus*

(C) *Coccidioides*

(D) *Microsporum*

68. Each of the following statements regarding *Mycobacterium tuberculosis* is correct EXCEPT:

(A) The predominant cells found in cavitary lesions are neutrophils

(B) It is transmitted by aerosol droplets

(C) In cavitary disease, the sputum contains rods that stain red with the acid-fast stain

(D) Multidrug therapy is required for months to treat cavitary disease

69. Comparing anaphylactic and immune complex hypersensitivities, which one of the following is MOST accurate?

(A) Complement participates in immune complex hypersensitivity, but not in anaphylactic hypersensitivity

(B) After contact with antigen, symptoms appear more rapidly in immune complex reactions than in anaphylactic reactions

(C) Less antigen is required for a reaction in immune complex hypersensitivity than in anaphylactic hypersensitivity

(D) IgE participates to a greater extent in immune complex hypersensitivity than in anaphylactic hypersensitivity

70. Regarding viruses that cause respiratory tract disease, which one of the following is LEAST accurate?

(A) Respiratory syncytial virus is an enveloped RNA virus that causes pneumonia primarily in infants

(B) Parainfluenza viruses are enveloped RNA viruses that cause croup primarily in infants

(C) Rhinoviruses are enveloped RNA viruses that cause pneumonia primarily in AIDS patients

(D) Coxsackieviruses are nonenveloped RNA viruses that cause myocarditis and pericarditis as well as respiratory tract disease

71. Each of the following statements regarding *Salmonella* species is correct EXCEPT:

(A) The fecal-oral route is the main mode of transmission

(B) They cause diarrhea by producing an exotoxin that activates adenylate cyclase

(C) They are non-lactose fermenters and form colorless colonies on EMB agar

(D) Their O antigen polysaccharides are an important means of classification

72. Regarding the nature of human immunodeficiency virus (HIV), which one of the following is LEAST accurate?

(A) Both the genome of HIV and the antigenicity of its envelope glycoprotein are remarkably stable compared with other retroviruses

(B) The genome of HIV contains sequences that enhance the transcription of other genes

(C) Host cell specificity is determined by the interaction of envelope glycoproteins of the virus with CD4 proteins on the surface of cells

(D) One of the cytopathic effects caused by HIV infection of CD4-positive T lymphocytes is giant-cell formation

73. Each of the following statements regarding *Nocardia asteroides* and *Actinomyces israelii* is correct EXCEPT:

(A) They are members of the normal flora of the mouth

(B) They are filamentous, branching rods

(C) *Actinomyces israelii* infections typically form sinus tracts that drain to the skin, whereas *Nocardia asteroides* infections do not

(D) *Actinomyces israelii* is an anaerobe whereas *Nocardia asteroides* is not

74. The family of herpesviruses contains members that infect both humans and various other animals. Which one of the following is LEAST accurate regarding these viruses?

(A) They are all enveloped viruses with a double-stranded DNA genome

(B) Animal herpesviruses are a source of new genes for human herpesviruses that allow them to evade our existing immunity

(C) Some herpesviruses are known to cause cancer

(D) Herpesviruses do not have a DNA polymerase in the virion

75. Each of the following statements regarding the PPD (tuberculin) skin test is correct EXCEPT:

(A) A positive test is judged by the amount of induration, ie, thickening, of the skin at the site of injection

(B) A positive test indicates that the person has formed a delayed-hypersensitivity response against certain proteins of *Mycobacterium tuberculosis*

(C) A positive test indicates that the person has been infected with *M tuberculosis* but may not have symptoms of disease at present

(D) A positive test indicates that the person should receive isoniazid (INH) and rifampin for 9 months

76. Each of the following statements regarding penicillin allergies is correct EXCEPT:

(A) The antibiotic is a hapten and must combine with one of our proteins to become immunogenic

(B) IgE antibodies mediate anaphylaxis, whereas IgG antibodies mediate serum sickness

(C) In autoimmune hemolytic anemia, penicillin is bound to the red cell surface

(D) Mast cells mediate serum sickness, whereas neutrophils mediate anaphylaxis

77. Each of the following statements regarding plague is correct EXCEPT:

(A) The causative organism, *Yersinia pestis*, is a gram-negative rod with a very low ID_{50}

(B) There is an animal reservoir for this disease, including rodents found in many areas of the western part of the United States

(C) The diagnosis must be made serologically because the organism does not grow in culture

(D) People should not handle dead wild animals since fleas associated with the animals can transmit the disease

78. Each of the following statements regarding poliovirus is correct EXCEPT:

(A) It is a nonenveloped virus with a single-stranded RNA genome

(B) It causes paralysis by inhibiting acetylcholine release by sensory neurons

(C) The most prominent site of viral replication is the gastrointestinal tract

(D) Complete protection against poliomyelitis requires that an individual have immunity against all three serologic types

79. Each of the following statements regarding *Bacteroides fragilis* is correct EXCEPT:

(A) It is a gram-positive, spore-forming rod
(B) Its natural habitat is the human colon
(C) Tissue infected by this organism typically contains foul-smelling pus and gas
(D) It is typically found in mixed infections, eg, with facultative bacteria such as *E coli*

80. Each of the following statements regarding poison oak is correct EXCEPT:
(A) The plant allergen is a hapten and must combine with one of our proteins to become immunogenic
(B) The reaction is due to activated CD4-positive T cells
(C) The reaction requires 1–2 days to appear after contact of a sensitized individual with the plant
(D) The skin reaction is caused by immune complexes that cause the release of histamine

81. Each of the following statements regarding *Mycobacterium leprae* is correct EXCEPT:
(A) Many patients have sensory nerve destruction and lose sensation
(B) Diagnosis involves culturing the organism on bacteriologic medium that contains a high concentration of lactose
(C) Cell-mediated immunity is the most important host defense
(D) Humans constitute the major reservoir

82. Measles and rubella vaccines share several characteristics. Which one of the following is NOT an attribute of BOTH vaccines?
(A) They both contain live, attenuated virus
(B) They both contain a single serotype of the virus
(C) Neither should be given to children younger than 15 months of age since maternal antibody can reduce the response to the vaccine
(D) They both should be given with immune globulins in order to reduce the side effects of the vaccine

83. Each of the following statements regarding tetanus is correct EXCEPT:
(A) The causative agent is a gram-positive anaerobic rod
(B) The antigen in the vaccine is tetanus toxoid, which is chemically modified toxin
(C) The natural habitat of the organism is the soil. Infection typically occurs when spores enter the body in contaminated wounds
(D) The toxin lyses red blood cells, causing severe anemia and kidney failure

84. Antibody synthesis involves a series of gene movements. Regarding these processes, which one of the following is LEAST accurate?
(A) The antibody-combining site of light chains is generated by the movement of a

variable (V) gene segment adjacent to a joining (J) gene segment
(B) Since the genes for the light and heavy chains are on the same chromosome, an antibody can contain one kappa and one lambda chain, which adds to antibody diversity
(C) Immunoglobulin molecules retain antibody specificity but acquire different biologic properties by switching the genes encoding the V portion of the heavy chain adjacent to the genes encoding a different constant (C) portion of the heavy chain
(D) A heavy chain gene is generated by recombining a V gene, a D (diversity) gene, and a J gene with a constant gene

85. In which one of the following infections do anaerobic bacteria NOT have an important role?
(A) Abdominal abscess
(B) Gas gangrene
(C) Impetigo (pyoderma)
(D) Pseudomembranous colitis

86. Each of the following statements regarding rabies is correct EXCEPT:
(A) The causative agent is an enveloped RNA virus that appears bullet-shaped in electron micrographs
(B) The virus has five serotypes; hence, the vaccine consists of five immunizations
(C) In the United States, skunks are a major animal reservoir of the virus
(D) In the pathogenesis of rabies, the virus spreads primarily via the nerves to the brain

87. Your patient has had severe diarrhea for the past 2 days, accompanied by fever and a shaking chill. From both the blood culture and the stool culture, a gram-negative rod was isolated that does not ferment lactose. Which one of the following organisms is the MOST likely cause?
(A) *Salmonella enteritidis*
(B) *Escherichia coli*
(C) *Helicobacter pylori*
(D) *Haemophilus influenzae*

88. Each of the following statements regarding arboviruses is correct EXCEPT:
(A) Humans and horses are "dead-end" hosts for encephalitis viruses because the concentration of virus in their blood is quite low
(B) Both yellow fever and dengue are mosquito-borne diseases
(C) Travelers to areas where yellow fever is endemic should receive the live, attenuated vaccine
(D) The main characteristic that links the various viruses in the arbovirus family is

that they are all double-stranded DNA viruses

89. Five days after major abdominal surgery, a 65-year-old man suddenly develops severe abdominal pain, fever, and shock. Examination of fluid removed from his peritoneum shows abundant leukocytes and many gram-negative rods, gram-positive rods, and gram-positive cocci. The major factor responsible for the fever and shock is MOST likely to be
   (A) collagenase elaborated by the gram-positive rods
   (B) enterotoxin produced by the gram-positive cocci
   (C) endotoxin associated with the gram-negative rods
   (D) intraperitoneal chemotactic factors produced by all three types of organisms

90. Each of the following statements regarding T cells is correct EXCEPT:
   (A) T cells originate in the bone marrow but must pass through the thymus to differentiate properly
   (B) Developing T cells typically express both CD4 and CD8 proteins, but mature T cells express only one or the other
   (C) Helper T cells play an essential role in delayed hypersensitivity reactions, eg, the tuberculin skin test
   (D) In the thymic education of T cells, clones of cells that react with self MHC and foreign antigen are deleted

91. Several diseases are caused by exotoxins that affect adenylate cyclase. Which one of the following diseases does NOT involve that enzyme in its pathogenesis?
   (A) Diphtheria
   (B) Traveler's diarrhea ("turista")
   (C) Whooping cough
   (D) Cholera

92. Interpretation of hepatitis B serologic tests provides important clinical information. If your patient was HbsAg negative, IgM core antibody negative, and Hbs antibody positive, which one of the following would be the BEST interpretation?
   (A) The patient is probably in the "window" phase
   (B) The patient probably has active signs and symptoms of hepatitis
   (C) The patient probably has chronic active hepatitis
   (D) The patient is immune to hepatitis B

93. Each of the following statements regarding *Pseudomonas aeruginosa* is correct EXCEPT:
   (A) It is commonly resistant to many antibiotics
   (B) It is an important cause of wound and burn infections

   (C) It produces neither exotoxins nor endotoxin
   (D) It is commonly associated with water sources

94. Regarding the major histocompatibility locus of genes (called HLA in humans), which one of the following is LEAST accurate?
   (A) These genes code for class I and class II proteins, which play a major role in the rejection of allografts
   (B) To generate sufficient diversity in these genes, the rearrangement of at least two gene segments is required
   (C) Class I proteins are expressed on virtually all human cells, whereas class II proteins are found only on certain cells, eg, macrophages and B lymphocytes
   (D) These genes have many different alleles at both class I and class II loci; hence, the corresponding proteins on the surface of human cells are very polymorphic

95. Which one of the following is MOST accurate regarding *Legionella pneumophila?*
   (A) It is a common cause of pneumonia because it is part of the normal flora of the oral pharynx
   (B) Human-to-human transmission is responsible for epidemic outbreaks
   (C) It is best visualized in freshly prepared Gram stains of clinical specimens
   (D) It can be isolated by growth on agar in the laboratory; ie, it is not an obligate intracellular parasite

96. Several viral infections occur primarily as inapparent, asymptomatic infections in young children rather than clinically apparent disease. Which one of the following viruses is LEAST likely to behave in this manner?
   (A) Hepatitis A virus
   (B) Poliovirus
   (C) Varicella-zoster virus
   (D) Epstein-Barr virus

97. Bacteria differ from viruses in several structural and chemical characteristics. Which one of the following is LEAST accurate?
   (A) Bacteria are cells, whereas viruses are not
   (B) Most bacteria have mitochondria, whereas viruses do not
   (C) Bacteria have ribosomes, whereas viruses do not
   (D) Most bacteria contain peptidoglycan, whereas viruses do not

98. Regarding the functions of antibodies, which one of the following is LEAST accurate?
   (A) Because IgM is made early in the primary response, it is a good indicator of current infection
   (B) Because IgG crosses the placenta, it is the main immunoglobulin in fetal blood

(C) Because the gamma heavy chain of IgG binds complement, IgG is frequently involved in diseases caused by immune complexes

(D) Because IgA is the main immunoglobulin found in respiratory tract secretions, it is frequently involved in respiratory allergies such as asthma

99. Regarding the movement of genes within a bacterium or from one bacterium to another, which one of the following is the LEAST accurate?

(A) Transposons can move antibiotic resistance genes from the bacterial chromosome to a plasmid

(B) Resistance plasmids (R factors) can be transferred from one bacterium to another by conjugation

(C) Lysogeny is the process by which genes are exchanged between one site on the bacterial chromosome and another site on the same chromosome

(D) Bacteria can acquire new genes when they are infected by viruses, a process called transduction

100. Some viral diseases occur once in a person, who then acquires lifelong immunity. These viruses typically have a single serologic (antigenic) type. Which one of the following viruses does NOT fit this picture?

(A) Measles virus

(B) Adenovirus

(C) Rubella virus

(D) Mumps virus

101. Two broth cultures were inoculated with 10^3 bacteria each and incubated at 37 °C under different conditions. The culture incubated anaerobically contained 10^8 bacteria/ml, but the number of organisms was 10-fold higher in the culture incubated aerobically. The MOST reasonable interpretation of this observation is that

(A) the bacteria are deficient in superoxide dismutase

(B) the bacteria lack a cell wall

(C) the bacteria contain metachromatic granules, a storage form of ATP

(D) the bacteria are facultative anaerobes

102. Each of the following statements regarding the T cell receptor is correct EXCEPT:

(A) It serves to internalize the antigen and present it to the B cell, which then is activated to produce antibody specific to the antigen

(B) It interacts with antigen when presented by either class I or class II MHC proteins

(C) When it binds antigen, the CD3 proteins transmit a signal to activate the T cell to produce interleukin-2

(D) The genes for its antigen-specific domains rearrange in a manner similar to that of immunoglobulin genes

103. Each of the following statements about staphylococci is correct EXCEPT:

(A) *Staphylococcus aureus* produces coagulase, whereas *Staphylococcus epidermidis* does not

(B) Some strains of *S aureus* produce an exotoxin which is an enterotoxin that causes vomiting and diarrhea

(C) Some strains of *S aureus* are resistant to penicillin due to production of β-lactamase

(D) Some strains of *S aureus* cause rheumatic fever as a result of an immunologic cross-reaction between the proteins of the organism and proteins of the myocardium

104. Some viruses are known to cause persistent infections during which virus is shed for a long time and therefore can cause infection in others. Which one of the following viruses fits this picture LEAST well?

(A) Influenza virus

(B) Cytomegalovirus

(C) Rubella virus

(D) Hepatitis B virus

105. Each of the following statements regarding the pathogenesis of disease by *Neisseria meningitidis* is correct EXCEPT:

(A) The polysaccharide capsule of this organism is an important virulence factor

(B) Many of the symptoms of meningococcemia can be attributed to endotoxin

(C) It is a gram-negative rod which produces an exotoxin that activates adenylate cyclase

(D) It colonizes the upper respiratory tract and evades secretory IgA by producing a protease specific for that immunoglobulin

106. Each of the following statements regarding complement is correct EXCEPT:

(A) The complement cascade can be initiated both by antigen-antibody complexes and by the surface components of bacteria

(B) When C3b is bound to microorganisms, phagocytosis is enhanced

(C) Patients who lack the inhibitor to the C1 component of complement typically have frequent bacterial infections

(D) Both C3a and C5a are anaphylotoxins; ie, they can cause the signs and symptoms of anaphylactic shock

107. Each of the following statements regarding *Streptococcus pyogenes* is correct EXCEPT:

(A) It is the most common bacterial cause of pharyngitis

(B) Patients can have multiple episodes of *S pyogenes* infections since there are multiple antigenic types of M protein

(C) Pathogenesis of acute glomerulonephritis involves antibodies formed against antigens of certain strains of *S pyogenes*

(D) Since it is commonly found as part of the normal flora of the colon, transmission typically involves fecal-oral spread

108. Prions have been postulated as the cause of certain central nervous system diseases. Which one of the following is the LEAST accurate statement about prions?

(A) They are particles that contain protein but no detectable nucleic acid

(B) They resemble papovaviruses in the electron microscope

(C) They are encoded by a cellular gene present in human cells

(D) They are highly resistant to inactivation by heat and UV light

109. Each of the following statements regarding toxin-mediated diseases is correct EXCEPT:

(A) Pseudomembranous colitis is a toxin-mediated disease caused by *Clostridium difficile*

(B) Tetanus toxin is a neurotoxin that acts at the level of the synapses in the central nervous system

(C) Trachoma is a toxin-mediated disease caused by *Coxiella burnetii*

(D) Botulism is characterized by muscle weakness and is caused by a toxin that inhibits the release of acetylcholine

110. Each of the following statements regarding autoimmune diseases is correct EXCEPT:

(A) In systemic lupus erythematosus, antibodies are formed against human DNA and other components of the nucleus

(B) In myasthenia gravis, antibodies are formed against the acetylcholine receptor, leading to muscle weakness

(C) In Graves' disease, antibodies are formed against the thyroid-stimulating hormone (TSH) receptor, leading to the release of thyroxine and, as a result, to hyperthyroidism

(D) In rheumatoid arthritis, IgE antibodies and mast cell mediators are the primary cause of the arthritis

111. Which one of the following statements regarding *Treponema pallidum* is MOST accurate?

(A) It is a spiral-shaped rod that appears gram-positive in Gram-stained smears

(B) Specimens cultured on blood agar plates reveal alpha-hemolytic colonies

(C) Since the lesions of primary syphilis are primarily due to an immune response against the organism, the lesions typically contain few *T pallidum* cells

(D) Despite the therapeutic use of penicillin for many years, no penicillin-resistant strains of *T pallidum* have been isolated

112. Each of the following statements regarding *Cryptococcus neoformans* is correct EXCEPT:

(A) It is a dimorphic fungus that forms septate hyphae in the soil and yeasts in the infected individual

(B) It is typically acquired by inhalation, and primary infections occur in the lungs

(C) It causes disseminated disease, eg, meningitis, more often in immunocompromised individuals than in the immunocompetent

(D) Diagnosis of cryptococcal disease can be made by detecting the polysaccharide capsular antigen in body fluids, eg, spinal fluid

113. Each of the following statements regarding immunodeficiencies is correct EXCEPT:

(A) In congenital thymic aplasia (DiGeorge's syndrome), the patient has no mature T cells and is particularly susceptible to severe viral infections

(B) Patients who lack the late-acting components of complement (C6–C9) have a high incidence of disseminated infections caused by *Neisseria*

(C) Since newborns with hypogammaglobulinemia cannot produce IgG, they contract severe bacterial infections within a few weeks after birth

(D) Patients with chronic granulomatous disease have defective phagocytes which cannot kill bacteria

114. Each of the following statements regarding *Neisseria gonorrhoeae* is correct EXCEPT:

(A) It produces an IgA protease that degrades secretory IgA, thereby enhancing the ability of the organism to colonize the urethral mucosa

(B) It grows poorly on bacteriologic media, so diagnosis is primarily made serologically

(C) Resistance to penicillin is mediated both by plasmid-encoded penicillinase and by changes in chromosome-encoded proteins that control the permeability of the drug

(D) The antigenicity of its pilus proteins varies significantly, thereby allowing the organism to evade the immune response

115. Certain viruses possess an outer structure called an envelope. Regarding the viral envelope, which one of the following is LEAST accurate?

(A) Proteins in the envelope determine host cell specificity

(B) Proteins in the envelope interact with neutralizing antibody

(C) Enveloped viruses are more easily inactivated by lipid solvents than are nonenveloped viruses

(D) When RNA polymerases are present in a virus, they are typically found as one of the envelope proteins

116. Which one of the following is NOT an obligate intracellular parasite?
   (A) *Coxiella burnetii*
   (B) *Mycobacterium avium-intracellulare*
   (C) *Chlamydia trachomatis*
   (D) *Rickettsia rickettsii*

117. During the latent period of the virus growth cycle, which one of the following events does NOT happen?
   (A) Production of extracellular virions
   (B) Synthesis of viral RNA
   (C) Synthesis of capsid proteins
   (D) Replication of the viral genome

118. Which one of the following is transmitted by an arthropod vector?
   (A) *Chlamydia psittaci*
   (B) *Coxiella burnetii*
   (C) *Brucella melitensis*
   (D) *Rickettsia rickettsii*

119. Each of the following statements regarding severe combined immunodeficiency disease (SCID) is correct EXCEPT:
   (A) Patients are very susceptible to infections by bacteria, viruses, and fungi
   (B) It can be diagnosed by skin testing with various antigens and measurement of serum immunoglobulin levels
   (C) It typically affects adult women
   (D) Patients typically lack both T cells and B cells

120. Some viruses possess a polymerase in the virus particle. Regarding virion polymerases, which one of the following statements is LEAST accurate?
   (A) Poliovirus possesses a polymerase that synthesizes double-stranded RNA
   (B) Hepatitis B virus possesses a polymerase that completes its double-stranded DNA genome
   (C) Measles virus possesses a polymerase that synthesizes mRNA
   (D) Retroviruses possess a polymerase that synthesizes double-stranded DNA

121. Regarding Rocky Mountain spotted fever, which one of the following is MOST accurate?
   (A) The disease is most prevalent in the western United States
   (B) Humans are the main reservoir of infection
   (C) The organism is transmitted by tick bite
   (D) Diagnosis is usually made by culturing the organism

122. One explanation for the remarkable ability of influenza virus to cause worldwide epidemics is the emergence of new antigenic strains of the virus. This is thought to be due to coinfection of cells with two different strains (perhaps a human strain and an animal strain). The emergence of the new strain is MOST probably due to
   (A) complementation
   (B) phenotypic mixing
   (C) production of defective interfering particles
   (D) reassortment of genome segments

123. Each of the following statements regarding *Candida albicans* is correct EXCEPT:
   (A) It is a budding yeast when it colonizes the mucous membranes of the mouth
   (B) The formation of germ tubes is an important diagnostic test
   (C) Because it does not grow well on laboratory media, the diagnosis of candidal infections is typically made by skin tests that detect a delayed hypersensitivity reaction
   (D) It causes thrush, a mucosal infection of the oropharynx, which occurs particularly in neonates and immunocompromised patients

124. There is reasonable evidence that certain viruses can cause cancer in humans. Regarding these viruses, which one of the following is LEAST accurate?
   (A) During infection by the retrovirus human T cell leukemia virus, a DNA copy of the viral genome is synthesized and becomes integrated into T cell DNA
   (B) When adenoviruses induce malignant transformation of cells, the RNA genome of the virus must be transcribed into DNA before the cells can become malignant
   (C) During infection by human papillomavirus, a protein encoded by the virus inactivates a cellular protein encoded by a tumor suppressor gene and this may be the mechanism by which the virus causes carcinoma of the cervix
   (D) The prevalence of hepatocellular carcinoma is high in areas where infection by hepatitis B virus is endemic

125. A young woman whose blood type is B Rh-negative mistakenly receives blood from an A Rh-positive donor after an automobile accident. She has a transfusion reaction but survives. Which one of the statements is LEAST accurate?
   (A) A subsequent fetus who is B Rh-positive might develop erythroblastosis fetalis
   (B) The transfusion reaction is related to naturally occurring antibodies against Rh antigen
   (C) A subsequent fetus who is B Rh-negative would not develop erythroblastosis fetalis
   (D) The woman would have detectable antibodies against blood group A before the transfusion

126. Each of the following statements regarding alpha interferon is correct EXCEPT:
 (A) It is induced efficiently by double-stranded RNA
 (B) It is produced primarily by macrophages
 (C) It is active against a wide variety of viruses
 (D) It induces a ribonuclease that degrades viral mRNA

127. Which one of the following statements is LEAST accurate about the mixed-lymphocyte culture (also known as the mixed-lymphocyte reaction)?
 (A) It is widely used as a test for matching organs from unrelated (cadaver) donors with potential recipients, since the test results are known within 24 hours
 (B) It measures the proliferative response of the recipient's T cells against the potential donor's white blood cells
 (C) The recipient's helper T cells are activated by class II MHC differences on the donor cells and produce interleukin-2, which promotes T cell proliferation
 (D) This in vitro test gives a good idea of the strength of the graft rejection response that the patient will mount against the engrafted organ

128. Live viral vaccines are used more commonly in the United States than killed viral vaccines. There are several reasons for this. Which one of the following is the LEAST accurate reason?
 (A) Live vaccines can be given to immuno-compromised patients since they induce mucosal (secretory) IgA
 (B) Live vaccines induce longer-lasting protection than killed vaccines
 (C) Live vaccines induce a more complete range of humoral and cell-mediated responses than killed vaccines
 (D) The virus in live vaccines can multiply in the portal of entry and exclude (interfere with) the "wild-type" pathogenic virus

129. Each of the following statements regarding oncogenes is correct EXCEPT:
 (A) There are genes in normal cells, many of which regulate growth control, that are homologous to genes in various cancer viruses
 (B) Certain cancer viruses do not contain oncogenes; they cause malignancy typically by insertional mutagenesis
 (C) In Burkitt's lymphoma, translocation of an oncogene adjacent to an immunoglobulin gene locus results in overproduction of the oncogene protein
 (D) Cellular proto-oncogenes are double-stranded circular DNA found in the cytoplasm of normal (nonmalignant) cells.

They typically code for proteins that block DNA synthesis

130. Rejection of organ transplants, eg, kidney, between different individuals is due PRIMARILY to which one of the following?
 (A) Macrophage-mediated lysis of the donor cells
 (B) Action of host CD4- and CD8-positive T cells induced by surface MHC molecules of the donor cells
 (C) Action of autoreactive T cells contained within the transplant
 (D) Action of alpha interferon on the donor cells

131. Each of the following statements regarding rhinoviruses is correct EXCEPT:
 (A) They typically cause infection in the upper respiratory tract, a phenomenon attributed to their inability to grow well at 37 °C
 (B) They do not infect the intestinal tract since they are killed by stomach acid
 (C) They are latent in the mucosal cells, and viral reactivation explains the high frequency of colds in the population
 (D) A rhinovirus vaccine is impractical because there are too many serologic types

132. Your patient is a man with a form of hemophilia due to a lack of clotting factor IX. As treatment, you prescribe preparations derived from human plasma that includes this clotting factor. You observe that he makes antibodies that react with and inactivate factor IX. Which one of the following is the MOST likely reason that these antibodies are made?
 (A) He has an autoimmune disease, in which tolerance to self has broken down
 (B) His inability to form blood clots properly interferes with regulation of antibody synthesis by helper T cells
 (C) He does not express any factor IX protein of his own, so his immune system sees factor IX as foreign
 (D) The repeated injection of the human plasma preparation is immunosuppressive

133. Each of the following statements regarding the influenza vaccine is correct EXCEPT:
 (A) It consists of killed virus of both influenza A and B strains
 (B) Boosters should be given every year
 (C) The main antigen in the vaccine is the hemagglutinin; antibody against the hemagglutinin neutralizes viral infectivity
 (D) Since the virus causes major epidemics each winter, the vaccine is recommended for everyone over the age of 2 years

134. Certain bacteria, eg, *Staphylococcus aureus,* cause severe infections in patients with C3 deficiency but not in those with C5 deficiency.

On the basis of these observations, which one of the following is MOST likely to be a critical mechanism for defense against this bacterium?

(A) The ability of the complement-mediated membrane attack complex to make holes in bacterial membranes

(B) The ability of neutrophils and macrophages to ingest bacteria coated with C3b

(C) The ability of C3b to attract phagocytic cells from the blood to the site of bacterial infection

(D) The ability of helper T cells to enhance the bactericidal potential of macrophages

135. Regarding herpes simplex virus type 1 and varicella-zoster virus, which one of the following is LEAST accurate?

(A) They both cause vesicular skin lesions

(B) They both cause disseminated disease in patients with reduced cell-mediated immunity

(C) They both cause multinucleated giant cells to form in the skin lesions

(D) They both have a reservoir in domestic animals that serves as a source of virus infection for humans

136. Regarding slow infections caused by conventional viruses, which one of the following is LEAST accurate?

(A) Progressive multifocal leukoencephalopathy (PML), which is caused by a papovavirus, occurs primarily in immunocompromised individuals

(B) Subacute sclerosing panencephalitis (SSPE) occurs in individuals who were infected with measles virus several years earlier

(C) In both PML and SSPE, the long latent period of the disease is attributed to integration of the viral DNA into the host cell DNA

(D) Human immunodeficiency virus (HIV) infects brain macrophages and causes a "slow infection" manifested by dementia

Directions (Questions 137–160): Select the ONE lettered option that is MOST closely associated with the numbered items. Each lettered option may be selected once, more than once, or not at all.

Questions 137–139:

You are an epidemiologist employed by the Public Health Service to investigate several outbreaks of disease. Which organism is MOST likely to cause each numbered scenario?

(A) *Yersinia pestis*
(B) *Brucella melitensis*
(C) *Rickettsia prowazekii*
(D) *Chlamydia psittaci*
(E) *Pasteurella multocida*

137. An outbreak in people who ate unpasteurized goat cheese

138. An outbreak in children who handled a dead squirrel while on a camping trip

139. An outbreak in people who purchased tropical birds smuggled from Central America

Questions 140–142:

You are a public health officer assigned to the sexually transmitted disease clinic in charge of tracing contacts. What is the BEST test to determine whether Sue M., John E., and Jane H. were the sources of the numbered sexually transmitted diseases?

(A) Stain epithelial cells with Giemsa stain and examine for cytoplasmic inclusions
(B) Perform the VDRL test
(C) Culture a specimen on Thayer-Martin medium

140. A patient with a purulent urethral exudate reports that he had intercourse with a prostitute, Sue M., 3 nights ago, and microscopic examination of the exudate revealed gram-negative diplococci within neutrophils

141. A patient with a papular rash on her trunk and palms and condylomata lata in her genital region reports that she had intercourse with John E. about 6 weeks ago

142. Jane H. gives birth to a baby, who develops conjunctivitis and pneumonia 4 days after birth

Questions 143–147:

Immunologic tests are used to diagnose or to aid in the treatment of a variety of diseases. Which one of the lettered tests is it MOST appropriate to perform in the following numbered illnesses or situations?

(A) Fluorescent antibody
(B) Radial immunodiffusion
(C) Agglutination
(D) Immunoelectrophoresis
(E) Flow cytometry

143. Acquired hypogammaglobulinemia

144. Herpes simplex virus infection of the patient's cells

145. ABO blood typing prior to giving a blood transfusion

146. Number of CD4-positive and CD8-positive T cells in a patient with AIDS

147. Multiple myeloma

Questions 148–151:

(A) Rotavirus
(B) Hepatitis D virus
(C) Epstein-Barr virus
(D) Rabies virus
(E) Human immunodeficiency virus

148. The genome of this virus does not encode its surface protein

149. This virus is a common cause of diarrhea in infants

150. This virus contains a DNA polymerase in the virion

151. This virus causes encephalitis characterized by cytoplasmic inclusions in neurons

Questions 152–160:

(A) *Giardia lamblia*
(B) *Entamoeba histolytica*
(C) *Plasmodium falciparum*
(D) *Trypanosoma cruzi*
(E) *Toxoplasma gondii*
(F) *Taenia solium*
(G) *Schistosoma haematobium*
(H) *Clonorchis sinensis*
(I) *Enterobius vermicularis*
(J) *Necator americanus*
(K) *Strongyloides stercoralis*
(L) *Trichinella spiralis*
(M) *Wuchereria bancrofti*
(N) *Onchocerca volvulus*
(O) *Toxocara canis*

152. Cysts with four nuclei are found in the stool

153. "Banana-shaped" gametocytes are seen in blood smears

154. The parasite is transmitted by cercariae penetrating the skin

155. Cysts in tissue contain an invaginated scolex with suckers and hooks

156. A 35-year-old man with AIDS, who has several cats at home, has a history of confusion and seizures; his CT scan now shows several "ring-enhancing" cavitary brain lesions

157. A 70-year-old farmer who enjoys making homemade pork sausages has periorbital edema, severe muscle pains, and marked eosinophilia

158. A 20-year-old woman, who has just returned from Africa where she was a Peace Corps volunteer, has had several episodes of high fever, shaking chills, and headache and has a hematocrit of 30%

159. The mother of a 4-year-old child who attends a day-care center notes that her child is sleeping poorly and scratching his anal area

160. A 24-year-old medical student who just returned from a camping trip in the mountains now has severe diarrhea consisting of nonbloody, foul-smelling fatty stools

Answers

1	(A)	17	(C)	33	(B)	49	(A)	65	(C)	81	(B)	97	(B)	113 (C)	129 (D)	145 (C)
2	(C)	18	(D)	34	(D)	50	(C)	66	(A)	82	(D)	98	(D)	114 (B)	130 (B)	146 (E)
3	(B)	19	(B)	35	(C)	51	(B)	67	(B)	83	(D)	99	(C)	115 (D)	131 (C)	147 (D)
4	(D)	20	(D)	36	(A)	52	(D)	68	(A)	84	(B)	100	(B)	116 (B)	132 (C)	148 (B)
5	(B)	21	(C)	37	(D)	53	(B)	69	(A)	85	(C)	101	(D)	117 (A)	133 (D)	149 (A)
6	(B)	22	(D)	38	(D)	54	(D)	70	(C)	86	(B)	102	(A)	118 (D)	134 (B)	150 (E)
7	(C)	23	(C)	39	(C)	55	(A)	71	(B)	87	(A)	103	(D)	119 (C)	135 (D)	151 (D)
8	(D)	24	(B)	40	(B)	56	(C)	72	(A)	88	(D)	104	(A)	120 (A)	136 (C)	152 (B)
9	(C)	25	(C)	41	(D)	57	(D)	73	(A)	89	(C)	105	(C)	121 (C)	137 (B)	153 (C)
10	(C)	26	(D)	42	(C)	58	(D)	74	(B)	90	(D)	106	(C)	122 (D)	138 (A)	154 (G)
11	(A)	27	(A)	43	(B)	59	(A)	75	(D)	91	(A)	107	(D)	123 (C)	139 (D)	155 (F)
12	(B)	28	(D)	44	(C)	60	(B)	76	(D)	92	(D)	108	(B)	124 (B)	140 (C)	156 (E)
13	(A)	29	(A)	45	(A)	61	(D)	77	(C)	93	(C)	109	(C)	125 (B)	141 (B)	157 (L)
14	(C)	30	(C)	46	(D)	62	(C)	78	(B)	94	(B)	110	(D)	126 (B)	142 (A)	158 (C)
15	(C)	31	(C)	47	(D)	63	(B)	79	(A)	95	(D)	111	(D)	127 (A)	143 (B)	159 (I)
16	(D)	32	(A)	48	(B)	64	(C)	80	(D)	96	(C)	112	(A)	128 (A)	144 (A)	160 (A)

Index

NOTE: Page numbers in bold face type indicate a major discussion. A *t* following a page number indicates tabular material, an *i* following a page number indicates an illustration, and an *s* following a page number indicates one of the brief summaries of medically important organisms. Drugs are listed under their generic names. When a drug trade name is listed, the reader is referred to the generic name.